W9-AAL-768

UNIT TWO

ADMINISTRATIVE PROCEDURES: PRACTICE FINANCE: ADVANCED ADMINISTRATIVE SKILLS

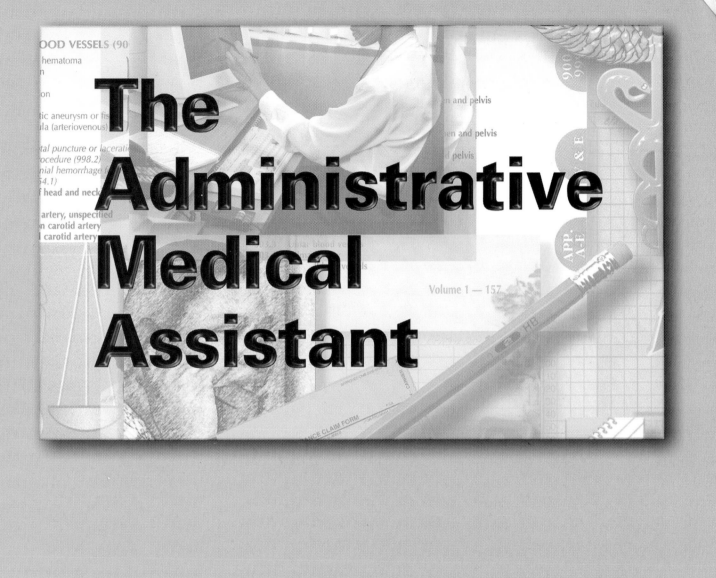

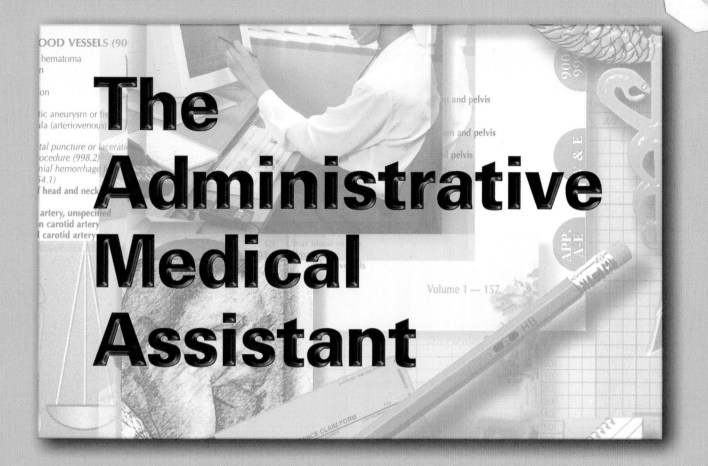

The Administrative Medical Assistant

MARY E. KINN, CPS, CMA-A

Assistant Professor, Health Technology, Retired
Long Beach City College
Long Beach, California

Past President, American Association of Medical Assistants

Former Chairman, American Association of Medical Assistants Certifying Board

4TH EDITION

W.B. SAUNDERS COMPANY
An Imprint of Elsevier Science
Philadelphia   London   New York   St. Louis   Sydney   Toronto

W.B. SAUNDERS COMPANY
An Imprint of Elsevier Science

The Curtis Center
Independence Square West
Philadelphia, Pennsylvania 19106

Library of Congress Cataloging-in-Publication Data

Kinn, Mary E.
The administrative medical assistant / Mary E. Kinn.—4th ed.

p. cm.

Includes bibliographical references and index.

ISBN 0–7216–7293–0

1. Medical assistants. 2. Medical offices—Management. I. Title.

R728.8.K49   1999

651'.961—dc21   99-17457

THE ADMINISTRATIVE MEDICAL ASSISTANT   ISBN 0–7216–7293–0

Copyright © 1999, 1993, 1988, 1982 by W.B. Saunders Company.

All rights reserved. No part of this publication may be reproduced or transmitted in any form or by any means, electronic or mechanical, including photocopy, recording, or any information storage and retrieval system, without permission in writing from the publisher.

Printed in China.

Last digit is the print number: 9   8   7   6   5

Contributors and Reviewers

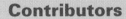

Contributors

SUE A. HUNT, MA, RN, CMA
Coordinator
Medical Assisting Program
Middlesex Community College
Lowell, Massachusetts
Health Insurance and Managed Care; Coding and Claims Processing

MARYANN WOODS, PhD, RN, CMA
Professor, Health Sciences and the Arts Division, and Director of Medical Assistant–Clinician Program, Fresno City College, Fresno, California; Member of California Association for Medical Assistant Instructors

Editorial Review Board

JUDITH BELL, BA, RT, CMA-C
Director, Allied Health
Midstate College
Peoria, Illinois

REV. DR. GENEVA BURCH
West Virginia Northern Community College
Benwood, West Virginia

KATHERINE BLANKENSHIP
San Antonio College
San Antonio, Texas

TRISH BOUDRIA, CMA-RMA
Department of Medical Assisting
Ultrasound Diagnostic School
Irving, Texas

BONNY MARIE BUTCHY, BA, MLT (ASCP), CMA (AAMA)
California Vocational Credentialed Teacher
Eden Area ROP
Hayward, California

PAMELA J. CARLTON
Director, Medical Assistant Program
Assistant Professor of Biology and Certified Paramedic
The College of Staten Island
Staten Island, New York

DEBBIE CUNNINGHAM
Medix School
Baltimore, Maryland

BARBARA M. DAHL, CMA
Whatcom Community College
Bellingham, Washington

VERA DAVIS, RN, CMA
Harper College
Palatine, Illinois

BONNIE DEISTER, MS, MA, BSN, RN, CMA-C
Broome Community College
Binghamton, New York

BARBARA F. ENSLEY, MS, RN, CMA-C
Haywood Community College
Clyde, North Carolina

LINDA FARRELL
Tidewater Tech–Virginia Beach
Virginia Beach, Virginia

MARGARET SCHELL FRAZIER, RN, CMA, BS

Program Chair, Medical Assisting
    Program
Ivy Tech State College, Northeast
Fort Wayne, Indiana

THERESA GAVAZZI, MS, BS, CMA

Delaware Technical and Community
    College
Dover, Delaware

MICHELLE GREEN, MPS, RRA, CMA

Alfred State College
Alfred, New York

DEBORAH HECHT

Akron Medical and Dental Institution
Cuyahoga Falls, Ohio

MARSHA HEMBY, BA, RN, CMA

Pitt Community College
Medical Assisting Department Chair
Greenville, North Carolina

JEANNE HOWARD, CMA, AAS

Department of Medical Assisting
    Technology
El Paso Community College
El Paso, Texas

SUE A. HUNT, MA, RN, CMA

Coordinator
Medical Assisting Program
Middlesex Community College
Lowell, Massachusetts

KAREN A. KITTLE, CMA, AAS

Department of Medical Assisting
Oakland Community College
Waterford, Michigan

CAROL LIGON, BS, RT (ARRT)(R), CMA

Ivy Tech State College
Evansville, Indiana

ANNE L. LILLY, RN, MVEd

Curriculum Consultant, Allied Health,
    Adult Education Professor, Retired
Santa Rosa Junior College
Santa Rosa, California

PATTY J. LYNCH, MEd

Bellingham, Washington

DEBORAH MONTONE, BS, RN, RMA

Dean of Academics
HoHoKus School of Medical Science
Ramsey, New Jersey

JANET R. SESSER, RMA (AMT), CMA, BS, Educational Administration

High Tech Institute, Inc.
Phoenix, Arizona

DIANE J. TRAMA, MT(ASCP)

Allied Medical and Technical Careers
Scranton, Pennsylvania

LORI WRIGHT, CMA, RMA, ART

Ultrasound Diagnostic School
Pittsburgh, Pennsylvania

CAROL ZEGLIN

Mt. Pleasant, Pennsylvania

Preface

In this fourth edition of *The Administrative Medical Assistant* you will find creative ideas and many interesting changes. The delivery of health care has been revolutionized in the past few years, and the changes that have occurred are recognized in this fourth edition. The newly developed AAMA Entry-Level Medical Assisting Curriculum, with its content and competency guidelines is utilized in each chapter, while throughout the text the author maintains the student-friendly level of presentation that has been the hallmark of this text since its inception in 1956.

As with all previous editions, this book remains designed for use in community colleges, vocational/technical schools, medical offices or clinic in-services, cross-training programs, and independent study programs. Key AAMA Curriculum content and competency guidelines are listed on the introductory page of each section and are covered in the appropriate chapters. Additionally, the book has been reorganized into a more logical presentation to be easier to use and better help the student in preparing for certification examination.

Each chapter opens with a detailed outline, followed by a vocabulary list and competency objectives, which provide a road map for the chapter. These objectives have been carefully edited to ensure that every administrative competency in the current Curriculum Content and Competency guidelines has been addressed and promotes the achievement of the basic entry-level skills. The chapter outline and competency objectives guide the instructor in preparing the material to be covered in the chapter and may also serve as a lecture outline for teaching the material. The Memory Joggers scattered throughout each chapter, along with the Critical Thinking challenges, assist the student in successful completion of the chapter objectives.

Unit I (Chapters 1 to 10) guides the student through the basics, beginning with professionalism, preparatory education, and the history from which modern medicine has evolved. The cornerstones of medical ethics, from historical codes to the AMA Principles of Medical Ethics, are presented in some detail. The legal responsibilities as well as the obligations and limitations of practicing medical assistants are addressed in each chapter. Unit I concludes with the importance of personal communications in every encounter.

Unit II (Chapters 11 to 25) addresses in detail the procedural steps in performing the administrative functions in a medical facility from the role of receptionist through appointment scheduling, telephone techniques, correspondence and mail processing, records management, professional fees, billing and collections, bookkeeping, insurance, and meetings and travel arrangements. Special attention is directed to the evolution of managed care and to the responsibilities of office management.

Finally, this fourth edition is accompanied by a complete supplemental package that has been developed with the major text to achieve two primary goals:

1. To assist students in mastering the essential skills and information needed

to secure a career as a medical assistant

2. To assist instructors in planning and implementing their programs for the most efficient use of time and available resources

The author hopes that the instructors, the students, and the practicing medical assistants who use this text will achieve the sense of fulfillment and professional achievement that the medical assisting profession provides.

MARY E. KINN, CPS, CMA-A

Acknowledgments

Over the span of more than 30 years that I have been involved with this text, hundreds of individuals have contributed ideas, knowledge, encouragement, praise, and—best of all—their hands in friendship. I acknowledge and express thanks to all of you.

Specifically I am deeply grateful to my editors:

Margaret Biblis and Shirley Kuhn for their innovative suggestions during the planning stage of this edition

Helaine Barron for her creative editing, patience, and devotion to the project

Adrianne Williams for her foresight, marketing talents, and personal touches.

I give special thanks to the Center for Women's Medicine in San Diego for the privilege of photographing in their beautiful facility, and especially to Arlene Saunders, Clinic Manager, for her cheerful cooperation.

I am grateful to:

Sue Hunt for rescuing the insurance and coding chapters

Bibbero Systems in Petaluma, California, and Colwell Systems, Inc., in Champaign, Illinois, for their continued support in providing sample forms for illustrating various administrative procedures

For the privilege of membership, for the sharing of their friendship and accumulated knowledge, and for fostering the challenge of excellence, I acknowledge the officers and members of the American Medical Writers Association (AMWA), the American Association of Medical Assistants (AAMA), the California Medical Assistants Association (CMAA), and the California Association of Medical Assistant Instructors.

I also wish to acknowledge the helpful and talented production team at the W.B. Saunders Company: Ellen Zanolle, designer, for the interior and cover designs; Sharon Iwanczuk, illustrator, for the creation of the collages and the interior art; Jeanne Carper, for copy editing; and Frank Polizzano, for overseeing the production process.

MARY E. KINN, CPS, CMA-A

The Publisher wishes to acknowledge the permission of the AAMA to use the interim language of the AAMA medical assisting curriculum. The language used for the curriculum content and competencies topics is adapted from the *AAMA Role Delineation Study: Occupational Analysis of the Medical Assisting Profession*, published by the American Association of Medical Assistants (AAMA), Chicago, IL. The AAMA does not endorse the language nor is the language the official, or taken from the official, AAMA medical assisting curriculum document.

Contents

SECTION 2
Understanding the Protocols of Medical Practice

UNIT TWO
ADMINISTRATIVE PROCEDURES: PRACTICE FINANCE: ADVANCED ADMINISTRATION SKILLS

SECTION 4
Written Communications and Record Keeping

11 Correspondence and Mail Processing 141

12 Dictation and Transcription 165

13 The Computer in Medical Practice 181

14 Filing Methods and Record Keeping 194

15 Health Information Management 208

SECTION 5
Financial Management

16 Professional Fees and Credit Arrangements 227

17 Managing Practice Finances 239

18 Banking Services and Procedures 263

19 Billing and Collecting Procedures 282

20 Health Insurance and Managed Care 301
Sue Hunt, MA, RN, CMA

NOTICE

Medical assisting is an ever-changing field. Standard safety precautions must be followed, but as new research and clinical experience broaden our knowledge, changes in treatment and drug therapy become necessary or appropriate. Readers are advised to check the product information currently provided by the manufacturer of each drug to be administered to verify the recommended dose, the method and duration of administration, and the contraindications. It is the responsibility of the treating physician, relying on experience and knowledge of the patient, to determine dosages and the best treatment for the patient. Neither the publisher nor the editor assumes any responsibility for any injury and/or damage to persons or property.

THE PUBLISHER

List of Procedures

TO THE STUDENT

Learning and mastering all the information in a textbook can seem like a daunting task. This is why the authors and editors have built in many helpful features throughout each chapter of the new The Administrative Medical Assistant, fourth edition. *These features, when used in conjunction with the* Student Mastery Manual *and* Virtual Medical Office CD-ROM, *are designed to enhance the lessons and assignments of your instructor to ensure a successful learning experience. Take a moment now to review these features, and keep them in mind as you move through the textbook and through your medical assisting curriculum.*

1 Section Openers

Each section opener identifies all the current Content and Competencies from the medical assisting entry-level curriculum that can be found in that section of the book. These are listed by chapter below the section title.

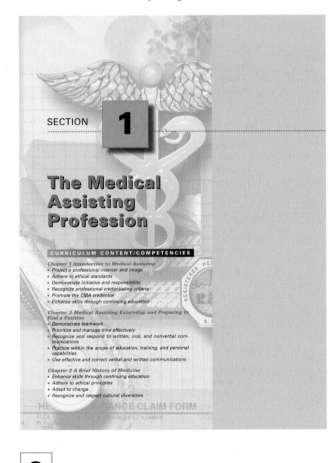

2 Chapter Openers

A detailed *Chapter Outline* introduces you to the material as a whole, allowing you to see at a glance how the subject material is organized. It will also help you focus on one topic at a time by showing you the relationship and placement of topics.

Learning Objectives list all the theoretical (cognitive) and procedural (performance) objectives you will be expected to meet on completion of the chapter.

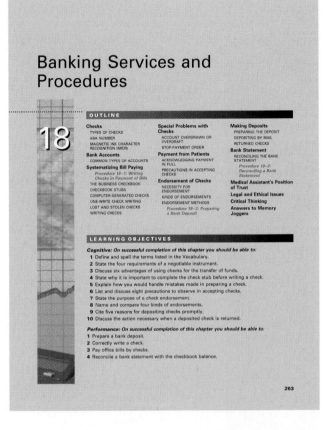

Vocabulary Lists define all pertinent medical terminology you will be expected to master throughout the chapter, in one easy-to-find location.

3 Special Focus

Sidebars contain information that focuses on professional topics that transcend chapters and reflect material that will be important to you as a student entering the real world of medical assisting. *Personal Qualities* highlight skills that are particularly essential to communicating and interacting effectively with people in general and patients and co-workers specifically. *Skills and Responsibilities* highlight important elements of your job that will be vital to your success and growth within the medical profession. *Patient Education* discussions offer tips and strategies for effectively implementing this important aspect of your job.

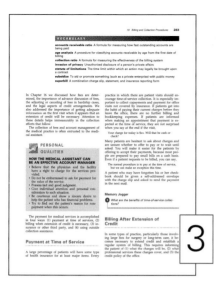

Legal and Ethical Issues (located at the end of each chapter) focus on areas of your job responsibility of which you will need to become keenly aware in order to protect yourself, your patients, and the practice for which you work.

Safety Alerts

These serve as a ready reminder of the many times when—and how—safety must be observed in order to protect you and others in the medical office.

Memory Jogger/How Did I Do?

Questions appear at intervals throughout the body of the text and are intended to intermittently check your understanding of the content. Answers to the questions are provided at the end of each chapter.

Examples

The highlighted examples bring the real world into your learning experience by discussing how the material you are mastering is directly and practically applied to the workplace.

Critical Thinking

Retaining content is not enough to completely master the material successfully. The scenarios presented in these boxes at the end of each chapter reinforce the content while also applying it to the real world through problem-solving and decision-making exercises of situations you could easily encounter on the job.

References

Located at the end of some chapters, references and resources provide you with a listing of other sources of information to help you further your understanding of chapter content.

Full Color Artwork

These pictures serve as a reminder of those important safety precautions that are required before performing the procedure.

Student Mastery Manual

This supplement to the fourth edition of *The Administrative Medical Assistant* tests your knowledge of chapter content, mastery of chapter skills, and ability to apply what you've learned in that chapter to a clinical situation.

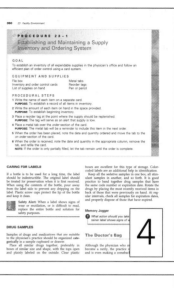

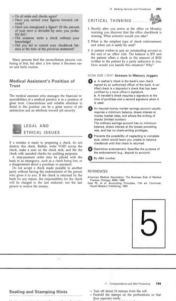

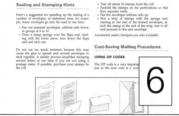

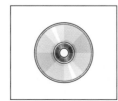

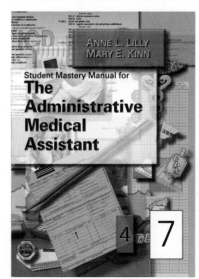

The Virtual Medical Office CD-ROM

Bound free in the back of the textbook, this innovative product lets you put it all together in a reality-based environment that makes learning challenging and fun.

PROFESSIONALISM: LEGAL CONCEPTS: COMMUNICATION SKILLS

The Medical Assisting Profession

CURRICULUM CONTENT/COMPETENCIES

Chapter 1 Introduction to Medical Assisting
- Project a professional manner and image
- Adhere to ethical standards
- Demonstrate initiative and responsibility
- Recognize professional credentialing criteria
- Promote the CMA credential
- Enhance skills through continuing education

Chapter 2 Medical Assisting Externship and Preparing to Find a Position
- Demonstrate teamwork
- Prioritize and manage time effectively
- Recognize and respond to written, oral, and nonverbal communications
- Practice within the scope of education, training, and personal capabilities
- Use effective and correct verbal and written communications

Chapter 3 A Brief History of Medicine
- Enhance skills through continuing education
- Adhere to ethical principles
- Adapt to change
- Recognize and respect cultural diversities

HEALTH INSURANCE CLAIM FORM

FECA OTHER INSURED'S I.D. NUMBER (FOR
N BLK LUNG
SSN

Introduction to Medical Assisting

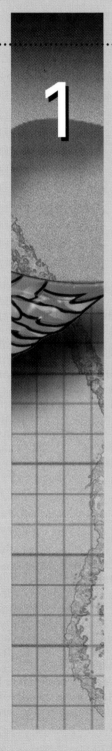

1

LEARNING OBJECTIVES

Cognitive: On successful completion of this chapter you should be able to:

1 Identify 10 career opportunities that are available to the trained medical assistant.
2 Identify at least five general knowledge areas in which the medical assistant should be proficient.
3 Differentiate between administrative and clinical responsibilities of a medical assistant.
4 List five personality traits that are beneficial to the successful medical assistant.
5 Briefly describe the training programs that are available for medical assistants.
6 Name four professional organizations that provide educational opportunities and certification examinations.

VOCABULARY

administrative Having to do with management duties; in medical assisting, refers to all "front office" activities

clinical Pertaining to actual observation and treatment of patients

discretion Quality of being discreet, tactful, or prudent

ethnic Pertaining to large groups of people classed according to cultural origin or background

externship The practice of receiving employment experience in qualified health care facilities under the cooperative supervision of the medical staff and the program instructor as part of the educational curriculum

freestanding emergency center An emergency facility not associated with a hospital

group practice The provision of services by a group of at least three practitioners

health maintenance organization (HMO) An organization that provides comprehensive health care to an enrolled group for a fixed periodic payment

mandatory In the nature of a mandate or command; obligatory

paradox A statement that seems to be contradictory and yet is perhaps true

regional Pertaining to a region or territory; local

rural Pertaining to the country, as distinguished from a city or town

solo private practice One physician practicing alone

urban Characteristic of or pertaining to a city or town

A career as a medical assistant is challenging and offers variety, job satisfaction, opportunity for service, commensurate financial reward, and possibility for advancement. It is open to both men and women. Entering the field of medical assisting is a significant decision. Medical assisting is a career requiring dedication, integrity, and a commitment to continuing education.

Past, Present, and Future

The first medical assistant was probably a neighbor of a physician who was asked to help when an extra pair of hands was needed. As the practice of medicine became more complicated, some physicians hired registered nurses to help in their office practices. Gradually, record keeping, data reporting, and an increasing number of business details began to be burdensome, and physicians realized a need for an assistant with business training. Community and junior colleges began offering training programs that focused on both administrative and clinical skills in the late 1940s.

Medical assistant organizations on county and state levels began developing around 1950. A national organization for medical assistants was formed in 1957, and, a few years later, national certification for medical assistants became possible. In recent years, legislation regarding the scope of practice of medical assistants has been enacted in some states.

Career Advantages

A trained medical assistant is equipped with a flexible, adaptable career. The skills acquired by the medical assistant can be carried throughout life, and employment is readily available anywhere in the world that medicine is practiced. Although medical assisting holds many opportunities for both men and women, it is one career that usually does not have a mandatory retirement age. Medical assisting attracts the nontraditional student who may be older than the average postsecondary student by a decade or more. Many medical assistants pursue their careers far beyond the usual retirement age because physicians realize the value of experienced, mature employees.

CAREER OPPORTUNITIES

The practice of medicine has changed dramatically in the past two decades. Increasing costs have created a trend away from hospital-based treatment and toward the delivery of care in physicians' offices and in outpatient centers. Although doctors have employed assistants in their practices for many years, computerization and technologic advances have created more opportunities for qualified medical assistants and increased their responsibilities. The result is an increase in the need for professional training. More clearly defined educational needs of medical assistants have resulted in improvement in both quality and accessibility of training courses. Medical assisting is recognized as an important allied health care profession. Employment opportunities in allied health for the medical assistant are abundant and extremely varied. More medical assistants are employed by practicing physicians than any other type of allied health care personnel.

Memory Jogger

1 *Why is it increasingly important for medical assistants to receive formal training before employment?*

A medical assistant's work can be **administrative** or **clinical.** Training for medical assisting has become a paradox. Leaders in the profession as well as employers are emphasizing the need for multiskilled medical assistants. At the same time, job descriptions are becoming more specialized. Employment can be as a receptionist in a hospital or physician's office, transcriptionist, insurance specialist, financial secretary, billing and collection specialist, clinical assistant involved in patient care, or emergency technician, to name just a few. The medical assistant may choose to work for a physician in **solo private practice,** for a medical partnership or **group practice,** for a **health maintenance organization (HMO),** for a hospital, or for a **freestanding emergency center.** The physician(s) may be engaged in general practice or a specialty such as surgery, internal medicine, dermatology, obstetrics, pediatrics, or psychiatry. The choices are almost limitless.

ADDITIONAL OPPORTUNITIES

Career opportunities abound in public health facilities, hospitals, laboratories, medical schools, research centers, voluntary health agencies, and medical firms of all kinds. Opportunities for work are also available with such federal agencies as the Department of Veterans Affairs, the United States Public Health Service, and Armed Forces clinics or hospitals.

This text is designed primarily for the student who is in training for employment in a private health care facility. It is also valuable as a reference after employment and as a review resource for the medical assistant in preparing for certification.

Earnings

What kind of earnings can the medical assistant expect? As in any other career field, there are **regional** differences, particularly between earnings in **rural** and in **urban** areas. Overall, the medical assistant

can generally expect a satisfactory return on the investment in training, experience, and skill. Most physicians realize that a good medical assistant is worth a good salary. Many have learned through bitter experience that "bargain help" is often the most expensive.

The job turnover among medical assistants is surprisingly low. This fact may show that medical assistants derive a high degree of satisfaction from their work. Many instances have been reported of medical assistants who were hired when a physician started practice and remained until the physician's retirement.

Knowledge and Skills

Ideally, the medical assistant should have both administrative and clinical skills, although he or she may have a personal preference for one or the other. The physician's staff must be able to handle all responsibilities of the office except those requiring the services of a physician or other licensed personnel. Where there are several assistants, each should be able and willing to substitute in an emergency for any of the others. Teamwork is a very important part of any occupation. Few physicians in private practice attempt to serve their patients without at least one assistant. The great majority have at least two assistants, and many have five or more.

Certain knowledge and skills are expected of a trained medical assistant. The skills listed here are not intended to be all inclusive but suggest what may be expected on entry to employment as a medical assistant.

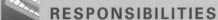 **SKILLS AND RESPONSIBILITIES**

GENERAL SKILLS
- Medical terminology usage and spelling
- Basics of medical law and ethics
- Human relations and personal communications
- Computer literacy
- Documentation of health information
- Cardiopulmonary resuscitation
- Emergency first aid
- Legible handwriting

ADMINISTRATIVE SKILLS
- Telephone skills and scheduling
- Proficiency in typing and keyboarding
- Communication, written and spoken
- Electronic dictation and word processing
- Health information management
- Patient and insurance billing

CLINICAL SKILLS
- Application of aseptic technique and infection control
- Testing for vital signs
- Interviewing and recording of patient history
- Patient instruction
- Specimen collection and handling
- Performance of selected tests

Memory Jogger

2 *Why is it important for a medical assistant to have both administrative and clinical skills?*

Personal Attributes

The professional services of a medical assistant are extremely personal. Therefore, the manner in which these services are performed can affect the health and welfare of a patient in either a positive or negative way.

PERSONAL
QUALITIES

HOW DO YOU INTERACT WITH PATIENTS?
- Do you have a friendly and pleasant attitude?
- Are you able to maintain confidentiality?
- Are you courteous?
- Are you considerate, respectful, and kind?
- Can you control your temper?
- Can you view a situation through the eyes of others?

You may be called on to assume charge of the office when the doctor is out. The doctor must depend on the medical assistant's good judgment when he or she is left alone.

PERSONAL
QUALITIES

CAN YOU TAKE CHARGE?
- Are you attentive to details?
- Are you accurate?
- Are you dependable?
- Can you remain calm and accept responsibility during an emergency?

Discretion and concern for the patient are very important. Patients might choose another physician because of the seeming lack of concern by a medical assistant. The patient who feels comfortable with the medical assistant will probably feel comfortable with the doctor.

Memory Jogger

3 *Name at least 10 desirable personal attributes that would enhance the medical assistant's success.*

Training

CLASSROOM EDUCATION

Medical assistants who were self-trained and already employed in the field were among the first to recognize the need for formally trained personnel in medical offices. Through chapters of the American Association of Medical Assistants (AAMA) and aided by local medical societies, established medical assistants have strongly influenced the rapidly accelerating development, refinement, and accessibility of such training. Formal training is essential for today's medical assistant.

Many community colleges and private vocational schools offer courses in medical assisting. After satisfactory completion of a program, the student receives a certificate, diploma, or, from some community colleges, an associate degree. Courses in a community college take 10 months to 2 years to complete. Students are usually admitted only once or twice per year. Private schools more frequently have open enrollment, and some programs are completed in 7 months. Currently, the trend is toward offering training in modules, thereby including the individual who may have limited time or who needs the opportunity for upgrading skills and specialty courses (Fig. 1–1).

ON-THE-JOB TRAINING

Effective training also includes an **externship** of at least several weeks to provide practical experience in physicians' offices, accredited hospitals, or other health care facilities. The success of a physician's practice is highly dependent on teamwork of the staff members. Furthermore, the physician, probably more than any other employer, expects employees to carry out their duties independently, with little or no direct supervision.

As a new employee, you should

- Be told exactly what your duties are
- Read your job description as it appears in an

TYPICAL CURRICULUM FOR MEDICAL ASSISTANT PROGRAM

anatomy and physiology
medical terminology
medical law and ethics
human relations
oral and written communications
computer skills, electronic transcription
financial record keeping
insurance coding and billing
health information management
clinical procedures, such as preparation, assisting, and follow-up of patients for medical
   examinations
first aid
principles of CPR
pharmaceutical principles and medication administration
specimen collection and processing
basic office diagnostic procedures

FIGURE 1–1 Typical curriculum for medical assistant program.

office procedure manual and then discuss it with the physician or your supervisor

- Ask for direction if it is not offered
- Show that you are responsible and dependable

The new employee brings many intangibles to the job that are not found in the job description. Courtesy toward others and a capacity for teamwork, a positive attitude, enthusiasm, initiative, and dedication are important personal attributes. After becoming comfortably acquainted with what is expected of your position, you will probably want to learn what other employees are doing so that you can offer them assistance when needed. In this way, you become a full member of the health care team.

CONTINUING EDUCATION

Education does not end with the completion of formal training. The amount of medical knowledge gained since the beginning of medical history is said to double every 5 years. The practicing medical assistant must keep current with the rapid changes within the profession. Most physicians appreciate the medical assistant who asks questions about unfamiliar conditions or procedures.

Much can be learned by reading or at least briefly reviewing the medical literature that arrives in the daily mail or the articles that appear in newspapers, news magazines, and specialized newsletters. The medical assistant who wishes to advance becomes an active member of a professional organization, has an inquisitive mind, and attends available professional seminars and workshops.

Memory Jogger

4 *Explain the statement "Education does not end with the completion of formal training."*

Responsibilities

The responsibilities of the medical assistant vary from one facility to another, because the position must be geared to the type of practice and the working habits of the individual physician. In the office with only one employee, the medical assistant's time is divided between administrative and clinical duties. In the multiple-employee office, positions generally are more specialized, but each employee has to have the ability to "pitch in" and help in any position.

SKILLS AND RESPONSIBILITIES

ADMINISTRATIVE RESPONSIBILITIES

The administrative (sometimes called *front office*) responsibilities of a medical assistant are similar to those of any administrative assistant to a top executive, but they have specific medical aspects.

- Answering telephones
- Scheduling appointments
- Interviewing and instructing new patients
- Explaining fees
- Opening and sorting mail
- Answering routine correspondence
- Transcribing electronic dictation
- Pulling patient charts for scheduled appointments
- Filing reports and correspondence
- Arranging for patient admission to a hospital and instructing the patient regarding admission
- Planning financial arrangements with patients
- Coding and transmitting insurance claims
- Maintaining financial records and files

- Preparing and mailing statements
- Collecting delinquent accounts
- Preparing checks for employer's signature
- Reconciling bank statements
- Maintaining files of paid and unpaid invoices
- Preparing and maintaining employees' payroll records (or supplying payroll information to an outside accountant)
- Supervising personnel
- Helping in the preparation of manuscripts or speeches
- Clipping articles from professional journals
- Assisting with the maintenance of the physician's professional library

CLINICAL RESPONSIBILITIES

The duties of a clinical assistant are also varied.

- Helping the patient prepare for examinations and other procedures
- Recording the medical history
- Assisting in the examination when requested to do so
- Cleaning and sterilizing instruments and equipment
- Instructing patients regarding preparation for radiologic and laboratory examinations
- Keeping supply cabinets well stocked
- Conforming with Occupational Safety and Health Administration (OSHA) requirements
- Supplying patient education
- Performing a variety of laboratory tests such as urinalysis and blood studies
- Performing electrocardiography and, depending on state regulations, assisting in radiography
- Taking of vital signs
- Preparing treatment or surgical trays

Professional Commitment

APPEARANCE

A well-groomed assistant in professional attire has a good psychologic effect on patients. The essentials of a professional appearance are good health, good grooming, and appropriate dress.

Good health requires getting adequate sleep, eating balanced meals, and exercising enough to keep fit. Medical assistants can set a good example by following a sensible and healthful lifestyle that includes regular checkups of their own physical condition. A radiantly healthy office staff promotes the best possible public relations image for the physician.

Good grooming is little more than attention to the details of personal appearance. Personal cleanliness, which includes taking a daily bath or shower, using a deodorant, and practicing good oral hygiene, is vital. Use of perfume or aftershave should be avoided; patients and co-workers may be allergic to some scents. The female medical assistant's makeup should be carefully selected and applied. Heavy or exaggerated makeup is out of place in the professional office. Subtle eye makeup and clear or natural shades of nail polish may enhance the assistant's appearance. Both male and female medical assistants should be sure that their hair is clean, neatly styled, and off the collar.

The medical assistant usually wears a uniform or laboratory coat, which not only presents a professional appearance but also identifies the assistant as a member of the health care team. Synthetic fabrics and fashionable styling make it possible for the medical assistant's uniform to be both practical and attractive.

Women may choose to wear pantsuits, which are available in white or a variety of colors; a two-piece dress uniform in white or a color; or an attractively styled traditional white uniform. Men usually wear white slacks with a white or light-colored shirt, jacket, or pullover top. A laboratory coat may be worn over casual street clothes by men or women if this is within the facility's dress code. Today's easy-care fabrics make it unthinkable to wear a uniform more than one day without laundering. Even accidental spills and spots that occur during the working day can usually be rinsed out immediately. Uniforms that are worn where people are ill should be considered contaminated.

The shoes the assistant wears should be appropriate for a uniform and be spotless and comfortable. White shoes must be kept white by daily cleaning. Remember that if a laced shoe is worn, the laces also need cleaning.

In some facilities, the physician prefers that the staff not wear uniforms. Some psychiatrists and some pediatricians, for example, believe that the clinical appearance of a uniform may affect patients adversely. Nevertheless, the medical assistant who does not wear a uniform should follow the dictates of good taste and propriety in choosing a professional wardrobe. The garments worn while on duty must be comfortable, allow easy movement, and still look fresh at the end of a busy day.

Whatever uniform style the assistant chooses, it should be personally becoming and worn over appropriate undergarments. The lines, colors, and ornamentation of undergarments should not be seen through the uniform; therefore, it is best to wear a neutral color without ornamentation. When wearing a uniform, jewelry should be limited to an engagement ring, wedding band, and professional pin (Fig. 1–2). A name badge worn on the right shoulder will help patients to identify each staff person by name.

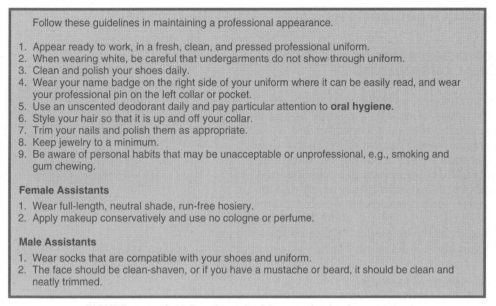

Follow these guidelines in maintaining a professional appearance.

1. Appear ready to work, in a fresh, clean, and pressed professional uniform.
2. When wearing white, be careful that undergarments do not show through uniform.
3. Clean and polish your shoes daily.
4. Wear your name badge on the right side of your uniform where it can be easily read, and wear your professional pin on the left collar or pocket.
5. Use an unscented deodorant daily and pay particular attention to **oral hygiene.**
6. Style your hair so that it is up and off your collar.
7. Trim your nails and polish them as appropriate.
8. Keep jewelry to a minimum.
9. Be aware of personal habits that may be unacceptable or unprofessional, e.g., smoking and gum chewing.

Female Assistants

1. Wear full-length, neutral shade, run-free hosiery.
2. Apply makeup conservatively and use no cologne or perfume.

Male Assistants

1. Wear socks that are compatible with your shoes and uniform.
2. The face should be clean-shaven, or if you have a mustache or beard, it should be clean and neatly trimmed.

FIGURE 1–2   Guidelines for maintaining a professional appearance.

ATTITUDE

Getting along with people is essential to success in the medical field. The person who can preserve his or her own positive self-image and the individual self-images of others has achieved the first step in human relations. Patients appreciate a reception that is polite and cordial. Establish rapport with the patient on the first encounter. In some areas a wide assortment of geographic and cultural customs exists throughout the population. The person suffering from an illness is often highly sensitive to any violation of ethnic customs, so violations should be avoided whenever possible.

TEAM DYNAMICS

The new employee must be exceptionally considerate of those who are experienced on the job. A natural tendency exists for the trainee just completing formal medical assisting training to want to share this new knowledge with others. This is not always what the established employee wants to hear. The new assistant should emphasize willingness to follow instructions and show appreciation for what others are doing until a firm relationship is in place. Team dynamics include working together, offering to do a colleague's work when he or she cannot be in the office, and being willing to help others when your work is caught up.

INITIATIVE AND RESPONSIBILITY

Responsibility is shown by arriving on time and being available for the full time agreed on. You should know what is expected in the regular course of employment and, if time permits, volunteer to help others who may have an overload if it is within your scope of education. Show a willingness to learn additional skills and show initiative by finding things to do when the office is less busy. Responsibility also includes calling your superior any time you will be unavoidably late or absent or alerting a co-worker when you will be absent from your work station.

Memory Jogger

5 *Can you recall an ethnic custom that would affect your contact with a patient?*

JOIN YOUR PROFESSIONAL ORGANIZATION

You may have become a student member of the local medical assistants association and advanced to an active member after your employment. Membership in your professional association shows a dedication to your career and establishes your identity as a medical assistant. Attending chapter meetings provides a source of continuing education. Participating in organization activities and being involved in the planning and action within the chapter develops your "people skills" and teaches leadership. Each individual can influence the future of the profession.

Being a medical assistant is more than just a job. It is a way of life.

Professional Organizations

BENEFITS OF MEMBERSHIP IN A PROFESSIONAL ORGANIZATION

By joining a professional organization and participating in the activities it affords, a medical assistant can grow personally and professionally and keep abreast of current trends. Most organizations give continuing education events resulting in continuing education units (CEUs) being recorded and reported that can be applied to a recertification program. Participation in a recognized professional organization shows that the employee is serious about his or her career and an asset to the employer. Dedicated medical assistants will attest to its rewards.

American Association of Medical Assistants

The AAMA was formally organized in 1956 as a federation of several state associations that had been functioning independently. In 1997, the AAMA had affiliated societies in more than 40 states, with national headquarters in Chicago, Illinois. It has been a continuing force behind establishing a national certifying program for medical assistants, the accrediting of medical assisting training programs in community colleges and private schools, and setting minimum standards for the entry-level medical assistant.

AAMA members have the opportunity to attend local, state, regional, and national meetings, where they can participate in workshops, learn of educational advances in their field, hear prominent speakers, and establish a networking system with other medical assistants.

The AAMA publishes a bimonthly journal, the *PMA (Professional Medical Assistant)*, which includes articles with tests that may be submitted for CEUs. Members may wear the AAMA insignia (Fig. 1–3). Since 1963, the AAMA has administered a certifying examination, with successful completion leading to a certificate and recognition as a certified medical assistant (CMA). Examinations are given in January

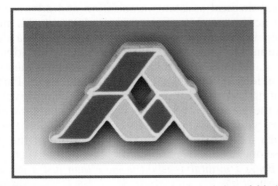

FIGURE 1–3 Insignia of the American Association of Medical Assistants. (Courtesy of the American Association of Medical Assistants, Chicago, IL.)

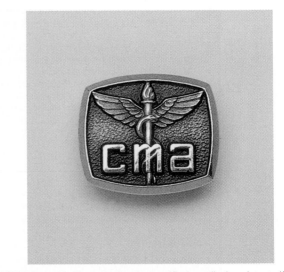

FIGURE 1–4 Pin worn by the certified medical assistant. (Courtesy of the American Association of Medical Assistants, Chicago, IL.)

and June of each year at designated centers throughout the United States. Certification is available to students or graduates of programs accredited by the Commission on Accreditation of Allied Health Education Programs (CAAHEP). Recertification is required every 5 years and can be accomplished through CEUs or reexamination. A certified medical assistant is permitted to wear the CMA pin (Fig. 1–4).

REGISTERED MEDICAL ASSISTANTS OF THE AMERICAN MEDICAL TECHNOLOGISTS In the early 1970s, the American Medical Technologists (AMT), a national certifying body for laboratory personnel since 1939, began offering an examination for medical assistants. The solid success of this project brought about the formulation of the registered medical assistant (RMA) program within AMT in 1976. Since that time, the RMAs have earned great respect in their own right. They have played an active role in public relations and professional recognition, protective legislation, improvements in training programs, and the provision of continuing education materials and opportunities.

The RMA certification examination is given in June and November of each year throughout the United States and as needed at schools accredited by the Accrediting Bureau of Health Education Schools (ABHES). Applicants must be graduates of a medical assisting course accredited by ABHES, a regional accrediting commission, or other acceptable agency or must meet certain experience requirements. All RMA members of the AMT Registry are certified medical assistants by examination and are entitled to wear the RMA insignia (Fig. 1–5). RMA headquarters is located in Park Ridge, Illinois.

Independent unaffiliated medical assistant organizations in some states offer professional participation at the local and state level as well as continuing education opportunities.

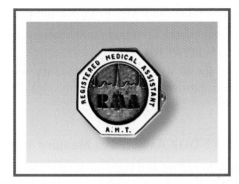

FIGURE 1–5 Pin worn by the registered medical assistant. (Courtesy of the RMA/American Medical Technologists, Park Ridge, IL.)

American Association for Medical Transcription

Many medical offices employ medical language specialists as medical transcriptionists; such professionals will find membership in the American Association of Medical Transcription (AAMT) valuable. The association was incorporated in 1978 with headquarters in Modesto, California. Voluntary certification by successful completion of an examination has been offered since 1981 and may be maintained through continuing education (Fig. 1–6). The AAMT publishes a professional journal six times per year. It offers outstanding education materials and holds an annual national convention.

Professional Secretaries International, the Association for Office Professionals

The administrative medical assistant may profit from membership in Professional Secretaries International (PSI), which was founded in 1942 as The National Secretaries Association (International) and is headquartered in Kansas City, Missouri. Through its Institute for Certifying Secretaries, PSI sponsors the Certified Professional Secretary (CPS) Examination, which covers Finance and Business Law (accounting, economics, business law); Office Systems and Ad-

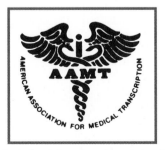

FIGURE 1–6 Insignia of American Association for Medical Transcription. (Courtesy of American Association for Medical Transcription, Modesto, CA.)

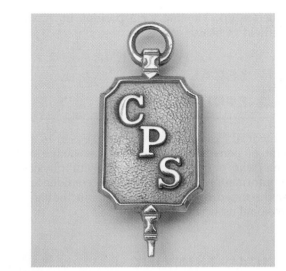

FIGURE 1–7 Pin worn by the certified professional secretary. (Courtesy of Professional Secretaries International.)

ministration (office technology, office administration, business communications); and Management (behavioral science in business, human resources management, organizations and management). The rating of CPS is obtained by meeting educational and work experience requirements and by passing the three-part examination (Fig. 1–7). The organization publishes *The Secretary* magazine nine times per year, sponsors Collegiate Secretaries International and the Future Secretaries Association in colleges and high schools, respectively, and holds an annual CPS seminar each June and an international convention each July.

Overview

This introductory chapter has presented the advantages of becoming a trained medical assistant and some of the many career opportunities available. Emphasis was placed on the necessary skills that must be developed and the general knowledge that must be acquired to function successfully in the medical arena. However, skills and knowledge alone do not bring success to the aspiring medical assistant. Therefore, personality traits and professional appearance have also been emphasized in this introductory chapter. The importance of getting the right start when entering new employment and the necessity for continuing education was discussed. Reviewing the development of the rapidly changing career of medical assisting highlights the importance of each individual in upholding the established professional standards.

Although this introduction to the profession precedes the presentation of performance skills, it is recommended that the student review it immediately before interviewing for a position in this fascinating field of health care.

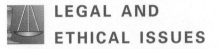

LEGAL AND ETHICAL ISSUES

As a medical assistant you will be exposed to a vast amount of personal and intimate knowledge of the patients who entrust their care to your physicians. Such information must be held in confidence and never discussed or relayed to others, including your professional associates.

CRITICAL THINKING

Medical assisting is a serious and rewarding career for both women and men. Persons involved in health care are highly respected in the community and provide an essential service. The expected qualifications are demanding but attainable. The woman or man who accepts this career must be willing to accept the responsibilities inherent in its standards.

1 Do you have a preference for either administrative or clinical duties? If you do, do you know why?

2 When is the last time you lost your temper?

3 Have you ever divulged information someone asked you not to tell?

4 Do you know any medical assistants who have attained certification status? How did they feel about it?

HOW DID I DO? Answers to Memory Joggers

1 Computerization and technologic advances in the practice of medicine require more training, and physicians expect this when hiring.

2 The physician's staff must be able to handle all responsibilities of the office except those requiring the services of licensed personnel.

3 Individual responses.

4 The practicing medical assistant must keep current with changes within the profession to function effectively.

5 *Example:* The Hmong people from Laos believe the head is sacred because that is where the soul resides. A Hmong child would be very distressed if you patted him or her on the head even in an affectionate way.

Medical Assisting Externship and Preparing to Find a Position

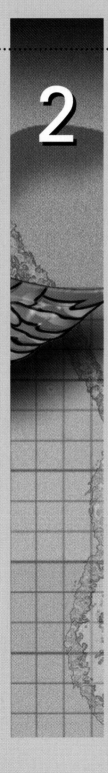

2

LEARNING OBJECTIVES

Cognitive: On successful completion of this chapter you should be able to:

1 Define and spell the terms listed in the vocabulary.
2 Explain the essentials of an externship.
3 Briefly explain four responsibilities of the student during externship.
4 Describe the responsibilities of an externship office or agency.
5 Explain how a student will benefit from externship experience.
6 List the three steps in applying for a position.
7 Identify the five essential parts of a personal inventory.
8 List seven basic items that should be included in every resumé.
9 Specify five items that must *not* be inserted in a resumé.
10 Cite five sources of leads for employment as a medical assistant.
11 List three avenues of evaluation that an interviewer may use in selecting an employee.

Performance: On successful completion of this chapter you should be able to perform the following activities:

1 Prepare a personal inventory.
2 Prepare two examples of a resumé.
3 Demonstrate a telephone request for an interview.
4 Write a letter in response to a newspaper help-wanted ad.
5 Compose a follow-up letter of thanks after an interview for a position.

VOCABULARY

avocational Pertaining to a subordinate occupation or a hobby

chronologic In the order of time

externship The practice of receiving employment experience in qualified health care facilities under the cooperative supervision of the medical staff and the program instructor as part of the educational curriculum

extracurricular Relating to those activities that form part of the life of students but are not part of the courses of study

format Shape, size, and general makeup of a publication, such as a resumé

objective Something toward which effort is directed; an aim or end of action

personal inventory A complete summary of pertinent information about oneself

re-entry student One who has been away from formal education or employment for several years and who is now preparing to re-enter the workplace

resumé A *selective* summary of one's education and employment record tailored to the position being sought

seminar A group of students meeting regularly and informally with a professor to discuss ideas and problems

Externship

As you progress in your training, you will be giving thought to just how and where you will fit into the health care world, and you will undoubtedly have acquired certain preferences.

One aid in defining and focusing your interests is experiencing an **externship** program that provides practical experience in a variety of qualified physicians' offices, accredited hospitals, or other health care facilities. Externship experience is included by most schools and colleges that have a complete curriculum for medical assisting. In those programs accredited by the Council on Accreditation of Allied Health Education Programs (CAAHEP) in collaboration with the American Medical Association and the American Association of Medical Assistants, an externship is mandatory. A minimum of 160 hours is recommended.

WHAT IS AN EXTERNSHIP?

The externship phase of your training may also be known as *work experience* or *on-the-job* training and is done without pay. The externship is planned and supervised by the instructor in collaboration with local employers. The medical offices and health care facilities serve as an extension of the college when physicians and administrators accept students for the externship. You may be expected to carry malpractice insurance during the externship. You will probably be required to undergo a physical examination, chest x-ray, appropriate serologic tests, and hepatitis vaccine.

During the very important weeks of your externship, you will have an opportunity to apply your administrative and clinical skills under the supervision of a practicing medical assistant. You will be expected to responsibly carry through with the assigned tasks. Your supervisor and the physician(s) at the externship site will be evaluating your personal qualities as well as the skills you have learned in the classroom.

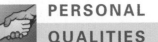 **PERSONAL QUALITIES**

- Grooming
- Poise
- Integrity
- Punctuality
- Relations with co-workers and patients
- Reaction to criticism and direction
- Respect for ethical standards
- Consideration for others

The on-site supervisor and physician assume responsibility for continual evaluation of your performance, as directed by your instructor, and this evaluation becomes a part of your student record.

DURATION AND TIME OF EXTERNSHIP

The duration of the externship and the time at which it is introduced into the program will vary, depending on the school or college. Some schools have the student spend 1 or 2 days in a health care

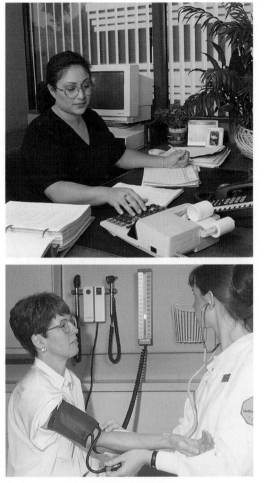

FIGURE 2–1 Medical assisting externship includes both administrative and clinical duties. (Bottom photo from Chester GA: Modern Medical Assisting. Philadelphia, WB Saunders, 1998, p 445.)

facility early in the training to provide a frame of reference for later instruction. Others combine work experience with classroom instruction throughout the training period. The majority of schools prefer a concentrated period of externship near the conclusion of the classroom instruction (Fig. 2–1).

STUDENT RESPONSIBILITIES

During the externship, both your appearance and actions must be according to accepted professional standards. You will report to work at a specified time on specified days, just as if you were a regular employee, but you will not be paid by the training facility. You may spend all your externship in one facility, but it is usually preferable to rotate among several types of practice for a well-rounded experience. Do not be surprised if you are expected to apply and be interviewed for the position just as you will later on when you are seeking employ-

ment. This is valuable experience and should be welcomed.

You, as a student, should recognize that a health care agency that cooperates with your education is accepting a great responsibility. You will require continual supervision, and your questions must be answered. You must be aware of ethical and legal concerns and of the potential for a claim of medical malpractice. One large concern is that of patient privacy. You must reveal no information concerning a patient or the practice to persons outside the facility. Some agencies may ask you to sign an oath of privacy while in that facility.

EXTERNSHIP SITES

The school or college will designate a specific individual to be your externship coordinator, who will carefully choose and screen suitable training facilities. The supervising staff at the health care facility must agree to complete an evaluation of your performance while providing ample opportunity for you to practice your skills. Quite often, the coordinator will seek out offices where former graduates of the program are employed. This ensures greater understanding and cooperation as well as the assurance that work habits and procedures meet the standards promoted in the classroom. In rare instances, a student may feel that the training facility is taking advantage of a situation and simply using the student to perform menial tasks. If you do have such an experience, it should be reported to your instructor.

The value of the externship is enhanced when the training program includes a weekly **seminar** at which all the students serving externship and their instructor may share experiences, problems, and solutions. All three parties to the agreement—the school, the externship agency or facility, and the trainee—benefit from the experience.

BENEFITS FROM AN EXTERNSHIP

- The school has a line of communication to the community and is better able to assess the needs and expectations of the public for which it is training prospective employees.
- The externship agency benefits from the new ideas and methods that the trainee may introduce. If the facility is looking for additional help, this is an ideal way to evaluate the performance of a trainee without involvement in the hiring process.
- The trainee benefits most of all by exposure to practical experience in a variety of settings. This experience in the real world removes a great deal of the anxiety that might otherwise be present in a first employment situation.

If the student performs well during the externship, he or she may be offered a permanent job with the facility, but it should not be assumed that this will happen. The externship facility may also be used as a reference when seeking a permanent position. When you are confident that you have performed well and have a comfortable relationship with the supervisory staff in the training facility, you may ask for a reference to be used later on when interviewing for employment.

Memory Jogger

1 *Explain the similarities and the differences between externship and regular employment.*

Finding the Right Position

After you have completed your classroom training and externship, the next step will be to find the right position. Your aptitudes and skills must be matched with the requirements of a physician or facility in need of an employee. Whether you are seeking your first position or are returning to the field after an absence of several years, or even if you are an experienced medical assistant preparing to change employers, the steps in applying for a position are essentially the same:

- Preparing for the interview
- Locating prospective employers
- Interviewing

Looking for work is a job in itself. Approach it as a job, establish a schedule, and stick to it.

PREPARING FOR THE INTERVIEW

Preliminary Steps

Before seeking an interview, you should give yourself a "preinterview" self-test:

- What type of work do I really want?
- Where can I function best?
- Do I prefer clinical or administrative functions?
- What are my best skills?
- Do I prefer to work in a small practice or in a large medical group?
- Would I enjoy the variety of a general practice or the concentration of a specialty?
- How important to me are salary, hours, and location?

In your externship experience, you may have formed some rather definite preferences, or you may feel absolutely certain of some things that would cause you to be dissatisfied. Include these judgments in your search.

Personal Inventory

It sometimes happens that your first position is so ideally suitable that you will accept and stay in it for the remainder of your working years. More than likely, however, you will have to make several changes of employment during your lifetime.

A **personal inventory,** to which you will add as you gain additional experience, will prove invaluable to you later as well as now. The personal inventory is for your own information and reference—rather like keeping a journal. It will be a ready source of information in preparing and updating your resumé. The personal inventory is *complete* information about your working life; a resumé is *selected* information tailored to the position you are seeking. Five steps are involved: (1) biographical data, (2) employment history, (3) educational data, (4) extracurricular interests, and (5) activities and personal goals.

Step 1. Start with a page for biographical data: your name, birth date, Social Security number, address, and telephone number.

BIOGRAPHICAL DATA
Name _____ Birth Date _____
Address _____
Tel. No. _____ Soc. Sec. No. _____

Step 2. Prepare a separate page for your employment history. This is especially important for the **re-entry student.** Not all students enter vocational training directly from high school or early in their employment careers. Many have spent intervening years as full-time homemakers or in other employment. The experience gained during these years should be included in your personal inventory. It could be important in future situations. If you have never been employed but have done volunteer work requiring personal responsibility, list that here. The employment history should include dates of employment, name of employer, type of business, your position title, and major duties. Because this will be a continuing record that you will add to as you gain experience, it is prepared in **chronologic** order, starting with the first major job you held. However, when you use this information in a resumé it will be listed in reverse chronologic order, beginning with the latest position.

EMPLOYMENT HISTORY

June   19xx   June   19xx
Month Year to Month Year

Employer _____ XXXXXXXXXX _____

Type of Business _____ Women's clothing _____

Position Held _____ Part-time sales clerk _____

Major Duties: Assisting customers in their selections, registering sales, closing out register at end of day.
Satisfactions: Enjoyed personal contacts
Learned to accept responsibility
Dissatisfactions: Not related to my goals

Step 3. Next, record your educational data, beginning with high school. List the dates, the institution attended, and the year of graduation, plus the diploma or degree earned. Make note of the areas of study you enjoyed most and list special competencies, awards, or honors. As time goes by, it may be difficult to recall these details, and you never know what will be important to an employer in the future. Remember, you are starting a permanent record for your own information and as a handy reference tool when needed. As with the employment history, the educational data are listed here in chronologic order but will appear in reverse chronologic order in a resumé, starting with the highest degree or certificate.

EDUCATIONAL DATA

Dates	Institution Attended	Year Graduated/ Degree
19xx–19xx	Valley High School Ola Vista	19xx Diploma
19xx–19xx	Ola Vista Community College	19xx Associate in Science, Medical Assisting

Special Competencies:
  Typing Certificate (70 wpm)
  Limited X-ray permit, 19xx
  CPR Certificate, 19xx, renewed annually
  Fluency in Spanish
Awards:
  Dean's list, all four semesters in college

Step 4. You may wish to include a page for your extracurricular interests and activities. List organization memberships and activities and any positions of leadership you held. Your volunteer activities and any significant hobbies might be included here if they are not in your employment record. Mention significant skills obtained while performing these activities. Many of these skills are important assets to a medical facility.

EXTRACURRICULAR INTERESTS AND ACTIVITIES

Organization Memberships	Year	Personal Participation
Associated Women Students	19xx	Secretary 19xx–19xx
American Association of Medical Assistants	19xx 19xx	Student Member Page, 19xx convention
Girl Scouts of the U.S.A.	19xx	Brownie group leader, 19xx
Hobbies Oil painting, backpacking		

Step 5. Have a page for your personal goals. What are your *immediate* goals? your *long-term* goals? What concessions are you willing to make in order to reach your goals (e.g., working nonconventional hours)?

PERSONAL GOALS

Date	Immediate Goals	Long-Term Goals
19xx	Medical assistant position preferably in pediatric practice	Bachelor of Science degree in Business Administration
Administrative position in large group practice or HMO

Resumé

The final and most important step in preparing for an interview is producing a **resumé** that will arouse the interest of a prospective employer.

THERESA O'SULLIVAN

233 Wentworth Street, San Diego, CA 92100   Telephone (619) 222-3333

EDUCATION	**Associate in Science**, Ola Vista Community College June 19xx (Dean's List, four semesters) **Diploma**, Valley High School, June 19xx
CERTIFICATES	**CPR** certificate (renewed annually since 19xx) **Certificate in Medical Assisting**, Ola Vista Community College
SPECIAL COMPETENCIES	Speak Spanish fluently Hold Limited X-ray Permit
EMPLOYMENT	**Part-Time Medical Assistant**, June 19xx to June 19xx Duties included: preparing patients for examination in general practice office; taking height, weight, and vital signs; answering the telephone and reception; and appointment scheduling. **Part-Time Sales**, Baxter Department Store, June 19xx to June 19xx Duties included: assisting customers in making their selections; registering sales; and closing out register at end of day.
AVOCATIONAL INTERESTS	**Student Member**, American Association of Medical Assistants **Secretary**, Associated Women Students OVCC
REFERENCES	Furnished upon request.

FIGURE 2–2   Sample chronologic resumé.

If you do not feel confident in doing this yourself, get help. If you are a student in a 2-year college, there is probably a career center on campus where you can ask for assistance. There are also many guidebooks in public libraries and in bookstores where you can find ideas (see the references at the end of this chapter). Computer software that provides guidelines, formatting, and suggestions for preparing the resumé is plentiful and easily located.

The purpose of the resumé is to get an interview, not to get a job. This should be kept in mind as you decide what to include. Using your personal inventory, you can select the information that applies to the position you have in mind. The **format** should be attractive, and the information typed on one sheet of paper with absolutely no errors or misspelled words (Figs. 2–2 and 2–3). Tinted paper will make the resumé more distinctive, but bright

THERESA O'SULLIVAN
233 Wentworth Street, San Diego, CA 92100   Telephone (619) 222-3333

**STATEMENT OF EMPLOYMENT ASSETS
FOR A CAREER IN MEDICAL ASSISTING**

GENERAL	Take pride in appearance Display professionalism Recognize and respond to verbal and nonverbal communication Apply legal and ethical concepts Work as a team member Speak Spanish fluently
ADMINISTRATIVE	Appointment scheduling, filing, pegboard and electronic billing systems, account collections, insurance billing, coding, record keeping, bank deposits and statement reconciliation, patient histories, medical terminology, machine transcription, word processing
CLINICAL	Understanding of anatomy and physiology, symptoms and diseases, collecting and handling specimens, procedures for assisting with physical examination, emergency first aid and CPR, injections, sterile techniques, ECG, inventory and supplies
REFERENCES	Furnished upon request.

FIGURE 2–3   Sample skills resumé.

colors or "arty" headings should be avoided. The resumé gives you an opportunity to display the qualifications that enhance your appeal to prospective employers. Anything that cannot help you or anything that would detract from your image should be omitted. Once you are in the interview, you can clarify any item not entirely explained on the resumé.

Memory Jogger

2 *Why is it better to have a prepared resumé rather than just a discussion of your qualifications during an interview?*

Writing the Resumé

There is no standard format for a resumé, but it should be typewritten on $8\frac{1}{2} \times 11$ good-quality paper. It should be concise and honest and have a professional look. Appearance and accuracy cannot be overemphasized. An employer may interview several acceptable candidates and will be looking for a reason to exclude one or more. Don't allow a "typo" to deny your possible acceptance.

HEADING At the top of the paper should be the necessary personal information: name, address, and telephone number. This is displayed prominently so that it stands apart and can be easily identified (it may be centered).

OBJECTIVE The current trend is to omit reference to an **objective**, particularly if your qualifications are vocationally specific. If you do include an objective, such words as *challenge* or *opportunity* should be avoided because this focuses on what the applicant wants instead of showing understanding of what the employer wants and needs.

EDUCATION AND EXPERIENCE If you are a recent graduate with little or no experience, your education should be listed first and then your employment, if any. College graduates need not include high school information. If you have a good history of recent employment, this is the first item, followed by education. In both cases, you should start with your most recent position and list the rest in *reverse* chronologic order. This is opposite to the order suggested for the personal inventory.

PROFESSIONAL LICENSES Any professional licenses or certificates are included along with memberships in professional organizations.

EXTRACURRICULAR ACTIVITIES Any **extracurricular** or **avocational** interests that would be applicable to the position sought are listed.

REFERENCES You should state on your resumé that references will be furnished on request. (Do not list names and addresses of references on the resumé.) Be prepared to furnish the names of at least three references at the time of your interview. These should have been typewritten on a separate page in the same style as your resumé. The permission of the persons you are listing should be obtained before you provide their names.

ITEMS TO EXCLUDE Do not include

- Your photograph
- Names of spouse and/or children
- Reasons for terminating previous position, if any
- Past salaries or present salary requirements
- Names and addresses of references

Memory Jogger

3 *List seven items to be included in your resumé and five items to exclude.*

LOCATING PROSPECTIVE EMPLOYERS If you are a student in an accredited school, your instructor or the school may be able to give you names of prospective employers. Other good sources for leads are the local medical society, other medical assistants, the local chapter of a professional medical assistants association, branches of the United States Employment Service, and state-operated employment offices.

You may also wish to check the classified advertisements in your local newspaper or place your name with an employment agency. Private employment agencies generally charge a fee equivalent to 2 to 4 weeks' salary to successful applicants. This fee is sometimes paid by the employer after a probationary period.

If you are responding to an advertisement that lists a telephone number, telephoning to request an interview is preferable to writing a letter, but an unsolicited telephone call may be disruptive and destroy the opportunity for an interview. If no telephone number is included in the advertisement, there will be an address listed (usually a box number) to which you may direct a letter requesting an interview. A cover letter responding to an advertisement should include

- A reference to the advertisement, including name of newspaper, date of publication, and position title. The employer may be running more than one recruitment ad.
- An enthusiastic expression of interest in the position.
- A comparison of your own qualifications with those of the position to be filled.
- Information about where you can be contacted.
- A request for a response or interview.
- Thanks for considering your request.

PROCEDURE 2–1

Preparing a Resumé

GOAL

To prepare a resumé of education and experience that will be informative to a prospective employer and create interest in arranging an interview for employment.

EQUIPMENT AND SUPPLIES

Summary of personal data
Quality stationery
Typewriter or computer

PROCEDURAL STEPS

1 Assemble all personal data necessary for resumé.

2 Arrange in reverse chronologic order.
   PURPOSE: To enable you to proceed in orderly fashion in preparing the resumé and to check accuracy of dates.

3 Typewrite heading that includes your name, address, and telephone number.
   PURPOSE: For easy identification by reader.

4 List highest education degree or diploma, including name of institution and year. Include high school if you are not a college graduate.
   PURPOSE: Training may be important to your employability.

5 List all work experience in reverse chronologic order.
   PURPOSE: To demonstrate transferable experiences toward future employment.

6 Include any professional licenses, certificates, and memberships in professional organizations.
   PURPOSE: Indicates employability and personal interest in profession.

7 List any extracurricular or avocational interests applicable to the position sought.

8 State that references will be furnished on request.
   PURPOSE: Prospective employers may wish to verify your experience and character. *Note:* Obtain permission before listing anyone as a reference.

9 Review resumé for accuracy, completeness, and attractive format.

10 If mailing, place in No. 10 envelope on which you have typed the address and your return address. Include a cover letter.

UNSOLICITED INTERVIEW REQUEST   You may decide to canvass a number of medical facilities to determine whether there are openings for a medical assistant. A letter such as the one shown in Figure 2–4 can be written and your resumé enclosed. Then you should follow up with a telephone call in about 1 week.

INTERVIEWING

Application Form

Completing an application for employment is not standard procedure in small medical practices, but you should be prepared for complying if requested (see Management Responsibilities). Larger health agencies such as hospitals and health maintenance organizations will definitely ask you to fill out their application form.

You should have readily available your Social Security number, driver's license, and telephone numbers where you can be reached. Your resumé should have the information you will need regarding education and employment. You need to be prepared to furnish telephone numbers for previous employers, if any, and have available the names, addresses, and telephone numbers of three references who have given you their permission to list them.

The appearance and completeness of your filled-in application will be considered in your overall evaluation. By law, employers cannot require you to answer questions regarding your place of birth, ethnic origin or religious preference, or your age, marital status, or number of children. If these questions are on the application, you may choose to leave them blank, but all allowable questions should be an-

PROCEDURE 2-2
Answering a Help-Wanted Advertisement

GOAL

To write a letter in response to a newspaper advertisement that will relay your qualifications and generate interest in arranging an interview.

EQUIPMENT AND SUPPLIES

Recent newspaper with classified
    employment ads
Stationery
Typewriter or computer
Pen

PROCEDURAL STEPS

1 Review letter writing information in Chapter 11, Correspondence and Mail Processing.

2 Draft a letter to include
  • Name of newspaper, date of publication, and title of position for which you are applying.
  PURPOSE: Employer may be running more than one advertisement.
  • Information about where you can be contacted.
  PURPOSE: To enable interested employer to reach you.

3 Express enthusiastic interest in the position offered, and state your qualifications.

4 Request a response to your letter by telephone or mail.
  PURPOSE: So that an interview can be arranged if position is still open and employer is interested in your qualifications.

5 End the letter with an expression of thanks for considering your request.
  PURPOSE: To demonstrate your knowledge of courtesy.

6 Review the letter for content and accuracy.
  PURPOSE: To make certain that you have included all essential information and that the letter is free of errors.

---

swered honestly and completely. Print your answers or write as plainly as possible. *Hint:* Have your own favorite pen with you.

Day of the Interview

Your appearance is extremely important. Clothing should be conservative, neat, and well pressed. Women should wear a dress or suit with a skirt. Slacks or pantsuits and open sandals are considered inappropriate for a job interview. Men should wear a suit and tie and appropriate dress shoes.

Hair should be well groomed and worn in a professional-looking style. Jewelry should be kept to a minimum and heavy scents of perfume or antiperspirants avoided. Women should be careful and conservative in applying makeup and should carry a modest purse that is not bulging with unnecessary items.

You should take a critical look at yourself in the mirror before leaving home and again just before entering the prospective employer's office (see Interviewing Tips).

PERSONAL QUALITIES

INTERVIEWING TIPS

• *Be prompt.* Arrive promptly for the interview. Under no circumstances should you be even so much as 1 minute late and then have to make a weak excuse.

• *Be prepared.* Bring two copies of your resumé, one to give to the interviewer and one to refer to in case you get nervous.

• *Be self-sufficient.* Go alone. You may want moral support, but you will be more relaxed if there is no one waiting for you.

• *Be poised.* Enter the office confidently and without appearing rushed.

• *Be polite.* Introduce yourself to the receptionist, and then express appreciation when you are asked to be seated.

• *Be patient.* If you must wait, try to relax, but avoid slouching in your chair.

• *Be considerate and composed.* Do not smoke or chew gum.

Theresa O'Sullivan
233 Wentworth Street, San Diego, CA 92100
Telephone (619) 222-3333

June 15, 19xx

Arthur M. Blackburn, MD
2200 Broadway
Any Town, US 98765

Dear Doctor Blackburn:

In a few weeks, I will complete my formal training in medical assisting with an Associate in Science degree from Ola Vista Community College.

The medical assisting program at Ola Vista includes theory and practical application in both administrative and clinical skills. My six-week supervised externship gave me additional practical experience in two specialty practices.

While studying at Ola Vista, I also worked part-time for a physician in family practice, while maintaining a 3.5 grade point average. My experience as Dr. Madden's employee is outlined on the enclosed resumé. I have enjoyed my work in Dr. Madden's office and am now seeking full-time employment.

If you will require a replacement or addition to your staff in the near future, may I be considered as an applicant? I will follow up with a telephone call within a week.

Sincerely yours,

Theresa O'Sullivan

Enc. Resumé

FIGURE 2–4 Sample cover letter.

When you prepared your resumé, you listed your job skills, your education, or both. The interviewer already knows how well you ought to be able to do the job. However, you will be judged in at least two other areas of evaluation:

- *What kind of co-worker you will be.* Working in a health care facility requires team effort, and your ability to work in cooperation and coordination with others bears heavily on how well you will do your job, apart from the excellence of your job skills.
- *What kind of employee you will be.* Dependability, trustworthiness, dedication, loyalty, and other personal characteristics are always important to an employer.

During the Interview

When you are ushered into the interviewer's room, wait to be seated until you are invited to do so. Let the interviewer lead the conversation. Be prepared to answer such questions as "Tell me about yourself," and "Why do you want to work here?" One reason for an opening such as this is to provide a little time to relax and get acquainted. You might start out by reviewing your professional background and training and then progress to personal interests, hobbies, and so forth (Fig. 2–5).

The interviewer will be observing your body language, your manners, poise, speech, alertness, and ability to give direct answers. A relaxed, friendly

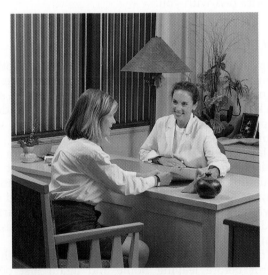

FIGURE 2–5 Student being interviewed for a job.

manner with good eye contact is important—look directly at the person to whom you are speaking. Your sense of humor may be tested as well, and questions may be directed to you that will test your common sense and frankness. You can promote yourself honestly and graciously by showing that you enjoy others, that you are willing to work and accept responsibility, and that you have an open mind about the position and are willing to learn.

Legislation affecting employment practices has influenced hiring practices nationwide. (See discussion of Americans with Disabilities Act of 1990 in Chapter 6.) Employers are restricted in the information that can be required on an application or asked in an interview. Although you may not be *required* to answer questions, such as your age, birthplace, and marital status, a prospective employer might appreciate your mentioning any such pertinent information in conversation. Remember that your objective is to obtain a position.

At the end of the interview, if the interviewer has not mentioned hours and salary, you may properly inquire about these subjects at this time. If you are not really interested in the position, do not bother to ask; but if the position sounds satisfactory and is one that you would like to accept, you may then ask if the interviewer wishes to discuss the salary. This should be enough of a lead, because it was probably an oversight on the interviewer's part. If the interviewer seems reluctant to discuss it, however, do not press the issue, because this may be an indication that your qualifications do not fit the position and there is no reason to pursue the interview further.

If you have been given a tour of the office, you may make some pleasant observations and comments but do not be falsely overenthusiastic. When you are introduced to the staff, be gracious and friendly. Try to remember their names so that you can thank them later. Show enthusiasm, but do not overdo it because it may appear to others that you are putting on an act.

Closing the Interview

The interviewer will usually take the initiative in closing the interview, perhaps by sliding back the chair and asking whether you have further questions. Do not show disappointment if the position is not offered to you at the time of the interview. There may be other applicants to see, or the interviewer may wish to check your references before making a commitment. Express your thanks for the interview as you leave, and remember, too, to thank the receptionist and say a friendly good-bye.

Follow-Up Activities

A brief, well-worded letter of thanks sent to the interviewer immediately after the interview could be crucial in deciding whether you will be hired. This is one of the most essential steps in the entire job-seeking process, and the one most overlooked by job-seekers. Simply write a brief note expressing appreciation for the interview and interest in the position (Fig. 2–6).

After a few days, you may call the office and ask if the position has been filled and tell them you are interested because you enjoyed your interview and the office staff. If the position is still open, ask

---

Theresa O'Sullivan
233 Wentworth Street, San Diego, CA 92100
Telephone (619) 222-3333

June 16, 19xx

Arthur M. Blackburn, MD
2200 Broadway
Any Town, US 98765

Dear Doctor Blackburn:

Thank you for taking the time to talk with me today about the medical assistant position in your office and for considering my qualifications for filling that position.

I would be pleased to accept your offer if you should decide that I meet your requirements.

Sincerely yours,

Theresa O'Sullivan

FIGURE 2–6 Sample of thank-you letter after interview.

whether you may inquire again in a few days. Be brief and thank the person with whom you are speaking.

If you are not hired, ask yourself some pertinent questions:

- Did I look my best?
- Did I show enthusiasm for the job?
- Did I listen carefully during the interview?
- Did I say or do something I should not have said or done?

Even if you are not hired, you should never feel that an interview is a waste of time. You learn from each experience, and with experience you are better able to promote your qualifications in future interviews.

If you are hired, ask the interviewer if you may borrow the office policy and procedure manual to review before you report to work. If this is allowed, jot down items that you find important to remember in your own notebook or questions that you need to ask when reporting to work.

On your first day of work, arrive promptly and eager for your new experience. And remember to bring your notebook!

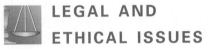

LEGAL AND ETHICAL ISSUES

Expect to observe all the office protocols of regular attendance, being on time and in appropriate attire. Do not expect or ask for payment for your services as an extern.

During your externship practice you are bound by the same regulations as the regular staff. Be punctual in your attendance. Restrict your performance to those areas in which you have been trained. If the state in which you live has a scope of practice for medical assistants, know the boundaries within which you can perform and do not exceed them. You may be expected to carry malpractice insurance.

Some schools provide a blanket policy for their students.

CRITICAL THINKING

Observe your surroundings and make a mental note of situations or practices that could be improved. Offer suggestions only when asked.

HOW DID I DO? Answers to Memory Joggers

1 *Similarities:*
Appearance and actions meet professional standards.
Regular hours are observed.
Differences:
Short term, may be part-time.
All activities will be supervised and evaluated.
No payment.
May report to several different agencies.

2 The purpose of the resumé is to provide preliminary information that will assist in arranging an interview. The resumé allows the interviewer to determine whether the applicant meets basic requirements.

3 *Include* name, address, telephone number, education, experience, licenses and certificates, and extracurricular activities.
Exclude photo, names of spouse and/or children, reasons for terminating previous position, past salaries or present salary requirements, and names and addresses of references.

REFERENCE

Bolles RN: What Color Is Your Parachute? Berkeley, CA, Ten Speed Press, revised annually. *Resumé Expert* software.

A Brief History of Medicine

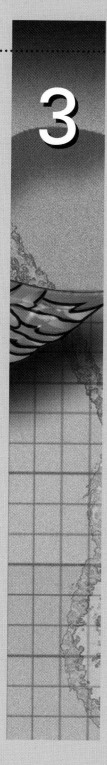

3

LEARNING OBJECTIVES

Cognitive: On successful completion of this chapter you should be able to:

1 Define and spell the terms listed in the Vocabulary.

2 Identify the two ancient mythologies that contributed a major portion of our medical terminology.

3 Distinguish between and describe the two medical symbols in general use today.

4 Name the oath that has been administered to new physicians for more than 2000 years.

5 Name the medical school that was the most famous in the world at the end of the 19th century.

6 Name a 20th century educator who played a major role in the development of medical education in the United States.

7 Identify the important discovery made by William Harvey that was only substantiated 200 years later.

8 Name the 18th century English surgeon who was declared the Founder of Scientific Surgery.

9 Name the Hungarian physician who earned the title Savior of Mothers.

10 List the names of five 19th century women who contributed significantly to medical history.

11 Name the surgeon who performed the first human heart transplant.

12 Name two agencies of the U.S. Department of Health and Human Services that play an important role in the advancement of health in the United States and the world.

VOCABULARY

anesthetic Agent that causes loss of sensation with or without loss of consciousness

anthrax An acute infectious disease caused by a bacillus. Humans contract the disease from animal hair, hides, or waste matter.

aphonia Loss of the ability to speak

aphrodisiacs Drugs that cause sexual arousal

attenuated Made thin or weaker

auscultation The act of listening for sounds within the body, normally with a stethoscope

bacteria Single-celled microscopic organisms

catheterization The act of passing a tube through the body for removing fluids or injecting them into body cavities

cervical vertebrae The upper seven bones of the spinal column; the skeleton of the neck

chemotherapy The treatment of disease using chemical agents

cholera An acute, infectious, bacillus-caused disease involving the entire small bowel; *chicken cholera*—cholera that affects chickens

contamination The act of soiling, staining, or polluting; especially the introduction of infectious materials or germs that produce disease

cyanosis A bluish discoloration of the skin

dissection The process of cutting apart or separating tissues for anatomic study

embryology The science or study of the development of living organisms during the embryonic stage

fallopian tubes The tubes that carry the ovum from the ovary to the uterus; the oviducts

hemiplegia Paralysis of one side of the body

histologist One who specializes in the study of the minute structure, composition, and function of the tissues

immunology A science that deals with the phenomena and causes of immunity and immune responses

innovation Act of introducing something new or novel

invulnerable Incapable of being injured or harmed

isolation The act of placing alone apart from others

ligation Something that binds

microorganisms Organisms of microscopic or ultramicroscopic size

millennia Thousands of years (*mille* = thousand)

mons veneris The rounded, elevated area overlying the symphysis pubis that is covered with hair after puberty

mysticism The experience of seeming to have direct communication with God or ultimate reality

mythology A branch of knowledge that deals with the interpretation of myths

neophyte A new convert or novice

oviducts The pair of tubes in the female that carry the egg from the ovary to the uterus; fallopian tubes

pandemic Affecting the majority of the people in a country or a number of countries

pathologic Altered or caused by disease

percussion The act of striking a part of the body with short, sharp blows as an aid in diagnosing the condition of the underlying parts by the sound obtained

perfusion The passing of a fluid through spaces

periphery The external surface or boundary of a body

phagocytosis The engulfing of microorganisms, other cells, and foreign particles by phagocytes

placenta The vascular structure that develops within the uterus during pregnancy and through which a fetus receives nourishment

protozoa Primitive animal organisms, each of which consists of a single cell

puerperal fever The fever that accompanies an infection of the birth canal following delivery of a child; childbed fever

purulent Consisting of or containing pus

pustule A raised pus-filled area or sac

putrefaction Decomposition of animal matter that results in a foul smell

rabies An acute infectious disease of the nervous system caused by a virus, usually communicated to humans through animal bite

rete mucosum The innermost layer of the epidermis (*rete* = network of nerves or vessels)

spermatozoa Mature male germ cells

statutory body A part of the legislative branch of a government

stethoscope An instrument for listening to sounds within the body

swine erysipelas A contagious disease affecting young swine in Europe

syphilitic chancre The primary sore of syphilis

vagina The canal in the female that extends from the vulva to the cervix

virulent Exceedingly pathogenic, noxious, or deadly

vivisection Operation or cutting on a living animal for research purposes

Learning the history of the development of modern medicine is not necessary to perform your duties as a medical assistant, just as a study of the genealogy of your family is not necessary for you to live a full life. However, both of these pursuits add interest and a uniqueness to the quality of life.

Modern medicine reflects its history in the names given to anatomic and physiologic phenomena, medications, diseases, instruments, and specialties. Even the latest medical discoveries often have names drawn from the ancients. When we live in the world of medicine and speak its language we are constantly touched by this fascinating past. The rich cultural heritage of medicine is interesting to study and provides a perspective and understanding of its impact on the present. It is also a history of hardships and disappointment that were pushed aside by determined men and women who wanted to pursue their dreams and goals. Learning about these pioneers (Table 3–1) is inspiring as we realize that we, too, can be a part of the heritage of caring and discovery that continues to improve health care throughout the world.

Medical Language and Mythology

Borrowing so liberally from ancient **mythology,** and so actively using the classical language that most civilizations abandoned centuries ago, may seem strange. Yet today's medicine uses words whose origins stem from the romance and fantasy of this long "dead" world. Anatomy, especially, seems to reach back to the dawn of history. Many early anatomic terms have reached modern times almost unchanged, although some terms are false when translated literally (because the ancients did not correctly understand body functions). *Example:* "artery," which comes from the Greek word *arteria,* literally "a windpipe"—the Greeks believed that the artery carried air, not blood.

Greek and Roman mythology have contributed a major portion of our medical terminology, but we have also borrowed liberally from Arabic, Anglo-Saxon, and German sources, with a heavy dash of the Bible added. A few of the many examples of medical terms derived from the classical past are presented.

ATLAS, the anatomic name for the first **cervical vertebrae** upon which the head rests, is aptly named for the famous Greek titan, who, according to mythology, was condemned by Zeus to bear the heavens on his shoulders. The tendon of ACHILLES (ah-kil′ēz) reminds us of the story of the youth whose mother held him by the heel and dipped him into the river Styx to make him **invulnerable.** This tendon was not immersed. Later, a mortal wound was inflicted in Achilles' heel. A common expression used today to show a point of weakness is "your Achilles heel." APHRODITE (af′ro-dī-te), the Greek goddess of love and beauty, gave her name to the sex-arousing drugs known as **aphrodisiacs.** The equivalent Roman goddess of love, VENUS (vē′nus), has distinctions paid to her not so much as the goddess of love but of lust. A portion of the female anatomy, the **mons veneris,** was dedicated to her memory. Venereal diseases are also named after Venus.

AESCULAPIUS (es″-ku-la′pe-us), the son of Apollo, was revered as the god of medicine. The early Greeks worshiped the healing powers of Aesculapius and built temples in his honor, where patients were treated by trained priests. His daughters were HYGEIA (hi-jé-ah), goddess of health, and PANACEA (pan″ah-se″-ah), goddess of all healing and restorer of health. Our modern word "hygiene," the science of health maintenance, has its origin in Hygeia, and the modern meaning of "panacea" is "a remedy for all ills or difficulties." The staff of Aesculapius, which is a staff encircled by one serpent, is used to signify the art of healing and has been adopted by the American Medical Association as the symbol of medicine. The mythological staff belonging to Apollo, the caduceus, which is a staff encir-

TABLE 3–1   Milestones in the History of Medicine

Dates	Person	Achievement	Dates	Person	Achievement
1205 BC	Moses (First "Public Health Officer")	Incorporated rules of health into the Hebrew religion	1749–1823	Edward Jenner	Discovered smallpox vaccine
460–377 BC	Hippocrates (Father of Medicine)	Gave scientific basis to medicine Hippocratic Oath	1781–1826	René Laënnec	Invented the stethoscope
131–201 AD	Galen (Father of Experimental Physiology)	First to describe cranial nerves and sympathetic system	1818–1865	Ignaz Philipp Semmelweis (Savior of Mothers)	Developed theory of childbed (puerperal) fever
1514–1564	Andreas Vesalius (Belgian anatomist; Father of Modern Anatomy)	Corrected some of Galen's errors Published *De Corporis Humani Fabrica* describing structure of human body	1820–1910	Florence Nightingale (Lady with the Lamp)	Founder of nursing
			1821–1912	Clara Barton	Founder of American Red Cross
1578–1657	William Harvey	Described pumping action of heart and circulation of the blood	1821–1910	Elizabeth Blackwell	First woman in United States to receive Doctor of Medicine degree from a medical school
1628–1694	Marcello Malpighi (First histologist)	Pioneered microscopic anatomy Identified the taste buds; described minute structures of brain and optic nerve	1822–1895	Louis Pasteur (Father of Bacteriology)	Developed germ theory of disease and destruction of microorganisms through use of heat
1632–1723	Anton van Leeuwenhoek	Discovered lens magnification First to observe bacteria and protozoa through a lens Made first accurate description of red blood cells	1827–1912	Joseph Lister	Applied Pasteur's theories and developed sterile techniques in surgery
			1843–1910	Robert Koch	Bacteriologist who developed culture-plate method for isolation of bacteria Set down Koch's postulates
1722–1809	Leopold Auenbrugger	Developed the use of percussion in diagnosis	1845–1922	Wilhelm Konrad Roentgen	Discovered x-ray in 1895
1728–1793	John Hunter (Founder of Scientific Surgery)	Introduced artificial feeding by insertion of flexible tube into stomach Made classic description of syphilitic chancre (hunterian chancre)	1854–1915	Paul Ehrlich	Began the use of injecting chemicals into the body to destroy a specific organism Developed drug used to fight syphilis
1745–1813	Benjamin Rush	Published first American treatise on psychiatry in 1812	1867–1940	Lillian Wald	New York City nurse who operated a visiting nurse service and helped establish the world's first public school nursing system

cled by two serpents, is the medical insignia of the United States Army Medical Corps and is often misused as a symbol of the medical profession (Fig. 3–1).

Memory Jogger

1 *How does the caduceus differ from the staff of Aesculapius?*

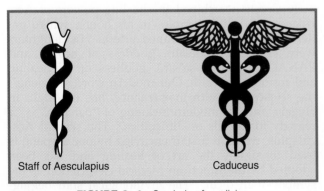

Staff of Aesculapius   Caduceus

FIGURE 3–1 Symbols of medicine.

Medicine in Ancient Times

Although religion and myth were the basis of care for the sick for **millennia,** there is evidence of drugs, surgery, and other treatments based on theories about the body from as early as 5000 to 2000 BC. In the well-developed societies of the Egyptians, Babylonians, and Assyrians, certain men acted as physicians and used their scant knowledge to try to treat illness and injury.

MOSES incorporated rules of health into the Hebrew religion around 1205 BC. He was thus the first

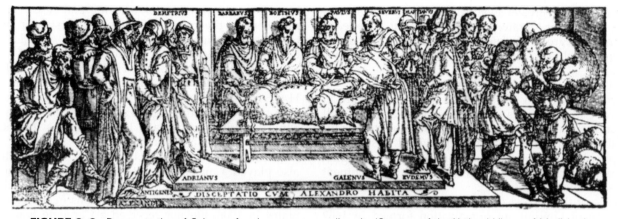

FIGURE 3–2 Demonstration of Galen performing surgery on a live pig. (Courtesy of the National Library of Medicine.)

advocate of preventive medicine and could even be called the first public health officer. Moses knew that some animal diseases might be passed on to humans and that **contamination** might linger on unclean dishes. Consequently, it became a religious law that no one was permitted to eat animals that were not freshly slaughtered or to eat or drink from dirty dishes, lest they become defiled and lose their souls.

HIPPOCRATES (hip-pok′rah-tēz) (460–377 BC) is the most famous of the ancient Greek physicians and is known as the Father of Medicine. He did much to separate medicine from **mysticism** and gave it a scientific basis. He is best remembered for the Hippocratic Oath (see Chapter 5) exacted from his pupils. This oath has been administered to physicians for more than 2000 years. Hippocrates' astute clinical descriptions of diseases and his voluminous writings on epidemics, fevers, epilepsy, fractures, and instruments were studied for centuries. He believed that the body tends to heal itself and that it is the physician's responsibility to help nature. In Hippocrates' time, very little was known about anatomy, physiology, and pathology, and no knowledge of chemistry existed. In spite of these handicaps, many of his classifications of diseases and his descriptions of symptoms are being used today.

Memory Jogger

2 *Why was Moses called the "first public health officer"?*

Many Greek physicians practiced, studied, and taught in Rome in the time after Hippocrates. One was GALEN (131–201 AD), who came to Rome in 162 AD and became known as the Prince of Physicians (Fig. 3–2). Galen is said to have written 500 treatises on medicine. He wrote an excellent summary of anatomy as it was known at that time. Nevertheless, his work was faulty and inaccurate, because it was based largely on the **dissection** of apes and swine. He is considered the Father of Ex-

perimental Physiology and the first experimental neurologist. He was the first to describe the cranial nerve and the sympathetic nervous system, and he made the first experimental sections of the spinal cord, producing **hemiplegia.** Galen also produced **aphonia** by cutting the recurrent laryngeal nerve, and he gave the first valid explanation of the mechanism of respiration.

The profound influence of the writings of Hippocrates and Galen on the course of medicine gives praise to these great thinkers, but their unquestioned authority actually had a negative effect on the progress of science throughout the Dark Ages. Their theories and descriptions were held to as law, so **innovation** was rarely attempted. Experimenters were scoffed at by their contemporaries. Later, the Christian religion taught people to care for the sick and encouraged the establishment of institutions where the sick could find help. This provided an opportunity for physicians to observe, analyze, and discuss the progress of a variety of patients. The establishment of universities led more to a study of theories of disease rather than to observation of the sick. It was not until the 16th century that Andreas Vesalius began to correct some of Galen's errors.

Early Development of Medical Education

In early times medical knowledge developed slowly, often in **isolation,** and distribution of knowledge was poor. Before the invention of the printing press there was very little exchange of scientific knowledge and ideas, and scientists were not well informed about the works of others.

In the middle of the 15th century, Johann Gutenberg's invention of movable type and adaptation of a certain kind of press for printing marked a turning point in history. Gutenberg's invention resulted in a faster way to produce multiple identical copies of any single text. Printing rapidly replaced the laborious method of scribes, who had to copy manuscripts by hand. The greater availability of books increased the number of literate people throughout Europe. In turn, ever greater refinements in the printing press were developed to meet the growing demand for books.

Another development important to science occurred in the 17th century with the establishment in Europe of academies or societies consisting of small groups of men who met to discuss subjects of mutual interest. The academies provided freedom of expression that, with the stimulus of exchanging ideas, contributed significantly to the development of scientific thought.

One of the earliest of the academies was the Royal Society of London, an organization formed in 1662 by the incorporation of several smaller groups under one royal charter. A significant aspect of these societies was their publications, such as the Royal Society of London's *Philosophical Transactions.*

The development of communications was improving. Society was becoming more complex and the need for regulation becoming greater. The passage of the Medical Act of 1858 in Great Britain was considered one of the most important events in British medicine. It established a **statutory body,** the General Medical Council, which controlled admission to the medical register and had great power over medical education and examinations.

In the United States, medical education was greatly influenced by the example set in 1893 by the Johns Hopkins University Medical School in Baltimore. It admitted only college graduates with a year's training in the natural sciences. Its clinical work was superior because the school was supplemented by the Johns Hopkins Hospital, which had been created expressly for teaching and research by members of the medical family. The first four professors at Johns Hopkins were SIR WILLIAM OSLER, professor of medicine; WILLIAM H. WELCH, chief of pathology; HOWARD A. KELLEY, chief of gynecology and obstetrics; and WILLIAM D. HALSTED, chief of surgery. Together, these four men transformed the organization and curriculum of clinical teaching and made Johns Hopkins the most famous medical school in the world.

ABRAHAM FLEXNER (1866–1959), an educator, also played a major role in the development of medical education in the United States. After publishing an appraisal of educational institutions in the United States in 1908, Flexner received a Carnegie Foundation commission to study the quality of medical colleges in the United States and Canada. The Flexner report, published in 1910, rated 155 schools according to the quality of instruction and facilities available to the students. The publication of this report resulted in the closure of many low-ranking schools and the upgrading of many others.

Memory Jogger

3 *Why did the Johns Hopkins Medical School become the most famous in the world?*

Early Pioneers

ANDREAS VESALIUS (an'drē-as ve-sa'le-us) (1514–1564), a Belgian anatomist, is known as the

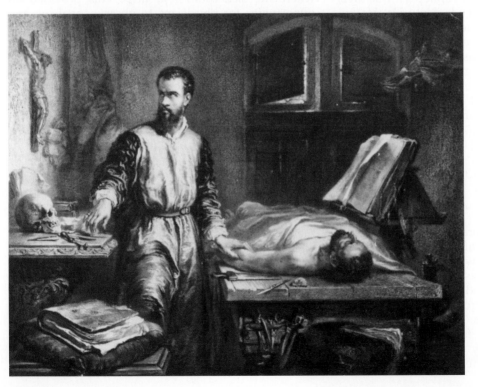

FIGURE 3–3 Andreas Vesalius. (Courtesy of the National Library of Medicine.)

Father of Modern Anatomy (Fig. 3–3). At the age of 29, he published his great *De Corporis Humani Fabrica,* in which he described the structure of the human body. This work marked a turning point by breaking with the past and throwing overboard the Galen tradition. Vesalius introduced many new anatomic terms, but because of his radical approach he was subjected to some persecution from his colleagues, his teachers, and his pupils. Despite his great contributions to the science of anatomy, his name is not used to identify any important anatomic structures.

GABRIELE FALLOPIUS (gā′brē-el fal-ōp′-e-us) (1523–1562), a student of Vesalius, was also an accurate and detailed dissector who described and named many parts of the anatomy. He gave his own name to the **oviducts,** known as the **fallopian tubes.** He also named the **vagina** and the **placenta.**

In 1628, WILLIAM HARVEY (1578–1657) made his pronouncement that the heart acts as a muscular force-pump in propelling the blood along and that the blood's motion is continual and continuous in a cycle or circle (Fig. 3–4). Harvey based his conclusion on his experimental **vivisection, ligation,** and **perfusion** as well as brilliant reasoning. The work of this English physician was not fully recognized until 1827, when the full importance of his work was substantiated. Harvey's writings were recognized in Germany before the English permitted their publication at home. Modern England now considers Harvey to be its medical Shakespeare.

Great advances in medicine were somewhat stilled for a century or so, but the unseen world of **microorganisms** was opened as ANTON VAN LEEUWENHOEK (än′tōn van lu′-en-hōk) (1632–1723), a Dutch linen draper and haberdasher by trade, pursued his hobby of grinding lenses. He ground over 400 lenses during his lifetime, most of which were very small—some no larger than a pinhead—and usually mounted between two thin brass plates that were riveted together. In grinding lenses Leeuwenhoek discovered how to use a simple biconvex lens to magnify the minute world of organisms and structures that had never been seen before.

Leeuwenhoek was the first man ever to observe **bacteria** and **protozoa** through a lens. His accurate interpretations of what he saw led to the sciences of bacteriology and protozoology. He described for the first time the **spermatozoa** from insects, dogs, and men. He studied the structure of the optic lens, striations in muscles, and the mouthparts of insects. Leeuwenhoek extended Marcello Malpighi's demonstration in 1661 of the blood capillaries by giving (in 1684) the first accurate description of red blood cells. From 1673 until 1723, he communicated by means of informal letters most of his discoveries to the Royal Society of England, to which he was elected as a fellow in 1680. Leeuwenhoek's advances have been further developed, and, with modern refinements, magnification now allows visualization of the smallest organisms with chemical structures.

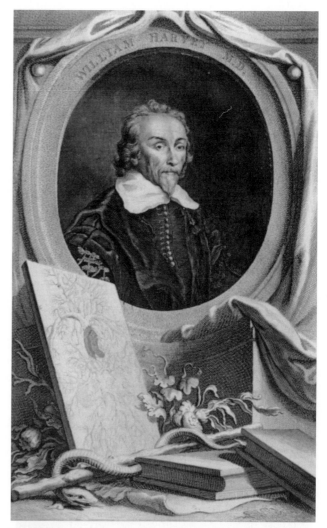

FIGURE 3–4 William Harvey. (Courtesy of the National Library of Medicine.)

Memory Joggers

4 *How were the lenses produced by Leeuwenhoek used in the advancement of medicine?*

MARCELLO MALPIGHI (mar-chel′-o mahl-pe′-ge) (1628–1694), the greatest of the microscopists, was born near Bologna, Italy; entered the University of Bologna in 1646; and, in 1653, was granted doctorates in both medicine and philosophy. Malpighi pioneered the use of the microscope in the study of plants and animals, after which microscopic anatomy became a prerequisite for advances in physiology, **embryology,** and practical medicine. He may be regarded as the first **histologist.** In 1661, he identified and described the pulmonary and capillary network connecting the small arteries with small veins, one of the most important discoveries in the history of science. When Malpighi found that the blood passed through the capillaries, it meant that Harvey was right—that blood was not transformed into flesh in the **periphery,** as the ancients had thought.

Malpighi continued to pursue his studies with the microscope while teaching and practicing medicine. He identified the taste buds and described the minute structure of the brain and the optic nerve. He was the first to see the red blood cells and to attribute the color of blood to them. He discovered the **rete mucosum** or malpighian layer of the skin. His work on the structure of the liver, spleen, and kidney is recalled today when we speak of the malpighian bodies of the kidney and spleen, Malpighi's pyramids (pyramides renales), and Malpighi's vesicles (alveoli pulmonis).

Scientific Advances (18th and 19th Centuries)

JOHN HUNTER (1728–1793), the famous English surgeon and anatomist, was born a few years after Leeuwenhoek's death (Fig. 3–5). Hunter has been given the title Founder of Scientific Surgery because his surgical procedures were soundly based on **pathologic** evidence. He was the first to classify teeth in a scientific manner. In 1778, he introduced artificial feeding by means of a flexible tube passed into the stomach. His description of the **syphilitic chancre** is classic, and the lesion is sometimes called the hunterian chancre.

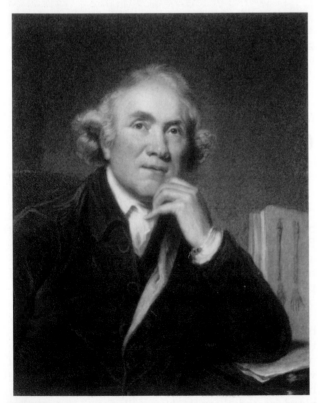

FIGURE 3–5 John Hunter. (Courtesy of the National Library of Medicine.)

In an unsuccessful attempt to differentiate gonorrhea from syphilis, Hunter inoculated himself with what he thought was gonorrhea, but instead he acquired syphilis. Hunter's results increased the confusion, because he concluded that gonorrhea was a symptom of syphilis. This confusion continued until the beginning of the 20th century.

Hunter's great collection of anatomic and animal specimens formed the basis for the museum of the Royal College of Surgeons. He was also a member of the Royal Society of Medicine and the Royal Academy of Surgery in Paris.

Memory Jogger

5 *Why was Hunter given the title "Founder of Scientific Surgery"?*

Hunter wrote many papers on anatomy and physiology; he was a brilliant lecturer and teacher. Among his many students was one who would become famous and well loved—Edward Jenner.

EDWARD JENNER (1749–1823) was a country physician in Dorsetshire, England (Fig. 3–6). He is listed among the immortals of preventive medicine for his discovery of the smallpox vaccine. The story goes that one day, while Jenner was serving as an apprentice in the office of Daniel Ludlow, a dairy maid was being given treatment. Smallpox was mentioned, and she said, "I cannot take that disease, for I have had cowpox." Smallpox at that time was a deadly **pandemic.** Jenner observed that farmers and dairy maids who once had cowpox never contracted smallpox. Later, as a practicing physician, Jenner continued investigating the relationship between cowpox and smallpox, to the extent that other medical society members became bored by him and threatened to expel him from their ranks.

On May 14, 1796, Dr. Jenner took some **purulent** matter from a **pustule** on the hand of Sarah Nelmes, a dairy maid, and inserted it through two small superficial incisions into the arm of James Phipps, a healthy 8-year-old boy. This was the first vaccination. Later, on July 1, a **virulent** dose of smallpox matter was given to young Phipps in the same arm. It had no effect: Phipps had been vaccinated and was safe from the dreaded disease. Edward Jenner's method of vaccination spread throughout the world. The results of his methods and experiments were published in 1798. He called this method of protection "vaccination" because the Latin word *vacca* means "cow." Cowpox was called vaccinia. Pasteur applied the term "vaccine" to suspensions of dead bacteria or **attenuated** bacteria. This term has come to be used in reference to other immunizing antigens not derived from cows. Today smallpox is extinct throughout the world due to a planned program of world vaccination.

Victor Robinson, in *Pathfinders in Medicine,* said of Dr. Jenner, "He died where an intellectual man

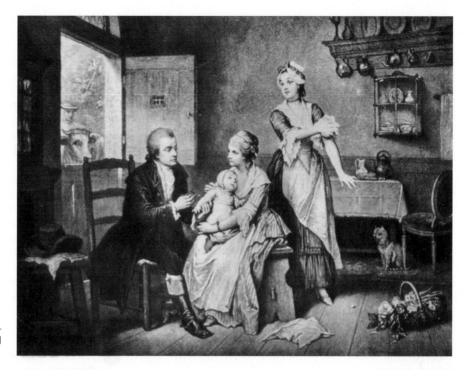

FIGURE 3–6 Edward Jenner vaccinating an infant. (Courtesy of the National Library of Medicine.)

should die (in his library)." The village that gave him birth received his illustrious ashes. When his worn-out body was laid to rest, it would not be surprising if some humble woman, whose child he had saved from smallpox, imagined that Edward Jenner had gone to heaven—to vaccinate the angels.

Memory Jogger

6 *What is the origin of the word* vaccination?

Percussion and **auscultation** have been the very basics of physical examination for many years. But no physician had a real understanding of what went on inside the body until anatomists had paved the way for an Austrian physician, LEOPOLD AUEN-BRUGGER (le'-a-pōld Ow-en-broog'-er) (1722–1809), who developed the use of percussion in diagnosis, and a French physician, RENÉ LAËNNEC (re-na' La'-en-nek) (1781–1826), who developed the **stethoscope.** Auenbrugger became physician-in-chief to the Hospital of the Holy Trinity at Vienna in 1751, and it was there that he tested his discovery, which afterward made him famous but which was generally ignored and scorned by his contemporaries. Laënnec invented the stethoscope in 1819, but at first it was only a cylinder of paper in his hands. His book concerning the stethoscope was readily accepted and translated into many languages. It is said to be the most important treatise in diseases of the thoracic organs ever written.

The first American treatise on psychiatry, *Medical Inquiries and Observations upon the Diseases of the Mind,* published in 1812, was written by BENJAMIN RUSH (1745–1813), a member of the Continental Congress in 1776 and a signer of the Declaration of Independence.

In the early 1800s, there were several men who are remembered for their fight against **puerperal fever** and for their concern for women's health. Puerperal fever, an infectious disease of childbirth, is also known as puerperal sepsis or childbed fever. This term is from *puerpera,* denoting a woman in childbed, from the Latin *puer,* a child, and *pario,* to bring forth. The word "puerperium" now designates the period from delivery to the time the uterus returns to normal size (about 42 days).

The best known of these men is the Hungarian physician IGNAZ PHILIPP SEMMELWEIS (ig'näts fil'-ip sem'-el-vīs) (1818–1865).* History has called him the Savior of Mothers. His fight against puerperal fever is a sad story of hardships, and resistance, especially from his instructor in Vienna, Professor Klein. Semmelweis noted the terrible results of puerperal fever in lying-in hospitals and observed that it occurred with special frequency in cases delivered by medical students who came directly from the autopsy or dissecting room. Semmelweis directed that in his wards the students were to wash and disinfect their hands with a solution of chloride of lime after leaving the dissection room and before going to the wards to examine a woman and deliver her child. This brought about a marked reduction of cases of childbed fever on his ward, but violent opposition was given by the hospital's medical men, and especially by Dr. Klein. As his theories were proven correct, Semmelweis began to feel the horror

---

*For a riveting novel about Semmelweis's life and career, read *"Not as a Stranger"* by Morton Thompson.

of the deaths that had been caused in the past by doctors themselves.

At the age of 47 years, Semmelweis died, ironically from the very infection he had fought, which was brought on by a cut in his finger while he was doing an autopsy. A monument to Semmelweis in Budapest is given great care, and it has been said that if people had been as tender to the man as they are to his statue, his career would have been happier.

Surely Semmelweis's death was a matter of tragic timing, for his grave had hardly been closed when the causes of this deadly disease were beginning to be understood as a result of the works of two great men, Louis Pasteur and Joseph Lister.

LOUIS PASTEUR (loo'is pas-ter') (1822–1895), a Frenchman, did brilliant work as a chemist, but his studies in bacteriology made him one of the most famous men in medical history and earned him the title of Father of Bacteriology (Fig. 3–7). He has also sometimes been honored with the name Father of Preventive Medicine. His skills and studies reached far beyond the outermost boundaries of the knowledge of the time. He pursued everything with the fire of genius.

Pasteur's adventures included studying the difficulties in the fermentation of wine. He saved the most important industry of France at that time from disaster by a process now called pasteurization, immortalizing his name. By this process of supplying enough heat to destroy microorganisms, wine was prevented from turning into vinegar. This made great improvements in spirit and malt liquors.

The French people called on Pasteur again to help the ailing silkworm industry. The silkworm epidemic in the south of France had reached such proportions that whole plantations were ruined. Pasteur devoted 5 years to the conquest of the two diseases that infected the silkworm. His work was interrupted only when he was stricken with hemiplegia. But after a long, difficult recovery when his mind was always fully active, he continued his work with a stiff hand and a limping foot.

With the conviction that the infinitely small world of bacteria held the key to the secrets of contagious diseases, Pasteur again left chemistry, this time to become a medical man. Many renowned scientists denied the germ theory of disease and devoted themselves to degrading Pasteur. In the midst of all this controversy he became involved in the prevention of **anthrax,** which threatened the health of the cattle and sheep of France as well as of the world. Pasteur's name was also honored for work on many other diseases, such as **rabies,** chicken cholera, and **swine erysipelas.** Pasteur died in 1895, with his family at his bedside. His last words were said to be, "There is still a great deal to do."

Memory Jogger

7 *Which of Pasteur's major accomplishments reflects his name?*

JOSEPH LISTER (1827–1912) was to revolutionize surgery through the application of Pasteur's discoveries. He saw the similarity between the infections that were taking place in postsurgical wounds and the processes of **putrefaction,** which Pasteur had proved were caused by microorganisms. Before this time, surgeons accepted infection in surgical wounds as inevitable. Lister reasoned that microorganisms must be the *cause* of infection and must, therefore, be kept out of wounds. Lister's own colleagues were

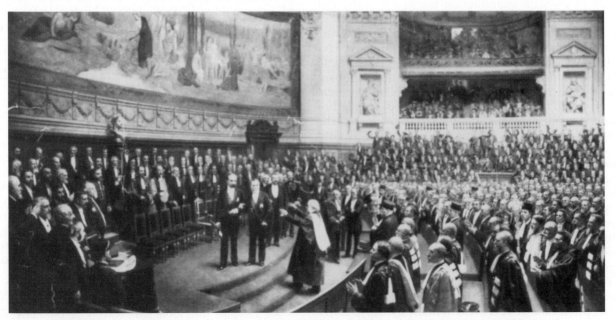

FIGURE 3–7 Louis Pasteur being honored at the Sorbonne. (Courtesy of the National Library of Medicine.)

quite indifferent to his theories, because they felt infections were God given and natural. Lister had once seen pain quelled by the administration of an anesthetic, and pain had been thought to be God given and inevitable also. He developed antiseptic methods by using carbolic acid for sterilization. By spraying the room with a fine mist of the acid, by soaking the instruments and ligatures, and by washing his hands in carbolic solutions, Lister proved his theory. He is honored with the title of Father of Sterile Surgery.

Pasteur and Joseph Lister met at the Sorbonne after years of great mutual admiration. The meeting was filled with emotion, and Robinson, in *Pathfinders in Medicine*, has said that a new star should have appeared in the heavens to commemorate the event. Only a small percentage of the human race entertains any adequate realization of how much we really owe to the combined labors of Louis Pasteur and Joseph Lister.

Memory Jogger

8 *What modern product reflects the name of Joseph Lister?*

ROBERT KOCH (Kok) (1843–1910) is a familiar name to all bacteriologists, because the first law learned as a **neophyte** in this microscopic world is Koch's postulates, which state rules that must be followed before an organism can be accepted as the causative agent in a given disease.

Koch was a German physician who truly earned great honors in bacteriology and public health. He gave the bacteriology laboratory many of its tools, such as the culture-plate method for isolation of bacteria. He discovered the cause of **cholera** and demonstrated its transmission by food and water. This discovery completely transformed health departments and proved the importance of bacteriology. It also established a place of great respect for Koch in the scientific world. A great disappointment in Koch's career was his failure to find a cure for tuberculosis. In this attempt, however, he isolated tuberculin, the substance produced by tubercle bacteria. Its use as a diagnostic aid proved to be of immense value to medicine.

Koch's work took him throughout the world. He traveled to America, Africa, Bombay, Italy, and anywhere nations sought his help in ridding themselves of feared diseases. He was investigating anthrax at the same time as Pasteur, but the ill-concealed animosity between the two men prevented any cooperative effort. In 1885, the University of Berlin created the Chair of Hygiene and Bacteriology in honor of Robert Koch. He became the Nobel Laureate in 1905.

Memory Jogger

9 *Define Koch's Postulates.*

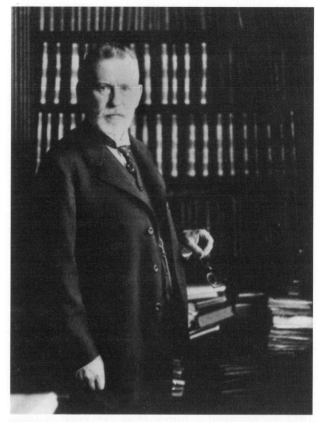

FIGURE 3–8 Paul Ehrlich. (Courtesy of the National Library of Medicine.)

While Robert Koch's brilliant career was nearing an end because of advanced age and illnesses, the work of PAUL EHRLICH (Ār'lik) (1854–1915) was reaching its zenith (Fig. 3–8). Ehrlich had been greatly honored when Koch had invited him to work in his laboratory. Koch had known Ehrlich well, since he had been a distinguished student of his and had already made a place for himself in scientific circles.

Ehrlich was a German physician, and one of the pioneers in the fields of bacteriology, **immunology,** and especially **chemotherapy,** a fairly new science. He was only 28 years old when he wrote his first paper on typhoid, but his greatest gift to humanity was to be called his *magic bullet,* or 606, which was designed to fight the terrible disease, syphilis. Only 3 years before, Bordet and Wasserman had identified the organism and devised a test that would smoke it out of hiding. With the offending germ identified, Ehrlich set out to find a chemical that would destroy the organism but not harm the germ's host, the human body. The search was long and tedious, and history tells us it was the 606th drug that Ehrlich tried that finally did the healing. He called the drug *salvarsan* because he believed it offered humankind salvation from this disease. This also was the beginning of the practice of injecting chemicals into the body to destroy a specific organism. Later, in 1912, Ehrlich discovered a less toxic drug, called neosalvarsan, to replace the original

606. The new drug bore the number 914. In 1908, Ehrlich shared the Nobel Prize with ELI METCHNI-KOFF, who is remembered for his theory of **phagocytosis** and immunology.

EMIL ADOLPH VON BEHRING (ba'ring) (1854–1917), a German bacteriologist and Nobel laureate, was born in Prussia (now Poland) and educated at the University of Berlin. In 1890, while working in the laboratory of German bacteriologist Robert Koch in Berlin, Behring and a Japanese bacteriologist Kitasato Shibasaburo discovered that injecting the blood serum of an animal that has tetanus into another animal produces an immunity against the disease in the second animal. On Behring's suggestion, and working with Paul Ehrlich, this principle was applied the following year to fight diphtheria in children, with highly successful results. Behring was awarded the first Nobel Prize in physiology or medicine in 1901.

CRAWFORD WILLIAMSON LONG (1815–1878) was the first to employ ether as an **anesthetic** agent. Early in 1842, after lectures on chemistry, a group of students would have a social gathering and inhale ether as a form of amusement. At one of these so-called "ether frolics," Dr. Long observed that people under the influence of ether did not seem to feel pain. After considerable thought, Dr. Long decided to use ether for a surgical operation. In March of 1842, he removed a tumor from the neck of James M. Venable after placing him under the influence of ether. Long did not report this operation or his discovery until 1848.

DR. HORACE WELLS, a dentist, reported discovering the use of nitrous oxide as an anesthetic in 1844. Another dentist, DR. WILLIAM T. G. MORTON, reported using ether in 1846 when he extracted a tooth from a patient, and also at Massachusetts General Hospital for a surgical procedure.

Surgery owes much to WILHELM KONRAD ROENTGEN (rent'gen) (1845–1922), a professor of physics at the University of Würzburg, Germany, who discovered the x-ray in 1895 while experimenting with electrical currents passed through sealed glass tubes (cathode-ray tubes). Roentgen was awarded the Nobel Prize in Physics in 1901. Although he called his ray the x-ray, science has honored him by calling it the roentgen ray.

Anyone who has had a radiograph or has received radium therapy should know the long struggle of MARIE and PIERRE CURIE leading to the discovery of radium in 1898.

Nineteenth Century Women in Medicine

Much attention is given to honoring great men in medical history, but women have also played important roles, which during those times was not an easy thing to do. Two famous women, in particular, are Florence Nightingale (1820–1910) and Clara Barton (1821–1912). You may notice that their careers overlap almost to the year.

FLORENCE NIGHTINGALE has been honored and known far and wide as "The Lady with the Lamp" and is immortalized as the founder of nursing (Fig. 3–9). She was of noble birth, and somewhat late in life she sought nurse's training in both England and Europe. By the time of the Crimean War in 1854, she already had a reputation for her work in hospital organization. She was invited by the Secretary of War to visit the Crimea to correct the terrible conditions that existed in caring for the wounded. She created the Women's Nursing Service at Scutari and Balaklava. The doctors at Scutari re-

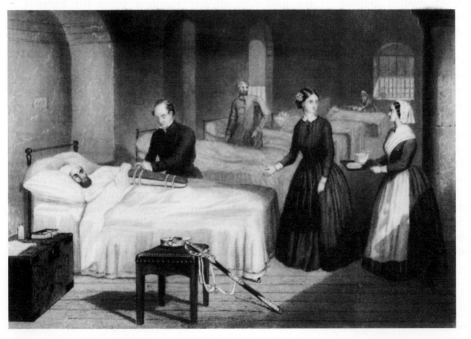

FIGURE 3–9 Florence Nightingale in the hospital at Scutari. (Courtesy of the National Library of Medicine.)

garded Florence Nightingale as a troublesome female intruder and treated her and her nurses quite shabbily. Only a crisis that brought thousands of wounded and sick soldiers to army hospitals persuaded the doctors to accept help from her and her nurses.

Miss Nightingale ruled her nurses with an iron hand. Aside from the practical work she did, it was she who insisted the nursing profession get public recognition and that nursing require special training and experience. From donated funds she organized a school of nursing that bears her name. The modern concept of nursing is based largely on the foundations laid by Florence Nightingale.

CLARA BARTON (Fig. 3–10) is the American counterpart to Florence Nightingale. Miss Barton was a nurse and philanthropist whose work during the American Civil War led her to recognize that very poor records, if any at all, were kept in Washington to aid in the search for missing men wounded or killed in combat. This led to the formation of the Bureau of Records. Clara Barton's fame spread as a result of her organization and recruitment of supplies for the wounded. In 1870, she observed the work of the Red Cross in the Franco-Prussian War; and in 1881, she organized a Red Cross Committee in Washington, forming the American Red Cross, of which she served as the first president from 1881 to 1904.

ELIZABETH BLACKWELL (1821–1910) was the first woman in the United States to receive the Doctor of Medicine degree from a medical school. Blackwell's family immigrated to New York from England in 1832. Young Elizabeth began her medical education by reading medical books and later on had private instruction. Medical schools in New York and Pennsylvania refused her applications for formal study, but, finally, in 1847, she was accepted at the Geneva (New York) Medical College. Ten years later, when Blackwell was practicing medicine in New York City, she established the New York Infirmary for Indigent Women and Children (now New York Infirmary), the first hospital staffed entirely by women. In 1869, Dr. Blackwell returned to her native England and became professor of gynecology (1875–1907) at the London School of Medicine for Women, of which she was a founder.

LILLIAN WALD (1867–1940), a social worker and nurse, made a great contribution to medical care when she founded the internationally known Henry Street Settlement at 265 Henry Street, New York City. Wald operated a visiting nurse service from this establishment. When one of her nurses was assigned to the city's public schools in 1902, the New York City Municipal Board of Health established the world's first public school nursing system.

MARGARET SANGER (1883–1966) was born in Corning, New York, on September 14, 1883, and trained as a nurse at the White Plains (New York) Hospital. Women all over the world can give thanks to Margaret Sanger, who became the American leader of the birth control movement. While work-

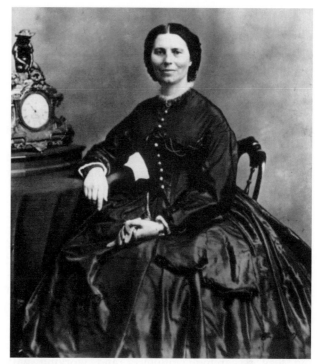

FIGURE 3–10 Clara Barton. (Courtesy of the National Library of Medicine.)

ing among the poor in New York City, she became aware of the need for information concerning contraception. She abandoned nursing to devote herself to the promotion of that objective. In 1873, federal legislation, known as the Comstock Law, had made it a crime to import or distribute any device, medicine, or information designed to prevent conception or induce abortion, or to mention in print the names of sexually transmitted diseases. Nurses and physicians were legally barred from providing this information to their patients. In 1914, Sanger was indicted for circulating through the mails a magazine called *The Woman Rebel*, in which she attacked the legislative restrictions of the Comstock Law. The case was dismissed 2 years later. In this same year she established the first American birth control clinic in Brooklyn, New York, for which she was charged and convicted and spent time in the county penitentiary. Sanger continued in her work, and when the Planned Parenthood Federation of America, Inc. was formed in 1941, she was named honorary chairperson.

Memory Jogger

10 a. Who founded the American Red Cross?
   b. What 19th century woman was called "the Lady with the Lamp"?
   c. Who was the inspiration for founding the first public school nursing system?
   d. Why should women all over the world give thanks to Margaret Sanger?

Twentieth Century Medicine

Coca-Cola was first used toward the end of the 19th century as a therapeutic agent and general tonic, containing cocaine. It also contained an extract of the kola nut, which is high in caffeine. When the Pure Food and Drug Law was passed in 1906 the makers of Coca-Cola were using decocainized coca leaves, but the caffeine remained.

WALTER REED, a United States Army pathologist and bacteriologist, in 1900, proved that yellow fever is transmitted by the bite of a mosquito. In 1901, action by U.S. military engineers in Cuba freed Havana from the disease by eliminating the mosquitoes.

Diabetics should be grateful to SIR FREDERICK GRANT BANTING, a Canadian physician, and CHARLES HERBERT BEST, a Canadian physiologist, both Nobel laureates, who isolated insulin for the treatment of diabetics in 1922.

In 1928, SIR ALEXANDER FLEMING (1881–1955), a British bacteriologist, discovered penicillin. This discovery came about accidentally while Fleming was researching influenza and working with staphylococcal bacteria. On investigation, he found a substance in the mold that prevented growth of bacteria even when the substance was diluted 800 times. He called it penicillin. His discovery remained a laboratory curiosity until World War II. In 1945, the Nobel Prize for Physiology and Medicine was awarded to Alexander Fleming, Howard Florey, and Ernst Chain for the "discovery of penicillin and its curative effect in various infectious diseases."

Children born with **cyanosis** due to a malformed heart (tetralogy of Fallot) owe thanks to HELEN B. TAUSSIG (tau′sig), of Baltimore, Maryland, who, together with ALFRED BLALOCK developed the lifesaving operation for so-called "blue babies." Although the Blalock-Taussig procedure, first performed in 1944 at Johns Hopkins University Hospital, may seem simple today, in 1944 it was revolutionary and led to a major change of direction in the treatment of heart disease.

During the 1950s the vaccines developed by JONAS EDWARD SALK and ALBERT SABIN almost eradicated poliomyelitis, once the killer or crippler of thousands in the United States. Dr. Salk's work in the 1940s on an anti-influenza vaccine led him and his colleagues to develop an inactivated vaccine against polio in 1952. Following wide-scale testing in 1954, the vaccine was distributed nationally and greatly reduced the disease. In the mid 1950s, Albert Sabin, an American virologist, developed an oral, live vaccine, which with Salk's discovery brought polio under control.

WEERNER FORSSMANN (fors′man) (1904–1979), a Berlin surgeon, originated a cardiologic technique, called **catheterization,** that is used in the diagnosis and treatment of heart disease, for which he was awarded a Nobel Prize in physiology or medicine.

He first demonstrated the technique by experimenting on himself by making an incision in a vein in his right arm and maneuvering a catheter up the vessel and into the right auricle of his heart while observing via a mirror the fluoroscoped image of the instrument as it traveled through his body.

CHRISTIAAN N. BARNARD (1922–), a South African surgeon, performed the first human heart transplant operation on December 3, 1967, when he transferred the heart of a 25-year-old woman into the body of a 55-year-old man. This patient died 18 days later. The second patient, who received a transplant on January 2, 1968, lived for 563 days after the operation. Since then bypass surgery has made thousands of hearts more functional and organ transplants are becoming almost commonplace.

In 1972, British engineers invented the computed tomography (CT) scanner; in 1978, the first test tube baby was born (in England); in 1982, the U.S. Food and Drug Administration approved the first drug developed with recombinant-DNA technology (a form of human insulin); in 1995, a Duke University surgeon successfully transplanted a heart from a genetically altered pig into a baboon; and in 1997, a sheep was cloned in Great Britain. What will follow?

National Institutes of Health

The National Institutes of Health (NIH) observed its centennial anniversary in the year 1987. It began as a one-room laboratory in the marine hospital on New York's Staten Island in 1887. Tuberculosis was the number-one cause of death at that time. There were few drugs that could alleviate or cure disease. There were no vaccines except for smallpox. There were no antibiotics. Doctors could diagnose some conditions but fell short on treatment. And there was not even aspirin. Morphine was injected for severe pain. In 1891, the laboratory moved from Staten Island to Washington, DC. In 1902 the Marine Hospital Service became the Public Health Service and in 1930 became the National Institutes of Health, an agency of the U.S. Department of Health and Human Services. As a part of the Public Health Service, it seeks to improve the health of the American people, supports and conducts biomedical research into the causes and prevention of diseases, and uses a modern communications system to furnish biomedical information to the health care professions.

The Institutes moved from Washington, DC, to Bethesda, Maryland, in 1938, where it occupied 3 buildings. It remains in Bethesda today but occupies more than 60 buildings covering 30 acres. It consists of 13 research institutes, four divisions, and the National Library of Medicine. Thousands of research projects are under way in NIH laboratories and clinics at any given time.

Centers for Disease Control and Prevention

The CDC is an agency of the United States Public Health Service, headquartered in Atlanta, Georgia. It was established in 1946 as the Communicable Disease Center, and became the Centers for Disease Control in 1970; "and Prevention" was added in 1992, but Congress requested that "CDC" remain the agency's initials. The agency conducts research into the origin and occurrence of diseases and develops methods for their control and prevention. Additionally, it develops immunization services, provides public health information, and aids in the training of health workers. The CDC also conducts international programs. In recent years the agency has been deeply involved in the battle against human immunodeficiency virus infection and acquired immunodeficiency syndrome (AIDS) through arranging educational programs to help prevent future outbreaks. The agency has developed guidelines that emphasize that *standard blood and body-fluid precautions* be consistently used for all patients in all situations where the risk of contamination by body fluids exists. The precautions are enforced by the Occupational Safety and Health Administration (OSHA).

Memory Jogger

11 *What is the basic purpose of the CDC?*

Overview

The nature of this text does not permit the exploration of every one of the medical miracles of the past century. It is tremendously exciting simply to be open to such advancements and to be aware of their potential. The supportive role of medical assisting is very important in maintaining the quality of medical service and in making today a strong foundation for the progress of tomorrow. If you have been enlightened by this brief history of medicine, further attention to medical discoveries as they occur will add an extra dimension to your study of medical assisting. Perhaps you will contribute some miracles of your own.

LEGAL AND ETHICAL ISSUES

As you advance in this exciting profession of health care, you will do well to review the efforts (sometimes lives) expended by those who pushed on to achieve today's level of care and to respect the standards achieved. Think positive, and expect a miracle.

CRITICAL THINKING

The historical legacy that is taken for granted by most people in our society represents enormous sacrifices by the discoverers of new principles and treatments in past centuries. The last half of the 20th century has completely changed the possibilities of diagnosis and treatment.

Let us be respectful of the efforts of our forefathers and be grateful for the added quality of life available at the beginning of the 21st century.

HOW DID I DO? Answers to Memory Joggers

1 The caduceus has two serpents; the staff of Aesculapius has only one.

2 Moses was called the "first public health officer" because he was an advocate of preventive medicine.

3 The university (a) acquired prior training in the natural sciences, and (b) had the advantages of Johns Hopkins Hospital close by as a training site.

4 The lenses ground by Leeuwenhoek magnified the minute world of organisms and led to the sciences of bacteriology and protozoology.

5 Hunter was given the title "Founder of Scientific Surgery" because his procedures were based on pathologic evidence.

6 The origin of the word *vaccination* is *vacca*, meaning "cow."

7 The process *pasteurization*.

8 Listerine.

9 Koch's postulates are laboratory rules that must be followed before an organism can be accepted as the causative agent in a given disease.

10 a. Clara Barton
b. Florence Nightingale
c. Lillian Wald
d. Sanger fought for the advancement of planned parenthood.

11 Research into the origin and occurrence of diseases and developing methods for their control and prevention.

REFERENCES

Bullock A, Woodings R (eds): Twentieth Century Culture, New York, Harper & Row, 1983.

Garrison FH: History of Medicine, 4th ed. Philadelphia, WB Saunders, 1929.

Magner LN: A History of Medicine. New York, Marcel Dekker, 1992.

Robinson V: Pathfinders in Medicine. New York, Medical Life Press, 1979.

SECTION 2

Understanding the Protocols of Medical Practice

CURRICULUM CONTENT/COMPETENCIES

Chapter 4 Medical Practice Systems
- Work as a team member
- Locate community resources and disseminate information

Chapter 5 Medical Ethics
- Practice within the scope of education, training, and personal capabilities
- Use appropriate guidelines when releasing information
- Maintain awareness of federal and state health care legislation and regulations
- Explain office policies and procedures

Chapter 6 Medicine and the Law
- Follow federal, state, and local legal guidelines
- Maintain and dispose of regulated substances in compliance with government guidelines
- Prepare and maintain medical records
- Document accurately
- Comply with established risk management and safety procedures

Medical Practice Systems

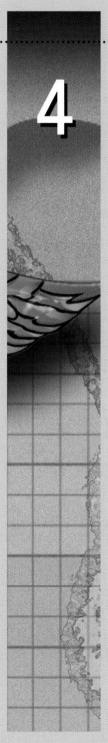

4

LEARNING OBJECTIVES

Cognitive: On successful completion of this chapter you should be able to:

1 Define and spell the terms listed in the Vocabulary.
2 Name the system of medical care delivery that has brought about a significant change in medical practice in the past decade.
3 State the principal difference between the training of the MD and the DO.
4 List the three medical practice business structures discussed in the chapter.
5 Name and compare the two principal methods of paying for medical care.
6 Identify 10 or more allied health occupations that might be represented in a medical practice.

accelerating Causing to act or move faster

maladies Diseases or disorders of the body

manipulative Treating or operating with the hands in a skillful manner

overutilization Excessive use

puerperium The period between childbirth and the return of the uterus to its normal size

rehabilitation Restoration of normal form and function after injury or illness

substantiated Having been established as true by proof of competent evidence; verified

The Business Structure of Medical Practices

Three general types of business structure exist in medical practice: sole proprietorship, partnership, and corporation. Sole proprietorship, or solo practice, consisting of one physician only, dominated medical practice until the last quarter of the 20th century. Solo practice is steadily declining.

SOLE PROPRIETORSHIP

A sole proprietor is an individual who holds exclusive right and title to all aspects of the medical practice. The sole proprietor may employ other physicians to participate in the practice. The employed physician is entitled to employee fringe benefits, but the owner is not so entitled. Additionally, the owner would be potentially liable for all of the acts of his professional employees. Earlier physicians enjoyed the flexibility and independence of practicing alone. Disadvantages are that the physician is totally responsible 24 hours a day, and the potential earnings are limited. In an unincorporated solo practice, the practice dies with the owner.

Memory Jogger

1 *Why do you think sole proprietorship is declining?*

Associate Practice

Often two or more physicians agree to share office space and employees but conduct their practice as sole proprietors. They have an agreement among themselves as to the manner in which the practice is to operate.

PARTNERSHIP

When two or more physicians elect to associate in the practice of medicine, they may draw up a partnership agreement, which should show all the rights, obligations, and responsibilities of each partner. The partners have more potential for profit than they would have if practicing as individuals. Each has more freedom by having another physician available in emergencies. One major disadvantage of partnership is the liability of each for the acts and conduct of other partners unless otherwise specified in the partnership agreement. In a partnership practice the death or retirement of a partner requires a new agreement.

PROFESSIONAL CORPORATION

A *corporation* may be defined as an artificial entity having a legal and business status that is independent of its shareholders or employees. Corporations are regulated by statutes of the state in which the incorporation takes place.

The physician shareholders are employees of the corporation. Even one physician in solo practice can incorporate. All employees of the corporation receive income and tax advantages. An attractive fringe benefit package is usually offered to the employees and may include pension and profit-sharing plans, medical expense reimbursement, life insurance, disability income insurance, and employee death benefit. Fringe benefits to the corporate employee are separate from salary; that is, they are tax deductible to the corporation and not taxable to the employee.

Professional employees of a corporation are liable only for their own acts. Another advantage of the corporate entity is the continuous life of the corporation. The corporation is an entity unto itself and does not end with a change in shareholders.

Group Practice

The governing bodies of the American Medical Association (AMA), the American Group Practice Association, and the Medical Group Management Association have formally adopted the following definition of medical group practice:

Medical Group Practice is the provision of health care services by a group of at least three licensed physician-practitioners, engaged full-time in a

formally organized and legally recognized entity; sharing the group's income and expenses in a systematic manner; and sharing facilities, equipment, common records, and personnel, involved in both patient care and business management.

A small or medium-sized group may be a single-specialty group with all the physicians engaged in the same specialty. Family practice and anesthesia services are two common examples. A large group would more likely be a multispecialty practice. Group practice usually takes the legal form of a partnership or a corporation.

Memory Jogger

2 *What are the three general business practice structures in medicine and how do they differ?*

Delivery of Medical Care

By the mid-20th century, medical practice was experiencing many changes. Rapid developments in medical science encouraged more specialization. The **accelerating** cost of maintaining an office was becoming prohibitive for a solo practitioner, especially the new graduate. Medical insurance for the patient became the rule rather than the exception. More government programs, with their accompanying regulations, were developing, and the management of a medical practice required more and better-trained personnel. These developments brought many changes in the delivery of medical care and the payment for those services.

FEE-FOR-SERVICE

Before July 1, 1966, when Medicare under Social Security for the patient older than age 65 years went into effect, payment for medical care was accomplished on a fee-for-service arrangement. The physician established the fee for his or her services. Fees for surgery or an extensive series of visits were usually discussed and agreed on by the patient before service. The patient was billed direct and was responsible for payment, irrespective of any reimbursement from insurance. Traditional fee-for-service plans now serve less than a fourth of insured workers in the United States.

MANAGED CARE

Managed care is difficult to define because it is still evolving. By general definition, the intent of managed care is a streamlining of the system of delivering medical care so that patients receive appropriate care in an appropriate setting at the least possible cost. In 1993, about half the Americans insured through employers were in managed care. That figure jumped to 73% by 1995 and is still rising. In 1997, there were 158 million members enrolled in managed care health plans.

Health Maintenance Organization (HMO)

An HMO is an organization that provides for comprehensive health care to an enrolled group for a fixed periodic payment. In the early 1970s, the federal government, which bears a great percentage of the costs of medical care, took action to contain the potential abuses of overtreatment and **overutilization** of health care services. The enactment of Public Law 93-222, the HMO Assistance Act, in December 1973, created Title XIII of the Public Health Service Act. Title XIII is intended to encourage and promote the growth of HMOs resulting in cost containment. HMOs function in a variety of ways within a federally regulated environment. The methods of delivering care vary, but the basic characteristics are similar.

As the name implies, the HMO concept emphasizes the maintenance of health and preventive medicine. Insured members of HMOs, because their contracts provide for comprehensive care, are more inclined to visit their physicians before major and more costly problems arise. An employer who provides health care benefits to employees may be required to offer federally qualified HMOs as an option. Managed care is discussed in more detail in a later chapter.

PREVENTIVE CARE AND PUBLIC HEALTH

The practice of medicine does not always involve patient care. General preventive medicine involves the relation of environment to health with special concern for the health requirements of population groups. The community is the public health physician's patient. Public health is a special field of preventive care embodying the use of medical and administrative methods to prevent disease and improve general health through community efforts in areas such as sanitation and education. The United States Public Health Service and the World Health Organization (WHO) are both concerned with preventive medicine. All branches of medicine are committed to preventive medicine.

SPECIALTY PRACTICE

Many physicians have a special interest in a specific branch of medical practice and eventually direct their efforts to becoming expert in their chosen field. Physicians who decide to limit their practice to a specialized field will spend an additional 3 to 6 years in a residency program after completion of internship and will probably seek certification by one of the specialty boards.

Memory Jogger

3 *Give a general definition of managed care.*

American Board of Medical Specialties

Twenty-four specialty boards exist under the umbrella of the American Board of Medical Specialties. These specialty boards help improve the quality of medical education by elevating the standards of graduate medical education and approving facilities for specialty training. The primary function of each approved specialty board is to evaluate the qualifications of candidates in its field who apply voluntarily for examination and to certify as diplomates those who are qualified. Qualifications vary with the various boards.

In accomplishing the described function, specialty boards determine whether candidates have received adequate preparation according to established educational standards; they provide comprehensive examinations to such candidates; and they issue certificates to those physicians who have satisfied the requirements. Those physicians who are board certified are known as diplomates of a specific specialty board (e.g., Fredrick B. Mears, MD, Diplomate of the American Board of Surgery).

A listing of the 24 specialty boards is shown here. The American Board of Medical Specialties is at One American Plaza, Suite 805, Evanston, IL 60201. It regularly publishes a directory listing all physicians certified as diplomates by the specialty boards, including biographical sketches detailing their educational qualifications. Many physicians consult the directory in making referrals.

APPROVED SPECIALTY BOARDS OF THE UNITED STATES

American Board of Allergy and Immunology
American Board of Anesthesiology
American Board of Colon and Rectal Surgery
American Board of Dermatology
American Board of Emergency Medicine
American Board of Family Practice
American Board of Internal Medicine
American Board of Medical Genetics
American Board of Neurological Surgery
American Board of Nuclear Medicine

American Board of Obstetrics and Gynecology
American Board of Ophthalmology
American Board of Orthopaedic Surgery
American Board of Otolaryngology
American Board of Pathology
American Board of Pediatrics
American Board of Physical Medicine and Rehabilitation
American Board of Plastic Surgery
American Board of Preventive Medicine
American Board of Psychiatry and Neurology
American Board of Radiology
American Board of Surgery
American Board of Thoracic Surgery
American Board of Urology

American College of Surgeons

The American College of Surgeons, located at 55 East Erie Street, Chicago, IL 60611 may also confer a degree on an applicant from a surgical specialty. The applicant is required to have completed a course of postgraduate training equivalent to "board requirements" and to have submitted 50 detailed, **substantiated** case reports of varied surgical procedures in which the applicant has been the chief surgeon during the past 3 years of practice before application. Successful applicants are identified as a Fellow of the American College of Surgeons (FACS).

American College of Physicians

The American College of Physicians issues a similar fellowship degree (FACP) to applicants who have completed approved postgraduate training and have exhibited special interest and competence in one nonsurgical specialty.

Osteopathic Medicine

Osteopathic medicine is a complete school of medical practice that began in the United States in the 19th century. Its founder was Andrew Taylor Still, an American Civil War army physician. Dr. Still established the first College of Osteopathic Medicine in 1892 at Kirksville, Missouri.

The Doctor of Osteopathy (DO) differs from the Doctor of Medicine (MD) in placing more emphasis on the relationship between the musculoskeletal structure and organ function. The use of **manipulative** therapy in diagnosis and treatment is an integral part of osteopathy. The DO is a graduate of a college of osteopathy and is a fully trained physician, qualified to be licensed as a physician and to practice all branches of medicine and surgery.

Colleges of osteopathy are accredited by the Bureau of Professional Education of the American Osteopathic Association (AOA), which is recognized by the U.S. Department of Education and the Council on Postsecondary Accreditation. Four academic years of study are required, which include the basic sciences of anatomy, physiology, biochemistry, pathology, microbiology, and pharmacology and a wide range of clinical subjects. Integrated throughout the curriculum is special instruction in osteopathic principles dealing with the interrelationship of all body systems in health and disease. After graduation, DOs participate in a 12-month rotating internship. Those who wish to become specialists serve an additional 2 to 6 years of residency or fellowship training.

Osteopathic physicians are licensed to practice medicine in all states of the United States. Requirements for licensure for both DOs and MDs are very similar, and after licensure both provide the same range of professional services. More than half of active DOs provide primary health care; the remainder are specialists practicing in such fields as internal medicine, surgery, psychiatry, and obstetrics. DOs are more prevalent in towns and cities having fewer than 50,000 inhabitants.

Memory Jogger

4 *How does the education of a DO differ from that of an MD?*

Specialties of Medicine

AEROSPACE MEDICINE Aerospace medicine is the specialty concerned with the physiologic, pathologic, and psychologic problems encountered by humans in space. This field is mostly confined to the space agencies of the federal government.

ALLERGY AND IMMUNOLOGY An allergy is an abnormal reaction to substances that are harmless to most people. Substances that frequently bother the allergic person include pollens from grass, weeds, and trees; molds; house and other dusts; dog and cat danders; certain foods and medications; and the stings of insects.

There are many kinds of medicines and treatments that can help relieve the allergic symptoms, but it is essential first to identify the cause. The allergist is specially trained to diagnose and treat allergy problems with a high degree of accuracy and success.

The American Board of Allergy and Immunology is a conjoint board of the American Board of Internal Medicine and the American Board of Pediatrics. To become an allergist, the pediatrician or internist must take several years of additional specialty training and pass another certifying examination.

ANESTHESIOLOGY An anesthesiologist is a physician who administers local and general anesthesia, usually to prepare and maintain a patient for surgery and in some cases for relief of pain. An anesthesiologist monitors the surgical patient through the surgical process until stable consciousness returns postoperatively.

DERMATOLOGY Dermatologists are medical doctors who have extensive specialized training in the medical and surgical treatment of disorders of the skin, hair, and nails.

Because of specific training, the dermatologist is able to determine the best treatment approach to skin disorders. This approach may involve the use of medicines, both internal and external, or it may involve skin surgery. In addition to common dermatologic procedures such as removal of moles, warts, cysts, benign tumors, and skin cancers, many dermatologists are also trained in certain surgical and cosmetic procedures. These include skin grafts and flaps, hair transplants, dermabrasion, and collagen implants.

EMERGENCY MEDICINE The emergency medicine specialist is a physician who specializes in the immediate recognition and treatment of acute illnesses and injuries. These specialists may also be involved in the administration, teaching, and research of systems designed to help patients seeking emergency care. Qualifications for this specialty include a formal emergency medicine residency training or experience and continuing medical education.

Traditionally, specialists in emergency medicine provide 24-hour coverage of emergency departments in acute care hospitals, making emergency care available at all times. These specialists also provide the authority and license under which paramedic prehospital care is provided.

FAMILY PRACTICE Family or general practice encompasses the care of all members of the family regardless of age or sex and covers a vast range of medical problems. This allows for continuity of care for the individual and integration of care for the family as a whole.

INTERNAL MEDICINE Internal medicine is the specialty concerned with the complete nonsurgical care of the adult. Internists are experts in the medical diagnosis and treatment of adult disorders as well as in the areas of health maintenance and wellness. General internists are responsible for a broad range of adult medical problems. Internal medicine comprises multiple subspecialties including allergy, cardiology, endocrinology, gastroenterology, gerontology, hematology, infectious disease, nephrology, oncology, pulmonary diseases, and rheumatology.

MEDICAL GENETICS The specialty of medical genetics is concerned with the study of heredity and its effects on individuals in health and disease.

NEUROLOGY Neurology is concerned with the nonsurgical management of neurologic disease. Generally, the neurologist manages infectious, metabolic, degenerative, and systemic involvement of the nervous system.

NUCLEAR MEDICINE Nuclear medicine is a specialty field in which radioactive substances are used for the diagnosis and treatment of disease.

OBSTETRICS AND GYNECOLOGY Obstetrics is the specialty involved in the care and management of women during pregnancy, labor, delivery, and the **puerperium.** Gynecology is the specialty devoted to the medical and surgical treatment of diseases of women, especially diseases affecting the reproductive organs and functions.

OPHTHALMOLOGY Ophthalmology involves the diagnosis and treatment of eye and vision disorders, utilizing surgery and other corrective techniques. The testing of visual acuity is a basic procedure. The ophthalmologist treats glaucoma, strabismus, astigmatism, and cataracts and is skilled in surgical procedures and laser techniques.

OTOLARYNGOLOGY Otolaryngology is professionally known as Otolaryngology/Head and Neck Surgery, whereas the community may think of the specialty as ENT. Otolaryngology is broadly based, encompassing medical and surgical treatment of ear, nose, and throat disorders, allergy therapy, facial cosmetic and reconstructive surgery, and tumor problems in the head and neck. Otolaryngology is advancing in the fields of microsurgery and laser surgery.

PATHOLOGY Pathology is the science that deals with the causes, mechanisms of development, and effects of disease. The pathologist seeks to detect the actual nature of disease—not just the physical symptoms or how it feels to the patient but what the disease is from a biologic standpoint, that is, what visible or measurable changes it produces in the cells, fluids, and life processes of the entire body.

The practice of pathology is divided into two major areas, Anatomic Pathology and Clinical Pathology, and these areas are further subdivided into many subspecialties. The function of the anatomic pathologist is to render a diagnosis based on examination of a tissue specimen and to learn as precisely as possible the extent of the disease. The clinical pathologist is in charge of the medical laboratory, in which a variety of diagnostic studies are done. Forensic pathology is a subspecialty dealing with various aspects of medicine and the law.

PEDIATRICS Caring for the health of children from birth to adolescence is the unique purpose of pediat-

rics. The pediatrician continually strives to prevent and treat all aspects of childhood diseases. The extent of the pediatrician's interest and responsibilities spans such areas as infectious diseases, newborn care, hospital care of children, environmental hazards, school health problems, nutrition, accident prevention, children with disabilities, drugs, allergy, cardiology, and pediatric pharmacology. The pediatric specialist can handle the problems of acutely ill children and provide guidance to parents regarding the development and preventive care of children who are well. The neonatologist treats the diseases and abnormalities of the newborn.

PHYSICAL MEDICINE AND REHABILITATION The specialty of Physical Medicine and Rehabilitation is concerned with the diagnosis and treatment of disorders and disabilities of the neuromuscular system. A physician in this specialty is called a *physiatrist.* The physiatrist uses the physical elements such as heat, cold, water, electricity, and exercise to help restore physical function and independence.

PREVENTIVE MEDICINE Preventive Medicine is concerned with preventing the occurrence of both mental and physical illness and disability. Analysis of present health services and planning for future medical needs are part of Preventive Medicine, as are Occupational Medicine and Public Health.

HOLISTIC HEALTH AND HOLISTIC MEDICINE Holistic health requires total cooperation of the patient. It is a philosophy of life that encompasses lifestyle, attitudes, and everyday events, all of which affect the physical response of the body—for good or for ill. Holistic medicine is not a specific method of treatment but includes all safe methods, as appropriate for the situation. The dominant factor is the acceptance, by the patient, of personal responsibility to cooperate with the chosen practitioner in achieving a reasonable state of well-being.

PSYCHIATRY A psychiatrist is a physician whose specialty is the diagnosis and treatment of persons with mental, emotional, or behavioral disorders. The psychiatrist is qualified to conduct psychotherapy and to prescribe medications when necessary. This allows the psychiatrist comprehensively to treat complex interactions of biologic, psychologic, and social factors that affect patients.

RADIOLOGY Radiology is a specialty in which x-rays (roentgen rays) are used for diagnosis and treatment of disease. A diagnostic radiologist specializes in using x-rays, ultrasound, nuclear medicine, computed tomography (CT), and magnetic resonance imaging (MRI) for detection of abnormalities throughout the body. Therapeutic radiology involves the use of ionizing radiation in the treatment of cancer and other tumors.

SURGERY Surgery is the correction of deformities, defects, diseases, or injured parts of the body by means of operative treatment. By making an incision into body tissue or by passing instruments through the skin, the diseased or injured tissues or organs can be corrected, modified, removed, or replaced. The various specializations contained within the broad field of surgery are listed below.

GENERAL SURGERY   General Surgery may include all aspects of surgery other than those included under special groups. Many general surgeons restrict their practice to surgery of abdominal conditions, traumatic situations, or tumor conditions. However, there is no restriction on the general surgeon's scope of activities, and many general surgeons take on additional fields as their training, interest, and capabilities dictate.

COLON AND RECTAL SURGERY   Colon and Rectal Surgery is a surgical subspecialty that concentrates on surgical treatment of the lower intestinal tract, which includes the colon and rectum.

NEUROSURGERY   A neurosurgeon specializes in the diagnosis and surgical treatment of the nervous system (the brain, spinal cord, and nerves) and the surrounding bony structures.

ORAL SURGERY   Oral Surgery is a branch of dentistry dealing with the extraction of teeth and the treatment of fractures of the jaws and adjacent facial bones. The oral surgeon may also do other surgical procedures on the jaws, oral tissues, and adjacent tissues to treat or correct abnormal conditions.

ORTHOPEDIC SURGERY   The orthopedic surgeon treats not only **maladies** of the musculoskeletal system but also congenital and acquired deformities, including spinal curvatures and arthritis. Orthopedic techniques are also used to treat sports injuries, including arthroscopic techniques, to maximize **rehabilitation.** Although orthopedics is a branch of surgery, many conditions are treated without surgery, including most fractures and muscle and tendon infirmities.

PLASTIC SURGERY   Plastic Surgery includes the operative repair of defects by graft, tissue transfer, or cosmetic alteration of tissue. A plastic surgeon specializes in burns, congenital defects, hand and extremity reconstruction, the treatment of skin wounds and lesions, the performance of aesthetic surgery of the face, and body contouring.

THORACIC (CARDIOVASCULAR) SURGERY   This surgical subspecialty is concerned with the operative treatment of the chest and chest wall, lungs, and respiratory passages. Specialists in this field are involved with heart surgery, including both valvular and coronary heart surgery.

UROLOGY   Urology is a medical specialty concerned with the treatment of diseases and disorders of the urinary tract of men, women, and children and of the male genitalia.

Related Health Care Specialists

CHIROPRACTOR (DC)   The practice of chiropractic is based on the premise that disease is caused by abnormal functioning of the nervous system. The chiropractor attempts to restore normal function by manipulation, especially of the spinal column. The practitioner earns the degree of Doctor of Chiropractic and is licensed by the state.

OPTOMETRIST (OD)   The optometrist is trained and licensed to examine the eyes to test visual acuity and to treat defects of vision by prescribing and adapting correctional lenses and other optical aids. He or she may also plan programs of exercise for the patient's eyes. An optician fills optical prescriptions for both ordinary eyeglasses and contact lenses.

PODIATRIST (DP)   Podiatrists are educated in caring for the feet, including the anatomy, pathology, medical, and surgical treatment. They earn the degree of Doctor of Podiatry and are licensed practitioners.

Support Personnel

In the complex delivery of 20th century medical care, the physician is the maestro, but for every practicing physician there are many behind-the-scenes support persons. As the delivery of medical

TABLE 4–1   Allied Health Professions for Which the AMA Has Collaborated in Establishing Accreditation of Educational Programs

Credential	Profession
AA	Anesthesiologist's Assistant
AT	Athletic Trainer
CVT	Cardiovascular Technologist
CLS	Clinical Laboratory Scientist
CLT	Clinical Laboratory Technician
CT	Cytotechnologist
DMS	Diagnostic Medical Sonographer
EEG-T	Electroneurodiagnostic Technologist
EMT-P	Emergency Medical Technician–Paramedic
RRA	Health Information Administrator
ART	Health Information Technician
HT	Histologic Technician/Technologist
CMA	Medical Assistant
MI	Medical Illustrator
NMT	Nuclear Medicine Technologist
OMT	Ophthalmic Medical Technician/Technologist
OP	Orthotist/Prosthetist
OT	Occupational Therapist
OTA	Occupational Therapy Assistant
PERF	Perfusionist
PA	Physician's Assistant/Surgeon's Assistant
RAD	Radiographer
RADT	Radiation Therapist
RRT	Respiratory Therapist
CRTT	Respiratory Therapy Technician
SBB	Specialist in Blood Bank Technology
ST	Surgical Technologist

TABLE 4–2 Health Care Occupations Accredited by the Commission on Accreditation of Allied Health Education Programs (CAAHEP)

Occupation	Credential	Brief Job Description
Anesthesiologist Assistant	AA	Functions under the direction of a licensed and qualified anesthesiologist. Assists in developing and implementing the anesthesia care plan.
Athletic Trainer	AT	Functions under supervision of attending and/or consulting physician. Provides a variety of services, including injury prevention, recognition, immediate care, treatment, and rehabilitation after physical trauma.
Cardiovascular Technologist	CVT	Performs diagnostic examinations at the request or direction of a physician in one or more of three areas: (1) invasive cardiology, (2) noninvasive cardiology, and (3) noninvasive peripheral vascular study.
Cytotechnologist	CT	Works with pathologist. Prepares cellular samples for study under the microscope and assists in the diagnosis of disease by examining the samples.
Diagnostic Medical Sonographer	DMS	Provides patient services using medical ultrasound under the supervision of a physician. Assists in gathering sonographic data necessary to diagnose a variety of conditions and diseases.
Electrodiagnostic Technologist	EEG-T	Works in collaboration with the electroencephalographer. Possesses the knowledge, attributes, and skills to obtain interpretable recordings of patients' nervous system function.
Emergency Medical Technician–Paramedic	EMT-P	Works under the direction of a physician—often through radio communication—and is able to recognize, assess, and manage medical emergencies of acutely ill or injured patients in prehospital care settings.
Health Information Administrator	RRA	Manages health information systems consistent with the medical, administrative, ethical, and legal requirements of the health care delivery system. Works with medical and hospital administrative staff involving medical records.
Health Information Technician	ART	Maintains components of health information systems in all types of facilities including hospitals and ambulatory health care centers. Processes, maintains, compiles, and reports patient data.
Medical Assistant	CMA	Multiskilled practitioner who works primarily in ambulatory settings such as physicians' offices and clinics, performing both administrative and clinical procedures.
Medical Illustrator	MI	Working with many different media, medical illustrators create visual material designed to facilitate the recording and dissemination of medical, biological, and related knowledge.
Ophthalmic Medical Technician/Technologist	OMT	Renders supportive services to the ophthalmologist. Administers diagnostic tests, takes ocular measurements, tests ocular functions, and performs other tasks assigned by the ophthalmologist.
Orthotist/Prosthetist	OP	Both the orthotist and the prosthetist work directly with the physician in the rehabilitation of the physically challenged. The orthotist designs and fits orthoses to provide care to patients who have disabling conditions of the limbs and spine. The prosthetist designs and fits devices for patients who have partial or total absence of limb.
Perfusionist	PERF	A perfusionist operates extracorporeal circulation equipment during any medical situation in which it is necessary to support or temporarily replace the patient's circulatory or respiratory function (e.g., cardiopulmonary bypass).
Physician Assistant	PA	The physician assistant is academically and clinically prepared to practice medicine with the supervision of a licensed doctor of medicine or osteopathy. The functions of the physician assistant include performing diagnostic, therapeutic, preventive, and health maintenance services.
Respiratory Therapist	RRT	The respiratory therapist working under the supervision of a physician evaluates all data to determine the appropriateness of the prescribed respiratory care and participates in the development of the respiratory care plan.
Respiratory Therapy Technician	CRTT	The respiratory therapy technician works under the supervision of the respiratory therapist and a physician in administering general respiratory care.
Specialist in Blood Bank Technology	SBB	Specialists in blood bank technology perform both routine and specialized tests in blood bank immunohematology in technical areas of the modern blood bank and perform transfusion services.
Surgical Technologist	ST/CST	Works in the surgical suite with surgeons, anesthesiologists, registered nurses, and other surgical personnel.

From Allied Health and Rehabilitation Professions Education Directory, 24th ed. American Medical Association, Chicago, IL, 1996–1997.

TABLE 4–3   Health Care Occupations Accredited by Agencies Other Than CAAHEP Under the AMA Umbrella

Occupational Therapist
Occupational Therapy Assistant
Dietetic Technician
Dietitian/Nutritionist
Dental Assistant
Dental Hygienist
Dental Laboratory Technician
Audiologist
Speech-Language Pathologist
Radiation Therapist
Radiographer
Nuclear Medicine Technologist
Clinical Laboratory Technician/Medical Laboratory
    Technician—Associate Degree
Clinical Laboratory Technician/Medical Laboratory
    Technician—Certificate
Clinical Laboratory Scientist/Medical Technologist
Histologic Technician/Technologist
Pathologists' Assistant

From Allied Health and Rehabilitation Professions Education Directory, 24th ed., American Medical Association, Chicago, IL, 1996–1997.

care has become more fragmented, the close relationship that formerly existed between family physician and patient has diminished, and the specialist often enters the picture as a complete stranger. The medical assistant is the professional who can bridge this gap. Familiarity with the training and scope of practice of other allied health occupations can help the medical assistant in this role.

For more than 50 years, the AMA has been involved in the setting of standards and the accreditation of allied health education programs. In 1935, the training of the occupational therapist was the first in allied health education to be accredited by the AMA. By 1997, the AMA Council on Medical Education was accrediting the training of nearly 30 health care professions (Table 4–1). The medical assisting program was accredited in 1969. Table 4–2 defines various members of the health care team and their functions. Table 4–3 lists health care occupations accredited by agencies other than the Commission on Accreditation of Allied Health Education Programs.

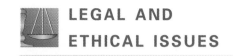

LEGAL AND ETHICAL ISSUES

During the era when sole proprietorship dominated medical care, practices were smaller and patients enjoyed an intimate climate of health care. Managed care has "depersonalized" the patient's care. The medical assistant has the unique opportunity to ensure that the patient feels comfortable and appropriately cared for.

CRITICAL THINKING

1 Briefly explain the two principal methods of paying for medical care and how it is changing.

HOW DID I DO? Answers to Memory Joggers

1 Sole proprietorship is declining because of the changes in the economic structure of medical practice.

2 *Sole proprietorship:* one individual holds exclusive ownership.
Partnership: two or more owners, with a legal agreement outlining their rights and responsibilities.
Corporation: the corporation is the legal owner, regulated by the state. The physician is an employee of the corporation.

3 A system by which patients receive appropriate care in an appropriate setting at the least possible cost.

4 A DO places more emphasis on the relationship between the musculoskeletal structure and organ function.

Medical Ethics

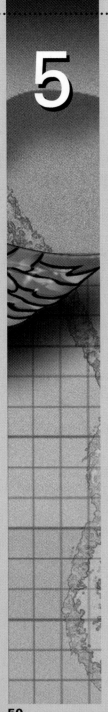

5

LEARNING OBJECTIVES

Cognitive: On successful completion of this chapter you should be able to:

1 Define and spell the terms listed in the Vocabulary.
2 Differentiate between the terms *ethics* and *etiquette*.
3 Identify the earliest written code of ethical conduct for medical practice.
4 Name the ancient Greek oath that remains an inspiration to physicians today.
5 Identify a code that was an example for the AMA Principles of Medical Ethics.
6 State a significant reason for the 1980 revision of the AMA Principles.
7 State the maximum penalty that a medical society can impose on a member for unethical conduct.
8 Discuss what and to whom information about a patient may be released.
9 Discuss the application of ethics in dealing with fees and charges.
10 Discuss the medical assistant's ethical obligations and restrictions.

VOCABULARY

abetting Encouraging or supporting

access Freedom to obtain or make use of

allocation Apportioned for a specific purpose or person

artificial insemination The introduction of semen into the vagina or cervix by artificial means

censure The act of blaming or condemning sternly

compulsory Obligatory; enforced

contingent Dependent on or conditioned by something else

culminate To reach a high or decisive point

deceptive Misleading; having the power to deceive

ethics A set of moral principles or values

expulsion Act of expelling or forcing out

fee splitting Sharing a fee with another physician, laboratory, or drug company not based on services performed

genetic Pertaining to the branch of biology dealing with heredity and variation among related organisms

ghost surgery A situation in which a patient has consented to have surgery done by one surgeon but, without the patient's knowledge or consent, the surgery is actually performed by another surgeon

preamble An introductory portion; a preface

precepts Practical rules guiding behavior or technique

public domain The realm embracing property rights that belong to the community at large and that are subject to appropriation by anyone

resident A graduate and licensed physician receiving training in a specialty in a hospital

suspension The act of interrupting or discontinuing temporarily, but with an expectation or purpose of resumption

Ethics concerns the thoughts, judgments, and actions on issues that have the greater implications of moral right and wrong. A morally right attitude is usually understood to be directed toward an ideal form of human character or action, which should **culminate** in the highest good for humanity. From the desire to achieve this good comes the sense of moral duty and a system of interpersonal moral obligations.

Medical ethics should not be confused with medical etiquette. *Etiquette* deals with courtesy, customs, and manners; *ethics* concerns itself with the underlying philosophies in the ideal relationships of humans. These relationships are often formally set forth in social contracts and codes.

Historical Codes

Ethics—judgments of right and wrong—have always been a concern of humans. It is not surprising that for centuries the medical profession has set for itself a rigid standard of ethical conduct toward patients and colleagues. The earliest written code of ethical conduct for medical practice was conceived around 2250 BC by the Babylonians and was called the Code of Hammurabi. It went into much detail regarding the conduct expected of a physician, even prescribing the fees that could be charged. Probably because of its length and detail, it did not survive the ages. See Evolution of Modern Code of Ethics.

About 400 BC, Hippocrates, the Greek physician known as the Father of Medicine, developed a brief statement of principles that has come down through history and remains an inspiration to the physician of today. The Oath of Hippocrates has been administered to medical graduates in many European universities for centuries (Fig. 5–1).

The most significant contribution to ethical history subsequent to Hippocrates was made by Thomas Percival, a physician, philosopher, and writer from Manchester, England. In 1803, he published his Code of Medical Ethics. Percival's personality, his interest in sociologic matters, and his close association with the Manchester Infirmary led to the preparation of a "scheme of professional conduct relative to hospitals and other charities," from which he drafted the code that bears his name.

In 1846, as the American Medical Association (AMA) was being organized in New York City, medical education and medical ethics were being

THE OATH OF HIPPOCRATES

I swear by Apollo, the physician, and Aesculapius, and Health, and Allheal, and all the gods and goddesses, that, according to my ability and judgment, I will keep this oath and stipulation, to reckon him who taught me this art equally dear to me as my parents, to share my substance with him and relieve his necessities if required; to regard his offspring as on the same footing with my own brothers, and to teach them this art if they should wish to learn it, without fee or stipulation, and that by precept, lecture, and every other mode of instruction, I will impart a knowledge of the art to my own sons and to those of my teachers, and to disciples bound by a stipulation and oath, according to the law of medicine, but to none other.

I will follow that method of treatment which, according to my ability and judgment, I consider for the benefit of my patients, and abstain from whatever is deleterious and mischievous. I will give no deadly medicine to anyone if asked, nor suggest any such counsel; furthermore, I will not give to a woman an instrument to produce abortion.

With purity and holiness, I will pass my life and practice my art. I will not cut a person who is suffering with a stone, but will leave this to be done by practitioners of this work. Into whatever houses I enter I will go into them for the benefit of the sick and will abstain from every voluntary act of mischief and corruption; and further from the seduction of females or males, bond or free.

Whatever, in connection with my professional practice, or not in connection with it, I may see or hear in the lives of men which ought not to be spoken abroad, I will not divulge, as reckoning that all such should be kept secret.

While I continue to keep this oath unviolated, may it be granted to me to enjoy life and the practice of the art, respected by all men at all times, but should I trespass and violate this oath, may the reverse be my lot.

FIGURE 5–1 The Oath of Hippocrates.

considered from a national point of view. At the first AMA annual meeting in Philadelphia in 1847, a Code of Ethics was formulated and adopted. It specifically acknowledged Percival's Code as its basic example and became a part of the fundamental standards of the AMA and of its component parts.

Memory Jogger

1 *How does ethics differ from etiquette?*

EVOLUTION OF MODERN CODE OF MEDICAL ETHICS

2250 BC	Code of Hammurabi
400 BC	Oath of Hippocrates
1803	Percival's Code of Medical Ethics
1847	First AMA Principles of Medical Ethics
1980	AMA Principles of Medical Ethics (latest revision)

AMA Code of Ethics

The AMA's Code of Ethics has four components:

- Principles of Medical Ethics
- Fundamental Elements of the Patient–Physician Relationship
- Current Opinions with Annotations
- Reports of the Council on Ethical and Judicial Affairs

The publication *Code of Medical Ethics, Current Opinions with Annotations*, contains the first three components, with discussion of more than 135 ethical

issues encountered in medicine. A separate publication, the *Reports of the Council on Ethical and Judicial Affairs*, discusses the rationale of the Council's opinions.

Principles of Medical Ethics

The AMA Principles of Medical Ethics has been revised on several occasions to keep it consistent with the times, but there has never been change in the moral intent or overall idealism. Major revisions were made in 1903, 1912, and 1947. In 1957, the AMA Principles of Medical Ethics was condensed to a **preamble** and 10 sections, a major change in format from the 1847 code. The 1980 revision of the code, which contains a preamble and seven sections, was done to clarify and update the language, to eliminate reference to gender, and to seek a proper and reasonable balance between professional standards and contemporary legal standards in our changing society (Fig. 5–2).

AMA Council on Ethical and Judicial Affairs

The Council on Ethical and Judicial Affairs of the AMA consists of nine active members of the AMA, including one resident physician member and one medical student member, and is charged with interpreting the Principles as adopted by the House of Delegates of the AMA. Although the code and the interpretations are directed specifically toward physicians, the medical assistant, as a member of the medical team, must be familiar with these principles and cooperate with the physician in practicing within their concepts.

Current Opinions with Annotations

The opinions of the Council elaborate and expand the **precepts** in the Principles of Medical Ethics. These opinions are continually updated to encompass developing situations, and they reflect the changing challenges and responsibilities of medicine.

Current Opinions with Annotations, 1996–1997, is presented in nine parts; selected portions are briefly summarized in the following pages. For a more detailed coverage, a copy of the publication may be ordered from the American Medical Association, 515 North State Street, Chicago, IL 60610.

INTRODUCTION

As stated in the Preamble, the AMA Principles are not laws but standards. Laws vary from state to state and from community to community. Ethical standards are universal and are never less than the standards required by law; frequently they are greater. Violation of the ethical standards of an association or society may result in **censure, expulsion,** or **suspension** of membership.

If a physician violates ethical standards involving a breach of moral duty or principle, the maximum penalty that the medical society can impose is expulsion. If there is alleged criminal conduct relating to the practice of medicine, the medical society is obligated to report it to the appropriate governmental body or state board. Violation of a law followed by conviction may result in punishment by fine, imprisonment, or revocation of license.

OPINIONS ON SOCIAL POLICY ISSUES

Abortion

The physician is not prohibited by ethical considerations from performing a lawful abortion in accordance with good medical practice and under circumstances that do not violate the law.

Abuse

Discovery that a patient is abusing a child, spouse, or parent creates a difficult situation for the physician. The patient may be the object of abuse but deny its existence in fear of further attacks. The law requires that such abuse be reported. If the physician does not report such suspected or discovered abuse, as required by the law, an added ethical violation is created that may result in continued abuse to the victim. The medical assistant is frequently the

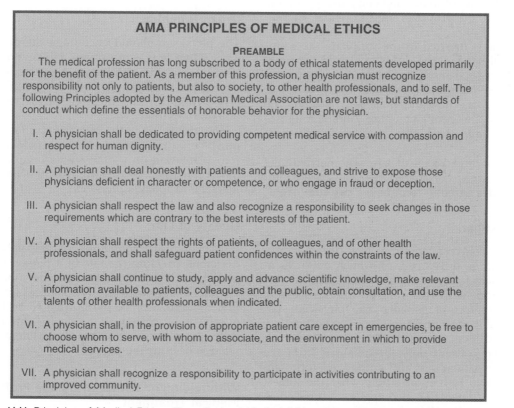

AMA PRINCIPLES OF MEDICAL ETHICS

PREAMBLE

The medical profession has long subscribed to a body of ethical statements developed primarily for the benefit of the patient. As a member of this profession, a physician must recognize responsibility not only to patients, but also to society, to other health professionals, and to self. The following Principles adopted by the American Medical Association are not laws, but standards of conduct which define the essentials of honorable behavior for the physician.

I. A physician shall be dedicated to providing competent medical service with compassion and respect for human dignity.

II. A physician shall deal honestly with patients and colleagues, and strive to expose those physicians deficient in character or competence, or who engage in fraud or deception.

III. A physician shall respect the law and also recognize a responsibility to seek changes in those requirements which are contrary to the best interests of the patient.

IV. A physician shall respect the rights of patients, of colleagues, and of other health professionals, and shall safeguard patient confidences within the constraints of the law.

V. A physician shall continue to study, apply and advance scientific knowledge, make relevant information available to patients, colleagues and the public, obtain consultation, and use the talents of other health professionals when indicated.

VI. A physician shall, in the provision of appropriate patient care except in emergencies, be free to choose whom to serve, with whom to associate, and the environment in which to provide medical services.

VII. A physician shall recognize a responsibility to participate in activities contributing to an improved community.

FIGURE 5–2 AMA Principles of Medical Ethics. (From Code of Medical Ethics. Current Opinions with Annotations of the Council on Ethical and Judicial Affairs of the American Medical Association. Copyright 1997, American Medical Association.)

first to notice symptoms of abuse and should report this to the physician or act as required by law.

Memory Jogger

2 *Why should the medical assistant report any symptoms of patient abuse to the physician?*

Allocation of Health Resources

Society must sometimes decide who will receive care, when serving all who need it is not possible. In organ transplantation, for example, several need the transplant and only one donor is available. Who shall be the recipient? Kidney dialysis is another situation in which the demand is greater than the supply. This creates a conflict for the physician, who has the duty to do all that can be done to benefit the patient. The attending physician must remain a patient advocate and therefore should not make **allocation** decisions. Procedures for such allocations are determined in an objective manner by the institutions involved.

Artificial Insemination

Informed consent for **artificial insemination** should include disclosure of risks, benefits, likely success rate of the method proposed, and potential alternative methods.

If the donor is married to the recipient, the resultant child will have all the rights of a child naturally conceived. Artificial insemination by an anonymous donor requires the informed consent of the recipient and consent of the husband if he is to become the legal father of the resultant child. Anonymous donors do not have the rights or responsibilities of parenthood.

If the donor and recipient are not married, the recipient would be considered the sole parent, unless both parties agree to recognize a paternity right.

Clinical Investigation

Without clinical investigation, no new drugs or procedures would be developed. However, all such investigation must follow a competently designed systematic program with due concern for the welfare, safety, and comfort of patients. The physician–patient relationship does exist in clinical investigation; and when treatment of the patient is involved, voluntary written consent must be obtained from the patient or the patient's legally authorized representative. Additional restrictions apply when the subject is a minor or a mentally incompetent adult. When participating in the clinical investigation of new drugs and procedures, physicians should show the same concern for the welfare and safety of the person involved as they would have if the person were a private patient.

Cost

Concern for the quality of patient care should be the physician's first consideration. However, the physician should be conscious of costs and not provide or prescribe unnecessary services.

Provision of Adequate Health Care

Access to an adequate level of health care for all members of our society is now a moral expectation. The following ethical principles should be considered in determining whether particular procedures or treatments should be included in an adequate level of health care:

- Degree of benefit
- Likelihood of benefit
- Duration of benefit
- Cost
- Number of people who will benefit

Genetic Counseling

Genetic counseling and organ transplantation may require personal and ethical decisions concerning the quality of the life that is to be saved.

Organ Donation

The physician should encourage the donation of organs when it is appropriate. However, it is considered unethical to participate in proceedings in which the donor receives payment, except reimbursement of expenses directly incurred in the removal of the donated organ.

The rights of both the donor and the recipient must be equally protected. In a case involving the transplantation of a vital, single organ, the death of the donor must be determined by a physician other than the recipient's physician.

Quality of Life

Physicians must sometimes participate or advise on decisions affecting the fate of a person whose future is dim, such as a deformed newborn or a person of advanced age with many physical problems. The first thought may be the burden to be borne by the family or by society in caring for this person. Ethically, the physician's primary consideration must be what is best for the patient.

Withholding or Withdrawing Life-Prolonging Medical Treatment

A physician is committed to *saving life* and *relieving suffering*. Sometimes these two goals are incompatible, and a choice between them must be made. If possible, the patient may decide. Often, the patient makes his or her wishes known to a responsible relative or other representative in the event that he or she becomes incapacitated. Patients who live in a state that has living will statutes may have some choice if a living will has been established. The living will is a document that states the wishes of that person in case of terminal illness. Usually, it is done to prohibit heroic measures being taken in a situation in which the patient would be unable or incompetent to make a decision. Without preplanning, the physician must act in the best interest of the patient. If it has been determined beyond a doubt that the patient is permanently unconscious, cutting off life-prolonging treatment is ethical.

Euthanasia

Euthanasia is the administration of a lethal agent by another person to a patient for the purpose of relieving the patient's intolerable and incurable suffering. Euthanasia is fundamentally incompatible with the physician's role as healer.

Memory Jogger

3 *What is the physician's primary consideration in deciding the fate of a deformed newborn?*

Interprofessional Relations

The interprofessional relations of the physician are mostly governed by ethics; however, some legal restrictions do exist. State laws may prohibit a physician from aiding and **abetting** an unlicensed person in the practice of medicine. Such laws also forbid aiding and abetting a person with a limited license in providing services beyond the scope of that license.

If a nurse or medical assistant recognizes or suspects an error in a physician's orders, it is his or her obligation to report this to the physician. Questioning a possible error is necessary even if it means risking the displeasure of the physician. It may possibly save a life or save the physician from a lawsuit if there is an error. For example, the person initiating a drug administration order should always check the dosage in the *Physician's Desk Reference (PDR)*.

 Safety Alert: If the dosage is suspected of being wrong, it should always be questioned.

Physicians often refer a patient to another physician for diagnosis or treatment when it is beneficial to the patient. The physician should make these referrals only when confident that the patient will receive competent treatment.

Lacking legal restrictions, a physician in private practice is free to choose whom to serve. Although private practitioners may refuse certain patients, patients who have already been accepted in the practice cannot be neglected.

The sports physician must keep in mind that the professional responsibility at a sporting event is to protect the health and safety of the participants, with personal judgments being governed only by medical considerations.

Hospital Relations

Most practicing physicians have staff privileges at one or more hospitals. It is considered unethical for a physician to charge a separate fee for the routine, nonmedical services performed in admitting a patient to a hospital. The physician may ethically bill a patient for services rendered the patient by a **resident** under the physician's personal observation, direction, and supervision, if the physician assumes responsibility for the services. The granting of hospital privileges should be based on the training, competence, and experience of the applicant—never on the condition of **compulsory** assessments for any purpose, such as a fee of $1000 for staff membership. Self-imposed assessments by vote of the medical staff are acceptable.

Confidentiality, Advertising, and Communications Media Relations

MINORS

When minors request confidential services, physicians should encourage them to involve their parents. If the minor does not wish to involve the parents, and the law does not require otherwise, physicians should permit a competent minor to consent to medical care and should not notify parents without the patient's consent.

For minors who are mature enough to be unaccompanied by their parents for their examination, confidentiality should be maintained, and information relayed to the parents only with consent of the patient.

ADVERTISING

The only restrictions on advertising by physicians are those that specifically protect the public from

deceptive practices. Standards regarding advertising and publicity have been liberalized over the years, but any advertisement or publicity must be true and not misleading. Testimonials of patients, for instance, should not be used in advertising, because they are difficult to verify or measure by objective standards. The physician can safely include information on educational background, fees, available credit, and any other nondeceptive information, but statements regarding the quality of medical services are highly subjective and difficult to verify.

Health maintenance organizations routinely seek members through advertising. Physicians who practice in such prepaid plans must abide by the same principles of ethics as do other physicians. Any deceptive advertising—for example, any that would be misleading to patients or prospective subscribers—is unethical.

COMMUNICATIONS WITH MEDIA

Although information regarding some patients, such as celebrities and politicians, may be considered news, the physician may not discuss a patient's condition with the press without authorization from the patient or the patient's lawful representative. The physician may release only authorized information or that which is public knowledge. Certain kinds of news are a part of the public record. News in this category is known as news in the **public domain** and includes births, deaths, accidents, and police cases.

Memory Jogger

4 *What about sharing information about a celebrity with just a few close friends?*

The medical assistant must be aware that only the physician is authorized to release information, and under no circumstances should the medical assistant violate the confidential nature of the physician–patient relationship.

An item of specific interest to the medical assistant is *what information may be revealed* by the physician's office to the representatives of insurance companies. The history, diagnosis, prognosis, and other information acquired during the physician–patient relationship may be disclosed to an insurance company representative only if the patient or the patient's lawful representative has consented to the disclosure by signing a release form. It is unethical even to certify that the individual was under the physician's care without the patient's permission. The same restriction applies to discussions with the patient's lawyer. However, a physician may testify in court or before a workers' compensation board in any personal injury or related case.

COMPUTERS

The expanding uses of computer technology permit the accumulation and storage of an unlimited amount of medical information. With the use of computers in the physician's office and the employment of computer service organizations, confidentiality becomes more difficult.

All individuals and organizations with some form of access to the computerized databases, and the level of access permitted, should be specifically identified in advance. Full disclosure of this information to the patient is necessary in obtaining informed consent to treatment. Patient data should be assigned a security level appropriate for the data's degree of sensitivity, which should be used to control who has access to the information.

Detailed guidelines have been developed by the AMA and are included in the *Current Opinions with Annotations.* These guidelines should be followed by physicians and any employed computer service organizations in maintaining the confidentiality of information in medical records when that information is stored in computerized databases.

Fees and Charges

Charging or collecting an illegal or excessive fee is unethical. Illegal charges may occur through ignorance of the law when billing for treatment of Medicaid or Medicare patients. A medical assistant has the responsibility to keep informed on current regulations and to see that they are conscientiously followed.

FEE SPLITTING AND CONTINGENT FEES

If a physician accepts payment from another physician solely for the referral of a patient, both are guilty of an unethical practice called **fee splitting.** Fee splitting, whether with another physician, a clinic or laboratory, or a drug company, is unethical.

Lawyers often accept cases on a contingency basis, that is, the fee is **contingent** on a successful outcome. A physician's fee is always based on the value of the service provided to the patient. Charging a fee based on the successful outcome of the medical care would be considered unethical.

INSURANCE FORMS

An attending physician should expect to complete one simplified insurance claim form for the patient without charge. Multiple or complex forms for the same patient may warrant a charge if this is in conformity with local custom.

INTEREST AND FINANCE CHARGES

Requesting that payment be made at the time of treatment is entirely appropriate, particularly if the patient has a history of making late payments. If the patient is notified in advance, adding interest or other reasonable charges to delinquent accounts is also proper. Advance notice can be accomplished by posting this information in the reception office or by notations on the billing statements. A more effective approach is the use of a Patient Information Folder that includes billing information; such a folder is provided for every new patient on the initial visit. Federal laws and regulations applicable to the imposition of interest charges are addressed in Chapter 16, Professional Fees and Credit Arrangements. Accounting and collection policies should be regularly reviewed with the physician to ensure that no patient's account is sent to collection without the physician's knowledge.

WAIVER OF INSURANCE COPAYMENTS

Physicians frequently write off or waive copayments to facilitate patient access to medical care. If access to care is directly threatened because the patient cannot make the copayment, the physician may forgive the copayment. Routine or consistent forgiveness or waiver of copayments may constitute fraud under state and federal laws. The forgiveness or waiver of copayments may violate the policies of some insurers, both public and private. Physicians should ensure that their policies on copayments are consistent with applicable law and with the requirements of their agreements with insurers.

PROFESSIONAL COURTESY

Professional courtesy (the provision of medical care to physician colleagues or their families free of charge or at a reduced fee) is a long-standing tradition. It is not an ethical requirement, and this decision is made on an individual basis.

Physician's Records

OWNERSHIP AND ACCESS

Notes made by the physician while treating a patient are made for the physician's own use and are considered the physician's personal property. On request of the patient, the physician should provide a summary of the record to the patient, to another physician, or to a person designated by the patient. Original records should not be released except on the physician's retirement or sale of the medical practice.

In some states, a patient is authorized by law to have **access** to his or her medical records. Health care professionals should familiarize themselves with the laws in their own states. Of primary concern regarding all records is the authorization of the patient before releasing any information, unless the release is required by law. A reasonable charge may be made for the cost of duplicating records.

RECORDS OF PHYSICIANS ON LEAVING A GROUP, RETIREMENT, OR DEATH

A patient may, for a variety of reasons, need access to his or her health records after a physician leaves a group, retires, or dies. The records may be necessary for employment, insurance, litigation, or other reasons.

The patients of a physician who leaves a group practice should be notified that the physician is leaving the group. They should also be notified of the physician's new address and offered the opportunity to have their medical records forwarded to the departing physician at his or her new address.

When a physician retires or dies, patients should be notified and encouraged to find another physician. They should be informed that, on their authorization, their records will be forwarded to the new physician. Records that are not forwarded to another physician should be retained by a custodian of the records in compliance with any legal requirements.

Practice Matters

APPOINTMENT CHARGES

May a physician charge for a missed appointment or one that was not canceled within a stated time? Yes, but only if the patient has been fully advised in advance that such charge will be made. Discretion should be used, however, in applying such charges.

CONSULTATION

Physicians should obtain consultation whenever they believe that it would be medically indicated in the care of the patient or when requested by the patient. When a patient is referred to a consultant, the referring physician should provide a history of the case to the consultant. The consultant should communicate the results of the consultant's examination to the referring physician.

DRUGS AND DEVICES: PRESCRIBING

A physician should not be influenced in the prescribing of drugs, devices, or appliances by a direct or indirect financial interest in the supplier. A physician may own or operate a pharmacy but generally may not refer his or her patients to the pharmacy. Patients should enjoy the same freedom of choice in deciding who will fill a prescription as they have in choosing a physician. A prescription is an essential part of a patient's record, and the patient is entitled to a copy.

HEALTH FACILITY OWNERSHIP BY A PHYSICIAN

A physician may ethically own or have a financial interest in a for-profit hospital or other health care facility such as a freestanding clinic. However, before admitting or referring a patient to that facility, the physician has an ethical obligation to reveal such ownership to the patient. In general, physicians should not refer patients to a health facility that is outside their office practice and at which they do not directly provide care or services.

GHOST SURGERY

The substitution of another surgeon without the patient's consent is called **ghost surgery.** The patient has a right to choose his or her own physician or surgeon. To make a substitution without consulting the patient is deceitful and unethical.

Professional Rights and Responsibilities

DISCIPLINE AND MEDICINE

A physician should expose incompetent, corrupt, dishonest, or unethical conduct on the part of members of the profession, without fear of loss of favor.

A physician may be subject to civil or criminal liability for violation of governmental laws. Expulsion from membership is the maximum penalty that may be imposed by a medical society for violation of ethical standards.

FREE CHOICE

The concept of free choice ensures the right of every individual generally to choose or change at will his

or her physician. Likewise, a physician in private practice may decline to accept that individual as a patient.

PATENTS

A physician may ethically patent a surgical or diagnostic instrument that he or she has discovered or developed, based on the doctrine that one is entitled to protect one's discovery. The patenting of medical procedures could pose substantial risk to the practice of medicine by limiting the availability of new procedures. It is unethical for a physician to patent medical procedures.

PHYSICIAN–PATIENT RELATIONSHIP

The physician–patient relationship is a form of contract. Both parties are free to enter into or decline the relationship. For example, a physician may decline to accept a patient whose medical condition is not within the physician's line of practice. However, physicians who offer their services to the public may not decline to accept patients because of race, color, religion, national origin, or any other discriminatory basis. The physician–patient relationship does not exist until the physician undertakes care of the patient (Fig. 5–3).

PHYSICIANS AND INFECTIOUS DISEASE

A physician who knows that he or she has an infectious disease, which if contracted by a patient would pose a significant risk to the patient, should not engage in any activity that creates an identified risk of transmission of that disease to the patient.

SUBSTANCE ABUSE

It is unethical for a physician to practice medicine while under the influence of a controlled substance, alcohol, or other chemical agents that would impair the ability to practice medicine.

Ethics for the Medical Assistant

The Code of Ethics of the American Association of Medical Assistants (AAMA) is an honorable standard for all medical assistants to observe. The Code is patterned after the AMA Principles and is adapted to the professional medical assistant who accepts this discipline as a responsibility of trust (Fig. 5–4).

FUNDAMENTAL ELEMENTS OF THE PATIENT-PHYSICIAN RELATIONSHIP

From ancient times, physicians have recognized that the health and well-being of patients depends upon a collaborative effort between physician and patient. Patients share with physicians the responsibility for their own health care. The patient-physician relationship is of greatest benefit to patients when they bring medical problems to the attention of their physicians in a timely fashion, provide information about their medical condition to the best of their ability, and work with their physicians in a mutually respectful alliance. Physicians can best contribute to this alliance by serving as their patients' advocates and by fostering these rights:

1. The patient has the right to receive information from physicians and to discuss the benefits, risks and costs of appropriate treatment alternatives. Patients should receive guidance from their physicians as to the optimal course of action. Patients are also entitled to obtain copies or summaries of their medical records, to have their questions answered, to be advised of potential conflicts of interest that their physicians might have, and to receive independent professional opinions.
2. The patient has the right to make decisions regarding the health care that is recommended by his or her physician. Accordingly, patients may accept or refuse any recommended medical treatment.
3. The patient has the right to courtesy, respect, dignity, responsiveness, and timely attention to his or her needs.
4. The patient has the right to confidentiality. The physician should not reveal confidential communications or information without the consent of the patient, unless provided for by law or by the need to protect the welfare of the individual or the public interest.
5. The patient has the right to continuity of health care. The physician has an obligation to cooperate in the coordination of medically indicated care with other health care providers treating the patient. The physician may not discontinue treatment of a patient as long as further treatment is medically indicated, without giving the patient reasonable assistance and sufficient opportunity to make alternative arrangements for care.
6. The patient has a basic right to have available adequate health care. Physicians, along with the rest of society, should continue to work toward this goal. Fulfillment of this right is dependent on society providing resources so that no patient is deprived of necessary care because of an inability to pay for the care. Physicians should continue their traditional assumption of a part of the responsibility for the medical care of those who cannot afford essential health care. Physicians should advocate for patients in dealing with third parties when appropriate.

FIGURE 5–3 Fundamental Elements of the Patient–Physician Relationship. (From Report of the Council on Ethical and Judicial Affairs of the American Medical Association. Updated June 1994.)

AAMA CODE OF ETHICS

The Code of Ethics of AAMA shall set forth principles of ethical and moral conduct as they relate to the medical profession and the particular practice of medical assisting.

Members of AAMA dedicated to the conscientious pursuit of their profession, and thus desiring to merit the high regard of the entire medical profession and the respect of the general public which they serve, do pledge themselves to strive always to:

A. render service with full respect for the dignity of humanity;
B. respect confidential information obtained through employment unless legally authorized or required by responsible performance of duty to divulge such information;
C. uphold the honor and high principles of the profession and accept its disciplines;
D. seek to continually improve the knowledge and skills of medical assistants for the benefit of patients and professional colleagues;
E. participate in additional service activities aimed toward improving the health and well-being of the community.

AAMA CREED

I believe in the principles and purposes of the profession of medical assisting.
I endeavor to be more effective.
I aspire to render greater service.
I protect the confidence entrusted to me.
I am dedicated to the care and well-being of all people.
I am loyal to my employer.
I am true to the ethics of my profession.
I am strengthened by compassion, courage and faith.

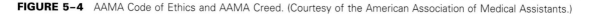

FIGURE 5–4 AAMA Code of Ethics and AAMA Creed. (Courtesy of the American Association of Medical Assistants.)

A PATIENT'S BILL OF RIGHTS

This policy document presents the official position of the American Hospital Association as approved by the Board of Trustees and House of Delegates

The American Hospital Association presents a Patient's Bill of Rights with the expectation that observance of these rights will contribute to more effective patient care and greater satisfaction for the patient, his physician, and the hospital organization. Further, the Association presents these rights in the expectation that they will be supported by the hospital on behalf of its patients, as an integral part of the healing process. It is recognized that a personal relationship between the physician and the patient is essential for the provision of proper medical care. The traditional physician-patient relationship takes on a new dimension when care is rendered within an organizational structure. Legal precedent has established that the institution itself also has a responsibility to the patient. It is in recognition of these factors that these rights are affirmed.

1. The patient has the right to considerate and respectful care.
2. The patient has the right to obtain from his physician complete current information concerning his diagnosis, treatment, and prognosis in terms the patient can be reasonably expected to understand. When it is not medically advisable to give such information to the patient, the information should be made available to an appropriate person in his behalf. He has the right to know, by name, the physician responsible for coordinating his care.
3. The patient has the right to receive from his physician information necessary to give informed consent prior to the start of any procedure and/or treatment. Except in emergencies, such information for informed consent should include but not necessarily be limited to the specific procedure and/or treatment, the medically significant risks involved, and the probable duration of incapacitation. Where medically significant alternatives for care or treatment exist, or when the patient requests information concerning medical alternatives, the patient has the right to such information. The patient also has the right to know the name of the person responsible for the procedures and/or treatment.
4. The patient has the right to refuse treatment to the extent permitted by law and to be informed of the medical consequences of his action.
5. The patient has the right to every consideration of his privacy concerning his own medical care program. Case discussion, consultation, examination, and treatment are confidential and should be conducted discreetly. Those not directly involved in his care must have the permission of the patient to be present.
6. The patient has the right to expect that all communications and records pertaining to his care should be treated as confidential.
7. The patient has the right to expect that within its capacity a hospital must make reasonable response to the request of a patient for services. The hospital must provide evaluation, service, and/or referral as indicated by the urgency of the case. When medically permissible, a patient may be transferred to another facility only after he has received complete information and explanation concerning the needs for and alternatives to such a transfer. The institution to which the patient is to be transferred must first have accepted the patient for transfer.
8. The patient has the right to obtain information as to any relationship of his hospital to other health care and educational institutions insofar as his care is concerned. The patient has the right to obtain information as to the existence of any professional relationships among individuals, by name, who are treating him.
9. The patient has the right to be advised if the hospital proposes to engage in or perform human experimentation affecting his care or treatment. The patient has the right to refuse to participate in such research projects.
10. The patient has the right to expect reasonable continuity of care. He has the right to know in advance what appointment times and physicians are available and where. The patient has the right to expect that the hospital will provide a mechanism whereby he is informed by his physician or a delegate of the physician of the patient's continuing health care requirements following discharge.
11. The patient has the right to examine and receive an explanation of his bill regardless of source of payment.
12. The patient has the right to know what hospital rules and regulations apply to his conduct as a patient.

No catalog of rights can guarantee for the patient the kind of treatment he has a right to expect. A hospital has many functions to perform, including the prevention and treatment of disease, the education of both health professionals and patients, and the conduct of clinical research. All these activities must be conducted with an overriding concern for the patient, and, above all, the recognition of his dignity as a human being. Success in achieving this recognition assures success in the defense of the rights of the patient.

FIGURE 5–5   A Patient's Bill of Rights. (Courtesy of the American Hospital Association.)

Patient's Bill of Rights

The Patient's Bill of Rights developed and approved by the American Hospital Association in 1973 should also be the credo of the practicing medical assistant (Fig. 5–5).

LEGAL AND ETHICAL ISSUES

The prime objective of the medical profession is to render service to humanity, and this must be the medical assistant's first concern as well. The importance of respecting the confidentiality of information learned from or about patients in the course of employment cannot be overemphasized. It is unethical to reveal patient confidences to *anyone*—this includes family, spouse, best friends, and other medical assistants. Do not even mention the names of patients outside the place of employment, because sometimes the doctor's specialty reveals the patient's reason for consultation.

Never discuss one patient's case with another patient; if curious patients ask questions about another, simply change the subject. A patient who asks questions of a medical nature about his or her own case should be referred to the physician for information. The medical assistant must avoid giving advice of a personal nature to any patient, because patients tend to identify remarks from any of the personnel as reflecting the advice of the physician. By remaining silent in these situations, the physician, the medical assistant, and the patient are protected. Confidential papers, case histories, and even the appointment book should be kept out of sight of curious eyes to protect the patient as well as the physician and office staff.

The medical assistant has an obligation to keep abreast of current developments that affect the practice of medicine and care of the patients. Membership in a professional organization provides access to continuing education for maintaining knowledge and skills pertaining to the performance of medical assisting.

In rare instances, a medical assistant is faced with a situation in which the physician-employer's conduct appears to violate established ethical standards. Before making any judgments, the medical assistant must be absolutely sure of all the information and circumstances. If there are, in fact, occurrences of unethical conduct, the medical assistant must then make some decisions.

Is it wise to remain under these circumstances? Would it be better to seek other employment?

Will a decision to remain adversely affect future opportunities for employment with another physician?

These decisions are difficult to make, especially if the relationship and employment conditions have been satisfactory and congenial. A medical assistant is not legally obliged to report questionable actions of the physician or to attempt to alter the circumstances. However, an ethical medical assistant will not wish to participate in the continuance of known substandard or unlawful practices that may be harmful to patients. The medical assistant is bound to ethical practices as are all health care providers.

CRITICAL THINKING

1 Give an example showing the difference between ethics and etiquette.

2 What symptoms of patient abuse would a medical assistant be likely to observe?

3 Have you read any articles in the news about "assisted suicide" or other ethical issues?

4 While assisting a patient in interpreting a prescription written by the physician you notice that the instructions specify taking the medication three times a day. Usually the drug is taken only once a day. How would you handle this?

5 A mother accompanies her teenage daughter to the doctor's office but remains in the reception area. While the patient is with the physician the mother engages you, the medical assistant, in discussion of the patient. How would you respond?

HOW DID I DO? Answers to Memory Joggers

1 Ethics concerns the issues of moral right or wrong. Etiquette deals with courtesy, customs, and manners.

2 The law requires that abuse noted must be reported.

3 The physician's primary consideration is what is best for the patient.

4 Only authorized information may be released. It is best to not even mention the case outside the office.

REFERENCE

American Medical Association: Code of Medical Ethics, Current Opinions with Annotations. Chicago, AMA, 1997.

Medicine and the Law

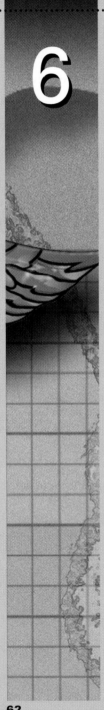

6

LEARNING OBJECTIVES

Cognitive: On successful completion of this chapter you should be able to:

1 Define and spell the terms listed in the Vocabulary.

2 State the purpose of medical practice acts and how they are established.

3 List the three methods by which licensure may be granted.

4 List the general categories of cause for revocation or suspension of a license.

5 Explain the difference between *criminal* and *civil* law.

6 Define a contract and explain its importance in a health care facility.

7 Outline the correct way for a physician to terminate the physician–patient relationship.

8 State the four "Ds of Negligence" as published by the American Medical Association.

9 Briefly describe the *arbitration* procedure, and identify three advantages.

10 List the six components of *informed consent*.

11 Explain the purpose of Good Samaritan Acts.

12 State two restrictions imposed on physicians by the Anatomical Gift Act.

13 Explain the medical assistant's role in claims prevention.

14 State the meaning of *administrative law.*

15 Discuss the importance of compliance with OSHA regulations.

16 Explain the essential difference between a living will and a durable power of attorney.

VOCABULARY

administering Instilling a drug into the body of a patient

administrative law Regulations set forth by government agencies

allegation A statement of what a party to a legal action will undertake to prove

arbitration The hearing and determination of a cause in controversy by a person or persons either chosen by the parties involved or appointed under statutory authority

arbitrator A neutral person chosen to settle differences between two parties in a controversy

assault An intentional, unlawful *attempt* of bodily injury to another by force

battery A willful and unlawful use of force or violence upon the person of another

biennially Occurring every 2 years

communicable Capable of being transmitted from one person to another

compensatory damages General or special damages without specific monetary value

concurrently Occurring at the same time

contagious Transmitted readily from one person to another by direct or indirect contact

contract law Enforceable promises

deposition Oral testimony taken from a party or witness to the litigation and is not limited to parties named in the lawsuit.

dispensing Giving drugs, in some type of bottle, box, or other container, to the patient. (Under the Controlled Substances Act of 1970, the definition of "dispense" includes the administering of controlled substances.)

emancipated minor A person under legal age who is self-supporting and living apart from parents or a guardian

endorsement To express approval publicly and definitely

exemplary Serving as a warning

expert witness Professional who belongs to a certifying or qualifying organization and who is called to testify in court

felony A crime of a graver nature than one designated as a misdemeanor; generally, an offense punishable by imprisonment in a penitentiary

infectious Capable of causing infection

informed consent A consent in which there is understanding of what treatment is to be undertaken and of the risks involved, why it should be done, and alternative methods of treatment available (including no treatment) and their attendant risks

infraction Breaking the law; a minor offense of the rules

liability Subject to some adverse action

litigation Contest in a court of justice for the purpose of enforcing a right

living will A document in which an individual expresses wishes regarding medical treatment at or near the end of life

malfeasance The doing of an act that is wholly wrongful and unlawful

malpractice Professional misconduct, improper discharge of professional duties, or failure to meet the standard of care by a professional that results in harm to another

misdemeanor A crime less serious than a felony

misfeasance The improper performance of a lawful act

nominal Existing in name only

nonfeasance The failure to do something that should have been done

perjured testimony Telling what is false when sworn to tell the truth

prescribing Issuing a prescription for the patient; directing, designating, or ordering use of a remedy

prudent Marked by wisdom or circumspection

punitive Inflicting punishment

quackery The pretension of curing disease

reciprocity A mutual exchange of privileges

respondeat superior Let the master answer

revoked Annulled by recalling or taking back

subpoena A writ commanding a person to appear in court

suspended Debarred temporarily from a privilege

tort law Governs acts that bring harm to a person or damage to property, caused negligently or intentionally

treason A crime against the United States

trespass To exceed the bounds of what is lawful, right, or just

A graduate of a medical school must be licensed before beginning the practice of medicine. Licensure is regulated by state statutes by their medical practice acts. It is important for the medical assistant to understand licensing and other laws and regulations that are intended to protect patients, physicians, medical assistants, and other health care workers.

Licensure and Registration

MEDICAL PRACTICE ACTS

Medical practice acts existed as early as colonial days. However, these acts were later repealed, and in the mid-19th century practically none of the states had laws governing the practice of medicine. As one might expect, a rapid decline in professional standards followed. The general welfare of the people was endangered by medical quackery and inadequate care; by the beginning of the 20th century, medical practice acts were established by statute and were again in effect in every state. Their purpose is to

- Define what is included in the practice of medicine within that state
- Govern the methods and requirements of licensure
- Establish the grounds for suspension or revocation of license

LICENSURE

A doctor of medicine (MD) degree or a doctor of osteopathy (DO) degree is conferred on graduation from medical school. The license to practice medicine is granted by a state board, frequently known as the Board of Medical Examiners or Board of Registration. Licensure may be accomplished by any of the following procedures:

- Examination
- Reciprocity
- Endorsement

EXAMINATION Every state requires medical doctors to pass a written examination. The Federation

of State Medical Boards and the National Board of Medical Examiners agreed in 1990 to establish a single licensing examination—the Federation Licensing Examination (FLEX)—for graduates of accredited medical schools.

RECIPROCITY Some states grant the license to practice medicine by **reciprocity;** that is, they automatically recognize that the requirements of the state in which the license was granted meet the standards required by the second state.

ENDORSEMENT Most graduates of medical schools in the United States have been licensed by **endorsement** of the National Board certificate. Licensure by endorsement is granted on a case-by-case basis. Those graduates who have not been licensed by endorsement are required to pass a state board examination.

In all states, graduates of foreign medical schools who are seeking licensure by endorsement must meet the same requirements as graduates of medical schools in the United States, in addition to various other qualifying factors.

EXEMPTIONS Some graduates may not wish to engage in the practice of medicine. Their interests may lie in research or administration, or even in the practice of law with a special interest in medical liability. In such instances licensure is not required. Licensed physicians in the Armed Forces, Public Health Service, or Veterans Administration facilities need not be licensed in the state where they are employed.

Memory Jogger

1 *What are the three ways by which a physician might seek licensure?*

REGISTRATION AND RE-REGISTRATION

After a license is granted, periodic re-registration is necessary annually or **biennially.** A physician can be **concurrently** registered in more than one state.

The issuing body notifies the physician when re-registration is due.

The medical assistant can aid the physician by being aware of when the registration fees are due, thus preventing a possible lapsing of the registration. Many states require proof of continuing education besides payment of a registration fee.

Continuing education units (CEUs) are granted to physicians for attending approved seminars, lectures, scientific meetings, and formal courses in accredited colleges and universities. A total of 50 hours a year is the average requirement for license renewal. The medical assistant may be expected to help the physician arrange for completing the required units for license renewal.

REVOCATION OR SUSPENSION

Under certain conditions, the license to practice medicine may be **revoked** or **suspended.** Grounds for revocation or suspension of the license to practice medicine generally fall within one of three categories:

1. Conviction of a crime. This may include felonies such as murder, rape, larceny, and narcotic violations.
2. Unprofessional conduct. Failure to uphold the ethical standards of the medical profession is indicated, for example, by betrayal of patient confidence, giving or receiving rebates, and excessive use of narcotics or alcohol.
3. Personal or professional incapacity. This is difficult to label or prove. For example, advanced age or an injury may reduce the apparent capacity of some physicians. Certain illnesses can affect the memory or judgment necessary to practice medicine.

Categories of Legal Environment

When the physician enters the practice of medicine certain medicolegal principles must be considered in the daily operation of the health care facility. Law is the system by which society gives order to our lives. For our purposes, the law may be divided into two general categories: criminal law and civil law.

CRIMINAL LAW

Criminal law governs violations of the law that are punishable as offenses against the state or government. Such offenses involve the welfare and safety of the public as a whole rather than of one individual. Criminal offenses are classified as

- **Treason**—A crime against the United States

- **Felony**—A major crime, such as robbery, arson, issuing bad checks, forgery, and using the mail to defraud. Conviction may result in imprisonment for 1 year or more.
- **Misdemeanor**—A lesser offense that might result in imprisonment for 6 months to 1 year. An example of a misdemeanor is possession of a hypodermic syringe or needle by an unauthorized person.
- **Infraction**—A minor offense, such as traffic or drug violations, that usually result in a fine only.

CIVIL LAW

This chapter is mainly concerned with civil law affecting the practice of medicine, which is explained in the following pages. Civil law is concerned with the relations of individuals with other individuals, with corporations or other organizations, or with government agencies. Classifications of civil law that might affect the practice of medicine are

- **Contract law,** which governs enforceable promises.
- **Tort law,** which governs acts, intentional or unintentional, that bring harm to a person or damage to property
- **Administrative law,** which involves regulations set forth by government agencies, for example, the Internal Revenue Service

Contract Law

The law of contracts touches our lives in many ways practically every day, but usually we do not give it much thought. The patient–physician relationship is governed by the law of contracts, and the medical assistant must be aware of what constitutes a contract.

A *contract* is an agreement creating an obligation. An *express contract* is a verbalized agreement between two or more parties, containing explicit terms of the agreement, either orally or in writing. An *implied contract* is a conclusion drawn from actions of the two parties, for example, when a patient seeks care by a physician and the physician undertakes care of the patient. To be valid or enforceable, a contract must have the following four basic elements:

1. Manifestation of assent (an offer and an acceptance). The parties to the contract must understand and agree on the intent of the contract. The party making the offer is known as the *offeror,* and the party to whom the offer is made is the *offeree.*
2. Legal subject matter. An obligation that requires an illegal action is not an enforceable contract.
3. Legal capacity to contract. Both parties to the

contract must be adults of sound mind. The emancipated minor may contract for medical care.

4. Consideration. There must be an exchange of something of value.

If any of these four elements is missing, there is no contract.

The physician–patient relationship is generally held by the courts to be a contractual relationship that is the result of three steps:

1. The physician invites an offer by establishing availability.
2. The patient makes an offer by arriving for treatment (offeror).
3. The physician accepts the offer by undertaking treatment of the patient (offeree).

Before accepting the offer, the physician is under no obligation, and no contract exists. However, once the physician has accepted the patient an implied contract does exist that the physician (1) will treat the patient, using reasonable care, and (2) possesses the degree of knowledge, skill, and judgment that might be expected of another physician in the same locality and under similar circumstances. It is extremely important that no express promise of a cure be made, for this then becomes a part of the contract.

The patient's part of the agreement includes the liability for payment for services and a willingness to follow the advice of the physician. Most physician–patient relationships are implied contracts. After the physician–patient relationship has been established, the physician is obligated to attend the patient as long as attention is required, unless a special arrangement is made. The physician–patient relationship may be terminated by the physician or the patient.

Memory Jogger

2 *What are the four basic elements of a binding contract?*

Termination by Physician

Before withdrawing from the relationship, the physician may wish to take into consideration the condition of the patient, the size of the community, and the availability of other physicians. When a physician does terminate the relationship, the patient must be given notice of the physician's intention to withdraw so that the patient may secure another physician.

The physician may write a letter of withdrawal from the case to the patient, similar to the one shown in Figure 6–1. The letter should state that

- Professional care is being discontinued
- The physician will turn over the patient's records to another physician
- The patient should seek the attention of another physician as soon as possible

The letter should be delivered by certified mail with a return receipt requested and a copy of the letter placed in the patient's medical record. When the return receipt is received, it should be attached to the copy of the letter and retained permanently.

To protect the physician against a lawsuit for abandonment, the details of the circumstances under which the physician is withdrawing from the case are included in the patient's medical record.

Termination by Patient

In the event that the patient terminates the relationship, the termination of the contract and the circum-

---

Date

Dear (Patient):

I find it necessary to inform you that I am withdrawing from providing you with medical care for the reason that _____

_____

As your condition requires medical attention, I suggest that you promptly place yourself under the care of another physician. If you do not know of other physicians, you wish to contact the county medical society for a referral.

If you so desire, I shall be available to attend you for a reasonable time after you have received this letter, but in no event for more than 15 days.

When you have selected a new physician, I would be pleased to make available to him or her a copy of your medical chart or a summary of your treatment.

Very truly yours,

FIGURE 6–1 Letter of withdrawal from a case.

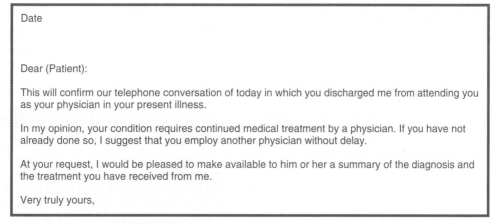

Date

Dear (Patient):

This will confirm our telephone conversation of today in which you discharged me from attending you as your physician in your present illness.

In my opinion, your condition requires continued medical treatment by a physician. If you have not already done so, I suggest that you employ another physician without delay.

At your request, I would be pleased to make available to him or her a summary of the diagnosis and the treatment you have received from me.

Very truly yours,

FIGURE 6–2   Physician confirmation of patient discharge.

stances surrounding it should be carefully documented in the physician's records. This may be accomplished by the physician's confirming the discharge by a certified mail letter similar to the one shown in Figure 6–2.

Statute of Frauds

In 1677, a statute was adopted in England aimed at reducing the evil of **perjured testimony,** by providing that certain contracts could not be enforced if they depended on the testimony of witnesses alone and were not evidenced in writing. The provisions of this English statute have been closely followed by statutes adopted in all the states of this country. Under the Statute of Frauds, some contracts, to be enforceable, must be in writing.

The promise to pay the debts of another is an example of this provision. If a third party who is not otherwise legally responsible for the person's debts agrees to pay a patient's medical bills, the agreement cannot be enforced unless it is in writing.

Another example is a contract that cannot be completed within a year. If the physician entered into an agreement to perform a series of treatments for a given sum, and this series covered a time span of more than 1 year, it would have to be in writing to be enforceable.

Tort Law

Medical professional liability is governed by the law of torts. The term *medical professional liability* encompasses all possible civil liability that can be incurred during the delivery of medical care. Medical professional liability is more easily prevented than defended.

All medical professional liability claims fall into one of three classifications:

- **Malfeasance**—the performance of an act that is wholly wrongful and unlawful
- **Misfeasance**—the improper performance of a lawful act

- **Nonfeasance**—the failure to perform an act that should have been done

Any and all of these situations are considered *professional negligence.*

Negligence Defined

When applied to the medical profession, negligence is called **malpractice.** *Negligence* is generally defined as the doing of some act that a reasonable and **prudent** physician or other health care provider would not do or the failure to do some act that such a person should or would do. The standard of prudent conduct is not defined by law but is left to the determination of a judge or jury.

A physician who performs an operation carelessly or contrary to accepted standards, or performs an unnecessary operation, or fails to render care that should have been given may be found guilty of negligence or malpractice.

A medical assistant whose responsibilities are clearly set forth in a policy and procedure manual may be found guilty of negligence through failure to carry out these responsibilities or to exercise reasonable and ordinary care in so doing. The medical assistant must also avoid rendering any care to a patient that might be construed as the practice of medicine, for example, giving an injection of penicillin without detaining the patient for several minutes in case of an allergic reaction.

Memory Jogger

3 *List the three classifications of professional liability.*

The Four Ds of Negligence

In a report by the Committee on Medicolegal Problems of the American Medical Association (AMA), it was stated that:

To obtain a judgment against a physician for negligence, the patient must present evidence of what has been referred to as the "four Ds." He must show: (1) that the physician owed a duty to the patient, (2) that the physician was derelict and breached that duty by failing to act as the ordinary, competent physician in the same community would have acted under the same or similar circumstances, (3) that such failure or breach was the direct cause of the patient's injuries, and (4) that damages to the patient resulted therefrom.

DUTY Duty exists when the physician–patient relationship has been established; that is, the patient has sought the assistance of the physician and the physician has knowingly undertaken to provide the needed medical service.

DERELICT (NEGLECTFUL OF OBLIGATION) Proof of dereliction, or proof of negligence of an obligation, must be shown in obtaining a judgment for malpractice.

DIRECT CAUSE There must be proof that the injury or death was directly caused by the physician's actions or failure to act and that it would not otherwise have occurred.

DAMAGES There are three kinds of damages recognized by the law:

- **Nominal** (existing in name only) damages are a token compensation for the invasion of a legal right in which no actual injury was suffered.
- **Punitive** (inflicting punishment) or **exemplary** (serving as a warning) damages require **allegations** and proof of willful misconduct and are unusual in lawsuits against physicians.
- **Compensatory** or actual **damages** are most frequently involved in professional liability cases and may be general or special. Compensatory or actual damages for injuries or losses that are the natural and necessary consequences of the physician's negligent act or omission are referred to as *general damages*. General damages include compensation for pain and suffering, for loss of a bodily member or faculty, for disfigurement, or for other similar direct losses or injuries. The fact of the losses must be proved—the monetary value need not be proved.

Memory Jogger

4 *What are the 4 Ds of negligence?*

Special damages are those injuries or losses that are not a necessary consequence of the physician's negligent act or omission. These may include the costs of medical and hospital care, loss of earnings, cost of travel, and so forth. Both the fact of these injuries or losses and the monetary value must be proved.

Some states limit the award amounts of nominal and punitive damages.

The Committee on Professional Liability of the California Medical Association in 1971 called these same four elements the "ABCDs" of negligence in medical practice.

ABCDs OF NEGLIGENCE IN MEDICAL PRACTICE

Acceptance of a person as a patient
Breach of the physician's duty of skill or care
Causal connection between the breach by the physician and the damage to the patient
Damage of a foreseeable nature—such as injury, pain, or loss of earnings—that could reasonably have been foreseen to result

Standard of Care

If a physician were to be held legally responsible for every unsuccessful result occurring in the treatment of a patient, no person would undertake the responsibility of practicing medicine. The courts hold that a physician must

- Use reasonable care, attention, and diligence in the performance of professional services
- Follow his or her best judgment in treating patients
- Possess and exercise the best skill and care that are commonly possessed and exercised by other reputable physicians in the same type practice in the same or a similar locality

Physicians who represent themselves as specialists must meet the standards of practice of their specialty. Whether or not they have met these requirements in treating a particular patient is generally a matter for the court to decide on the basis of testimony provided by an **expert witness.** Expert witnesses are members of the profession involved—in this case, medicine. To be considered an expert witness, the person must belong to a certifying or qualifying organization against which the qualities of the defendant may be compared. *Negligence is not presumed; it must be proved.*

Physicians are not required to possess extraordinary learning and skill, but they must keep abreast of medical developments and techniques, and they cannot experiment. They are also bound to advise their patients if they discover that the condition to be treated is one beyond their knowledge or technical skill.

Importance of the Physician–Patient Relationship

When injury results to a patient as a result of a physician's negligence, the patient can legally initiate a malpractice suit to recover financial damages. However, experience has shown that the incidence of malpractice claims is directly related to the personal relationship existing between the physician and the patient. Deterioration of the physician–patient relationship is a frequently demonstrated reason for a patient's initiating a malpractice suit, even though there was no real injury to the patient.

Medical Assistant's Role in the Physician–Patient Relationship

The medical assistant acts as the physician's agent and has an important role in forming and maintaining a favorable physician–patient relationship. For example, a patient who is kept waiting for an inexcusably long time without explanation or reassurance has developed some feeling of hostility before ever seeing the physician. A few words from the medical assistant at the appropriate time may forestall hostility and promote understanding.

When reassuring an apprehensive patient, the medical assistant must be very careful in the choice of words. Rather than saying, "I'm sure you will soon be entirely well," a friendly smile will comfort the patient but be noncommittal. Any time a medical assistant has reason to believe that a patient is dissatisfied, it is the medical assistant's duty to pass along such information to the physician.

Administrative Law

Administrative law involves the rights and powers of government agencies. The Workers' Compensation Insurance laws and the Family and Medical Leave Act are examples related to employees.

Workers' Compensation

Workers' compensation insurance is mandated by federal and state law. It becomes effective when a worker is injured on the job or suffers an incapacity as a result of the employment. The purpose of the insurance is to provide medical care and compensation during the period of disablement and to provide rehabilitation if necessary.

Family and Medical Leave Act, 1993

The Family and Medical Leave Act requires employers covered by the act to provide 12 weeks per year of unpaid, job-protected leave to eligible employees for some family and medical reasons. Employees must have worked for the employer at least 1 year and for 1250 hours during the previous 12 months. The reasons for the leave and conditions of employment are clearly outlined in the law. The United States Department of Labor is authorized to settle any violation.

There are many other mandated regulations, for example, the Internal Revenue Service, Social Security Act of 1935, and state medical practice acts.

Other more recent federal regulations are discussed more fully later in this chapter.

When the Physician Is Sued

Malpractice suits are far from rare, and every physician faces the probability of being sued at least once during his or her career. When a suit is filed, the medical assistant may become involved in scheduling depositions or court appearances and in preparing materials for court.

INTERROGATORY

Before the trial, the physician may be requested to complete an *interrogatory*, which is a list of general questions from another party to the lawsuit. Answers to the interrogatory must be provided within a specified time and must be answered under oath. Interrogatories are limited to parties named in the lawsuit.

DEPOSITION

There may be a request for a **deposition.** A deposition is oral testimony taken from a party or witness to the litigation and is not limited to parties named in the lawsuit. A witness who is not a party to the lawsuit will be summoned by **subpoena** for the deposition. The deposition is usually taken in an attorney's office in the presence of a court reporter and must be taken under oath to tell the truth, just as in a court of law. The person giving the deposition is called the *deponent*. The transcribed deposition is sent to the deponent for review, and the deponent is at liberty to make any necessary changes or corrections. Only deponents who are not parties to the suit are compensated for their time.

SUBPOENA

A subpoena is a document issued by the court requiring the person to whom it is directed to be in court at a given time and place to testify as a witness in a lawsuit.

SUBPOENA DUCES TECUM

A subpoena duces tecum is an order to provide records or documents of some sort and is usually addressed to the custodian of the records. This may be the medical assistant. The custodian of the records may expect to be compensated for the time spent in compiling the records and for photocopying charges. The fee must be demanded at the time the

Physician's Copy

PATIENT-PHYSICIAN ARBITRATION AGREEMENT

1. It is understood that any dispute as to medical malpractice, that is as to whether any medical services rendered under this contract were unnecessary or unauthorized or were improperly, negligently or incompetently rendered, will be determined by submission to arbitration as provided by California Law and not by a lawsuit or resort to court process except as California Law provides for judicial review of arbitration proceedings. Both parties to this contract, by entering into it, are giving up their constitutional right to have any such dispute decided in a court of law before a jury, and instead are accepting the use of arbitration.

2. I have read and understood Article 1 above and I voluntarily agree, for myself and all persons identified in Article 3 below, to submit to arbitration any and all claims involving persons bound by this Agreement whether those claims are brought in tort, contract or otherwise. This includes, but is not limited to, suits for personal injury, actions to collect debts, or any other kind of civil action.

3. I understand and agree that this Arbitration Agreement binds me and anyone else who may have a right to assert a claim on my behalf. I further understand and agree that if I sign this Agreement on behalf of some other person for whom I have responsibility (including my spouse or children, living or yet unborn) then, in addition to myself, such person(s) will also be bound, along with anyone else who may have a right to assert a claim on their behalf. I also understand and agree that this Agreement relates to claims against the physician and any consenting substitute physician, as well as his/her partnership, professional corporation, employees, partners, heirs, assigns or personal representatives. I also hereby consent to the intervention or joinder in the arbitration proceeding of all parties relevant to a full and complete settlement of any dispute arbitrated under this Agreement, as set forth in the Medical Arbitration Rules and/or CHA-CMA Rules for the Arbitration of Hospital and Medical Fee Disputes.

4. I agree to accept medical services from the undersigned physician and to pay therefor. I UNDERSTAND THAT I DO **NOT** HAVE TO SIGN THIS AGREEMENT TO RECEIVE THE PHYSICIAN'S SERVICES, AND THAT IF I DO SIGN THE AGREEMENT AND CHANGE MY MIND WITHIN 30 DAYS OF TODAY, THEN I MAY REVOKE THIS AGREEMENT BY GIVING WRITTEN NOTICE TO THE UNDERSIGNED PHYSICIAN WITHIN THAT TIME STATING THAT I WANT TO WITHDRAW FROM THIS ARBITRATION AGREEMENT. I further understand that after those 30 days, this Agreement may be changed or revoked only by a written revocation signed by both parties.

5. On behalf of myself and all others bound by this Agreement as set forth in Article 3, agreement is hereby given to be bound by the Medical Arbitration Rules of the California Hospital Association and California Medical Association and the CHA-CMA Rules for the Arbitration of Hospital and Medical Fee Disputes, as they may be amended from time to time, which are hereby incorporated into this Agreement.

6. I have read and understood the attached explanation of the Patient-Physician Arbitration Agreement and I have read and understood this Agreement, including the Rules. I understand and agree that this writing makes up the entire arbitration agreement between me and/or the person(s) on whose behalf I am signing and the undersigned physician and/or consenting substitute physicians.

NOTICE: BY SIGNING THIS CONTRACT YOU ARE AGREEING TO HAVE ANY ISSUE OF MEDICAL MALPRACTICE DECIDED BY NEUTRAL ARBITRATION AND YOU ARE GIVING UP YOUR RIGHT TO A JURY OR COURT TRIAL. SEE ARTICLE 1 OF THIS CONTRACT.

Dated: _____, 19 ___   _____
                                                                        (Patient)

Physician's Agreement to Arbitrate

In consideration of the foregoing execution of this Patient-Physician Arbitration Agreement, I likewise agree to be bound by the terms set forth in this Agreement and in the Rules specified in Article 5 above.

Dated: _____, 19 ___   _____
                                                                        (Physician)

_____   _____
        (Name of partnership or   (Title—e.g., Partner, President, etc.)
        professional corporation)

© California Medical Association, 1977, 1981

FIGURE 6–3 Arbitration agreement between patient and physician. (Copyright, California Medical Association. Reprinted by permission of the Western Journal of Medicine.)

subpoena is served, or it is considered to be waived. The medical assistant never copies or releases records without physician approval. Often private services bring the subpoena duces tecum and make an appointment to copy the records.

Some states have laws that permit patients to obtain a copy of their records on request, although a photocopying charge may be made. It is never wise to release the original records.

Memory Jogger

5 *How does a* subpoena *differ from a* subpoena duces tecum?

Arbitration

Arbitration is the settlement of a dispute by a third party or parties who have been selected because of their familiarity with the practices involved. It is common in modern business life. **Arbitration** is established by statute and is available to the medical profession in many states. It affords an alternative method of resolving legal disputes between doctor and patient. Many physicians and lawyers see it as one way to help solve the malpractice crisis. Instead of taking the disagreement through the long and expensive process of court litigation, which may take as long as 7 or 8 years, the patient and the physician (or hospital) agree in advance to submit the dispute informally to a neutral person or persons. After an informal hearing, a binding decision is rendered by the arbitrator(s) based on very specific rules of arbitration, as to any award. Arbitration applies essentially the same rights and the same measure of damages as a court. Arbitration is fair, less expensive, faster, and more confidential than court litigation.

DEVELOPING AN ARBITRATION AGREEMENT

An arbitration agreement is a contract and is subject to the judgment of the courts only as to the fairness of the agreement. The agreement is precisely worded by an attorney and should not be paraphrased when explaining it to a patient (Fig. 6–3). Signing the agreement is a voluntary act on the part of the patient, who has a period of grace in which to revoke the agreement if he or she later decides against it.

SELECTING AN ARBITRATOR

Both the patient and the physician have the opportunity to agree on who will arbitrate the case, so

that it does not favor one side over the other. By prior agreement, the **arbitrator(s)** may be appointed by or from the American Arbitration Association, which is a neutral, private, nonprofit association dedicated solely to the advancement of out-of-court remedies. Its panels of arbitrators are made up of persons from business, the professions, and public interest groups.

THE MEDICAL ASSISTANT'S ROLE IN ARBITRATION

If an arbitration statute exists in your state, you should get details of the procedure from your state or local medical society. If a physician elects to implement the procedure, every member of the physician's staff should know the details of the agreement, how to sign up patients, and how to answer the patient's questions. The fairness with which the physician's personnel present the program to the patient and the willingness with which the personnel answer the patient's questions largely determine whether the court will uphold the arbitration agreement. Furthermore, when the physician's personnel "speak for the physician," any representations made by the personnel could be held against the physician.

Securing a Patient's Informed Consent or Informed Refusal

A physician must have consent to treat a patient even though this consent is usually implied by virtue of the patient's having come to that physician for treatment. This implied consent is sufficient for common or simple procedures that are generally understood to involve little risk. A blood screen, chest radiograph, and electrocardiogram are examples. When more complex procedures are anticipated, the physician must obtain the patient's **informed consent** for each procedure. A physician who fails to secure some formal expression of consent could be charged with **trespass** or with **assault** and **battery**.

A number of states have passed specific laws that require the written informed consent of a patient before a test for the acquired immunodeficiency virus (AIDS) antibody may be performed by a health care facility, physician, or other health care provider.

Even in cases in which the treatment was not negligent, the physician can be sued for failing to obtain an informed consent. Under such circumstances, the physician must be prepared to prove in court that a full explanation was given to the patient before obtaining the patient's consent. Informed consent implies an understanding of

- What is to be done
- Why it should be done
- The risks involved

- Expected benefits of recommended treatment
- Alternative treatments, including the failure to treat
- Attendant risks of alternative treatment

The informed consent is not satisfied merely by having the patient sign the form. A discussion must occur during which the physician provides the patient or the patient's legal representative with enough information to decide whether to undergo the proposed therapy. After such a discussion, the patient either consents or refuses to consent to the proposed therapy and may be required to sign a consent form. If the patient signs with an "X," the medical assistant should write beside the "X" the words "patient's mark" and have a family member witness the signature. In any event, the discussion should be fully documented in the patient's medical record. If a form is used, a copy of the signed form should also be included in the patient's record. Treatment may not exceed the scope of the consent.

Forms on which a patient can grant written consent for operations or other procedures are kept in most physicians' offices. Many procedures are performed in the medical office that may require a consent form.

Who May or May Not Give Consent

MENTALLY COMPETENT ADULTS

If a mentally competent adult expressly indicates assent to a particular form of treatment, then consent has been obtained. If the act consented to is unlawful—for instance, an abortion in states where abortion is prohibited—the consent is invalid. The consent is also invalid if it is given by a person unauthorized to do so or if it is obtained by misrepresentation or fraud.

IN EMERGENCIES

In an emergency, one may render aid or care to prevent loss of life or serious illness or injury. However, implied consent in this circumstance lasts only as long as the emergency, and formal consent must be obtained for follow-up procedures done after the emergency has passed.

Good Samaritan Acts

The purpose of a Good Samaritan Act is to provide immunity from liability to volunteers at the scene of an accident for any civil damages as a result of rendering emergency care. Physicians are sometimes reluctant to fulfill an ethical obligation to render aid in an emergency to someone who is not their patient for fear they may later be charged with negligence or abandonment by a total stranger. In 1959, California passed the first *Good Samaritan Act*, and today all 50 states have Good Samaritan statutes. Although there are minor variations in the state statutes, their purpose is to provide immunity from liability to volunteers at the scene of an accident for any civil damages as a result of rendering emergency care to accident victims, provided that such care is given in good faith and with due care under the circumstances. There is no creation of a contract in giving emergency care (Fig. 6–4).

INCOMPETENT ADULTS

Adults who have been found by a court to be insane or incompetent usually cannot consent to medical treatment. Consent must be obtained from the guardian.

MINORS

Generally, when the patient is a minor, consent for surgery or treatment must be obtained from a parent or guardian except in an emergency requiring immediate treatment. If the parents are legally separated or divorced, consent should be obtained from the parent who has legal custody. There are exceptions to necessary consent.

Consent for treatment is not required when

- Consent may be assumed, such as in a life-threatening emergency
- A certain treatment is required by law, such as vaccination or x-ray for school entry or safety
- A court order has been issued, as in a situation in which parents withhold consent for a necessary treatment because of religious reasons

Treatment of sexually transmitted disease, drug abuse, alcohol dependency, or pregnancy usually does not require parental consent.

Emancipated Minors

Emancipation is defined by statute and varies from state to state. An emancipated minor is a person younger than the age of majority (usually 18 or 21 years) who meets one or more of the following conditions:

- Is married
- Is in the armed forces
- Is living separate and apart from parents or a legal guardian
- Is self-supporting

Some statutes include a minimum age for emancipation.

Unless a statute declares otherwise, a minor who has the right to consent to treatment is entitled to

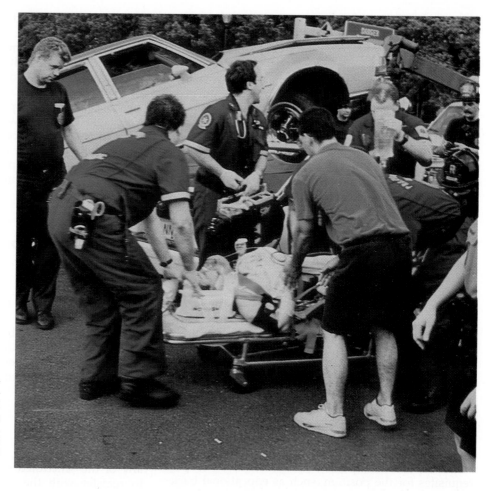

FIGURE 6–4 The Good Samaritan Act protects medical professionals from liability for any civil damages as a result of rendering emergency care. (From Henry M, Stapleton ER: EMT Prehospital Care, 2nd ed. Philadelphia, WB Saunders, 1997.)

the protection of his or her confidences, even from parents.

Memory Jogger

6 *What is the purpose of the Good Samaritan Act?*

Federal Regulations

The following is a brief overview of laws and regulations affecting the medical office environment. A fuller discussion will be found in the clinical coverage in Unit 3.

OCCUPATIONAL SAFETY AND HEALTH ACT (OSHA)

The Occupational Safety and Health Act was established by the federal government in 1970 to set standards and protocols for occupational health and safety. OSHA is a part of the Department of Labor. The involvement of OSHA with medical practices

accelerated during the 1980s, partly because of the risk of exposure to the hepatitis B virus and later because of the spread of AIDS. As a result of the increasing danger of exposure to the AIDS virus, bloodborne pathogen regulations were introduced in 1991.

OSHA regulations are critically important to all health care facilities. Medical office managers must know the regulations and follow them explicitly. The regulations include

- A hazard communications plan
- An exposure plan
- A medical waste management plan
- Housekeeping facilities
- Personal protective measures
- General safety precautions
- Fire safety plan
- Staff development/in-service training program

Training sessions must be provided to every employee who is at risk of exposure to blood or other infectious materials. The training session must be provided during working hours and before a new employee begins the job.

The health care facility is subject to an OSHA compliance inspection at any time during regular office hours.

CLINICAL LABORATORY IMPROVEMENT AMENDMENTS OF 1988 (CLIA '88)

The Clinical Laboratory Improvement Act was first enacted in 1967, then amended in 1988. Its purpose was to establish performance requirements for all laboratories within the United States and its territories. In-office laboratories are subject to both state and federal regulations. Inspections of the laboratories are conducted by regional surveyors from the Health Care Financing Administration (HCFA) and state agency representatives. Physicians' office laboratories are included under these regulations.

AMERICANS WITH DISABILITIES ACT OF 1990 (ADA)

Employers with 15 or more employees are subject to ADA regulations. The ADA prohibits covered employers from discriminating against a person with a mental or physical disability in any aspect of employment merely because the person has such a disability. This affects the employment process, hiring, job training, promotion or advancement, compensation, termination, and any other aspect of the employment relationship.

The ADA protects all *qualified* individuals with a disability from employment discrimination. A qualified individual is a person (1) who satisfies the prerequisites for the position, such as educational background, employment experience, skills, or licenses and (2) who, *with or without reasonable accommodation*, can perform the essential functions of the job. An example of reasonable accommodation is *making all facilities readily accessible to, and usable by, individuals with disabilities*. The act also includes a *public access* requirement for service establishments, for example, a health care provider, that would focus on making the place physically accessible from public sidewalks, public transportation, or parking areas. Examples of structural and nonstructural alterations might be adding grab bars, lowering telephones, creating a ramp, adding raised letters or braille markings to elevator control buttons, and widening doors.

PATIENT SELF-DETERMINATION ACT, 1991

This law requires that medical care facilities such as hospitals, nursing homes, personal care facilities, hospices, home health care agencies, and health maintenance organizations ask patients whether they have prepared an advance directive for guidance in the event they are terminally ill or in a vegetative state. The directive may be a living will or a durable power of attorney for health care.

The term **living will** generally refers to any document in which an individual expresses his or her wishes regarding medical treatment at or near the end of life. A durable power of attorney for health care (DPAHC) must meet certain statutory requirements. A valid DPAHC document must specifically authorize the agent to make health care decisions for the patient.

Each state has its specific regulations on what is acceptable and the wording that must be used. Some states do not accept the living will. The health care facility performs a service for its patients by having copies of acceptable forms available for patients and being willing and informed enough to explain them.

Controlled Substances Act of 1970

On May 1, 1971, the Controlled Substances Act of 1970 became effective, replacing the former Narcotic Acts and the Drug Abuse Control Amendments. In October 1973, the regulatory agency became known as the Drug Enforcement Administration (DEA) within the U.S. Department of Justice.

REGISTRATION

Before **administering, prescribing,** or **dispensing** any of the scheduled drugs, a physician is required to register with the Registration Branch, Drug Enforcement Administration, PO Box 28083, Central Station, Washington, DC 20038-8033, or with the nearest regional office. The registration is renewable every 3 years. The medical assistant should take note of the renewal date and make certain that the renewal is filed. If a physician administers or dispenses any of the drugs listed in the five schedules at more than one office, he or she must register each office. Regulations regarding the writing, telephoning, and refilling of prescriptions vary according to which schedule is involved.

SCHEDULES

Under the Controlled Substances Act, drugs are categorized into Schedules I, II, III, IV, and V. Drugs in schedule I have the highest potential for abuse and addiction, and those in Schedule V have the least potential.

Schedule I substances are those that have no accepted medical use in the United States and have a high potential for abuse. Examples include heroin and LSD. Only the physician who is involved in conducting research with such drugs is concerned with Schedule I substances.

Schedule II substances have a high abuse potential with severe psychic or physical dependence liability. They include certain narcotic, stimulant, and depressant drugs. Examples are opium, morphine, and codeine. Controlled substances in Schedule II can be obtained only with a Federal Triplicate Order form obtained from the DEA. A special inventory must be maintained on controlled substances and retained for 2 years. Some states require the inventory to be kept 3 years. When a controlled substance is removed from the inventory it must be recorded. The record must show the date, the name of the drug, the dosage, and the names of the patient, the physician, and the employee involved.

Schedule III substances have an abuse potential that is lesser than that of the first two schedules. They include compounds that contain limited quantities of certain narcotic drugs combined with non-narcotic substances. Paregoric, Empirin Compound with Codeine, and Tylenol with Codeine are examples.

Schedule IV substances have still less potential for abuse. Phenobarbital, diazepam (Valium), and propoxyphene (Darvon) are examples.

Schedule V substances have less abuse potential than those in Schedule IV but still warrant control. They include preparations that contain moderate quantities of certain narcotics such as may be found in cough medicines and antidiarrheal products.

WRITTEN PRESCRIPTIONS

Schedule III, IV, and V substances do not require triplicate forms but are subject to the following prescription requirements.

PRESCRIPTION REQUIREMENTS FOR SCHEDULE III, IV, AND V SUBSTANCES

- The prescription must be signed and dated by the prescriber.
- It must contain the name and address of the person for whom the controlled substance is prescribed, the name and quantity of the substance, and the directions for its proper use.
- For all controlled substances classified in Schedules III and IV, the signature, date, and information described above must be written in ink or indelible pencil in the handwriting of the prescriber.
- These substances may not be refilled in an amount exceeding a 120-day supply unless the prescription is renewed by the prescriber.
- The prescription must contain the name, address, telephone number, category of professional license, and DEA registration number of the prescriber.

Schedule V prescriptions must be signed and dated by the prescriber and must also include the name of the patient, name and quantity of the con-

trolled substance prescribed, and the directions for use.

Memory Jogger

7 *Which schedule of controlled substances has the highest potential for abuse?*

ORAL PRESCRIPTIONS

The physician may dispense any Schedule III, IV, or V controlled substance by an oral prescription, but the prescription must be put in writing by the pharmacist who fills it. With permission from the physician, any employee may orally transmit a prescription for controlled substances *only* in Schedules III, IV, or V, again with the prescription being put in writing by the dispensing pharmacist. An employee cannot, under any circumstances, orally transmit a prescription for a controlled substance classified in Schedule II.

NONNARCOTIC DRUGS

A physician who regularly engages in dispensing any of the nonnarcotic drugs listed in the schedules as a regular part of the professional practice and who charges for the drugs either separately or together with other professional services must keep records of all such drugs received and dispensed. The records must be kept for a period of 2 years and are subject to inspection by the DEA. If the physician only occasionally dispenses a nonnarcotic controlled drug to a patient (such as a physician's sample), he or she is not required to maintain a record of such dispensing.

SECURITY

Stored controlled substances must be kept in a locked cabinet or safe. Any loss of controlled drugs by theft must be reported to the regional office of the DEA at the time the theft is discovered. If a physician discovers that his or her DEA number is being used in the unauthorized prescribing of controlled substances, he or she should report the incident to the DEA, the state regulatory agency, and to the local police authorities.

DISCONTINUANCE OF PRACTICE

A physician who discontinues medical practice must return his or her registration certificate and any unused order forms to the nearest office of the DEA. The regional DEA office will advise on the disposition of any controlled drugs still on hand.

Uniform Anatomical Gift Act

The Uniform Anatomical Gift Act was approved by the National Conference of Commissioners on Uniform State Laws in 1968. Although many states had passed laws before this time that permitted living persons to make a gift of their body or portions of it after death, the laws were so different from state to state that arrangements for a donation in one state might not be recognized in another. All states have adopted the Uniform Anatomical Gift Act or similar legislation.

Essentially, the model law for donation states that

- Any person of sound mind and 18 years of age or older may give all or any part of his or her body after death for research, transplantation, or placement in a tissue bank.
- A donor's valid statement of gift is paramount to the rights of others except when a state autopsy law may prevail.
- If a donor has not acted during his or her lifetime, his or her survivors, in a specified order of priority, may do so.
- Physicians who accept organs or tissues, relying in good faith on the documents, are protected from lawsuits. The physician attending at the time of death, if acquainted with the donor's wishes, may dispose of the body under the Uniform Anatomical Gift Act.
- The time of death must be determined by a physician who is not involved in the transplantation, and the attending physician cannot be a member of the transplant team.
- The donor may revoke the gift, or the gift may be rejected.

The most important clause permits the donation to be made by a will (without waiting for probate) or by other written or witnessed documents, such as a card designed to be carried on the person (Fig. 6–5). The Uniform Donor Card is considered a legal document in all 50 states.

The provisions of the Uniform Anatomical Gift Act are so designed that the offer is exercised only after death. Therefore, the donors should reveal their intentions to as many of their relatives and friends as possible and to their physician. Because the human body or its parts are not commodities in commerce, no money can be exchanged in making an anatomic donation.

Legal Disclosures

The physician is charged with safeguarding patient confidences within the constraints of the law, but according to state laws, which vary somewhat throughout the nation, certain disclosures must be made. Frequently it is the medical assistant who has the responsibility of reporting these events.

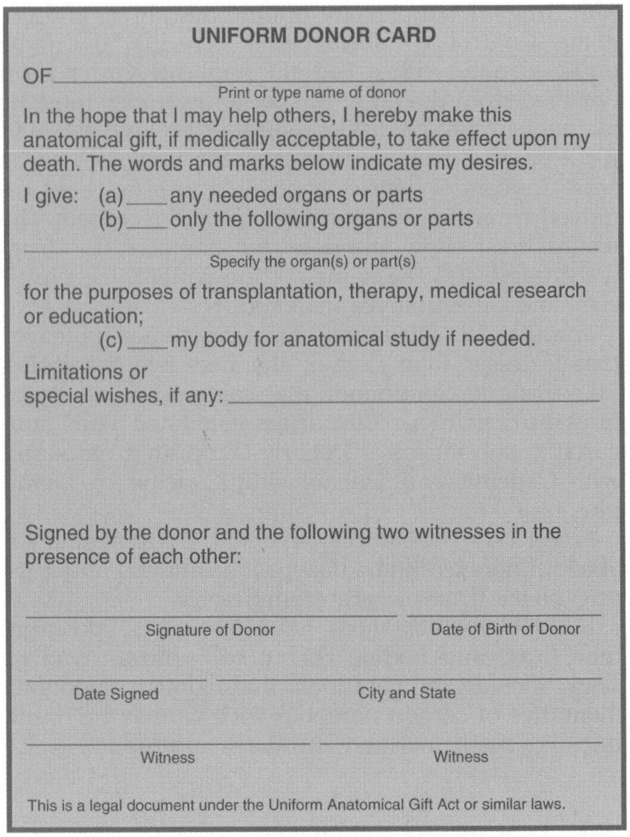
UNIFORM DONOR CARD

OF ____________________

Print or type name of donor

In the hope that I may help others, I hereby make this anatomical gift, if medically acceptable, to take effect upon my death. The words and marks below indicate my desires.

I give: (a)____ any needed organs or parts
(b)____ only the following organs or parts

____

Specify the organ(s) or part(s)

for the purposes of transplantation, therapy, medical research or education;
(c)____ my body for anatomical study if needed.

Limitations or
special wishes, if any: ____________________

Signed by the donor and the following two witnesses in the presence of each other:

Signature of Donor | Date of Birth of Donor

Date Signed | City and State

Witness | Witness

This is a legal document under the Uniform Anatomical Gift Act or similar laws.

FIGURE 6–5 Uniform Donor Card.

Births and deaths must be reported. Births out of wedlock must be reported on special forms in some states; some states require detailed information about stillbirths.

Physicians are required to report cases that may have been a result of violence, such as gunshot wounds, knife injuries, or poisonings. They must also report deaths from accidental or unexplained causes.

In some states, occupational diseases must be reported within specific time lines.

Sexually transmitted diseases are reportable in every state. All fifty states require that confirmed cases of AIDS be reported to state public health officials. In at least 13 states, a seropositive test result is also a reportable condition. Individuals are reported either by name or by patient identifiers.

Child abuse is a leading cause of death among children younger than 5 years of age, and health care professionals are required by law to report any suspected cases of child abuse. This should be done as soon as evidence is discovered. Suspected elder abuse often creates a dilemma for the physician and other health care personnel. The older adult may deny the abuse in fear of further mistreatment if it is made known. The law requires that suspected cases of physical abuse to children, the elderly, or any others at risk be reported to the authorities.

The physician must report any cases of **contagious, infectious,** or **communicable diseases.** Local health departments publish lists of diseases that are reportable as well as the method of reporting. Often, the report may be made by telephone. When reporting by mail, the appropriate forms, which are supplied by the health department, must be used. In many areas, the county health department issues regular bulletins that are sent to all physicians in the county. Check with the local authorities for specific procedures in your area.

Memory Jogger

8 *How many required legal disclosures of patient information can you list?*

Legal Responsibilities of the Medical Assistant

Generally, the law holds that every person is liable for the consequences of his or her own negligence when another person is injured as a result. In some situations, this liability also extends to the employer. Physicians may be held responsible for the mistakes of those who work in the health care facility, and sometimes they must pay damages for the negligent acts of their employees.

Physicians are legally responsible for the acts of their employees when the employees are acting within the scope of their duties or employment. Physicians are also responsible for the acts of assistants who are not their own employees if they commit acts of negligence in the presence of the physician while under the physician's immediate supervision. For example, a medical assistant who is a clinic employee makes an error in a procedure while acting under a physician's direction. The court

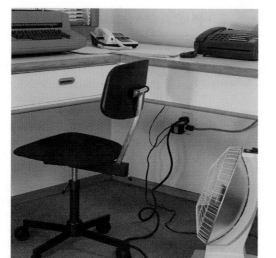

FIGURE 6–6 Example of potential hazard from exposed electrical cord.

may determine that the medical assistant came so completely under the direction and supervision of the physician that the physician is liable for the medical assistant's negligence. This is known as the doctrine of **respondeat superior** (let the master answer). On the other hand, if a registered nurse is employed by the patient, the physician is not usually held liable for negligent acts of the registered nurse. When physicians practice as partners, they are liable not only for their own acts and those of their partner but also for the negligent acts of any agent or employee of the partnership. The medical assistant, while acting within the scope of the employment contract, is considered an agent of the employer.

A physician who properly writes a prescription is not liable for a pharmacist's negligence in compounding it but may be liable in cases in which there is misunderstanding as to the ingredients when the prescription is ordered over the telephone.

NEED FOR EXTREME CARE

Medical assistants who are guilty of negligence are liable for their own actions, but the injured party generally sues the physician because there is a better chance of collecting damages. However, even an assistant who has no money can still be liable for any negligent action. This fact illustrates the continuing importance of exercising extreme care in performing all duties in the professional office.

While working under pressure, there is always the danger of interchanging blood, serum, or medications or of mixing names or improperly preparing labels. Medication and treatment solutions should be labeled clearly and their expiration dates checked. Never proceed with administration of a medication or treatment without checking all details at least three times. It is an accepted rule that the medication label should be read three times: (1) when you remove the container from its storage place; (2) when you are preparing the medication; and (3) when you return the medication to the storage place before patient administration.

RECHECKING EQUIPMENT

One person in the facility should be designated to make periodic safety checks of reception room and treatment room furniture and of the condition of instruments and supplies. Every person on the staff should be alert for potential hazards, such as slipping rugs, exposed telephone and light cords, highly waxed floors, and protruding objects, because patients who are harmed as a result of these conditions can sue for damages (Fig. 6–6).

ILLEGAL PRACTICE OF MEDICINE

A physician studies many years to learn the profession before becoming licensed by the state to practice medicine. The medical assistant is not licensed to practice medicine and must never prescribe or attempt to diagnose a patient's ailment. This is the *illegal practice of medicine*. For this reason, it is not good policy for the medical assistant to discuss patients' complaints with them because patients tend to identify the medical assistant's remarks as being the opinion of the physician.

ASSISTING AT PATIENT EXAMINATIONS

Except in an actual emergency, the male physician should not examine a female patient unless a third person is present. Allegations of sexual misconduct are made against physicians of all specialties. The charge of undue familiarity against a physician is very damaging. For this reason, the assistant generally stands by during examinations.

EMERGENCY AID

The question sometimes arises of whether a medical assistant should give emergency care to a patient brought into the office during the physician's absence. In a medical emergency, the medical assistant, like any other layperson, may do whatever is reasonably necessary, provided the action taken is within that person's skill and competence. The physician should instruct the medical assistant regarding what course of action to take in such instances. The medical assistant must immediately get in touch with a physician to care for the patient once any emergency measures have been performed.

The Medical Assistant's Role in Claims Prevention

The majority of patients never entertain the thought of taking legal action against their physicians, and the medical assistant should not develop an attitude of skepticism. However, the medical assistant can play a role in preventing legal claims.

SKILLS AND RESPONSIBILITIES

PREVENTION OF LEGAL CLAIMS AGAINST THE PRACTICE

Give scrupulous attention to the needs of each patient.

Avoid leaving patients alone (especially children and elderly patients).

Avoid destructive and unethical criticism of the work of other physicians.

Do not give out information either orally or in writing without the patient's consent.

Verify the identity of anyone requesting information.

Use discretion in telephone and office conversations.

Be aware of your tone of voice and attitude during spoken communications.

Communicate office policies and procedures to patients in advance of treatment whenever possible.

Keep records that clearly show what was done and when it was done.

Record all patient interactions on the patient's chart.

Make no promises as to outcome of treatment.

Record canceled appointments.

Record the facts if a patient discontinues treatment or fails to follow instructions.

Avoid making any statement that might be construed as an admission of fault.

Check the office equipment regularly to see that it is operating properly and safely.

Make periodic safety inspections of furniture.

Keep toxic substances out of reach of patients and clearly labeled.

Keep drug samples and prescription pads out of sight.

Never diagnose, prescribe, or offer a prognosis.

Perform only those tasks that are within your scope of knowledge and training.

Keep abreast of new procedures and technical advances in health care.

Correctly follow all federal and state record-keeping and reporting requirements.

LEGAL AND ETHICAL ISSUES

Both the physician and the medical assistant must be thorough when giving instructions to patients. Written instructions should be provided whenever possible. A patient might forget oral instructions, resulting in drug-related injuries stemming from poor understanding of the proper use of the medications, their limitations, and their contraindications.

An efficiently operated medical practice will have a policy and procedure manual describing the office policies and including a designated procedure section for each personnel position in the practice. A medical assistant who fails to carry out the written instructions or who failed to exercise reasonable and ordinary care in doing so may be found guilty of negligence. The medical assistant who renders any care to a patient that might be deemed the practice of medicine is also subject to malpractice liability.

A physician must have consent to treat a patient. When complex procedures are planned, a discussion must occur between the patient and the physician whereby the physician provides enough information for the patient to decide whether or not to go ahead with the proposed therapy. Discussion between the patient and the medical assistant is not sufficient to satisfy this requirement.

Regulations of the Drug Enforcement Administration require a federal triplicate order and prohibit the oral transmittal of prescriptions for Schedule II substances, which have a high abuse potential.

If you will be at risk of exposure to blood or other infectious materials, make certain that you go through a training session in OSHA regulations before you begin the job.

A "medical assistant" is an unlicensed health professional who performs noninvasive routine technical support services under the supervision of a licensed physician and surgeon or a licensed podiatrist in a medical office or clinic setting.

"Technical supportive services" means simple routine medical tasks and procedures which may be performed by a medical assistant with limited training who functions under the supervision of a physician or podiatrist. For example, a medical assistant may administer certain medications; perform electrocardiograms or electroencephalograms; apply and remove bandages and dressings; apply orthopedic appliances; select crutches; perform automated visual field testing; remove sutures, and so forth.

CRITICAL THINKING

1 For what reasons might a medical assistant be accused of negligence?

2 What is the meaning of *prudent* conduct? How is it determined?

3 Why would the attending physician of a deceased patient whose organs are being donated be prohibited from being a member of the transplantation team?

4 Who is responsible for a mistake made by a medi-

cal assistant during the course of his or her employment? Give examples.

5 Why is it dangerous for a medical assistant to discuss a patient's complaint with the patient?

HOW DID I DO? Answers to Memory Joggers

1 A physician may be licensed by
a. Examination
b. Endorsement
c. Reciprocity

2 The basic elements of a binding contract are
a. Offer and acceptance
b. Legal subject matter
c. Legal capacity to contract
d. Consideration

3 The three classifications of professional liability are
a. Malfeasance
b. Misfeasance
c. Nonfeasance

4 The four Ds of negligence are
a. Duty
b. Derelict
c. Direct cause
d. Damages

5 A *subpoena* requires a person to appear in court. *Subpoena duces tecum* is an order to provide records or documents.

6 The Good Samaritan Acts are designed to provide immunity from liability to volunteers at the scene of an accident for any civil damages as a result of rendering emergency care.

7 Schedule I drugs have the highest potential for abuse.

8 State laws vary, but many are common to all states (e.g., births, deaths, out of wedlock births, injuries resulting from violence, gunshot, knifings, poisonings, venereal diseases).

REFERENCES

Andress A: Saunders Manual of Medical Office Management. Philadelphia, WB Saunders, 1996.
Flight MR: Law, Liability, and Ethics. Albany, NY, Delmar Publishers, 1988.

3

Communicating with Patients and Colleagues

CURRICULUM CONTENT/COMPETENCIES

Chapter 7 Interpersonal Skills and Human Relations
- *Treat all patients with compassion and empathy*
- *Recognize and respect cultural diversities*
- *Recognize and respond to verbal and nonverbal messages*
- *Serve as liaison*

Chapter 8 Patient Reception
- *Adapt communications to individual's ability to understand*
- *Promote the practice through positive public relations*
- *Instruct patients according to their needs*

Chapter 9 Telephone Techniques
- *Use professional telephone techniques*
- *Project a professional manner and image*
- *Use medical terminology appropriately*
- *Receive, organize, prioritize, and transmit information*

Chapter 10 Appointment Scheduling and Time Management
- *Schedule, coordinate, and monitor appointments*
- *Schedule inpatient/outpatient admissions and procedures*
- *Use professional telephone techniques*
- *Prioritize and perform multiple tasks*
- *Explain office policies and procedures*

Interpersonal Skills and Human Relations

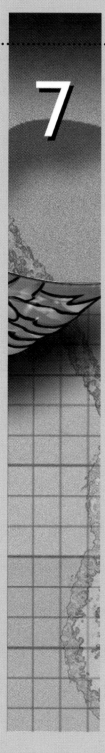

7

LEARNING OBJECTIVES

Cognitive: On successful completion of this chapter you should be able to:

1 Define and spell the terms listed in the Vocabulary.
2 State the factors that most influence the formation of a first impression.
3 List three distinct steps in communicating with the patient.
4 Name the three components of listening.
5 List four possible barriers to communication.
6 Briefly describe the paths of communication.
7 List seven rules of good team cooperation.
8 List and briefly describe the three styles of management.
9 Explain the meaning of being a patient advocate.

VOCABULARY

advocate A person who leads the cause of another

authority The quality of being in command

autocratic Ruling with unlimited authority

barrier A factor that restricts free movement

body language Gestures and mannerisms that influence communication

categorically Applied to a limited classification

caustic remark Biting comment

congruency The quality of agreeing

conversely Something reversed in order

democratic Relating to social equality

discernible To see or understand a difference between two or more things

discrimination Different treatment on a basis other than individual merit

empathy Intellectual and emotional awareness of another person's thoughts, feelings, and behavior

feedback Letting people know how you feel about them at a given moment

gesture The use of motions as a means of expression

harmony Having an atmosphere of cordiality

impartiality The quality of treating or affecting all equally

laissez-faire Management style of "hands off" when dealing with employees

listening An active process of receiving information and examining one's reaction to the messages received

litigious Tending to engage in lawsuits

nonconsensual Not having received consent

observation An inference from what has been seen or heard

physical impairment A lessening of physical capabilities

pitch Highness or lowness of sound

response Something constituting a reply or reaction

self-concept A mental picture of one's self

steepling Upward position of hands together with fingertips touching

---

The interpersonal skills of the medical assistant set the tone of the human relations in the medical establishment. Greeting the patient pleasantly starts the process. Every ensuing encounter of the patient with a staff member adds to that first impression. If these encounters are consistently pleasant and positive, the patient will tell the world how wonderful the doctor is. The medical assistant is the key person in helping the physician make the patient feel comfortable and important.

First Impressions

Physical appearance is the first attribute to be noticed and is probably the most influential factor in forming that first impression. The successful medical assistant presents the best appearance that he or she can. A clean appropriate uniform, good grooming and personal hygiene, and a warm greeting, all combined with a healthful energetic attitude, set the stage for a positive patient experience.

Communicating with the Patient

To be an effective communicator you must understand the underlying cause-and-effect process. Several steps are involved.

OBSERVATION

Notice how the patient approaches the first station, which is probably a "sign-in" window or reception desk. Look the patient in the eye when you extend your greeting. Does the patient seem apprehensive, seriously ill, or carefree?

LISTENING

True listening includes hearing, understanding, and responding. The main reason for the patient's appointment has probably been noted on the daily schedule. Acknowledge to the patient that you are aware of his or her needs, while at the same time preserving the patient's privacy. Speak quietly. Give the patient an opportunity to ask questions or convey any problems. If there are questions to be answered, make sure that the patient understands.

> PATIENT: Will you be billing my insurance?
> MEDICAL ASSISTANT: We will be glad to do that, but first you must sign this form.
> PATIENT: Why do I need to sign a form?
> MEDICAL ASSISTANT: This is called a consent form. By signing here you give us permission to release confidential information to your insurance company.

A good listener helps the speaker to clarify or modify his or her ideas in the course of expressing them, by responding with meaningful questions and comments, eye contact, and appropriate smiles.

RESPONSE

Responding is both verbal and nonverbal. There needs to be an exchange of information. Is the patient responding in the way you expected? Does he or she seem hesitant? Try to find a way to ensure there is no lack of understanding.

Every patient should be treated with **empathy** and **impartiality.** This does not mean that every patient is treated exactly the same.

Memory Jogger

1 *As an appointed patient approaches the reception desk, what observations should the medical assistant make?*

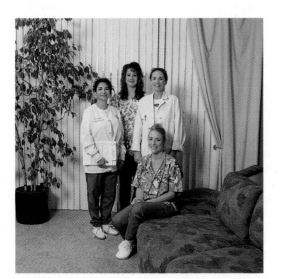

FIGURE 7–1 Colleagues who represent an ethnic mix.

Barriers to Communication

PHYSICAL IMPAIRMENT

Does the patient have a vision problem? This need is usually readily discernible. Try to use more descriptive language in your communication with this patient.

The person with diminished hearing may be very sensitive and in denial of this condition. Be certain that you have his or her attention and that you are face to face with the person while speaking. The hearing impaired are often very dependent on lip reading for comprehension.

Being elderly is not an impairment. Many of your older patients will be physically able and mentally alert and will not expect special treatment.

LANGUAGE

With non–English-speaking patients you may need to use **gestures** and body language to convey your message. In such cases you must be extra alert to the possibility of misunderstanding. Confirm that the message you are sending is the message that the listener is receiving. A response with **feedback** is necessary.

BIAS

Personal and social bias brings about discrimination. **Discrimination** is a word that is used to **categorically** describe unfair treatment of a person because of race, gender, religious affiliation, or handicap. Discrimination is unethical, morally and socially wrong, and in many situations illegal. It prevents us from effectively communicating.

Another type of discrimination is often referred to as *subtle discrimination*. It is not obvious and seldom expressed openly. Subtle discrimination is based on a person's appearance, values, or lifestyle or on some other personal factor. Examples include discrimination against obesity, divorce, homosexuality, welfare recipients, and victims of sexually transmitted diseases. Sometimes we may not even be aware that our words or actions reflect subtle discrimination against another.

Recognize your personal prejudices in order to change them. Medical personnel are exposed to a great variety of persons who need care. You cannot allow prejudice to affect the care of any individual (Fig. 7–1).

Memory Jogger

2 *Describe what is meant by "subtle discrimination."*

Communication Paths

In the medical arena, much of the communication is accomplished through talking. We also communicate through writing, by gesturing, by facial expression, and much more. *Verbal communication* in its strictest sense means "relating to or consisting of words." In this chapter we will use verbal communication in the context of talking (Table 7–1).

VERBAL COMMUNICATION

Verbal communication depends on words and sounds. The messages are conveyed by the use of language, which may be written or spoken. While you may function comfortably in your familiar surroundings, try to put yourself in the place of the new patient who is entering unknown territory. As the "resident" medical assistant you are in familiar surroundings and already have some information about the new patient but he or she knows nothing of you or the other staff members. The very best first step in breaking that barrier is to have all staff members wear name badges, with letters large enough to be read at a distance of three feet. Include the staff position if there are several divisions of responsibility (e.g., medical assistant, nurse, laboratory assistant). When the patient approaches, even though you are wearing a name badge, stand and introduce yourself in the way you wish to be addressed. If your badge reads DOROTHY OWEN and you like to be on a first name basis, say, "Good morning, Mr.—, my name is Dorothy," while you smile with both your mouth and your eyes. This small effort will put the patient at ease in your environment.

The **pitch** of the voice is a part of verbal communication. The voice lifts at the end of a question. It drops at the end of a statement. Usually, when a speaker intends to continue a statement, the voice will hold the same pitch, the head will remain straight, the eyes and hands will be unchanged. This is not an appropriate time to interrupt. If the message is interrupted before its time, it may never be completed. The tone of voice and choice of words also affect the message.

Medical assistants must become aware of how they express themselves and how they affect the feelings of others. There is no place for sarcasm or a **caustic remark** in the medical facility. For example, "I hope you can manage to be on time for your next appointment," "I don't understand why you are late," or "Late people lose their appointment times."

NONVERBAL COMMUNICATION

Nonverbal communications are messages conveyed without the use of words. They are transmitted by

TABLE 7–1 Therapeutic Communication Techniques

Technique	Therapeutic Value
Acknowledgment	Emphasizes the importance of the patient in the communication process
Establishing guidelines	Helps patients to know what is expected of them
Focusing	Directs the conversation toward important topics
Listening	Communicates your interest in the patient
Open-ended comments	Helps patients to decide what is relevant and encourages them to continue discussion
Reducing distance	Communicates your involvement to the patient
Reflecting	Shows the patient the importance of his or her ideas and feelings
Restating	Lets the patient know how you interpreted the message that he or she communicated
Seeking clarification	Demonstrates your desire to understand what the patient is communicating
Silence	Communicates your acceptance of the patient

body language, which is partly instinctive, partly taught, and partly imitative. Nonverbal communication, or **body language,** as it is sometimes called, involves grooming, dress, eye contact, facial expression, hand gestures, space, tone of voice, posture, the way we walk, ethnic customs, and much more. We are usually unaware of our own nonverbal signals and recognize only a small number of the signals sent by others. Our ability to help others increases greatly as we increase our own skills in interpreting nonverbal communication.

Appearance is a part of nonverbal communication. This emphasizes the message presented in an earlier paragraph that your appearance is influential. The successful person expresses self esteem, confidence, and ability to perform the job by appropriate clothing, stance, vocabulary, facial expression, and a caring attitude.

If you have ever had the experience of speaking to a person who does not make eye contact, you will realize the importance of greeting the patient with your eyes as well as your voice or body language. Facial expressions usually convey our true feelings and are not masked by the words we use.

Our need for personal space is demonstrated by how patients in the reception area will choose a seat. You will seldom see a person sit in an adjoining seating space with a stranger, if there is an option. Although the need for space varies with the individual culture, some might even remain standing to satisfy the need for personal space. Imagine how those patients feel when you touch them, especially when the patient does not know your name.

GENERALLY ACCEPTED PERSONAL AND SOCIAL SPACE DISTANCES

Intimate: physical contact
Personal: 1.5 to 4 feet
Social: 4 to 12 feet
Public: 12 to 25 feet

Posture can signal depression, excitement, anger, or even an appeal for help. When the physician sits at the front of the chair and leans forward, he or she is giving the message of caring.

Positioning is also important. Sitting behind a desk gives the message of **authority.** Standing or sitting across a room may convey a negative message of denying involvement.

The interchange of warmth by touching can have a dynamic effect on people. Until recent years, touching was acceptable in a medical setting. In the **litigious** atmosphere of the modern world, any nonconsensual touching may be deemed battery, and it is best avoided or used with discretion.

Congruency

Nonverbal and spoken language are dependent on each other. They must be in harmony to convey a definite message. If they are not harmonious, the nonverbal is usually dominant and expresses the true message.

Some believe that crossed arms mean "I will not let you in" and that **steepling** of the fingers means a feeling of superiority. Sometimes these gestures are true and sometimes they are not. They are only true in the context of the entire behavior pattern of the person (Table 7–2).

WRITTEN COMMUNICATIONS

The medical assistant may be asked to give instructions to a patient regarding medication, exercise, diet, and many other topics. This is best done through written instructions that are read and orally

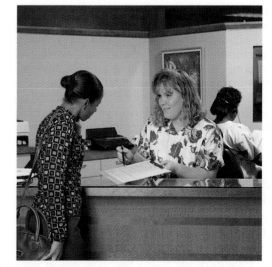

FIGURE 7–2 Medical assistant explaining instructions to a patient.

explained to the recipient. Use common uncomplicated language that is not likely to be misinterpreted or confusing. Make certain that the instructions are correctly understood before the patient leaves the premises (Fig. 7–2).

MEDICAL ASSISTANT: (handing prescription to patient) Dr. . . . wants you to take this medication for 2 weeks.
PATIENT: When do I take it?
MEDICAL ASSISTANT: Under the directions, you see "1 tab h.s." This means that you will take one tablet at bedtime.
PATIENT: Do I take it every night?
MEDICAL ASSISTANT: Yes, the prescription is for 14 tablets. You will take one each night until they are all gone.

CULTURAL DIFFERENCES

Body language is not universal in the messages conveyed. Cultural differences are responsible for many misunderstandings unless we make an attempt to understand them. As a medical assistant you need to be aware of the nonverbal messages being sent by

TABLE 7–2 Nonverbal Communication

Message	Low-Level Behavior	High-Level Behavior
Empathy	Frown resulting from lack of understanding	Positive head nods; facial expressions that reflect the content of the conversation
Respect	Mumbling; patronizing tone of voice	Devoting one's full attention
Warmth	Apathy; fidgeting; signs indicating a desire to leave	Smiling; physical contact
Genuineness	Avoidance of eye contact	Congruence between verbal and nonverbal behavior
Self-disclosure	Bragging gestures; pointing to oneself	Gestures that minimize references to oneself
Confrontation	Pointing a finger or shaking one's fist; speaking in a loud tone of voice	Speaking in a natural tone of voice

the persons with whom you interact, as well as of the messages you are returning. In our society a simple up-and-down nod of the head means yes and a side-to-side shake means no, but in Bulgaria and among the Eskimos these signals have the opposite meaning. See Examples of Various Cultural Traditions for other traditions that illustrate the importance of being sensitive to and aware of beliefs of the many cultures that will be represented in your patient population.

EXAMPLES OF VARIOUS CULTURAL TRADITIONS

- A husband speaks for his wife. The wife does not speak to the physician.
- The palm of the hand, facing down, is used to beckon someone. The hand motion signaling one to come or follow, performed with the back of the hand toward the patient, is used only when calling an animal. An open hand is used to point, rather than one finger.
- A female's clothing is not removed without the presence of another female family member.
- Emotional crying and sobbing denote femininity.
- Going to the doctor is a sign of weakness.
- The female medical assistant never touches the male patient.
- Acquaintances are not permitted to stand within 3 feet of the patient; only immediate family members are permitted to stand within this space.
- The Chinese do not like to be touched by people they do not know.
- The Laotian's "yes" response may not mean "yes," because it is considered rude to say "no" to others or to cause conflict.
- A native of Cambodia, as well as a Laotian, will not look into the eyes of the person being addressed because long eye contact means disrespect and is impolite.
- Cambodians do not like to have their blood drawn because they believe it will weaken them.
- Afghans and Mexicans have a concept of time that is less precise than in the United States.
- Vietnamese consider the head to be a sacred part of the body and are offended by being touched on the head or shoulders. Only the elderly may touch the head of a child without giving offense.

If you work in a practice that predominantly serves a distinct ethnic group, discuss possible cultural differences with the physician and with influential people within the cultural group. Learning to under-

stand cultural differences helps you to gain the confidence and respect of patients.

Memory Jogger

3 *Can you list additional signs of nonverbal communication not discussed previously?*

Communicating with Staff Members

SETTING THE TONE

Patients are usually quite sensitive to the degree of **harmony** that exists in the medical facility, and it is important to their well-being that they be treated in a harmonious atmosphere. The tone of the medical establishment is determined by the interpersonal skills demonstrated by the employees toward one another. When personality problems exist among staff members, these problems should be openly discussed so that they can be resolved. Care must be taken to avoid constantly criticizing others and participating in office gossip. Liking a person is not a requirement for acceptance of that person as a working colleague. Try addressing yourself to the situation rather than to the person's character or personality.

A successful medical assistant must have the knowledge to understand what he or she is expected to do and the skills to perform the assigned tasks. This is essential in today's busy and multiskilled offices. With this assumption, the success of the medical assistant is almost always dependent on how he or she responds to patients, staff, and the physicians.

SELF-CONCEPT

Your self-concept is composed of all the attitudes you have about yourself. Understanding yourself and feeling good about yourself are important. Confidence and self-esteem can affect your success, and feeling down on yourself can lead to failure. When you expect to fail, it is almost inevitable that you will. However, when you believe in yourself and expect to succeed, the likelihood of your success is greatly improved.

Many of the perceptions you have about yourself are based on the feedback you have received from others. Keep in mind that you, too, affect others in the way they perceive themselves. This is especially true when people are involved in a team effort, as you will be in the medical facility. In other words, the self-concept has a circular effect.

COOPERATION

Cooperation is the ability to work with others effectively. It requires your extending yourself to be helpful to others. You learn cooperation not by thinking of your immediate comfort but rather of the ultimate success of your medical facility and of your patients. Cooperation is actually an expression of self-interest and unselfishness. It demands that you adjust your own immediate pleasure to benefit the interests of others.

As a medical assistant, you will be expected to cooperate often and in many ways. You will need to keep your work place and belongings neat and orderly, assume additional duties and responsibilities without complaint, work overtime when there is a need, and *offer your services even when you are not obligated to do so.* Share ideas and listen when others are trying to help you. Work harmoniously with others to advance the interests of the medical facility.

Teamwork is based on the ability of one worker to depend on another. Every person on the team is important and must complete his or her share of the workload if the team is to succeed.

PERSONAL QUALITIES

BEING A TEAM MEMBER

* Act with initiative about getting the job done; don't wait to be told what to do.
* Avoid being rigid about procedures; be flexible and receptive to doing things the way another person might want them done.
* Try never to take advantage of co-workers.
* Think before you speak.
* Never let your emotions take control over you.
* Don't make hasty judgments about others.
* Share the sense of accomplishment from a job well done.
* Don't expect others to do things "your way."

Little phrases such as *please, thank you, good morning,* and *good night* are very powerful in the work environment. Comments of politeness let others know that you care about them and appreciate them. A simple "good morning" may minimize the impact of an unpleasant event that occurred the previous workday and contribute to a cooperative working atmosphere.

Not everyone catches on to new ideas and routines at the same rate. It is important that you remain calm when helping a co-worker perform a new routine. Be patient when you are asked questions. A negative attitude can quickly lead to conflict and a breakdown of communication. Remember that someone took the time to teach you, so when the time comes for you to be the teacher, you should do the very best job you can.

When you have a difficult situation, or do not know how to solve a problem, invite your co-workers to assist in the solution. Be prepared to share the successful resolution when it occurs. A word of caution—ask for advice only when you are willing to consider hearing something with which you may disagree. If all you are seeking is confirmation of what you already have decided, you are not being fair to ask for advice. When you do receive help, be certain to say *thank you* and be sincere when saying it.

FEEDBACK

Feedback is letting people know how you feel about them at a given moment. When a co-worker does something you like, tell him or her. It will make both of you feel good. **Conversely,** sometimes you will need to give negative feedback. A co-worker does something that is not acceptable. Instead of harboring ill feelings, be open and honest about it. Your comments should refer to the situation—not to the co-worker's character.

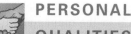
PERSONAL QUALITIES

RULES IN CONVEYING NEGATIVE FEEDBACK

* Give it as soon as possible after the event at a mutually agreeable time.
* Keep it friendly and nonthreatening.
* Give it in the appropriate place, in private.
* Deal only with facts, and how the behavior affects you.
* Avoid appearing judgmental.

If you are the recipient of negative feedback, learn to accept it in the same manner as you would any constructive information. The goal for every staff member is to deliver the best possible health care.

Relating to Management Style

A medical facility with three or more employees usually has a supervisor who manages the staff under the direction of the physician(s). In a few instances this may be an informal arrangement, but inevitably someone must be in charge. The supervisor may be one of the medical assistants. In any event, a supervisor has personality traits, strengths and weaknesses, good days and bad days, hopes and fears, just as you do. Learn to respect the manager's style and respond to him or her as another human being.

The three basic styles of management are **autocratic, democratic,** and **laissez-faire.** An awareness of these different management styles will aid your relationship. Remember that you cannot change the supervisor's style of management. After you discover which style of management inspires your best efforts, you should direct any future search for employment toward a facility that has the management style you prefer.

AUTOCRATIC

This supervisor is a strong leader who dictates procedure, policy, and assignments, including directions for when and how things should be done. The autocrat does not delegate easily and seldom welcomes initiative or creativity in the staff. If your supervisor fits into this category, be sure to follow directions and strictly adhere to the rules.

DEMOCRATIC

In contrast to the autocrat, the democratic supervisor encourages participation in the management process and exercises only a moderate degree of control over the employees' performance. This supervisor will be quick to explain policies and procedures when needed. Staff members will be encouraged to make suggestions and participate as a member of the management team. A democratic environment will allow you to "stretch your wings."

LAISSEZ-FAIRE

The highly confident medical assistant will blossom under this supervisor, who provides only general guidance and allows staff members to work independently. Initiative and creativity are encouraged. Employees are free to complete their tasks relying on their own training and past experience. The "down side" is that it requires more self-discipline from the employee. People may not work together because there is little direction. If you are not a self-starter you may not succeed in this environment.

Memory Jogger

4 *Name the three basic styles of management.*

 # PATIENT EDUCATION

The medical assistant has the opportunity to provide an educational service to every patient who enters the medical facility. If patients feel uneasy about asking the physician questions, let them know that you are available to transmit their questions to the physician. You might suggest that they prepare a list of their questions before their appointments and that they give this list to the physician when they come to the office.

When patients experience anxiety about why a procedure is necessary or how it will be accomplished, the medical assistant can often explain. He or she can help by alerting the physician to the patient's concerns or by encouraging the patient to speak to the physician directly. By acting as the patient's **advocate,** the medical assistant helps to establish a positive rapport between the patient and the physician.

Patients have many questions about medical care facilities and providers of medical services such as laboratories, therapeutic facilities, and hospitals. Medical information and new treatment methods are favorite topics for coverage by the news media. Patients often ask questions about medical news that they have heard.

The entire staff should work as a team to create an atmosphere of patient confidence and trust. Offer information regarding appointment schedules, billing, insurance services, telephone hours, office hours, and emergency coverage. Information about fees for services, office policy, and Medicare should be readily available to patients.

The medical assistant is the front door to the practice. In this role, expect to have contact with outside physicians, staff members, salespersons, supply company representatives, and service representatives. Courtesy, patience, and effective communication skills help to promote a positive public image of the facility.

LEGAL AND ETHICAL ISSUES

The physical appearance of the medical assistant has a profound effect on the patient's appraisal of medical care received.

When personality problems exist among staff members, an attempt should be made to resolve them. Address yourself to the existing situation—not to the person's character or personality.

Study the cultural differences of ethnic groups served by your facility for a better understanding of their behavior.

CRITICAL THINKING

1 Patients often will express their fear of a situation by exhibiting anger. A patient is early for his appointment but is becoming abusive and making unreasonable demands. In your position as medical assistant, how will you react to this patient?

2 The patient often loses the sense of privacy while in a health care facility. As a medical assistant, what can you do to diminish this loss to the patient?

3 List some possible reasons that a patient might feel apprehensive about visiting the physician.

4 Have you ever been a victim of discrimination? Have you felt discrimination toward another person? Describe your feelings.

5 Which of the three described management styles would you find most comfortable as a working environment? Why?

HOW DID I DO? Answers to Memory Joggers

1 Is the patient relaxed? Apprehensive? Obviously ill? Assertive? Defensive? Add your own suggestions.

2 Subtle discrimination is based on the observer's personal experience and expectations.

3 Some additional signs of nonverbal language: playing with a finger ring, moving restlessly, tapping of the foot, a wink of the eye, crossing the legs, turning the head, pulling one's hair.

4 Autocratic, democratic, laissez-faire.

REFERENCES

Dresser N: Multicultural Manners. New York, John Wiley & Sons, 1996.
Fast J: Body Language. New York, Pocket Books, 1970.
Peterson A, Allen R: Human Relations for the Medical Office. Chicago, AAMA, 1978.

Patient Reception

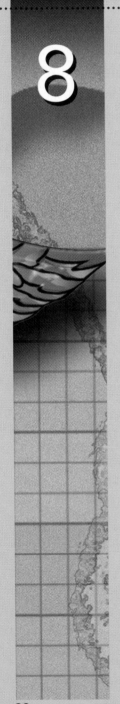

8

LEARNING OBJECTIVES

Cognitive: On successful completion of this chapter you should be able to:
1 Define and spell the words listed in the Vocabulary.
2 List six considerations in keeping a reception room comfortable for patients.
3 State two reasons for checking supplies at the beginning of each day.
4 Identify and discuss the importance of the three components of greeting an arriving patient.
5 Instruct a new patient about providing personal data for the records and completing a registration form.
6 List three actions a medical assistant might take to reduce stress caused by a delayed schedule.
7 Discuss ways a medical assistant might help a physically impaired, uncomfortable, or ill patient.
8 Suggest a way to successfully handle an angry patient.

Performance: On successful completion of this chapter you should be able to perform the following activities:
1 Follow correct procedure for reviewing patient charts for the day's appointments.
2 Supervise completion of a new patient's registration form.

VOCABULARY

augment To make greater or more effective

flagged Using something to signal or attract attention

harmonious All parts are agreeably related or in accord

intercom (intercommunication system) A direct telephone line from one station to another

pediatrician A physician who specializes in the care of children

perception A mental image

phonetic Alteration of ordinary spelling that better represents the sounding of a word

responsible person One who is responsible for payment, usually the patient if an adult

sequentially Following one another in an orderly plan

A first impression is lasting. Nowhere is this more important than in the health care facility, where the environment must appear orderly and faultlessly clean. The facility may be a physician's office, a hospital, a health maintenance organization, an insurance company, or one of the many other health care sources. No matter what facility is involved, the appearance of the reception room and the front desk, and a cordial greeting by the receptionist, influence a patient's **perception** of the entire facility and the care that he or she will receive.

The Reception Room

The *reception room* is just that—a place to *receive* patients. The area should be planned for the patients' comfort, made as attractive and cheerful as possible, and kept clean and uncluttered (Fig. 8–1). Often the medical assistant has the opportunity to assist in decorating or re-decorating this very important room.

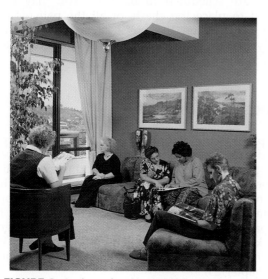

FIGURE 8–1 A comfortable, tasteful reception room.

Fresh **harmonious** colors and cleanliness are the basis of an attractive room. Add comfortable furniture that is adequate to accommodate the peak load of patients seen each day and arrange it in conversational groups. Individual chairs are best. People sometimes prefer to stand rather than sit next to a stranger on a sofa. Provide good lighting, ventilation, and a regulated temperature for additional comfort, and you have the essentials of an attractive reception room that tells the patient you care. A place to hang coats, rainwear, and umbrellas helps reduce reception room clutter. Professional designers can be consulted regarding reception room improvements when there is a problem area. See Features of Reception Area.

FEATURES OF RECEPTION AREA

Cleanliness
Restful colors
Adequate seating
Lighting to read by
Good ventilation
Regulated temperature

Most physicians' offices are well supplied with recent magazines in washable plastic covers. Patients seem to enjoy looking at pictures rather than something that requires concentrated reading. Pictorial travel books and magazines with short items of popular interest are favorites. The reception room, incidentally, is *not the place* for the physician's professional journals.

A writing desk and writing paper in the reception area for the convenience of patients are a nice touch, as is restful music via a concealed speaker. Even such additions as a television, available coffee or a cool drink, a lighted aquarium, or an educational display of some sort will enhance the attractiveness and individuality of the reception area of the professional practice. See Added Attractions for Reception Area.

For the **pediatrician,** a children's corner, equipped with small-scale furniture and some playthings, works well. Youngsters who might otherwise get into mischief are kept pleasantly occupied. Toys should be easily cleanable; plastic washable items are especially good. Take extra care to ensure that no toy has sharp corners that could injure a child, and that it has no small parts that could be swallowed. Also, in selecting toys, make certain that they will not stimulate the child toward noisy activity. And no rubber balls, for obvious reasons!

Take an objective look around the reception room periodically. Could it use a little brightening or freshening up? Try to look at it as if you were seeing it for the first time. The receptionist is at least partly responsible for the appearance of the area by making certain that the room remains neat and orderly throughout the day. Check the temperature and lighting for comfort. Scanning the room at intervals during the day and 1 to 2 minutes devoted to putting the room in order aid in keeping it at its best.

If the medical assistant's desk is in the reception area or in open view of the patients, it should be free of clutter. In particular, patients' charts and financial records should not be in sight. Personal articles, coffee cups, and so forth should not be on the receptionist's desk. Computer monitors should not be in view of patients, to protect the confidentiality of records (Fig. 8–2).

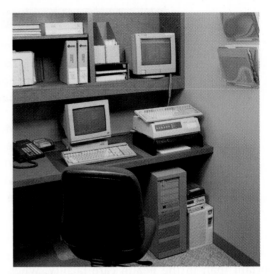

FIGURE 8–2   A neat, well-organized reception desk.

in the morning to be prepared to greet patients by name, and to know whether the patient is *new* or *established*. Patients should not be expected to provide details of the reason for their visit in a public area. Remember to ask *about the patient* before you ask about insurance.

REVIEW THE PATIENTS' CHARTS

Pull the charts for the day, checking the patient's name on your day list for accuracy (see Procedure 8–1). Occasionally, more than one patient may have the same or a similar name. Review each chart to verify that any recently received information, such as laboratory reports and radiograph readings, has been correctly entered and that each chart is current. Arrange the charts **sequentially** in the order the patients are scheduled to be seen. You may be expected to place the charts of all the patients to be seen that day on the physician's desk. It is more likely that the physician will prefer to receive a patient's chart just before seeing him or her.

ADDED ATTRACTIONS FOR RECEPTION AREA

Plants, fresh or artificial; if artificial arrangements are used, make sure they are dusted and cleaned
Pictures
Travel posters
Bulletin board displays
Recent general interest magazines
Pictorial travel books
Coffee, or cool drink
Aquarium (built-in for safety)
Safe toys for children's corner

Preparing for Patient Arrival

Advance preparation helps to make the day go smoothly and contributes toward a more relaxed atmosphere for all concerned.

KNOW WHO THE PATIENTS ARE

Patients like to be acknowledged when they arrive. All staff members should review the day's schedule

REPLENISH SUPPLIES

Supplies at the reception desk need to be replenished regularly. Stationery, appointment cards, charge slips, sharpened pencils, and any items likely to be needed during the day should be on hand when the day begins. Discovering depleted supplies during a busy day can seriously interrupt the flow of patient care. One person can be in charge of checking the inventory of supplies on a regular basis and of ordering as necessary (see Inventory Control in Chapter 23).

In a multiple-employee practice, a clinical assistant usually has the responsibility of checking clinical supplies. However, in a small practice there may be

PROCEDURE 8–1

Preparing Charts for Scheduled Patients

GOAL

To prepare patient charts for daily appointment schedule and have them ready for the physician before patients' arrival.

EQUIPMENT AND SUPPLIES

Appointment schedule for current date
Patient files
Clerical supplies (e.g., pen, tape, stapler)

PROCEDURAL STEPS

1 Review the appointment schedule.

2 Identify full name of each scheduled patient.

3 Pull patients' charts from files, checking each patient's name on your list as each chart is pulled.
   PURPOSE: To determine that the correct charts have been pulled and that none have been omitted.

4 Review each chart.
   PURPOSE: To reaffirm that:
   • All information has been correctly entered.
   • Any previously ordered tests have been performed.
   • The results have been entered on the chart.

5 Annotate the appointment list with any special concerns.
   PURPOSE: To alert the physician regarding matters that should be checked or discussed with the patient.

6 Arrange all charts sequentially according to each patient's appointment.

7 Place the charts in the appropriate examination room or other specified location.

---

only one assistant in charge. Before patients start arriving, *everything should be ready for the day* so that the physician and medical assistant can give undivided attention to the patients' needs.

Check all rooms to make certain that

• Everything is clean
• Cabinets are well stocked
• Drugs have been counted with narcotics checked off and locked if appropriate

Memory Jogger

1 *Why is it important to preview the day's schedule of patients to be seen that day?*

Greeting the Patient

Every patient has the right to expect courteous treatment in the physician's office. No matter what the patient's economic or social status may be, each individual who enters the reception room should receive a cordial, friendly greeting. Using the personal touch in receiving patients is important.

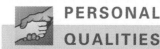

PERSONAL QUALITIES

GREETING THE PATIENT

Cultivate the habit of greeting each patient immediately in a friendly, self-assured manner. Establish eye contact, smile, and introduce yourself to the *new patient*, giving your name and job title: "Good morning, I'm Elizabeth Parr, Dr. Wade's medical assistant."

Greet the *established patient* by name. Learn how to pronounce each patient's name correctly, because incorrect pronunciations may offend and irritate some people. If the name is unusual, write the **phonetic** spelling on the record for reference.

Try to remember the patients' names and something personal about each one. Jot down key words on the patient's chart that will provide reminders for future conversations. Most patients appreciate the interest of the physician and the staff in their families, hobbies, and work.

The reception desk is usually placed for a clear view of all visitors who come into the office. If there is only one medical assistant, it is sometimes impossible for each new caller to be welcomed personally. In this situation, some announcement system must be worked out. The patient who enters an empty reception room does not know whether to sit down,

knock on the glass partition, or try to announce his or her presence in some way. A bell at the desk or window that the patient can ring is one solution.

Sometimes a register is placed in the reception room with a sign above it reading:

PLEASE SIGN THE REGISTER WHEN YOU ARRIVE. THE DOCTOR WILL SEE YOU SHORTLY.

This is a makeshift arrangement and *should be avoided* because patient confidentiality is violated when others can read the register. It is preferable to hand the register to the patient if this system must be used.

PROCEDURE 8–2
Registering a New Patient

GOAL
To complete registration form for a new patient with information for credit and insurance claims, and to inform and orient patient to facility.

EQUIPMENT AND SUPPLIES
Registration form
Clerical supplies (pen, clipboard)
Private conference area

PROCEDURAL STEPS

1 Determine whether the patient is new.

2 Obtain and record the necessary information:
   • Full name, birth date, name of spouse (if married)
   • Home address, telephone number (include ZIP and area codes)
   • Occupation, name of employer, business address, telephone number
   • Social Security number and driver's license number, if any
   • Name of referring physician, if any
   • Name and address of person responsible for payment
   • Method of payment
   • Health insurance information (photocopy both sides of insurance ID card)
   • Name of primary carrier
   • Type of coverage
   • Group policy number
   • Subscriber number
   • Assignment of benefits, if required
   PURPOSE: This information is necessary for credit and insurance claims

3 Review the entire form and confirm patient eligibility for insurance coverage
   PURPOSE: To verify that information is complete and legible

4 Determine that required referrals have been received if applicable.
   PURPOSE: Insurance coverage may not be valid without referral.

5 Explain medical and financial procedures to patient.
   PURPOSE: Patient develops comfort level and knows what to expect

6 Collect copays or balance payment charges.
   PURPOSE: Keeps accounts current and prevents the necessity of mailing statements

Today's Date _____

PATIENT INFORMATION SHEET

Patient's Name				Date of Birth
First	Middle	Last		Mo / Day / Year

Responsible Person's Name _____

First	Middle	Last	Relationship

Address _____

Number	Street	City	State	Zip	Area / Phone

Employer _____ Department or Occupation _____

Address _____

Number	Street	City	State	Zip	Area / Phone

Social Security Number _____ Driver's License Number _____

Spouse of Resp. Person _____

First	Middle	Last	Area / Phone

Employer _____ Department or Occupation _____

Address _____

Number	Street	City	State	Zip	Area / Phone

Social Security Number _____ Driver's License Number _____

Nearest relative (not living with you) _____

Relationship

Address _____

Number	Street	City	State	Zip	Area / Phone

Patient referred to this office by _____

AUTHORIZATION TO PAY BENEFITS TO PHYSICIAN: I hereby authorize payment of any insurance benefits covering these medical charges directly to the physician/surgeon.
Signature of the Insured _____ Date _____

AUTHORIZATION TO RELEASE INFORMATION: I hereby authorize the physician/surgeon to release any medical information to my insurance company.
Responsible person's signature _____ Date _____

STATEMENT OF FINANCIAL RESPONSIBILITY: I, _____ , do hereby agree to pay all medical charges incurred by the above listed patient. I further understand that these charges are my responsibility regardless of insurance coverage.
Responsible person's signature _____ .

FIGURE 8–3   Patient information sheet and credit application. (Courtesy of Credit Service Systems, Anaheim, CA.)

Introductory Procedures

REGISTRATION

Certain introductory procedures are required on a patient's first visit to the facility (see Procedure 8–2). Most physicians use a Patient Information Form of some kind to gather subjective information about the patient (Fig. 8–3). The medical assistant may complete the form while interviewing the new pa-

tient or have the patient complete the form on arrival for the first appointment. The form may be attached to a clipboard and handed to the patient with instructions to complete all parts of the form, with assurance that the assistant is ready and willing to answer any questions.

The patient's name and date of birth should appear prominently at the top of the form, followed by the name of the **responsible person** and pertinent facts in logical order. See Information Contained in a Patient Information Form.

INFORMATION CONTAINED IN A PATIENT INFORMATION FORM

- Patient's name and date of birth
- Responsible person's name

  Relationship to patient
  Address and telephone number
  Name, address, and telephone number of
  employer
  Occupation
  Social Security number
  Driver's license number

- Name of responsible person's spouse

  Related information, same as for responsible
  person (in some community property states,
  both spouses are equally responsible)

- Nearest relative not living with patient, and
  his or her relationship
- Source of referral, if any

When the completed form is returned to the medical assistant, it must be checked carefully to verify that all the necessary information has been included.

Memory Jogger

2 *It is not uncommon to find a patient registration form at the reception desk for patients to sign in. Why is this practice discouraged?*

OBTAINING PATIENT HISTORY

The personal and medical history, and the patient's family history, may be obtained by asking the patient to complete a questionnaire; the physician can augment this information during the patient interview. The *experienced medical assistant* may be expected to conduct the interview for the patient's personal and medical history, family history, and chief complaint. This is a very specialized procedure, and the interviewer must be specifically trained for the individual practice.

Consideration for Patients' Time

Once the preliminaries have been completed, the patient will expect to see the physician or practitioner at the appointed time. The medical assistant should get the patient in for treatment or consultation as near the appointment time as possible or explain any potential delay to the patient. All patients want to be kept informed about how long to expect to wait. Almost all patients will respond positively when the physician or the assistant comes to the reception area to apologize for any delay. *Consideration for the patient's time* is the keyword.

Most experts will agree that in a solo or small practice, there should seldom be more than three to five patients in the reception room. "Too long a wait in the doctor's office" is one of the most frequently heard criticisms of the medical profession. The patient who complains about medical fees or the care received may actually be complaining about the long wait or discourteous service. Most patients are fearful and tense, but the medical assistant can often put them in a better frame of mind with just a friendly smile and a show of concern.

A crowded reception room is not always an indication of a physician's popularity. It may simply mean that the physician or the assistant is inefficient in scheduling patients. Business people, for example, who are in the habit of making the most of their time, are particularly displeased at what may appear to them to be inefficient scheduling of appointments. Any delay of longer than 15 minutes should be explained to the person waiting. Some personal attention, such as offering a drink of water, a cup of coffee, or a new magazine, may help to calm a patient who appears irritated with the delay.

Patients with Special Needs

Some patients will be physically challenged, some will be very ill, and some will be severely uncomfortable. There may be language or cultural barriers.

Observe the patient's appearance and behavior. Is the patient pale or drawn looking? Do the eyes or voice reflect pain or discomfort? Find out how the patient is feeling before you suggest that he or she be seated to wait for the physician. The patient may need to lie down in a cool room or perhaps should be seen as an emergency.

The patient who is in a wheelchair or using a walker or crutches may need personal attention. Some patients may need help in disrobing even when a disability is not obvious. Ask if you can be of assistance. The medical assistant must use good judgment in helping disabled patients, perhaps even bypassing some of the usual routines.

Escorting and Instructing the Patient

Sometimes we become so accustomed to our own surroundings that we forget that the stranger may be confused or disoriented by all the hallways, doors, and rooms. Uncertainty creates anxiety. Do take the time to personally escort the patient to the appropriate examination or treatment room. This is usually the responsibility of the clinical medical assistant. If a urine specimen is to be obtained, direct the patient to the rest room.

If the patient is to disrobe, explain what garments, if any, can be left on, whether shoes are to be removed, that he or she must remove jewelry if an x-ray film is to be taken, and so forth. If a gown is to be worn, specify whether the opening should be in front or back, and tell the patients where they can hang their clothes if this is not obvious. All instructions must be clear. *Do not assume* that patients will know what you want if you have not told them.

Be equally clear when the examination has been completed: "You can get dressed now and return to the consultation room," or "After you are dressed, please stop by the desk to make your next appointment," or "Have you any questions?"

The medical assistant can help keep the schedule operating smoothly by immediately tidying each examination room and moving the next patient in so that the physician need have no idle moments waiting for a patient to be prepared. Try not to place a patient in an examination room just to clear out the reception area. It is especially inconsiderate to keep the patient waiting after being gowned, draped, and positioned on the examining table. A magazine rack on the wall of the treatment room is a welcome addition in some practices.

Handling Complaints

Even under the best of conditions, there will at times be complaints from patients. Remember that the practice of medicine is a personal service for individual personalities, and the medical assistant must cultivate the skill of listening (see Chapter 7). Each patient is a very important person, and any complaint should be taken seriously. Try to resolve the matter if it is within your realm of responsibility. Otherwise, assure the patient of your concern and explain that you will try to find a solution. Then be sure to carry through.

Problem Situations

THE TALKER

There can be certain problem patients in any professional office. The *talker*, for example, takes up far more of the physician's time than is justified. An alert medical assistant can usually spot this tendency during the initial interview. The patient's history can be **flagged** with a symbol to alert the physician. A prearranged agreement to contact the physician on the **intercom** at the end of the allotted

time, with the message that the next patient is waiting, gives the physician an opportunity to conclude the interview. Once you have learned which patients take extra time, you can book them for the end of the day or simply allow more time for them.

CHILDREN

Children sometimes present special management problems. It is often advisable to escort the younger patients into the treatment room *without the parent.* This, of course, should be at the discretion of the physician.

While this practice of separating children from their parents to treat their needs is not always feasible, it sometimes can be applied with great success. In some offices, a token of the physician's friendship, such as a trinket or toy, is given to the child at the completion of the visit.

THE ANGRY PATIENT

Every medical assistant at some time will be confronted by an angry patient. The anger may simply be a reflection of the patient's pain or fear of what the physician may discover on the examination. If possible, invite the patient into another room out of the reception area. Usually it is best to let the patient talk out his or her anger. A calm attitude on the part of the medical assistant, with a few remarks interjected in a low voice, will often pacify the patient. Under no circumstances should the assistant return the anger or become argumentative.

PATIENT'S RELATIVES

A patient will sometimes be accompanied by a relative or well-meaning friend who may become restless while waiting for the patient and attempt to discuss the patient's illness. The medical assistant should sidestep any discussion of a patient's medical care, except by direction of the physician. Also avoid a too casual attitude, such as "I'm sure there's nothing to worry about." A show of moderate concern and offering reassurance that "the patient is in good hands" usually takes care of the situation.

Friendly Farewell

As soon as the visit with the physician has been completed the medical assistant should be ready to take charge by assisting the patient in dressing, if necessary, and by making sure that any questions that the patient may have are answered. In a small practice, this may be the responsibility of the administrative medical assistant.

If the patient has *nontechnical* questions that the assistant can capably and ethically answer, the assistant should answer them clearly and note this on the patient's chart. Some questions can be answered only by the physician; in such cases the assistant can offer to get answers for the patient.

The assistant can help convey the impression of *caring* by terminating the patient's visit cordially. If the patient is returning for another visit, the assistant can say something like "We'll see you next week." If it is the patient's last visit, a pleasant "I certainly hope you'll be feeling fine from now on" is appropriate. The assistant may wish to tell a patient on his (or her) last visit that he has been a fine patient and that it has been a pleasure to serve him. Whatever words of good-bye are chosen, all patients should leave the facility with the feeling that they have received top-quality care and were treated with friendliness and courtesy.

LEGAL AND ETHICAL ISSUES

Use the personal touch in receiving patients.

Try to remember the patients' names and something personal about each one.

Greet the established patient by name.

The registration form may be considered an application for credit and is subject to the regulations of the Equal Credit Opportunity Act of 1975. If you ask for the marital status, avoid using the terms *divorced* or *widowed*.

When a patient complains, listen carefully and resolve the problem or assure the patient that you will try to find a solution.

If someone other than the patient asks for information regarding that patient, refrain from discussion except by direction of the physician.

CRITICAL THINKING

1 Role-play with another student in the various patient situations (talker, children, angry patient, relatives) described in this chapter.

2 Calm an angry patient who is complaining about a long wait. The physician has been delayed by an emergency at the hospital.

3 Recall your latest visit to a medical facility and consider how the reception area could have been more attractive or more comfortable.

4 Based on your own experience or other information, describe what you believe to be a good system of handling patient arrival.

HOW DID I DO? **Answers to Memory Joggers**

1 Patients like to be acknowledged on arrival. You need to be able to identify *new patients* who will usually require more time and attention.

2 A sign-in sheet at the reception desk violates patient confidentiality.

Telephone Techniques

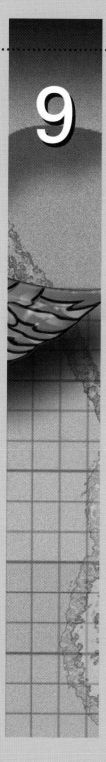

9

LEARNING OBJECTIVES

Cognitive: On successful completion of this chapter, you should be able to:

1 Define and spell the terms in the Vocabulary.

2 Discuss the importance of telephone communications.

3 List ways by which the medical assistant can develop a pleasing telephone personality.

4 Cite seven items to be included in taking a complete telephone message.

5 Identify 10 kinds of telephone calls that the medical assistant should be able to handle successfully.

6 Identify six kinds of telephone calls that will need to be referred to the physician for response.

7 Explain what is involved in monitoring telephone calls.

8 Explain what is meant by *preplanning a call.*

9 Explain the ways in which an operator-answered telephone answering service can benefit a medical practice.

Performance: On successful completion of this chapter, you should be able to:

1 Demonstrate the appropriate method of placing and receiving telephone calls.

2 Using a multiple-line telephone, demonstrate the correct handling of two incoming calls, one of which must be transferred to another person.

3 Correctly record a telephone message from a laboratory facility reporting test results on a patient.

4 Respond to a call from a pharmacist regarding a request for a prescription refill, demonstrating appropriate precautions and completing necessary information.

5 Using a list of local social service agencies, respond to telephone calls for emergency treatment (at a poison or burn center) and for nonemergency services (at a facility for crippled children or a cancer-screening center).

VOCABULARY

appease To make peaceful or quiet

clarity The quality or state of being clear

confidential Containing information that requires authorization for disclosure

copay A flat fee payable by the insured in most health maintenance organization plans

diction Choice of words to express ideas, especially with regard to correctness, clearness, or effectiveness

enunciation The act of pronouncing words distinctly

flourishing Achieving success

inflection Change in pitch or loudness of the voice

monitor To listen to a matter transmitted by telephone as a third party

noncommittal Not revealing any specific attitude or opinion

overaccentuate Greatly emphasize

pitch The vibratory frequency of a tone or sound

practitioner One who practices a profession

pronunciation The act or manner of pronouncing words

salutation Expression of greeting (e.g., *good morning*)

screen The act of determining to whom a telephone call is to be directed

tedious Tiresome because of length or dullness

transmitter The part of telephone into which one speaks

General Guidelines

The telephone is the lifeline of a medical practice as well as a powerful public relations instrument. Ninety percent of the patients who are seen in a medical facility make their initial appointments by telephone. When used appropriately, the telephone can help build a beginning medical practice; if used inappropriately, it can do much to destroy even a **flourishing** practice. A physician's office without one or more telephones is impossible to imagine, and the medical assistant who regards the telephone as a nuisance has no place in a medical practice.

The majority of telephone contacts are incoming calls from

- Established patients calling for appointments or to seek advice
- Individuals reporting emergencies
- Other physicians who are making referrals
- Laboratories reporting vital information regarding a patient
- New patients making a first contact

Although great emphasis is placed on rules for speaking, the importance of active listening is often overlooked. The same attention should be given a telephone conversation that would be given a face-to-face conversation. Concentration is not always easy; it must be practiced. Effective active listening is vital to the medical assistant.

YOUR TELEPHONE PERSONALITY

When you receive a telephone call from a stranger, you probably try to visualize that person's appearance. You also form some opinion of his or her personality (e.g., he or she is a mature adult, is somewhat worried, thinks quickly, is well educated). The caller responds to your voice in the same way. To the caller, your voice is your entire personality. The caller cannot see you, your smile, or your facial expression. The caller's total impression of you and of the facility is formed from hearing your voice. What image do you create with your telephone personality?

PERSONAL
QUALITIES

IS THIS YOUR TELEPHONE PERSONALITY?

- Your voice is warm and friendly.
- Your tone is confident.
- Your conversation is courteous and tactful.
- Your words are well chosen.

Every caller should be made to feel that you have time to attend to his or her wishes. A small mirror, placed near the telephone, will remind you to smile. Smiling helps to relax your facial muscles and improves your tone of voice. If you are rushed when you pick up the telephone, wait a few seconds until you are able to answer graciously without seeming breathless or impatient.

CONFIDENTIALITY

Keep in mind that all communications in a health care facility are **confidential.** This means that if others are within hearing range of your voice, you are to use discretion when mentioning the name of the caller. You must also be careful about being overheard when you repeat any symptoms or other information you are receiving by telephone.

> **EXAMPLES OF SENSITIVE PHONE CALLS**
> A woman calls about being struck by her husband, resulting in injuries that need to be treated.
> An established patient believes he may have been exposed to the human immunodeficiency virus.

HOLDING THE TELEPHONE HANDSET CORRECTLY

You may have developed some very casual personal habits when using the telephone that will need correction in the professional office. How do you hold the telephone handset? Is it placed so that your voice is relayed distinctly and accurately?

Practice holding the handset around the middle, with the mouthpiece about 1 inch from your lips and directly in front of your teeth. Never hold it under your chin. You can check the proper distance by taking your first two fingers and passing them

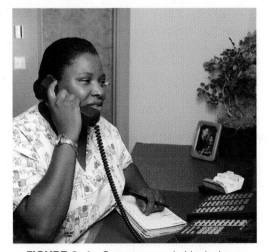

FIGURE 9–1 Correct way to hold telephone.

through sideways in the space between your lips and the mouthpiece. If your fingers just squeeze through, your lips are the correct distance from the telephone and your voice will go over the line as close to its natural tone as possible (Fig. 9–1).

Speak directly into the telephone immediately after removing it from its cradle. If you turn to face a window or another part of the room, make sure the telephone transmitter moves, too; otherwise, your voice will be lost.

DEVELOPING A PLEASING TELEPHONE VOICE

What are the qualities of a good telephone voice? How do you cultivate good voice quality? Some general tips are presented.

 PERSONAL QUALITIES

TIPS ON DEVELOPING A PLEASING TELEPHONE VOICE

- Stay alert. Be alert and interested in the person who is calling. Let the caller know that he or she has your full attention
- Be pleasant. Build a pleasant, friendly image for you and your office. Be the voice with a smile.
- Talk naturally and be yourself. Use your own words and expressions. Avoid repetition of mechanical words or phrases (e.g. "you know," "uh huh," "like"). Avoid the use of professional jargon, such as referring to *otalgia* when the patient is reporting an *earache*.
- Speak distinctly. Clear, distinct pronunciation and enunciation are vital. Move the lips, tongue, and jaw freely. Talk directly into the transmitter. Never answer the telephone when you are *eating, drinking,* or *chewing gum.*
- Be expressive. A well-modulated voice carries best. Use a normal tone of voice, neither too loud nor too soft. Talk at a moderate rate, neither too quickly nor too slowly. Vary your tone. It will bring out the meaning of sentences and add color and vitality to what you say.

HOW IS YOUR DICTION?

Everyone should have the experience of hearing his or her own voice; it reveals immediately the importance of careful **diction.** Try putting your voice on tape and listening to a playback. Each word and each sound must be given individual attention to achieve **clarity.** Slurring your words or dropping

TABLE 9–1   Key Words to Verify Letters

A as in Adams	J as in John	S as in Samuel
B as in Boston	K as in Katie	T as in Thomas
C as in Charles	L as in Lewis	U as in Utah
D as in David	M as in Mary	V as in Victor
E as in Edward	N as in Nellie	W as in William
F as in Frank	O as in Oliver	X as in x-ray
G as in George	P as in Peter	Y as in Young
H as in Henry	Q as in Queen	Z as in Zebra
I as in Ida	R as in Robert	

your voice too much at the end of a sentence can place a strain on your listener.

Memory Jogger

1 *There will be days when you are not feeling your best. What one exercise can you use to relax facial muscles and improve the tone of your voice?*

Do not **overaccentuate;** it causes you to sound artificial. Use a friendly natural style. Few words need to be spelled over the telephone if a person speaks slowly and clearly. Table 9–1 lists key words commonly used when it is necessary to verify letters in spelling over the telephone.

Try to avoid the habit of dropping "ers," "uhs," and long pauses into your conversation. Also, remember that it is seldom necessary to raise the **pitch** of your voice to be heard. If you have trouble being understood on the telephone you probably are

- Speaking too fast
- Enunciating poorly
- Failing to speak into the transmitter

Incoming Telephone Calls

You will be receiving many calls during the course of a single day. Each one deserves your most competent attention. See Procedure 9–1, Answering the Telephone, and also Professional Office Telephone Communication for a summary of how to communicate effectively on the telephone. Carefully review Pitfalls to Avoid to help you side-step problems with telephone communications.

PERSONAL CALLS

Because the telephone is so vital to the medical practice, personal calls should not be allowed to keep a line busy. Physicians usually are understanding about occasional urgent calls from the medical assistant's family, but casual calls should be discouraged.

PROCEDURE 9 – 1
Answering the Telephone

GOAL

To answer the telephone in a physician's office in a professional manner, respond to a request for action, and accurately record a message.

EQUIPMENT AND SUPPLIES

Telephone
Message pad
Pen or pencil

Appointment book
Script for conversation

PROCEDURAL STEPS

1 Answer the telephone on the first ring, speaking directly into the transmitter, with the mouthpiece positioned 1 inch from the mouth.
   PURPOSE: Answering promptly conveys interest in the caller. Proper positioning of the handset carries the voice best.

2 Speak distinctly with a pleasant tone and expression, at a moderate rate, and with sufficient volume for the calling party to understand every word.

3 Identify the office and yourself.
   PURPOSE: The caller will know that the correct number has been reached and the identity of the staff member.

4 Verify the identity of the caller.
   PURPOSE: To confirm the origin of the call.

5 Provide the caller with the requested information or service, if possible.
   PURPOSE: The medical assistant can handle many calls and conserve the time and energy of the physician or other staff members.

6 Take a message for further action, if required.
   PURPOSE: Not all calls can be responded to immediately.

7 Terminate the call in a pleasant manner and replace the receiver gently.
   PURPOSE: To promote good public relations.

A medical assistant who is active in a professional organization sometimes finds it necessary to take calls from colleagues or others involved in the profession. Although these communications are not considered entirely personal, they, too, should be kept to a minimum. The physician's telephone lines should be clear to receive all professional calls.

 PERSONAL QUALITIES

PROFESSIONAL OFFICE TELEPHONE COMMUNICATION

- Answer promptly.
- Visualize the person to whom you are speaking.
- Hold the instrument correctly.

- Develop a pleasing telephone voice.
- Identify your office and yourself.
- Identify the caller.
- Offer assistance.
- Screen incoming calls.
- Minimize waiting time.
- Identify the caller when transferring a call.
- When answering a second call, identify the caller, then return to the first call.
- End each call pleasantly and graciously.

PITFALLS TO AVOID

- **Having too few telephone lines.** On request, the telephone company will do a traffic survey to determine how many busy signals are occurring and advise you as to whether you need additional lines. If collections and insurance processing require extensive use of the telephone, a special line just for this purpose may be advisable.

- **Having too few assistants to handle the existing lines.** One assistant can handle two incoming lines, but three lines are probably too many for one person. Another assistant should be assigned to pick up the phone after a specified number of rings.
- **Wasting time looking up frequently called numbers.** Keep these in a personal directory where they can be quickly and easily located or use speed dialing.
- **Incoming or outgoing personal calls by employees, except in emergencies.** Most physicians have an unlisted private line to take care of their own personal and priority calls.
- **Using the telephone to give travel directions to new patients** (except for short notice appointments). This information should be included in a patient information sheet or folder sent to every new patient.
- **Taking extensive patient histories by telephone.** This can be done more efficiently at the time of the patient visit.
- **Diagnosing or giving medical advice without authorization from the physician.**
- **Releasing patient information without authorization.**

ANSWERING PROMPTLY

Whenever possible, answer the telephone on the first ring, and always by the third ring. If your facility has several incoming lines or more than one telephone, it will sometimes be necessary for you to interrupt a conversation to answer another call. It is courteous to

- Excuse yourself by saying, "Pardon me just a moment; the other line is ringing."
- Answer the second call, determine who is calling, and, if it is not an emergency, ask that person to hold while you complete the first call. Do not make the mistake of continuing with this call while the first caller waits.
- Return to your first call as soon as possible, and apologize briefly for the interruption.

Think of what you would do if there were a face-to-face conversation. You would not allow a second person to just interrupt a conversation and then ignore the *one you* were speaking with first.

If the second call is an emergency, you can still take a moment to return to the first line and alert the caller that you will have to keep him or her waiting or call back.

Never answer a call by saying, "Hold the line, please," without first finding out who is calling. It could be an emergency, and it is extremely discourteous. It takes only a moment to be courteous, and this courtesy could save a life.

Memory Jogger

2 *Recall at least 7 of the 12 rules for Professional Office Telephone Communication.*

PERSONALIZING THE CALL

Try to use the caller's name three times during the conversation. Use other courtesy expressions, such as *thank you, please,* and *you're welcome,* as often as possible.

IDENTIFYING THE FACILITY AND YOURSELF

Your response to an incoming call should be to *first identify the facility* and then *yourself.* Numerous telephone greetings can be used. You will probably wish to discuss which are best with the physician or office manager. Your response might be something like this:

"This is Dr. Black's office—Miss Anderson."

Answering a professional office telephone merely by repeating the telephone number or saying "Hello" is unsatisfactory. The caller will invariably ask:

"Is this Dr. Black's office?"

Rarely can a person immediately recall the number that he or she has just dialed. Time is wasted, the caller is psychologically rebuffed, and you have lost another opportunity to create a favorable impression of your facility.

The use of a **salutation** in telephone identification is optional. Sometimes the addition of "Good morning" or "Good afternoon" to the identification is awkward. A rising **inflection** or a questioning tone in your voice indicates interest and a willingness to assist and eliminates the need for an additional greeting.

When you have decided on the greeting to be used, practice it until you can say it easily and smoothly without having to think about what you are saying.

IDENTIFYING THE CALLER

If the caller does not identify himself or herself, you should ask to whom you are speaking. Repeat the caller's name by using it in the conversation as soon as possible; if patients are within the range of your voice, remember that the caller's privacy should be respected.

OFFERING ASSISTANCE

You can offer assistance both by the *tone of your voice* and by the *words you use.*

"May I help you?" or "How may I help you?" will open the conversation and assure the caller that you are both willing and capable of being of service.

SCREENING INCOMING CALLS

Most physicians expect the medical assistant to **screen** all telephone calls. Good judgment in deciding whether to put a call through to the physician comes with experience.

Do put through calls from other physicians at once. If your physician is busy and cannot possibly come to the telephone, explain this briefly and politely and then say that you will ask the physician to return the call as soon as possible.

Many callers will ask, "Is the doctor in?" Avoid answering this question with a simple "Yes" or "No" or by responding with the question, "Who is calling, please?" *If the physician is not in,* say so *before* asking the identity of the caller. Otherwise, you may create the impression that the physician is just not willing to talk with this person.

If the *physician is away* from the office, the rule of offering assistance still holds. You can say

"No, I am sorry, Dr. Black is not in. May I take a message?" *or*

"No, I am sorry, but Dr. Black will be at the hospital most of the morning. May I ask her to return your call after 1 o'clock?"

If the *physician is in* and is available for telephone calls, a typical response would be

"Yes, Dr. Black is in; may I say who is calling, please?"

When physicians prefer to keep telephone calls to a minimum, you might say

"Yes, Dr. Black is here, but I am not sure whether she is free to come to the phone. May I say who is calling, please?"

By responding in this way, the physician is not committed to taking the call.

During the time that a physician is examining a patient, he or she will not wish to be interrupted with a routine call. In such cases, you might say

"Yes, Dr. Black is in but is with a patient right now. May I help you?" *or*

"Yes, Dr. Black is in but is with a patient right now. Is there anything you would like me to ask her?"

Try to guard against being overprotective. A patient should be able to talk with the physician when necessary; but unless it is an emergency, the patient is probably willing to do so at the convenience of the physician. Don't let it be said of your physician, "He's a good doctor, but you can never talk to him." The medical assistant who answers the telephone acts as a screen, not a roadblock.

Find out exactly how calls are to be handled when the physician is out of the office and under what circumstances you can interrupt when the physician is on the premises. Be firm in your commitment to those preferences and cultivate a reputation for being helpful and reliable. You will save the physician many interruptions if patients develop confidence in your ability to help them and have faith in your promise to take their messages and deliver them properly.

MINIMIZING WAITING TIME

When a call cannot be put through immediately, ask

"Will you wait, or shall I call you back when Dr. Black is free?"

If the caller elects to wait, remember that waiting with a silent telephone can be **irritating** and **tedious.** The waiting time, no matter how brief, always seems long. *Let no more than 1 minute pass* without breaking in with some reassuring comment, for instance

"I'm sorry, Dr. Black is still busy."

If the wait is longer than expected, the caller may wish to reconsider and call back at another time or have the call returned, but he or she needs to communicate this to you. By going back on the line at frequent intervals, you give the caller an opportunity to express such concerns. In fact, you may ask the caller if he or she wishes to continue waiting. Say something like the following:

"I'm sorry to keep you waiting so long, Mr. Hughes. Would you prefer to have me return your call when Dr. Black is free?"

Try to give the caller some estimate of when he or she may expect the return call. In any event, irritation can be lessened by your consideration in saying

"Thank you for waiting, Mr. Hughes."

When it is necessary that you leave the telephone to obtain information, ask the caller

"Will you please wait while I get the information?"

Wait for a reply. If it will take longer than a few seconds to get the information, give some estimate of the time required and offer to call back. When you return to the telephone, thank the caller for waiting. Requests that might require pulling the patient's chart from the files may best be handled with a call back to the patient.

Memory Jogger

3 *What is the maximum time a caller should wait on a telephone line without being able to communicate?*

TRANSFERRING A CALL

Always identify the person who is calling when you transfer a call to the physician or another person in the facility. Any person who refuses to give a name should not be put through unless you have been instructed to do so.

When the caller is a patient, the physician will probably need the patient's chart at hand during the conversation. If there is no concern about others hearing your conversation, you can announce the caller's name on the intercom and tell the physician that you will bring the chart. If there are others within hearing range, you might simply take the chart to the physician and say

"Dr. Black, this party is waiting on the telephone to speak with you."

In this way, the patient's right to privacy is protected.

ENDING A CALL

When a caller's requests have been satisfied, do not encourage needless chatting or permit the call to monopolize your time unnecessarily. The telephone lines should be cleared for other calls.

 PERSONAL QUALITIES

HOW TO END A CALL

- End the call pleasantly.
- Allow the person who placed the call to hang up first.
- Thank the person for calling.
- Close the conversation with some form of good-bye; do not just abruptly hang up.
- Replace the telephone on its cradle as gently as if you were closing a door.

Taking a Telephone Message

BE PREPARED

Always have a pen or pencil in your hand and a message pad nearby when you answer the telephone. You may be answering several calls before you have an opportunity to relay a message or carry out a promise of action. The *written message* is vital.

What kind of message pad will you use? An ordinary spiral-bound stenographer's notebook is inexpensive, sturdy, and well proportioned; lies flat on a desk; and can be filed for future reference if desired. Never use small scraps of paper for messages. They are too easily lost.

Date the bottom of the first blank page in your notebook at the beginning of each day. You will then have a permanent record that can be referred to later if the need arises. If you will draw a half-inch column down one side of each page, you can use this area to check off each message as it is delivered or taken care of. This creates a good reminder system.

MINIMUM INFORMATION REQUIRED FROM EACH CALL

- Name of the person to whom the call is directed
- Name of the person calling
- Caller's daytime telephone number
- Reason for the call
- Action to be taken
- Date and time of the call
- Your initials

TRANSMITTING AND RECORDING THE MESSAGE

Messages that are to be transmitted to another person may be rewritten on individual message slips and delivered or posted on a message board later. Message pads that provide for a carbon copy of each page are good insurance that no message will be forgotten. The nature of the message will determine whether you must report it immediately. Figure 9–2 illustrates a model message log that can be adapted to the practice by inserting the patient symptoms and requests you hear most often. The person who completes the call must sign and date it. If the call is from a patient and relates in any way to the medical history, or if any instructions were given or queries answered, this information should be placed in the patient's chart. Message forms that have a self-adhesive backing and can be placed permanently in the patient's case history (Fig. 9–3) are readily available.

TAKING ACTION

The message procedure is not complete until the necessary action has been taken. Notations on the memo pad should be carried over to the following day if they have not been attended to. Just place an

TELEPHONE MESSAGE LOG

Date: _____ Time: _____ Taken by: _____

Caller: _____ Patient: _____ Age: _____
Phone # Day: _____ Evening: _____
Address: _____

Complaint: _____ How long: _____
Pain: _____ Location: _____
Any treatment: _____
Temperature: _____

____ Cough   ____ Lab results
____ Sore throat   ____ Rx refill
____ Vomiting   ____ Appointment
____ Diarrhea   ____ Insurance
____ Bleeding   ____ Billing

____ Return call   ____ Will call back

Message: _____

_____

_____

Action taken: _____ Date: _____ Signature: _____

FIGURE 9–2 Telephone message log.

"X" in front of the item and move it onto the next page. Sometimes a notation will be carried over for several days until action can be completed. Do not trust to memory messages unattended to from previous days; always carry them forward in writing.

Make brief notations of patients' reactions while you are talking to them on the telephone. The physician does not require a character study, but it is helpful to know when a patient appears fearful, apprehensive, or nervous. If a patient shows such symptoms, it may be wise to transfer the call to the physician.

When your employer is talking to another physician about a referral, you may sometimes be requested to take down a brief outline of the patient's case history by listening on the extension telephone. This information can be typewritten and incorporated with the patient's chart and handed to the physician before the patient is seen.

Memory Jogger

4 *List the seven bits of information that are basic in recording a telephone memorandum.*

Incoming Calls the Medical Assistant Can Handle

One reason for having a medical assistant answer the incoming calls is to spare the physician unnecessary interruptions during visits with patients. Addi-tionally, many calls relate to the administrative aspects of the office and can actually be better handled by the medical assistant. The policy regarding how calls are to be handled should be clearly set forth in the office procedure manual. Figure 9–4 shows how the instruction page might be arranged in the manual. Listed below are some kinds of calls that can be handled by the medical assistant in most offices.

NEW PATIENT AND RETURN APPOINTMENTS

Procedures for handling appointments for new patients and scheduling return appointments are discussed in the previous chapter.

INQUIRIES ABOUT BILLS

A patient may request to speak with the physician about a recent bill. Ask the caller to hold for a moment while you pull the ledger. If you find nothing irregular on the ledger, you can return to the telephone and say

"I have your account in front of me now. Perhaps I can answer your question."

Most likely, the caller will have some simple inquiry, such as

"Is that my total bill?"

"Has my insurance paid anything?"

"May I wait until next month to make a payment?"

Not all patients realize that the medical assistant

PRIORITY ☐

PATIENT	AGE
CALLER	
TELEPHONE	
REFERRED TO	
CHART #	
CHART ATTACHED ☐ YES ☐ NO	

DATE / /	TIME	REC'D BY

Copyright © 1978 Bibbero Systems, Inc.
Printed in the U.S.A.

TELEPHONE RECORD ☎

MESSAGE

		TEMP	ALLERGIES

RESPONSE

PHY/RN INITIALS	DATE / /	TIME	HANDLED BY

PRIORITY ☐

PATIENT	AGE
CALLER	
TELEPHONE	
REFERRED TO	
CHART #	
CHART ATTACHED ☐ YES ☐ NO	

DATE / /	TIME	REC'D BY

Copyright © 1978 Bibbero Systems, Inc.
Printed in the U.S.A.

TELEPHONE RECORD ☎

MESSAGE

		TEMP	ALLERGIES

RESPONSE

PHY/RN INITIALS	DATE / /	TIME	HANDLED BY

FIGURE 9–3 Message form with self-adhesive backing. (Courtesy of Bibbero Systems, Inc., Petaluma, California, (800) 242-2376, Fax (800) 242-9330.)

STANDARD PROCEDURE FOR TELEPHONE CALLS IN THE OFFICE OF

_____ :

CALLS THE ASSISTANT CAN HANDLE:

Appointments for New Patients

Office Administration Problems

CALLS TO BE PUT THROUGH IMMEDIATELY:

Calls from Other Physicians

Emergency Calls

CALLS TO BE REFERRED TO PHYSICIAN:

Unsatisfactory Progress Reports

Third Party Requests for Information

FIGURE 9–4 Page from procedure manual showing standard procedure for incoming telephone calls.

usually makes such decisions and is the best person with whom to discuss these matters.

INQUIRIES ABOUT FEES

In some offices, the medical assistant is instructed *not to quote fees.* For example, a caller may inquire

"How much does Dr. Arnold charge for an examination?"

He or she may not be pleased to hear

"That's impossible to say—it depends on how extensive an examination is required."

The following response is equally noncommittal but far more satisfying to the caller.

"Mr. Barker, the fee usually varies with the nature of the problem. An uncomplicated physical examination without any laboratory tests or x-rays might run as low as $ _____. On the other hand, the fee could be considerably higher if special tests are required."

If fees are regularly discussed on the telephone, write a suggested script in the policy manual. Do not be evasive. Have a schedule of fees available.

REQUESTS FOR INSURANCE ASSISTANCE

Not too many years ago, many patients completed and mailed their own insurance claims. In today's environment of managed care, copay, Medicaid, and Medicare, insurance claims will more than likely be completed and filed by the health care facility. Still, patients may call to inquire about their coverage or ask whether there has been any response to the filing of the claims. The medical assistant or a member of the staff whose sole responsibility is filing of insurance claims will have the knowledge to answer these inquiries.

RADIOLOGY AND LABORATORY REPORTS

Laboratory and radiologic findings may be telephoned to the physician's office on the day the procedures are performed when they are urgent. The medical assistant can take these reports and relay them to the physician. More often the report is faxed to the physician if it is a stat report. Original reports will be delivered by mail for the permanent record. Some facilities are equipped to receive laboratory results directly from the laboratory via computer and electronic media.

SATISFACTORY PROGRESS REPORTS FROM PATIENTS

Physicians sometimes ask a patient "Phone and let me know how you are feeling in a few days." The medical assistant can take such calls and relay the information to the physician if the report is satisfactory. Assure the patient that you will inform the physician about the call by saying, for example,

> "I will relay this information as soon as Dr. Wright is available."

ROUTINE REPORTS FROM HOSPITALS AND OTHER SOURCES

There may be routine calls from a hospital and other sources reporting a patient's progress. If it is only a reporting procedure, take the message carefully, make sure that the physician sees it, and then place the message in the patient's medical record.

OFFICE ADMINISTRATION MATTERS

Not all calls concern patients. There may be calls from the accountant or auditor or calls regarding banking procedures, office supplies, or office maintenance, most of which the medical assistant can handle or refer to the appropriate person. For some of these calls, the medical assistant may need to gather additional information and return the call.

REQUESTS FOR REFERRALS

Physicians who are liked and respected by their patients frequently will be called for referrals to other specialists. If the physician has furnished the medical assistant with a list of practitioners for this purpose, these inquiries can usually be handled without consulting the physician. However, the physician should always be informed of such requests.

PRESCRIPTION REFILLS

If the physician has placed a note on the patient's chart indicating that a prescription may be filled a certain number of times, the medical assistant can give an okay to the pharmacist after determining the number of times it has already been filled. This information should appear on the patient's chart, but it is always best to double check. If there is any

question, tell the pharmacist that you will have to check with the physician and call back.

Memory Jogger

5 *Name 10 categories of calls that a medical assistant should be able to handle without assistance.*

Incoming Calls That Require Transfer to the Physician or Call Back

PATIENTS WHO WILL NOT REVEAL SYMPTOMS

Occasionally, patients will call and wish to talk with the physician about symptoms that they are reluctant to discuss with a medical assistant. Do not make the mistake of pressing for details. Even though you may not be embarrassed, patients have the right to privacy. Put these calls through or offer to have the physician call back.

UNSATISFACTORY PROGRESS REPORTS

If a patient under treatment reports that he or she "still is not feeling well" or that the "prescription the doctor gave me makes me feel sick," do not try to practice medicine by telling the patient that this is to be expected. Even though you think the physician will say the same thing, the patient should hear it directly from the physician for reassurance.

REQUESTS FOR TEST RESULTS

When the physician orders special tests for the patient, the patient may be told to call the office in a couple of days for the results. Never assume that the patient will call for results. It is ultimately the responsibility of the physician to notify the patient of test results. Be certain that the physician has seen the results and has given you permission to tell the patient before giving out any information. Particularly if the result is unfavorable, the physician should be the one to inform the patient and give further instructions. This call must be handled tactfully; otherwise, the patient may get the feeling that you are concealing information.

Patients do not always understand that the medical assistant does not have the privilege of giving out information without the permission of the physician. You might answer an inquiry in this manner:

"Dr. Wright has not seen the report yet; will you please call back after 2 o'clock? I will try to have the information for you then."

Alternatively, you might offer to call the patient as soon as you have the necessary information. Never call the patient with laboratory results unless specifically directed to do so.

THIRD-PARTY REQUESTS FOR INFORMATION

If there is no legal requirement for disclosure of information, you must have the written permission of the patient before giving information to third-party callers. This includes insurance companies, attorneys, relatives, neighbors, employers, or any other third party.

COMPLAINTS ABOUT CARE OR FEES

You may be able to offer a satisfactory explanation to a patient who complains about the care he or she received or the fee charged. If a patient seems angry, you may say that it will take a few moments to pull the chart and offer to call back. This reassures the patient that someone is willing to talk about the problem and also gives the patient a chance to cool off. However, if you are unable to appease the patient easily, the physician would probably prefer to talk directly to the patient.

UNIDENTIFIED CALLERS

Although it will rarely happen, you will sometimes encounter individuals who refuse to give you their name or business but are insistent on speaking with the physician. Such callers frequently are salespersons who are fully aware that if their identity is revealed they will never get the opportunity to speak to the physician. Your own course in such instances is to say firmly,

"Dr. Jones is very busy with a patient and has asked me to take all messages. If you will not give me a message, I suggest you write a letter to Dr. Jones and mark it *personal*."

CALLS FROM FAMILY AND FRIENDS

Personal calls to the physician from family members or friends are handled in accordance with instructions from the physician. If the physician does not wish to take the calls, the medical assistant must deal with it. You can say,

"Dr. Wilson is with a patient now and cannot be disturbed. We are booked rather heavily this afternoon,

and you may have more time to talk with Dr. Wilson if you call at home this evening."

Occasional Situations

ANGRY CALLERS

No matter how efficient you are on the telephone or how well liked your employer may be, sooner or later you will have an angry caller on the line. There may be a legitimate reason for the anger, or it may have resulted from a misunderstanding. It is a real challenge to handle such calls. First, take the required action—even if it is to say that you will take the matter up with your employer as soon as possible and call back later. If answers are not readily available, a friendly assurance that you will find the answer and call back will usually calm the angry feelings.

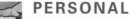 **PERSONAL QUALITIES**

HOW TO RESPOND TO AN ANGRY CALLER

- Avoid getting angry yourself.
- Try to find out what the real problem is.
- Provide the answers, if possible.
- Actively listen while you let the caller talk.
- Express interest and understanding.
- Do not pass the buck.
- Take careful notes.
- Maintain your own poise.

MONITORING CALLS

Occasionally you may be asked to **monitor** a telephone call. You will be expected to listen from an extension phone and take notes on the conversation. It is possible to record both sides of a telephone call by placing a tape recorder close to the telephone receiver. However, you should be aware that this is illegal unless the other person is told that the conversation is being recorded.

REQUESTS FOR HOUSE CALLS

Scheduling house calls is discussed in Chapter 10. In responding to a telephone request for a home visit, be sure to inquire as to the nature of the illness. Certain conditions are impossible to treat at home, and time will be saved if the patient is sent directly to the hospital where the doctor can meet him or

EMERGENCY CALL PROCEDURES

When the physician is not in the office, follow these emergency procedures:

Patient Complaint	Refer to Physician Below	Call RN	Call Paramedics	Have Patient	
				Go to Hospital	Come to Office
Severe bleeding Head injury Severe chest pain Broken bone Severe laceration Unconscious High fever Difficulty in breathing					

FIGURE 9–5 Form for instructions on emergency call procedures (when physician is not in office).

ASSISTANT'S GUIDE FOR HANDLING ROUTINE TELEPHONE CALLS	Refer immediately to physician	Physician will call back	Refer to clinical personnel: RN, CMA, PA	Other
New patient—ill and wants to talk to physician				
Established patient—wants to talk to physician				
Patient—request for lab results				
Family requesting patient information				
Patient or pharmacy—regarding Rx refill				
Another physician—wants to talk to physician				
Hospital—regarding a patient				
Insurance carrier or attorney requesting patient information				
Business calls for physician (attorney, accountant, broker)				
Professional society calls for physician				
Personal calls for physician (family, friends)				

FIGURE 9–6 The new assistant needs a guide for handling even routine calls.

her. Alternatively, you might urge the patient to come to the office. You can point out that the health care facility is better equipped to give the best medical care and that office visits are more economical.

Consult the physician, if possible, before scheduling a house call. In most cases, you can explain to the patient that you will check with the physician and call back immediately. If making the house call is not possible, you should attempt to find other assistance for the patient. It is easier for one of the office staff to call another physician than it is for the distraught patient to do so. One of the most common complaints of patients about the medical profession is that patients are unable to get help in an emergency. In communities that have paramedic teams, this is not such a problem.

RESPONDING TO EMERGENCY CALLS

The handling of telephone calls involving possible emergency situations is briefly discussed in Chapter 10. According to the American Medical Association's *The Business Side of Medical Practice:*

> Many emergency calls are judgment calls on the part of the person answering in the medical practice. Good judgment only comes from proper training by the physician in what constitutes a real emergency in your type of practice and how such calls should be handled. If you are not immediately available, what should your staff do?

The person answering the telephone should first determine, "Is it urgent?" If the physician is in, the call should probably be transferred immediately. Some plan for the action to be taken when the physician is not present should be agreed on (Fig. 9–5). The physician and medical assistant may also jointly develop typical questions to ask the caller to determine the validity and disposition of an emergency.

EXAMPLES OF QUESTIONS TO ASK TO DETERMINE AN EMERGENCY CALL

- At what telephone number can you be reached?
- What are the chief symptoms?
- When did they start?
- Has this happened before?
- Are you alone?
- Do you have transportation?

TRIAGE GUIDELINES

In the facility with multiple employees, the physician may designate one individual as the triage nurse or assistant. Within the environment of man-

aged care, the physician would be wise to have a written telephone protocol for handling urgent situations and emergencies. The protocol should state that the employees are bound by the written guidelines and that any giving of advice by unauthorized personnel may be grounds for dismissal.

A special sheet of instructions listing specific medical emergencies such as chest pain, heavy bleeding, fainting, seizure, and poisoning should be posted by each telephone. Include the phone number for the nearest poison control center, hospital, and ambulance. Such calls would be routed to a physician immediately. Additional instructions should include what action to take if no physician is available, for example, sending the patient to an emergency department or calling an ambulance or 911.

Routine but Troublesome Calls

Many of the so-called routine calls coming into the physician's office will be difficult for a new medical assistant to handle (Fig. 9–6). Although no stock answer can be phrased for these calls, a gracious and prompt reply paves the way for a quicker handling of a call, because it lets the caller know that you are capable, pleasant, and willing to offer assistance.

Following are a few typical calls that any medical assistant might receive:

APPOINTMENT CHANGES

THE CALL: "I have an appointment with the doctor this morning and I cannot keep it. May I come in this afternoon?"

THE ANSWER: Even though this type of call throws the appointment book into confusion, showing irritation with the patient will not help the situation. Make a sincere effort to help the caller make a new appointment.

STATEMENTS

THE CALL: "I received my statement this morning, and I don't understand why it is so high."

THE ANSWER: If billing matters are handled by another employee, tell the patient that you will transfer his or her call to the billing office. If you are responsible for billing, politely *ask the patient to hold the line* while you pull the patient ledger. When you return to the line, *thank the patient* for waiting and *explain the charges* carefully. If there is an error, apologize and say a corrected statement will be sent out at once. *Thank the patient for calling.* If patients are properly advised about charges at the time that services are rendered, the number of these calls will be considerably reduced.

PRESCRIPTION REFILL

THE CALL: "The last time I had an office visit, the doctor gave me a prescription for some sleeping tablets. Please call the druggist and okay a refill."

THE ANSWER: Ask the patient for the *prescription number and date,* the *name* and *telephone number of the pharmacy,* and the *patient's phone number.* Explain that you will give the message to the physician as soon as possible. Pull the patient's chart and have it ready with the message when the physician is available. If the physician okays the refill, you may be asked to phone the pharmacy and the patient with the information.

PHYSICIAN "SHOPPING"

THE CALL: "Does the doctor treat stomach trouble?"

THE ANSWER: The answer depends on the physician's field of practice. Many people do not understand the various medical specialties, and this call may come from a person referred to the physician by a friend who did not explain that your physician is an orthopedist. In situations in which your physician would be unable to handle the case, you may have to refer the patient to another physician. Give the patient the *names of at least three physicians,* when possible; these should be only names that your employer has had you place on the referral list. Do not presume to make a diagnosis when a patient calls in with bizarre complaints; transfer the call to the physician or take the caller's name and number and have the physician return the call later.

UNAUTHORIZED INQUIRY

THE CALL: "My next-door neighbor is a patient of the doctor's, and I am quite concerned about her. Could you tell me what is wrong with her?"

THE ANSWER: Confidentiality is a legal and ethical issue here. It is not the role of the medical assistant to give out any information about a patient's condition, except information that the physician has specifically okayed for release. The caller in this case may be merely curious or may actually be a kindly neighbor who wishes to help a friend. Your possible response might be

"I'm unable to answer your question because information about a patient cannot be released without that person's authorization. I will relay your message of concern to the doctor if you wish."

Telephone Answering Services

Because a physician's telephone is an all-important tool of the practice, it must be constantly *covered;* that is, there must be someone to answer it at all times—day and night, weekends and holidays. This presents no problem during weekdays, but nights and weekends require special attention. Most physicians subscribe to telephone answering services that provide round-the-clock coverage. Alternatively, the physician may use an automatic answering device.

OPERATOR-ANSWERED SERVICES

There are two types of operator-answered services.

Type 1

Doctor-subscribers leave messages with, or obtain patients' messages from, a service whose number appears in the local telephone directory in this way,

After _____ PM, call _____ (number) *or*
If no answer, call _____ (number).

Such listings are placed immediately below the physician's own telephone number in the directory. This form of service is somewhat inconvenient for the patient but is far better than no coverage at all.

Type 2

The answering service has a direct connection with the office telephone. When the telephone rings in the physician's office or at home, it also signals on the switchboard of the answering service. As long as the telephone is ringing, it will continue to signal at the answering service. If no one answers within a certain agreed-on number of rings, the answering service operator takes the call. This method provides continuous live telephone coverage.

Even during the day, such an answering service can function effectively. There may be times when you are assisting the physician and it is impossible for you or anyone else to answer the telephone. Not answering the telephone is extremely poor policy, but if you have an agreement with the answering service (sometimes referred to as "the exchange"), its operators will accept calls for you in such situations. With this direct-wire answering method, the operator answers the telephone in your employer's name, as you would in the office, explaining "This is Dr. Wilson's exchange. May I take a message?"

The answering service will greatly appreciate your cooperation if you call them every day before leaving the office and tell them where the physician will be during the evening or give them other special messages. Then, in the morning when you return to the office, call the exchange and ask for any messages they may have taken. Usually there will be messages from patients who called after office hours but whose calls were not urgent enough to merit an emergency call to the doctor. An exchange can act as a buffer for the physician and help eliminate too frequent, unnecessary calls during the late evening or night hours.

Here is how the system works: During the hours that the office is closed, the exchange will answer the telephone, take a message, and relay it to the physician. If it is urgent, the physician will then return the call to the patient; if not, the exchange will call the patient and explain that the physician will call the first thing in the morning. Emergency calls, of course, are immediately put through by the exchange to the doctor.

Occasionally, it is a good idea to check up on your answering service by placing a few random calls at various hours. It may be that now and then the service does not answer the calls or the response may not meet your standards. The service may be enhanced by inviting the manager of the answering service in to see the office or by the medical assistant going to the exchange facility to meet with the manager and staff. This personal contact frequently improves the rapport and quality of service you may expect.

ELECTRONIC ANSWERING DEVICES

Some physicians use an answering device after office hours. Callers who dial the office number hear a recorded message either telling them how to reach the physician (or a colleague who may be covering the practice) or inviting the caller to leave a message. The caller's message is recorded for later checking by the physician or a staff member.

Most electronic answering devices are equipped with remote control to allow the subscriber to operate them from any Touch-Tone telephone. By using a personal code number, it is possible to

- Retrieve messages, including the times at which they were recorded
- Reset the tape for future messages
- Change the outgoing message when necessary

VOICE MAIL

Voice mail is a computer system that operates much like the answering devices that we have incorporated into our home telephone systems. In large facilities it is an integral part of the private system. For individuals or small groups voice mail is available by subscribing to a service. By dialing a personal code, the subscriber can record, send, or receive messages.

AUTOMATIC ROUTING

The call is answered by an automated operator that presents a list of options, such as *If you are calling about your account, push 1; to make an appointment, push 2;* and so forth. The impersonal nature of auto-

mation does not lend itself well to answering the telephone in a private physician's office, but the medical assistant will encounter it frequently when placing outgoing calls.

Placing Outgoing Calls

PREPLANNING THE CALL

Before placing a call, make certain you have the correct telephone number and the information you will need during the call at your fingertips.

If you are reporting a patient's history, have the complete record before you, including all the latest laboratory and radiology reports.

If you are placing a call to order supplies, have the catalog in front of you, along with any previous order sheets or invoices. Also have a list of the items desired, the specifications for the items, and any questions you may have regarding them.

Apply this rule to every call you make. You will save a great deal of time and prevent errors.

PLACING THE CALL

Lift the receiver, listen for the dial tone, and then start dialing your number. It sometimes happens that just as you pick up the telephone to place a call, an incoming call has reached your line but you lifted the receiver before the telephone had time to ring. If you start dialing without listening for the dial tone, you will not only fail to reach your number, you will have offended the ear of the party trying to reach you.

CALLING ETIQUETTE

When placing a call, at your employer's request, to a patient or any other person, your physician should be ready to speak as soon as the call goes through. Physicians, because of their busy schedules, sometimes are negligent in this respect. The telephone company's courtesy rule is that the person placing the call should be on the line and ready to speak when the called party answers.

If you are calling a patient to change an appointment, be ready to offer a new appointment time. Also, give the patient a logical reason for the inconvenience of having to change the original appointment. This change may cause considerable disruption of plans, and the patient is fully entitled to an explanation.

Remember that if your telephone is within hearing range of office patients, you should be careful when mentioning names or diagnoses.

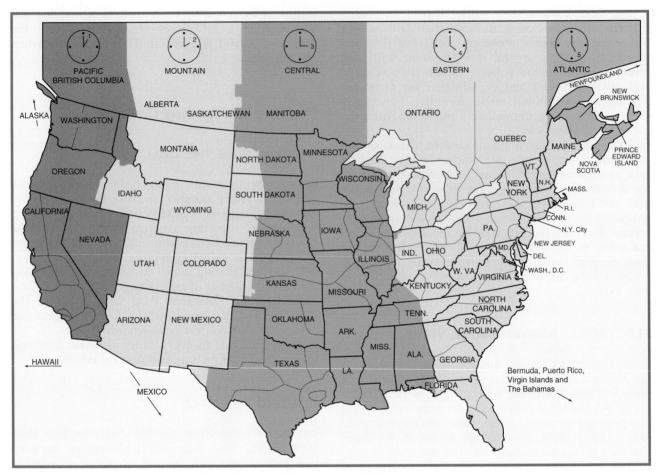

FIGURE 9–7 Time zones across the United States.

LONG DISTANCE SERVICE

Long distance calls are simple to place, inexpensive, and efficient. When information is needed in a hurry, it is much more expedient to telephone rather than wait for an exchange of letters.

Before placing a long distance call, have the correct number ready. This number often may be obtained from a letterhead or from other records. If you do not have the number, you may obtain directory assistance by dialing the area code of the party you are calling, followed by 555-1212. In some areas you must dial 1 before the area code. Directory assistance is now an automated service and you will be asked for the name of the city and the person you are calling.

TIME ZONES

The continental United States is divided into four standard time zones: Pacific, Mountain, Central, and Eastern (Fig. 9–7). When it is noon Pacific time, it is 3 PM Eastern time. If you are calling from San Francisco to New York, you will probably plan to make the call no later than 2 PM when calling a business or professional office. When it is 2 PM on the West Coast it is 5 PM on the East Coast.

DIALING DIRECT

By dialing your own long distance calls, you will pay the lowest rate and pay for only the minutes you talk (minimum, 1 minute). Use direct dialing when you are willing to talk with anyone who answers the phone and you want the call charged to the number from which you are calling.

OPERATOR-ASSISTED CALLS

Operator-assisted calls include calls such as

- Person-to-person
- Bill to a third party
- Collect calls
- Requests for time and charges
- Certain calls placed from hotels

There is a 1-minute initial period charge through most servers. The rates are equal to the direct-dial rates plus a service charge.

INTERNATIONAL SERVICE

International Direct Distance Dialing (IDDD) is available in many areas. International dialing codes are the same for all companies offering IDDD. Depending on your long distance company, additional numbers or codes may preface the international access, country, and city codes. IDDD is still not available in all areas. If it is available, you may place international station-to-station calls by dialing in sequence

1. International Code 011
2. Country Code
3. City Code
4. Local telephone number
5. # button if your telephone is Touch-Tone

If you were to place a call to London you would dial:

International Access Code		Country Code		City Code
011	+	44	+	1

plus the local telephone number and # if Touch-Tone dialing

After dialing any international code, allow at least 45 seconds for the ringing to start.

WRONG NUMBERS

One slip in direct distance dialing can give you Los Angeles or New York instead of Dallas. If you reach a wrong number when dialing long distance, be sure to obtain the name of the city and state you have reached. By reporting this information promptly to the operator in your own city, you will not be charged for the call. If you are cut off before terminating your call, this, too, should be reported to the operator, who will either reconnect your call or make an adjustment of the charge.

CONFERENCE CALLS

Conference telephone service is of great value to the medical profession in notifying and explaining to a family how a patient is progressing. It has exceptional value in family conferences, at which a quick decision by the entire family regarding a patient's condition is required.

This service can connect from 3 to 14 points for a two-way conference in which each person can hear or talk to all others participating. Conference calls may be local or long distance. Charges are added for the number of places connected, mileage, and the length of the conversation.

To place a call, dial the operator and say you wish to make a conference call. Give the operator the names and telephone numbers of the people you want to connect. If prior arrangements are made with all parties, there is a better chance of reaching everyone at a given time.

Telephone Equipment and Services

NUMBER AND PLACEMENT OF TELEPHONES

Familiarity with a multiple-line telephone is a must for the medical assistant. Few health care facilities can get along with just one telephone line. Two incoming lines along with a private outgoing line with a separate number for the physician's exclusive use is the minimum recommended.

One medical assistant can handle no more than two incoming lines, so the addition of more lines may also involve additional staffing. If there is a staff member assigned solely to dealing with insurance and billing, a separate line and listing in the telephone directory for this service may considerably lessen the load on the main incoming lines.

Telephones should be placed where they are accessible but private. Rather than placing telephones in the examining rooms, many practices have a wall telephone placed near a stand-up desk top outside the examining room. Some facilities place a telephone in the reception room for the convenience of patients and to prevent their asking to use the facility's phones.

Recent trends suggest a separate telephone line with a limited calling area for the convenience of patients who need to call out. This telephone should not be in the reception room but in an area available to patients on request. It should be placed low enough for use by patients in wheelchairs. Wherever possible, telephones should be placed on the wall to conserve desk space.

EQUIPMENT SELECTION

Selection of telephone equipment and services offers many options. The *six-button key set* with several incoming lines, an intercom line, and a hold button has been the standard business phone for decades. It is still being used in many offices. Lights within the buttons flash slowly for incoming calls and blink rapidly to remind of calls being held; a steady light indicates that the line is in use.

A popular modern system is the two-line speaker phone that has distinctive ringing and flashing indicators that let you know which line is receiving a call. It also has other features, including:

- Last number redial
- Volume control on the receiver, ringer, and speaker

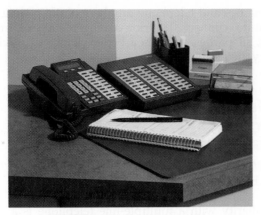

FIGURE 9–8   Multi-line telephone.

- Memory for frequently dialed numbers
- Intercom paging

Another available feature, *ring back on HOLD*, allows the caller who dials a busy number to place it on hold. When the called line is free, the connection is completed and the caller is reminded.

Larger facilities tend to select small switchboard-type equipment. One system can start with as few as 2 lines and 6 extensions and expand to a maximum of 8 outside lines and 24 extensions (Fig. 9–8).

HEADSETS

A popular headset is a very lightweight plastic earphone and microphone combination that allows the wearer to move about the room and to have the hands free. One brand name is StarSet. Originally designed for the astronauts, it weighs less than 1 ounce and is worn behind the ear or clipped to the wearer's glasses. The headset can be equipped with a cord up to 10 feet long for easy mobility. It also has an optional quick-disconnect feature that allows the user to separate the headset even during a call without breaking the connection.

FACSIMILE (FAX) MACHINES

A FAX machine can be a great time and labor saver in conveying patient information from physician to physician or from physician to hospital. It allows its user to send and receive copies of printed documents over telephone lines to other facilities that have FAX machines. Most offices find this machine indispensable. Unless precautions are taken to ensure security of information arriving by FAX, there is some danger of loss of confidentiality. When sending sensitive material it is wise to telephone ahead to alert the receiver that this information will be arriving so that the appropriate person will be on hand to receive it (Fig. 9–9).

CELLULAR PHONES AND PAGERS

Many physicians have a mobile phone installed in their automobiles for communication with their office or the hospital while they are traveling by car. Most carry a personal pager that can be activated by the medical assistant or the answering service by calling a special number.

Using the Telephone Directory

The primary purpose of the telephone directory, of course, is to provide lists of those who have telephones, their telephone numbers, and, in most cases, their addresses. Additionally, the directory is an aid in checking the spelling of names and in locating certain types of businesses (through the yellow pages). Some directories are color coded (e.g., residences are on white pages, business numbers on pink pages, business by categories and advertisements on yellow pages). Directories are usually organized into three sections:

- Introductory pages
- Alphabetical pages (white pages)
- Yellow pages

The introductory pages are sometimes entirely overlooked by the subscribers. This section precedes the white alphabetic pages and provides basic information concerning the telephone services in the area, including

- Emergency services (fire, police, ambulance, and highway patrol)
- Service calls
- Dialing instructions for local and out-of-town calls
- Area codes for some cities

The introductory pages may also include

- A survival guide
- Community service numbers
- Prefix locations

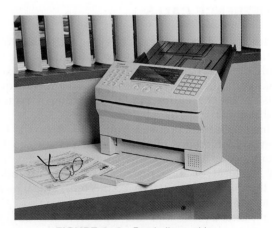

FIGURE 9–9   Facsimile machine.

- Rates
- Long distance calling information
- International calling information
- Time zones
- Government listings

Some directories include ZIP code maps for the local area. Take a few moments to familiarize yourself with your local directory; then use it frequently for getting information fast.

The white pages are an alphabetical listing of telephone subscribers with their telephone numbers and, in most cases, their addresses.

The yellow pages directory, sometimes published separately, contains listings for businesses arranged by the product or services they sell. Physicians are listed alphabetically, usually under the heading *Physicians and Surgeons,* and have the option of another listing by type of practice.

In some metropolitan areas, a street address telephone directory is published that is arranged by street address, followed by the name and telephone number of the person or business at that address.

Organizing a Personal Telephone Directory

Organize your telephone numbers in an indexed 3 × 5-inch desktop file or a rotary file. Emergency numbers might be typed on a colored card or flagged with a color tab. Your personal directory of telephone numbers should include all the numbers that you frequently call.

FREQUENTLY CALLED NUMBERS

- Specialists to whom your employer refers patients
- Professional facilities, such as hospitals, the Poison Control Center, pharmacies, ambulance companies, and laboratories
- Special duty nurses, along with their specialties and other pertinent information
- Administrative contacts, such as stationers, equipment dealers and repair services, laundry and maintenance services, and surgical supply houses
- Personal numbers, such as the physician's family, special friends, insurance agent, stockbroker, accountant, and lawyer

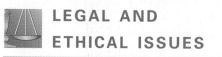

LEGAL AND ETHICAL ISSUES

Use discretion when mentioning the name of a caller. All communications in a health care facility are confidential. Discourage personal phone calls. Encourage friends and family to call you at home. When answering an incoming call, identify the facility and then yourself. Transfer calls from other physicians at once if possible. If you are requested to furnish names of other specialists, refer these requests to the physician unless you have been given a list of preferred practitioners from which to choose. When a patient calls for results of a test, the physician should be the one to inform the patient unless you have been given permission to do so. Never give unfavorable results to a patient over the telephone.

CRITICAL THINKING

1 Develop a dialogue for responding to a telephone call from a patient who is complaining about a fee.

2 Use a situation to illustrate the meaning of triage.

HOW DID I DO? Answers to Memory Joggers

1 Smile

2 Seven of these 12 rules:
Answer promptly.
Visualize the persons to whom you are speaking.
Hold the instrument correctly.
Develop a pleasing telephone voice.
Identify your office and yourself.
Identify the caller.
Offer assistance.
Screen incoming calls.
Minimize waiting time.
Identify the caller when transferring a call.
When answering a second call, identify the caller, then return to the first call.
End each call pleasantly and graciously.

3 One minute

4 Name of person to whom call is directed
Name of the person calling
Caller's daytime telephone number
Reason for the call
Action to be taken
Date and time of the call
Your initials

5 New patient and return appointments
Inquiries about bills
Inquiries about fees
Requests for insurance assistance
Radiology and laboratory reports
Satisfactory progress reports from patients
Routine reports from hospitals and other sources
Office administration matters
Requests for referrals
Prescription refills

Appointment Scheduling and Time Management

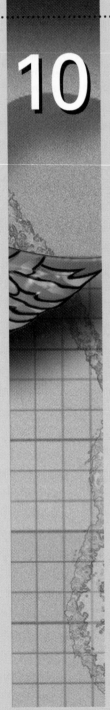

10

LEARNING OBJECTIVES

Cognitive: On successful completion of this chapter, you should be able to:

1 Define and spell the terms listed in the Vocabulary.
2 Describe four important features of an appointment book.
3 List and explain the three basic guidelines to follow in scheduling appointments.
4 Identify and discuss the advantages of wave scheduling.
5 Cite three common situations that would require adjusting the appointment schedule.
6 Describe how you would determine whether a request for an appointment is an emergency.
7 State the reason for recording a failed appointment in the patient's chart.

8 Discuss the handling of cancellations and delays brought about by office situations.

9 List the seven points of information that will be necessary in scheduling surgery with a hospital.

10 State four items of information that must be available before arranging an outside laboratory appointment for a patient.

Performance: On successful completion of this chapter, you should be able to:

1 Select an appropriate appointment book to suit a given type of practice.

2 Demonstrate the advance preparation that must be done before using a new appointment book.

3 Schedule patients according to the urgency of their complaints and the anticipated treatment time.

4 Rearrange the schedule in the event that the physician's arrival is delayed.

5 Explain the physician's unavailability to patients in the reception room.

6 Arrange a referral appointment for a patient.

7 Schedule a patient for a diagnostic test as indicated by the physician.

8 Schedule a surgery with the hospital, notifying all the persons and departments concerned.

9 Instruct a patient regarding preadmission requirements, hospital stay, and insurance information needed.

10 Arrange for a patient's admission to a hospital as ordered by the physician.

VOCABULARY

disruption A breaking down or upset

expediency A situation requiring haste or caution

integral Essential; being an indispensable part of a whole

interaction A two-way communication

intermittent Coming and going at intervals, not continuous

matrix Something in which something else originates, develops, takes shape, or is contained; a base upon which to build

no-show A person who fails to keep an appointment without giving advance notice of that failure

proficiency Competency as a result of training and practice

socioeconomic Relating to a combination of social and economic factors

stat report An immediate report (from the Latin *statim,* meaning "at once"

tickler (file) A chronologic file used as a reminder that something must be taken care of on a certain date

triage Responding to requests for immediate care and treatment after evaluating the urgency of the need and prioritizing the treatment

---

The most valuable asset within a medical practice is the physician's time. It follows that the person who schedules this time must understand the practice, be familiar with the working habits of the physicians, and have clear guidelines for time management within the practice.

Management of Office Hours

Appointment scheduling is the process that determines which patients will be seen by the physician, dates and times of the appointments, and how much time will be allotted to each patient based on his or her complaint and the practitioner's availability. Time management involves the realization that there will always be unforeseen interruptions and delays. Most providers of medical care find that efficient scheduling of appointments is one of the most important factors in the success of the practice. There are many approaches to scheduling and each facility must find what suits it best.

OPEN OFFICE HOURS

Few health care facilities in metropolitan areas have open office hours with no *scheduled* appointments, but this system is still found in some rural areas, where the way of life is governed not so much by the clock as by the sun and the seasons. With *open office hours*, the facility is open at given hours of the day or evening, and the patients are "scheduled" by the physician or the medical assistant by saying something such as, "Come back in a couple of weeks." At a convenient time, the patients come in, knowing in advance that they will be seen in their order of arrival. Physicians who use this method say that it eliminates the annoyance of broken appointments and of the office "running late." The open office hours method has been referred to as *tidal wave scheduling*. There can be many disadvantages to open office hours:

- The office may already be crowded when the physician arrives, resulting in extremely long waits for some patients.
- There is danger of rushing some patients through without giving them full attention.
- Few, or possibly no, patients will arrive before noon, and both the physician and the staff will need to stay late to accommodate everyone.
- Without planning, the facilities as well as the staff can be overburdened.

Other types of practices that have open hours are emergency centers, many of which are open on a 24-hour basis. Although they are frequently referred to as "emergicenters," they may in reality deal with many general practice types of care.

SCHEDULED APPOINTMENTS

Studies have shown that practitioners are able to see more patients with less pressure when their appointments are scheduled. If appointments are made by telephone, that first telephone interaction creates the patient's impression of the practice (Fig. 10–1). Un-

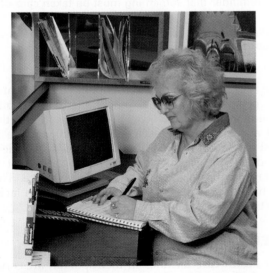

FIGURE 10–1 Receptionist with appointment book.

fortunately, the skill required for the scheduling of appointments is often not fully appreciated by the practitioner or practice manager, resulting in this responsibility being delegated to perhaps the least qualified medical assistant. But while the skill and attitude of the assistant who manages the appointment schedule is very important, the ultimate success of the system lies in the cooperation of the practitioner(s).

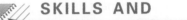

SKILLS AND RESPONSIBILITIES

GUIDELINES FOR EFFICIENT SCHEDULING

Understand the nature of the practice.
Consider the personality and habits of the medical staff.
Be aware of the time needed for each patient.
The key to planning appointments efficiently is planning realistically.
Scheduling with this in mind (1) pleases the patients, (2) results in economic gain, and (3) ensures a more regular schedule for the staff and the physicians.

FLEXIBLE OFFICE HOURS

Most scheduling practices are carryovers from the days when expectant mothers or families with young children relied on one wage earner—the father. Today, families commonly have two working parents. As a result, many health care providers, especially family practice, pediatricians, obstetricians, gynecologists, and ophthalmologists, are turning to *extended-day* and *flexible office hours*. Staff hours are affected by these changes.

EXAMPLE OF A FACILITY'S SCHEDULE	
Monday	7 AM–3 PM
Tuesday	8 AM–5 PM
Wednesday	8 AM–5 PM
Thursday	NOON–8 PM
Friday	8 AM–5 PM

Evening and weekend hours are frequently scheduled, as well. With a schedule such as this, a variety of options are made available to patients.

Memory Jogger

1 *Why is efficient scheduling of patient appointments so important? What one factor most influences the success of the scheduling?*

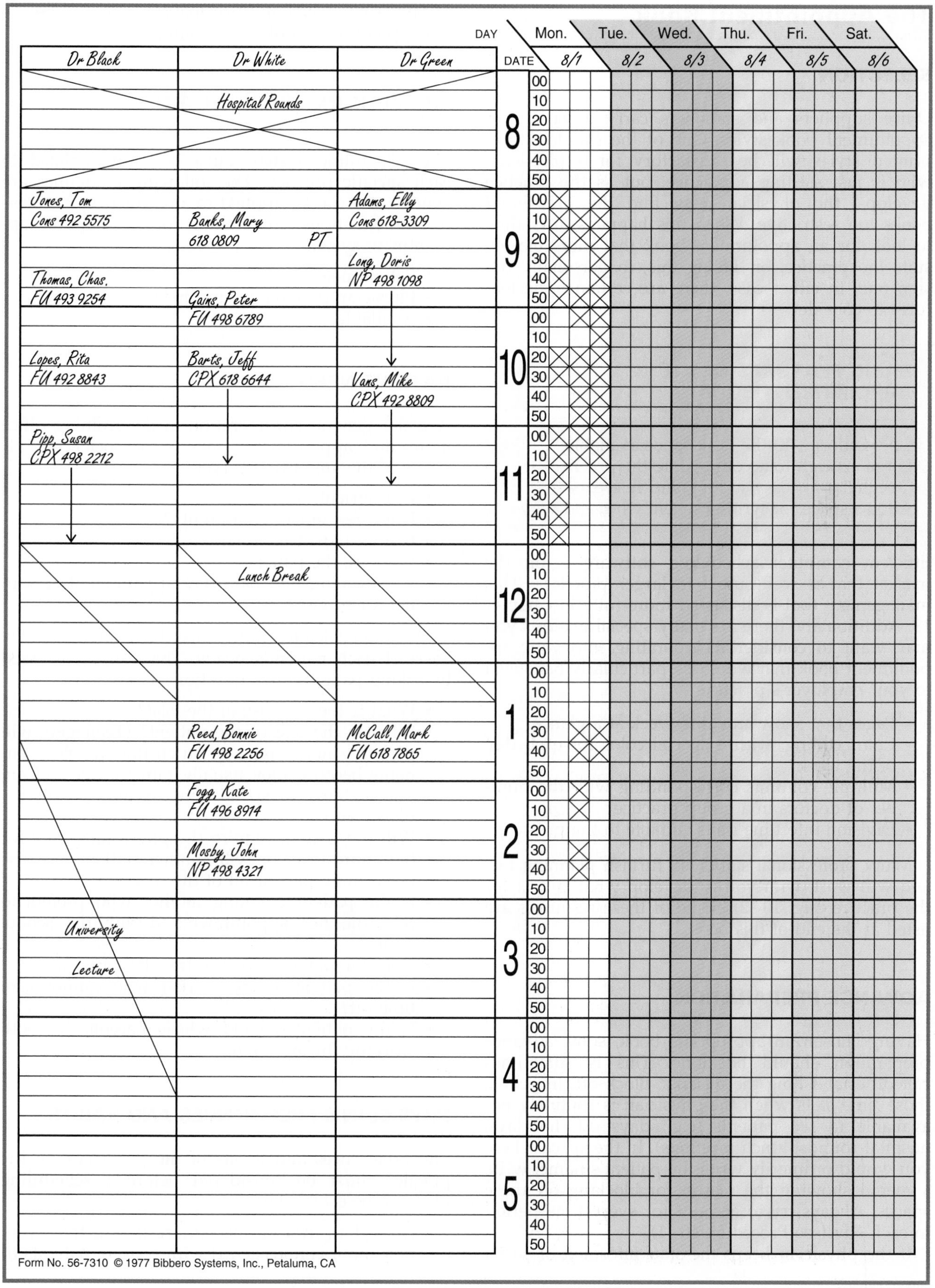

Dr Black	Dr White	Dr Green	DAY	Mon. 8/1	Tue. 8/2	Wed. 8/3	Thu. 8/4	Fri. 8/5	Sat. 8/6

8 — Hospital Rounds

9
Jones, Tom — Cons 492 5575
Banks, Mary — 618 0809 — PT
Adams, Elly — Cons 618-3309
Long, Doris — NP 498 1098
Thomas, Chas. — FU 493 9254
Gains, Peter — FU 498 6789

10
Lopes, Rita — FU 492 8843
Barts, Jeff — CPX 618 6644
Vans, Mike — CPX 492 8809

11
Pipp, Susan — CPX 498 2212

12 — Lunch Break

1
Reed, Bonnie — FU 498 2256
McCall, Mark — FU 618 7865

2
Fogg, Kate — FU 496 8914
Mosby, John — NP 498 4321

3 — University Lecture

4

5

Form No. 56-7310 © 1977 Bibbero Systems, Inc., Petaluma, CA

FIGURE 10–2 Sample appointment book. (Courtesy of Bibbero Systems, Inc., Petaluma, California, (800) 242-2376, Fax (800) 242-9330.)

The Appointment Book

SELECTION

Office suppliers and stationers carry a variety of appointment book styles. One of the standard pre-printed styles will be satisfactory for a physician who is just starting a practice, but as the practice develops, the physician may find the preprinted books too restrictive. When this happens, it is time to look for an appointment book that more closely suits the practice, or, failing this, to personally design one. In either case, there are certain basic features to consider.

BASIC FEATURES OF AN APPOINTMENT BOOK

Size conforms to the desk space available
Large enough to accommodate the practice
Opens flat for easy writing and reference
Allows space for writing when, who, and why

Efficient computer scheduling software is on the market that is well suited to larger practices. This management tool is discussed more fully in Chapter 13. Additionally, there are many special features you may want to consider incorporating into your appointment book that would be particularly beneficial to your employer's practice.

- Pages that show an entire week at a glance
- Color coding, with a special color for each day of the week
- Multiple columns corresponding with the number of doctors in a group practice
- Division into time units suitable to the practice

Many professional stationers furnish planning kits and will work with you to develop what is best for the practice (Fig. 10–2). Some of these resources are listed at the end of this book.

ADVANCE PREPARATION

Having chosen an appropriate book, some advance preparation should be done. This is sometimes called "establishing the matrix." Block off, in pencil, those time slots when the physician is routinely not available to see patients (e.g., days off, holidays, hospital rounds, lunch meetings). In the space where you would ordinarily write the patient's name, write a memo showing the reason for blocking off these spaces. Always try to account for every time period in each day (see Procedure 10–1).

If the physician keeps the staff informed of social

or family engagements, also make a note of these on the appointment book as a reminder.

Guidelines for Scheduling

The scheduling system must be individualized to each specific practice. The following guidelines are general and can be applied to any practice. All these recommendations are similar for a computer appointment system.

- Patient need
- Physician preferences and habits
- Available facilities

PATIENT NEED

A major general consideration in determining office hours and appointment times is the socioeconomic status of the area being served.

- Is it agricultural?
- Is it a retirement community?
- Is it an industrial area?
- Who are the patients?
- Are evening and Saturday appointments essential for some?

More specifically, time must be allotted on the basis of each patient's needs. This can be assessed by asking patients such questions as

- What is the purpose of the visit?
- What is the age of the patient? (Teenagers will probably not require as much time as older patients because they usually move faster and are less inclined to spend time speaking with the physician.)
- Will the patient require the physician's time for the entire visit, or will another staff member be performing part or all of the service?
- Is the patient a young mother who prefers to schedule her appointments during the school hours?
- Does the patient object to traveling after dark?
- Is the patient a day worker who cannot take time off?
- Is the patient a child whose parents are both working during the day?

PHYSICIAN'S PREFERENCES AND HABITS

The preferences and habits of the physicians in the practice must be considered before a scheduling plan can be established.

- Does the physician become restless if the reception room is not packed with waiting patients or

PROCEDURE 10-1
Preparing and Maintaining the Appointment Book

GOAL
To establish the matrix of the appointment page, arrange appointments for 1 day, and enter information according to office policy

EQUIPMENT AND SUPPLIES
Page from appointment book
Office policy for office hours, and
    doctor' availability
Clerical supplies

Calendar
Description of patients to be
    scheduled

PROCEDURAL STEPS

1 Determine the hours that the physician will not be available.
    PURPOSE: To block out those hours on the appointment page.

2 Establish the matrix of the appointment page for the day.
    PURPOSE: To leave available only those time slots that can be used for patient appointments.

3 Identify each patient's complaint.
    PURPOSE: This information is necessary in allotting time and space for the appointment.

4 Consult guidelines to determine the length of time necessary for each patient.

5 Allot appointment time according to the complaint and facilities available.

6 Enter information in the appointment book.
    NOTE: A telephone number must follow the patient's name. If the patient is new, add the letters N.P. (new patient) after his or her name.

7 Allow buffer time in the morning and afternoon.
    PURPOSE: To allow the physician and staff a short rest period and catch-up time.

---

does the physician worry if even one patient is kept waiting?

- Is the physician methodical and careful about being in the facility when patient appointments are scheduled to begin, or is the physician habitually late?
- Does the physician move easily from one patient to the next, or does the physician require a "break time" between patients?
- Would the physician rather see fewer patients and spend more time with each one?

All of these preferences and habits become an **integral** part of the scheduling process.

Keep in mind that the physician cannot spend every moment of the day with patients. There are telephone calls to make and receive, reports to examine and dictate, meetings to attend, mail to answer, and many other business items that require the physician's attention. The experienced staff can handle many, but not all, of these tasks.

AVAILABLE FACILITIES

There is no point in getting a patient into the office at a time when no facilities are available for the services needed. For example, suppose that in a two-physician office there is only one room that can be used for minor surgery. You would not schedule two patients requiring minor surgery for the same time block even though both doctors could be available. If there is only one electrocardiograph, you would not book two electrocardiograms at the same time. As you gain proficiency in scheduling, you should be able to pair patients' needs with the available facilities.

Memory Jogger

2 *What are the three basic guidelines that determine the system of scheduling? Why are they important?*

APPOINTMENT TIME ANALYSIS

NAME	ARRIVED	BEGIN TREATMENT	END TREATMENT	SERVICE CODE

SUMMARY

SERVICE	AVERAGE WAITING TIME	AVERAGE TREATMENT TIME

FIGURE 10–3 Form for determining appointment pattern.

Planning a Time Pattern

The physician is the person who should decide how much time each type of visit usually requires, and an estimated time schedule should be posted at the appointment desk. The physician who has been in practice for years knows how much time he or she needs for the various kinds of office visits: complete physical, presurgery workup, well-child visit, eye examination, and so forth. However, because a physician's timing does change through the years owing to experience or changes in the practice, an annual review of the scheduling pattern should be made to accommodate these changes as well as changes in the patient profile.

It may be that a time pattern has never been determined. The medical assistant can do the preliminary work on this through an informal practice analysis, noting the arrival time, treatment or conference time, departure time, and service performed (Fig. 10–3). After a few weeks, a definite time pattern should be distinguishable for each type of service. When possible, smooth out the schedule by having some long and some short appointments and go over the schedule with the physician at the beginning of each day.

BUFFER TIME

Every medical practice should have at least one, or preferably two, appointment slots open each day. These slots are usually referred to as *buffer time*. Family practitioners may leave as much as 25% of

their time open for emergencies and walk-in patients. Many find that reserving one time slot at the end of the morning and one at the end of the afternoon works well and causes the least **disruption** of a schedule.

Time studies have shown that in the average medical practice, Mondays and Fridays are the most hectic days of the week. Patients may have waited the whole weekend to call for an appointment and expect to be seen immediately on Monday. Similarly, toward the end of the week, small problems that could magnify if left unattended over the weekend may prompt anxious emergencies on Friday. Consequently, incorporating more buffer time on these 2 days can be worthwhile.

Time Management

WAVE SCHEDULING

Many scheduling systems lack flexibility. *Wave scheduling* is an attempt to include short-term flexibility within each hour by allowing for such variables as

- Late arrival of one patient
- A patient who needs more time or less time than expected
- Failed appointments
- Unscheduled interruptions

When all patients are assigned the same length of time, for instance, 20 minutes each, the schedule might look like this:

**EXAMPLE OF WAVE SCHEDULING
APPOINTMENTS EVERY 20 MINUTES**

10:00 Barker, Alicia
10:20 Davies, Colleen
10:40 Farber, Edna
11:00 Havens, Gertrude
11:20 Jackson, Irene
11:40 Lambert, Katherine

Barker, the first patient is late, arriving at 10:15. The physician has already lost 15 minutes. The patient needs 25 minutes instead of the allotted 20 minutes.

Davies, the second patient, also arrived at 10:15, five minutes early for her appointment, but is kept waiting until 10:40, the time that Farber, the third patient, was to have been seen.

Farber is on time but will also be kept waiting. Fortunately, Davies actually needs only 10 minutes, so Farber can be seen at 10:50, but if she requires the allotted 20 minutes, Havens, the fourth patient, will also have to wait, and so on throughout the day.

Wave scheduling assumes that the actual time needed will average out. If the average time is 20 minutes per patient, three patients will be scheduled for each hour and will be seen in order of arrival. Thus, one person's late arrival will not disrupt the entire schedule. The appointment schedule would then look like this:

**EXAMPLE OF WAVE SCHEDULING
AVERAGING OUT**

10:00 Barker, Alicia
　　　 Davies, Colleen
　　　 Farber, Edna
11:00 Havens, Gertrude
　　　 Jackson, Irene
　　　 Lambert, Katherine

Given the circumstances illustrated above, Davies would have arrived first (5 minutes early), Farber would be next (on time), and Barker would be third (15 minutes late). All could have been seen within the hour, with no delay affecting the patients scheduled for the next hour.

MODIFIED WAVE SCHEDULING

There are several ways of modifying the wave schedule. One method is to have two patients scheduled to come in at 10:00 and the third at 10:30, with this hourly cycle repeated throughout the day. Another application is to have patients scheduled to arrive at given intervals during the first half of the hour, and none scheduled to arrive during the second half of the hour.

DOUBLE BOOKING

Booking two patients to come in at the same time, both of whom are to be seen by the physician, is poor practice. Of course, if each is expected to take only 5 minutes or so, there is no harm in telling both to come at 2:00 and in reserving a 15-minute period for the two. This is one application of wave scheduling. However, if each patient requires 15 minutes, two will require 30 minutes; this should be reflected in the scheduling. It is not considered double booking if a patient comes to the office to receive a treatment or injection from a member of the staff other than the physician.

GROUPING PROCEDURES

Another method of time management that appeals to some practitioners is the grouping or *categorization* of procedures

---

EXAMPLES OF GROUPING CATEGORIES

An internist might reserve all morning appointments for complete physical examinations.

A surgeon whose practice depends on referrals might reserve 1 day of each week or specific hours of each day for referrals.

A pediatrician might have well-baby hours.

By experimenting with different groupings, the plan that works best for the practice will eventually become evident. In applying a grouping system of appointments, the medical assistant may find it helpful to lightly color-code those sections of the appointment book being reserved for special procedures.

ADVANCE BOOKING

When booking appointments weeks or months ahead, make it a policy to leave some open time during each day's schedule. Then, if a patient calls with a special problem that is not an immediate emergency, you will be able to book the patient for at least a brief visit. A busy physician will always be able to fill these open slots, and the patients will appreciate being able to book an appointment within a reasonable time when the circumstances warrant it. Some authorities recommend that appointments not be scheduled more than 3 months in advance.

If possible, set aside time in the morning and afternoon for a *breather*, or work break. Even 15 minutes will give the physician an opportunity to return calls from patients, verify prescription calls, or answer questions you may have that were not an emergency.

Details of Arranging Appointments

ARRANGEMENTS BY TELEPHONE

It is as important for the medical assistant to express pleasantness and a desire to be helpful when using the telephone as it is when meeting patients face to face. This is especially essential in the arranging of appointments. It is often the manner in which the booking is made rather than the convenience of the appointment time that makes a lasting impression.

Be especially considerate if you must refuse an appointment for the time requested. Explain why and offer a substitute time and date. It should also be determined whether the patient has been in before and whether any necessary insurance information has been obtained. Comply with the patient's desires as much as possible and do not show annoyance if a patient is not understanding of the problems involved in scheduling appointments. Most people do appreciate the need for a well-managed office and are willing to cooperate.

End the conversation pleasantly with something like this:

"Thank you for calling, Mrs. Albright. Dr. Wright will see you next Wednesday, August 28, at 2:30. Goodbye."

This little courtesy adds to the patient's feeling of esteem and additionally reinforces the time of the appointment. While you are saying this, you should be rechecking your appointment page to be certain that you have written it in the right time slot on the right day.

SKILLS AND RESPONSIBILITIES

PROFESSIONAL APPROACH TO TELEPHONE APPOINTMENTS

- Write legibly when making entries in the appointment book.
- Check off the patients' names as they arrive.
- Note any appointment failure or cancellations in ink on the appointment schedule.
- Always *immediately* write the patient's name in full, last name first, together with the reason for the appointment. *Do not trust the information to memory.*
- Reserve sufficient time for the appointment.
- Form the habit of entering the patient's daytime telephone number after every entry in the appointment book. It may become necessary to cancel or rearrange that day's schedule in a hurry, and many precious minutes can be saved if you have the telephone number handy.

APPOINTMENTS FOR NEW PATIENTS

Arranging the first appointment for a new patient requires time and attention to detail (see Procedure 10–2). At this first encounter you are, in a sense, extending a welcome to the practice. The patient will form a first impression of the office, of you, and of the physician from that first telephone contact. Tact and courtesy are extremely important.

ESSENTIAL QUESTIONS TO ASK WHEN SCHEDULING A NEW PATIENT

- Patient's full name (verify the spelling)
- Date of birth
- Complete address
- Daytime telephone number
- Pager number, if appropriate
- Source of referral, if any
- General type of examination required
- Insurance coverage, especially in a managed care practice

During this conversation request preliminary information to assist you in deciding how much time to allot on the appointment schedule. The physician may also expect you to give general instructions to patients seeking care for specific complaints; for example, to request the patient to bring in a urine specimen or to make certain that laboratory work is done before the appointment.

After you have recorded the necessary data, you may ask the patient, "Do you prefer morning or afternoon?" and then offer the first available date. Make certain that the patient knows where the office is located and, if necessary, how to get there. If there are special parking conveniences, tell the patient. Before concluding the conversation, repeat the appointment date and time agreed on and thank the person for calling.

If the appointment is several days away, mail to the patient a patient information brochure (see Chapter 24), a registration form, and a "welcome" letter. The brochure should provide advance information to the patient about the nature of the practice, introduce the medical staff, and explain appointment policies and financial arrangements.

If another physician has referred the patient, the medical assistant may need to call the referring physician's office and obtain additional information before the patient's appointment. This information should be printed out and given to the attending physician in advance of the patient's arrival.

In some offices, the medical assistant calls all patients the day before their appointment as a reminder. This takes time but can be done during slow periods, and many patients appreciate this service.

PROCEDURE 10 – 2
Scheduling a New Patient

GOAL
To schedule a new patient for a first office visit.

EQUIPMENT AND SUPPLIES
Appointment book   Appointment card
Scheduling guidelines   Telephone

PROCEDURAL STEPS

1 Obtain the patient's full name, birth date, address, and telephone number.
NOTE: Verify the spelling of the name.

2 Determine whether the patient was referred by another physician.
PURPOSE: You may need to request additional information from the referring physician, and your physician will want to send a consultation report.

3 Determine the patient's chief complaint and when the first symptoms occurred.
PURPOSE: To assist in determining the length of time needed for the appointment and the degree of urgency.

4 Search the appointment book for the first suitable appointment time and an alternate time.

5 Offer the patient a choice of these dates and times.
PURPOSE: Patients are better satisfied if they are given a choice.

6 Enter the mutually agreeable time in the appointment book followed by the patient's telephone number.
NOTE: Indicate that the patient is new by adding the letters "N.P."

7 If new patients are expected to pay at the time of visit, explain this financial arrangement when the appointment is made.
PURPOSE: The patient will be aware of the payment policy and can come prepared to pay at the time of the visit.

8 Offer travel directions for reaching the office as well as parking instructions.
PURPOSE: To relieve any anxiety about being able to find the medical facility.

9 Repeat the day, date, and time of the appointment before saying good-bye to the patient.
PURPOSE: To verify the patient understands the date and time of the appointment.

SCHEDULING RETURN APPOINTMENTS

In Person

Many return appointments are arranged while a patient is in the office. The physician will probably ask the patient to stop at the desk and make another appointment before leaving. While you reach for your pencil and the appointment book, look at the patient and say something such as

"We have Tuesday and Thursday morning or evening available. Do you have a preference?"

If the patient asks for a time that is not available, this places the medical assistant in a negative position by having to refuse a request.

Enter the patient's name and telephone number in the slot agreed on and give the patient a completed appointment card that you have verified with the book entry, along with your best smile. Give the patient any necessary instructions at this time.

By Telephone

Usually it is necessary only to determine when the patient is expected to return and then to find a suitable time on the schedule. It is not necessary to give extensive explanations about the location of the office and parking facilities. However, if there has been a lengthy interval since the patient's last visit, the medical assistant should recheck certain information and enter any changes on the patient's chart.

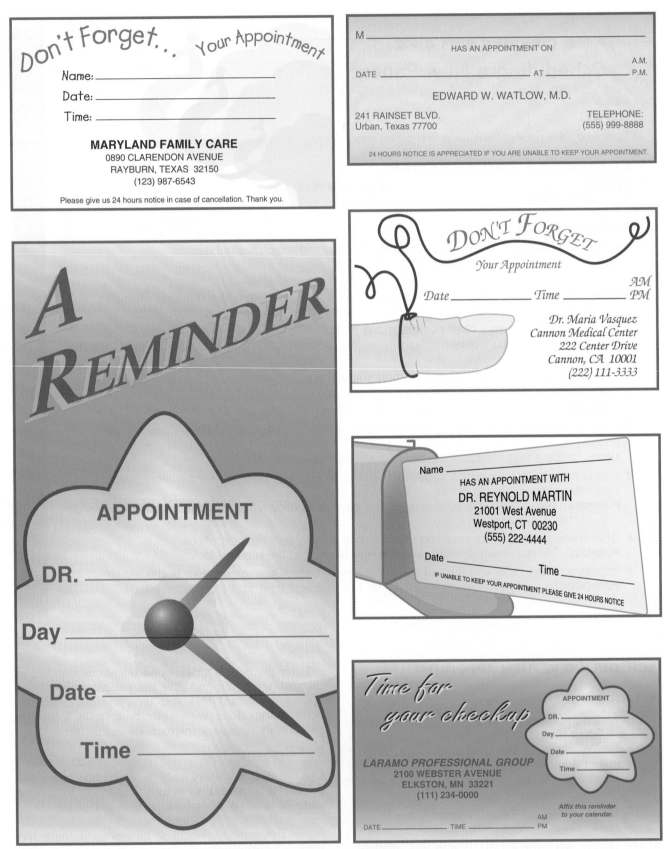

FIGURE 10–4 Examples of appointment cards.

ESSENTIAL QUESTIONS TO ASK A PATIENT BETWEEN LENGTHY INTERVALS

- Patient's current address
- Daytime telephone number
- Current insurance coverage
- Employment information
- Nature of the current complaint

Memory Jogger

3 *What are the seven items of information that you must obtain from each new patient?*

Appointment Cards and Reminders

APPOINTMENT CARDS

Most health care facilities use cards to remind patients of scheduled appointments, as well as to eliminate misunderstandings about dates and times (Fig. 10–4).

Make a habit of reaching for an appointment card while writing an entry in the appointment book. After you have written the date and time on the appointment card, double-check with the book to see that the entries agree. Patients who have made appointments in advance may be sent a reminder card or notified by telephone near the time of the appointment.

REMINDERS

A patient who is due for an appointment but has not yet arranged a date and time may be sent a *recall reminder*. A simple way of handling this is to have a supply of postal cards on hand; while the patients are still in the office, have them write their name and address on a card. Then place the card in a file box under the date it is to be mailed.

Special Circumstances

LATE PATIENTS

Probably every medical practice has a few patients who are habitually late for appointments. This seems to be a problem for which no cure has been found; consequently, you must find a way of booking such patients as the last appointments of the

day. Then, if closing time arrives before the patient does, you need feel no obligation to wait. Some medical assistants simply tell the patient to come in 30 minutes earlier than the time they actually write in the book. The point to remember is that you must learn to work around this patient, with the realization that in all likelihood he or she is not going to change.

RESCHEDULING A CANCELED APPOINTMENT

Sometimes changes must be made in the appointment schedule. For example, the patient who has a 3 PM appointment next Monday calls and asks to have this postponed to 1 week later. You find an opening at 3 PM on the following Monday and write in the patient's name, but in your haste you fail to cross out the first appointment. Someone else looking at the appointment book (or possibly even yourself a couple of days later) will either expect the patient on both days or be unable to determine which day is correct. Avoid this embarrassing situation by making it a habit to cross out the first appointment before writing in the new one.

You may have a patient who requires a series of appointments, for example, at weekly intervals. Try to set up the appointments on the same day of each week at the same time of day, if possible. This considerably reduces the risk of a forgotten appointment. A calendar that shows the dates several months in advance at a glance is useful to have on or near the appointment desk.

EMERGENCY CALLS

Calls for appointments may be categorized as *emergencies, urgent,* or *routine.* **Triage** in responding to requests for immediate care and treatment puts the responsibility of evaluating the urgency of the need and prioritizing the treatment on the medical assistant who answers the telephone. Triage is an extremely important function that requires experience and tact.

Emergencies may include emotional crises as well as the more obvious physical problems, and patients having emergencies generally should be seen the same day. The calling patient may have an emotionally charged issue such as "I just found a lump in my breast" or "I can't urinate or get an erection." The urgency of the call can be initially determined by having available a list of questions previously prepared with the help of the physician and posted near the telephone for easy reference. The physician should define what is to be considered *urgent* as well as the time frame for scheduling urgent appointments (probably within 1 to 4 days). Try to have a list of questions to ask the caller appropriate to the situation.

RESPONDING TO AN EMERGENCY CALL

1 Is there bleeding?
2 From where is the blood coming?
3 What is the patient's temperature?
4 Are there chills?
5 Is there nausea or vomiting?
6 If there is pain, is it steady or intermittent?
7 Is the pain severe? sharp? dull?
8 How long have the symptoms been present?

In many cases the caller will consider the situation more urgent than his or her responses to the medical questions would indicate. Skillful handling of these situations requires considerable tact by the medical assistant. Maintaining a caring and reassuring response will frequently alleviate the fear being evidenced by the caller.

ACUTELY ILL PATIENTS

Patients cannot always give advance notice of when they will need medical care. There is sometimes a very fine line between an emergency patient and the acutely ill patient, but the latter should be seen as soon as possible. At the very least, let the physician decide whether the patient should be seen immediately or whether an appointment should be made for another day.

For example, a patient may report having had flu symptoms for several days and now has an elevated temperature. The physician will probably want more information before deciding whether the patient should be seen immediately or whether some other course of action is appropriate. The 15- to 20-minute breather time you saved in the middle of the morning and the afternoon may rescue your schedule. Patients with symptoms of contagion should be placed so as to discourage patient cross-contamination.

PHYSICIAN REFERRALS

If another physician telephones and requests that a patient be seen by your physician today, this is another exception you will have to make. Most physicians recognize the importance of keeping a schedule and will not be inconsiderate in this respect.

Memory Jogger

4 *How can the medical assistant determine the urgency of a call when the physician is not present?*

Failed Appointments

REASONS FOR FAILED APPOINTMENTS

Why do patients fail to keep appointments? Some are simply forgetful. If you detect this tendency in a patient, form the habit of telephoning a reminder the day before the appointment or send a postcard timed to arrive 1 or 2 days in advance of the appointment.

If your office consistently runs behind schedule, with patients being kept waiting for more than 20 to 30 minutes, the patient whose own time is well planned may simply elect not to run the risk of losing so much valuable time. Perhaps you gave a patient an appointment at a time that really was not agreeable to him.

A patient who has been pressed for payment may stay away because of being unable to pay on that day.

It is extremely important that you determine the reason for failed appointments and do what you can to remedy the situations. Telephone the patient to be sure there was no misunderstanding. If the patient's health is such that medical treatment must continue, write a letter explaining this to the patient. Send the letter by certified mail with return receipt requested and keep this letter in the chart for legal protection.

NO-SHOW POLICY

Some patients may not realize the importance of keeping their appointments. A busy practice must have a very specific policy on appointment no-shows and enforce it effectively. A suggested **no-show** policy may be as follows: The first time a patient fails to show, note the fact on the medical record or ledger card. The second time this happens, you'll have a warning, and if the patient is more than a half-hour late, call his or her home. The third time a patient fails to show without good reason, consider dropping the patient by using the customary methods that avoid legal problems.

CHARGING FOR FAILED APPOINTMENTS

Legally, a patient may be charged for failing to keep an uncanceled appointment if the patient was informed in advance about this policy and if it can be shown that this time was not used for another patient. However, few physicians attempt to collect for such occasions. The risk of poor public relations is too great; it generally results in a lost patient. Some other way must be found to handle failed appointments if they become a problem.

RECORDING THE FAILED APPOINTMENT

Whenever a patient fails to keep an appointment, a notation should be made in the patient's chart as well as in the appointment book. If the patient is seriously ill, the physician should also be told about the failure. This may be a legal consideration at some later date. In some cases, it may be necessary for the physician or the medical assistant to call and remind the patient that an unkept appointment may have serious effects on the patient's health.

Handling Cancellations and Delays

WHEN THE PATIENT CANCELS

Inevitably some cancellations will occur. If you keep a list of patients with advance appointments who would like to come in sooner, get busy on the telephone and try to get one of them in to fill the available opening. By placing a colored dot alongside their names in the appointment book where the first appointment was made, you can readily identify which patients to call to fill the vacancy.

WHEN THE PHYSICIAN IS DELAYED

There will be days when the physician(s) is delayed in reaching the office. If you have advance notice of the delay, you can start calling those patients with early appointments and suggest that they come later. If some patients have already arrived before you learn of the delay, you will have to explain that an emergency has detained the physician.

Show concern for the patient, but avoid being overly apologetic, which might imply some degree of guilt. Most patients realize that a physician has certain priorities. The patient who is in the office may be *inconvenienced*, but it is not a *life-or-death* matter. If this kind of situation occurs frequently, however, you may have to devise a different scheduling system.

WHEN THE PHYSICIAN IS CALLED OUT ON EMERGENCIES

Physicians are conscious of their responsibilities for responding to medical emergencies, and most patients will be sympathetic to such occurrences if the medical assistant takes the time to explain what has happened. You may say something like,

> "Dr. Wright has been called away to answer an emergency. She asked me to tell you she is very sorry to keep you waiting. There will be at least a 1-hour delay."

Ask the patient,

> "Do you wish to wait? If it is inconvenient, I'll be glad to give you the first available appointment on another day. Or perhaps you'd like to have some coffee or do some shopping and return in an hour."

As quickly as possible, call the patients who are scheduled for a later hour. In many offices, especially those of obstetricians, surgeons, and general practitioners, it sometimes is necessary to cancel a whole day's appointments. For this reason, it is particularly important that you have the daytime telephone number of each patient available so that you can cancel the appointment and make a new one without delay. If it is at all possible, cancel appointments *before* the patient arrives in the office to find that the doctor is not available.

WHEN THE PHYSICIAN IS ILL OR IS CALLED OUT OF TOWN

Physicians get ill, too, and the patients who are scheduled to be seen during the course of the physician's expected recovery period must be informed of this. They need not be told the nature of the illness. When the physician is called out of town for personal or professional reasons, the appointments will have to be canceled or rescheduled. It is customary to give the patient the name of another physician, or possibly a choice of several, who will be providing care during such absences. For security reasons, it is best to merely state that the doctor is unavailable. Stating over the telephone that the physician is out of town could lead to attempted burglary or other unauthorized intrusion of the premises.

Patients Without Appointments

What will you do with *walk-in* patients, that is, those who arrive without a scheduled appointment? There must be a policy agreed on by the physician and then carried out by the medical assistant.

The patient who requires immediate attention will most likely be accommodated into the schedule somehow. If the patient does not need immediate care, a brief visit with the physician and a scheduled appointment at a later time may be the answer. You may simply have to turn down the request. Follow the established office policy.

The medical assistant should always make it clear, even when accommodating patients without appointments, that the office runs on an appointment basis. You might say, for example:

> "Dr. Wright will be able to see you today, but we would appreciate it very much if you would make an appointment for your next visit."

Or,

> "Dr. Wright can see you now and I am sorry you had to wait so long. Perhaps it would be possible for you to make an appointment the next time."

Try to convey the message that appointments save not only the physician's time but also the patient's time. Emphasize that the physician is able to give the patient full attention and more time if an advance appointment is made.

Preplanning for the Next Day

Before leaving at the end of the day, look over the appointments scheduled for the next day. Review the charts for scheduled patients. If laboratory tests or other procedures were scheduled on the patient's last visit, determine that the reports are available in the chart. If the patient is scheduled for specific procedures on this visit, make certain that everything that will be needed for the procedure is on hand and available. Preplanning can save many precious moments at the time of the patient visit.

Scheduling Outside Appointments

There are other appointments that the medical assistant will make and that will appear on the appointment book, such as *scheduled surgery* at a hospital, *consultations* at a hospital or at another physician's office, and *house calls* at extended-care facilities or in the home. The physician must have time to get from one place to another, so allowance must be made for traveling time when arranging these appointments.

SURGERIES

You may be responsible for scheduling surgeries. In scheduling with most hospitals, you should call the secretary in surgery first when your physician plans an operation. Give the surgical secretary the necessary information. Explain any special requests the physician may have, such as the amount of blood to have available. Be certain that you have all this information at hand before placing the call.

> **ESSENTIAL INFORMATION TO GIVE FOR SCHEDULING SURGERY**
>
> - Preferred date and time
> - Type of surgery to be scheduled
> - Approximate time required

> After the date and hour have been established, give
>
> - Patient's full name
> - Sex
> - Age
> - Telephone number

Some hospitals request that the patient complete a preadmittance form so that all records can be processed before the patient is admitted. In such cases it may be the medical assistant's responsibility to see that this is done. These are general guidelines only, because procedures will vary in different areas and different hospitals.

HOUSE CALLS

If the physician regularly makes *house calls* or sees patients in *convalescent homes,* you will probably set aside a special block of time for this on your appointment schedule. In arranging such appointments, be sure to get all the pertinent details.

> **ESSENTIAL INFORMATION TO GIVE PHYSICIAN**
>
> - Name and address of patient
> - Telephone number
> - Best route to reach the home
> - Nearest cross street
> - Name of person making the request

Again, traveling time must be allowed for. Many physicians never make house calls, believing that the patient can best be examined and treated in the medical facility or in a hospital.

OUTSIDE APPOINTMENTS FOR PATIENTS

The medical assistant is often requested to arrange laboratory or x-ray appointments for patients (see Procedure 10–3). Before calling you need to know certain facts.

> **ESSENTIAL INFORMATION IN ARRANGING LABORATORY APPOINTMENTS**
>
> - Exact procedure required
> - Whether **expediency** is a factor
> - Whether the insurance plan requires notification and determination of medical necessity

PROCEDURE 10 – 3
Scheduling Outpatient Diagnostic Tests

GOAL

To schedule a patient for outpatient diagnostic test ordered by physician within the time frame needed by physician, confirm with the patient, and issue all required instructions.

EQUIPMENT AND SUPPLIES

Diagnostic test order from physician
Name, address, and telephone
number of diagnostic facility

Patient chart
Test preparation instructions
Telephone

PROCEDURAL STEPS

1 Obtain an oral or written order from the physician for the exact procedure to be performed and the time frame for results.
PURPOSE: The urgency of the test results affects the time and date of the appointment needed.

2 Determine the patient's availability.
PURPOSE: To be certain that the patient will be able to comply with the arrangements for the test.

3 Telephone diagnostic facility:
 * Order the specific test needed.
 * Establish the date and time.
 * Give the name, age, address, and telephone number of the patient.
 * Determine any special instructions for the patient.
 * Notify the facility of any urgency for test results.

4 Notify the patient of arrangements, including:
 * Name, address, and telephone number of the diagnostic facility
 * Date and time to report for the test
 * Instructions concerning preparation for the test (e.g., eating restrictions, fluids, medications, enemas)
 * Ask the patient to repeat the instructions.
PURPOSE: To be certain that the patient understands the preparation necessary and the importance of keeping the appointment. If time permits, issue written instructions to the patient.

5 Note arrangements on the patient's chart.
PURPOSE: To ensure follow-up on diagnosis and/or treatment.

6 Place reminder on a tickler or desk calendar.
PURPOSE: To check whether the appointment was kept and report was received from the testing facility.

 * Which laboratory or facility must be used to qualify for insurance payment
 * Whether a **stat report** is necessary
 * Patient's availability

With this information before you, you can set up the appointment with confidence. When you inform the patient of the time and place for the appointment, you can also relay any special instructions that may be necessary. Then note these arrangements on the patient's chart and place a follow up reminder on your **tickler** or desk calendar.

Other Callers

There will be a wide range of other unscheduled callers with whom the physician will need to meet.

PHYSICIANS

Another physician dropping in to your facility should be ushered in to see the physician as soon as possible regardless of the appointment schedule. If your physician is seeing a patient, explain the situation and, if possible, take the visiting physician into a private room to wait. Then notify your employer as soon as possible. Visits from other physicians are usually brief and do not appreciably affect your schedule.

PHARMACEUTICAL REPRESENTATIVES

Also known as *detail persons* or *reps*, representatives from pharmaceutical houses are frequent visitors to physicians' offices and are generally welcomed when the schedule permits. They are well trained and bring valuable information on new drugs to the physician. The medical assistant is often expected to screen such visitors and turn away those whose products would not be used in that practice. If you do not know the representative or the pharmaceutical company, ask for a business card, then check with the physician, who will decide whether or not to see the caller.

Specialists usually limit their conferences with pharmaceutical representatives to their line of practice. The medical assistant, together with the physician, can prepare a list of those representatives with whom the physician is willing to spend time, and then let the list be the determining factor in future conferences.

The medical assistant can say whether the physician will be available that day and give an estimate of the waiting time or suggest a later time at which to return. The caller can then make a decision regarding whether to wait or return later. The pharmaceutical representative is usually quite understanding and cooperative and is willing to wait patiently a long while for just a brief visit with the physician. The medical assistant should in turn treat the representative with courtesy, showing as much cooperation as possible.

In some cases, the representative will just leave literature or materials for the physician with the medical assistant. The detail person who is not on the calling list for a particular physician will also appreciate the saving in time by knowing this in advance. Most representatives say they would rather be told outright if the physician does not wish to see them than to be given some evasive reply.

SALESPERSONS

Salespersons from medical, surgical, and office supply houses call regularly at physicians' offices. Sometimes they will want to see the physician, but the office manager or the medical assistant who is in charge of ordering supplies usually is able to handle these calls.

Unsolicited salespersons can sometimes present a problem in the professional office. If the physician does not wish to see such callers, the medical assistant must firmly but tactfully send them away. You can suggest that they leave their literature and cards for the physician to study and say that the physician will contact them if further information is desired. Persistent callers who ignore a polite "No" can be discouraged by the suggestion that perhaps they would like to schedule an appointment, at the physician's customary fee.

MISCELLANEOUS CALLERS

From time to time, other callers appear in the medical office. Some are civic leaders seeking the physician's aid in community projects. Others may be church leaders, insurance representatives, solicitors for fund drives, and so forth. A general policy regarding seeing such callers should be established so that each incident does not require a separate discussion and decision.

Civic leaders should be treated with courtesy and consideration when they telephone or come into the office. Most physicians feel a responsibility to take an active part in community affairs, but no one can participate in all activities. The responsibility for accepting or refusing such community appointments is sometimes delegated to the office manager or medical assistant. In this event, one should use discretion and exercise great tact and courtesy. Turning away community leaders with a blunt refusal does not create good medical public relations.

When it is necessary to refuse requests for community projects, the medical assistant can explain that the physician is already participating in such community projects as, for example, the Boy Scouts, Girl Scouts, Kiwanis, and the Health Council (naming specific activities or organizations) and cannot accept additional responsibilities at this time. The practice of tact, courtesy, and consideration applies to *every caller* in the health care facility.

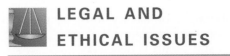 # LEGAL AND ETHICAL ISSUES

When scheduling appointments be especially considerate of complying with the patient's wishes when possible. Explain any refusal and offer a substitute time and date.

If a patient fails to appear for a scheduled appointment, note this in the patient's chart and in the appointment book. Always determine the reason for failed appointments and attempt to remedy anything that can be changed.

CRITICAL THINKING

1 List the three premises that determine an efficient scheduling system.

2 When entering an appointment in the daily schedule, what two items will you include in addition to the patient's name?

3 Recall some of the reasons that patients fail to keep appointments and describe how you would handle each situation.

4 Discuss the meaning and reason for buffer time?

HOW DID I DO? Answers to Memory Joggers

1 Efficient scheduling is important because the most valuable asset within the medical practice is the

physician's time. Its success ultimately depends on the cooperation of the physician.

2 The nature of the practice, the personality and habits of the medical staff, and time needed by each patient. Be able to discuss the reasons for their importance.

3 Patient's full name, date of birth, complete address, daytime telephone number, source of referral, if any, general type of examination required, and insurance coverage.

4 Refer to a list of questions approved by the physician and the action to follow based on the answers.

REFERENCES

American Medical Association: Managing the Medical Practice. Chicago, AMA, 1996.

Conomikes Associates: Medical Office Management Institute, 1996.

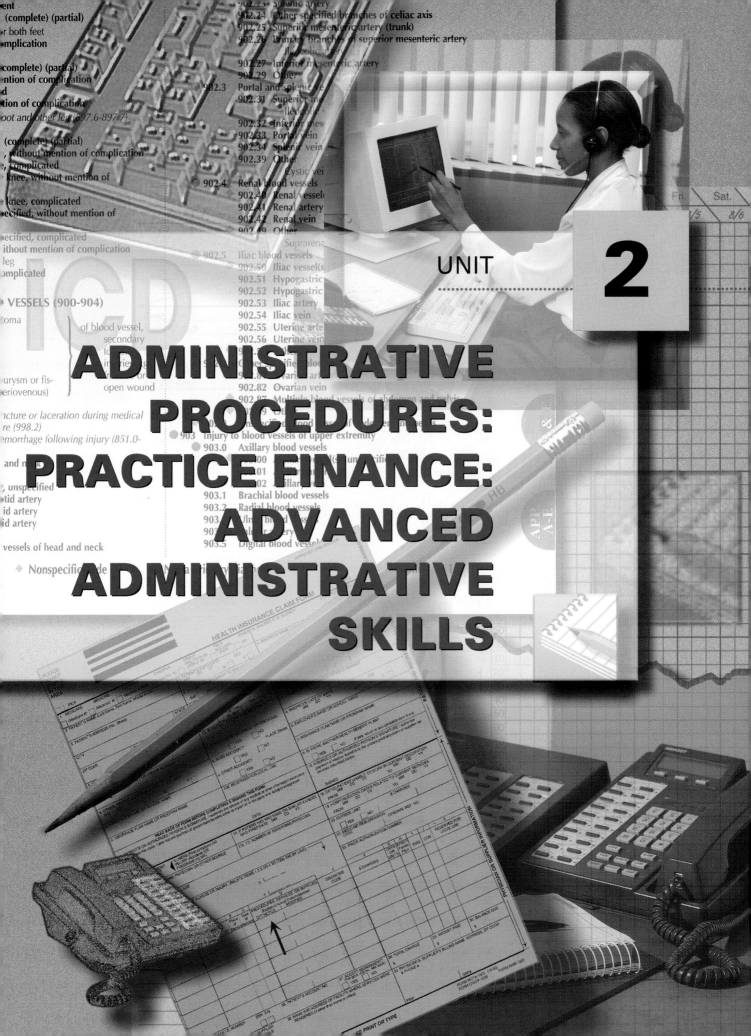

UNIT

2

ADMINISTRATIVE PROCEDURES: PRACTICE FINANCE: ADVANCED ADMINISTRATIVE SKILLS

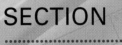

SECTION 4

Written Communications and Record Keeping

CURRICULUM CONTENT/COMPETENCIES

Chapter 11 Correspondence and Mail Processing
- Perform basic clerical functions
- Recognize and respond to verbal and nonverbal communications
- Receive, organize, prioritize, and transmit information
- Promote the practice through positive public relations

Chapter 12 Dictation and Transcription
- Perform medical transcription
- Manage time effectively
- Use medical terminology appropriately
- Prepare and maintain medical records

Chapter 13 The Computer in Medical Practice
- Apply computer techniques to support office operations
- Obtain reimbursement through accurate claims submission
- Practice within the scope of education, training, and personal capabilities
- Evaluate and recommend equipment and supplies

Chapter 14 Filing Methods and Record Keeping
- Receive, organize, and prioritize information
- Document accurately
- Perform basic clerical functions

Chapter 15 Health Information Management
- Prepare and maintain health information records
- Document accurately
- Maintain confidentiality
- Perform basic clerical functions
- Use appropriate guidelines when releasing information

Correspondence and Mail Processing

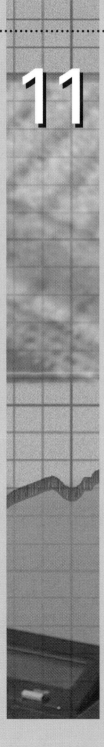

11

LEARNING OBJECTIVES

Cognitive: On successful completion of this chapter, you should be able to:

1 Define and spell terms listed in the Vocabulary.

2 Discuss the responsibility of the medical assistant with respect to office equipment.

3 Select stationery suitable for producing professional correspondence.

4 List the three basic sizes of letterhead stationery.

5 Name three types of essential references for the medical assistant's library.

6 Explain the five steps in getting ready to answer a letter.

7 Discuss the process of developing and the value of a correspondence portfolio.

8 Name four letter styles and discuss their differences.

9 List the four standard parts of a business letter.

10 Explain how using ZIP codes can save money for the mailer.

Performance: On successful completion of this chapter, you should be able to:

1 Open, sort, and annotate incoming mail.

2 Prepare a response to an inquiry letter.

3 Compose original letters.

4 Correctly address envelopes for optical scanning.

5 Fold outgoing mail for insertion into three styles of envelopes.

VOCABULARY

academic degree A title conferred by a college, university, or professional school on completion of a program of study

annotating To furnish with notes, which are usually critical or explanatory

categorically Placed in a specific division of a system of classification

clarity The state of being clear or lucid

concise Expressing much in brief form

continuation pages The second and following pages of a letter

intrinsic Inward; indwelling

portfolio A set of documents either bound in book form or loose in a folder

Correspondence and mail processing can consume a large part of the administrative medical assistant's day. Many physicians, when queried about the skills they most desire in an administrative assistant, have said, "Send me someone who can write a good letter." Or they may say, "My spelling is atrocious; I need help!" When a physician delegates to the medical assistant the responsibility of composing letters or reports that have the potential to reflect positively or negatively on the practice, he or she is expressing confidence in the assistant.

Public Relations Value

Written communications offer the perfect opportunity for making a good impression on others, but they don't just happen. They require thought, preparation, skill, and a positive attitude. Written communications take many forms in the medical office. The medical assistant may be required to be skilled in creating various forms of communication.

SKILLS AND RESPONSIBILITIES

WRITTEN COMMUNICATION SKILLS

- Transcribe from machine or shorthand dictation
- Type consultation and surgical reports
- Compose original letters
- Reply to inquiries
- Respond to requests for information

- Write collection letters
- Order supplies
- Write instructions for patients
- Process a variety of other communications

The form and process of letter writing are discussed in this chapter. Transcription will be covered in Chapter 12.

Written communications should be *courteous* to the reader, *correct* in content, and **concise** without being curt. Communication is an art as well as a skill: The ability to communicate effectively is extremely important to the administrative medical assistant who wants to succeed and advance in his or her career.

Equipment and Supplies

To create a good impression with your letters, you must use good equipment and quality supplies.

EQUIPMENT

Whatever kind of equipment is available for your use, it is your responsibility to know how to use it to the best advantage and keep it in good working condition. If the equipment manual is available, study it and keep it handy for reference when problems occur. Know how to maintain your equipment so that your best efforts always result in a quality appearance.

COMPUTER OR WORD PROCESSOR If you are unfamiliar with the specific model supplied, study the manual so that you know how to format documents, make corrections, and print the necessary copies.

TYPEWRITER Most typewriters use correctable film ribbon that passes through the spool only one time. However, if your typewriter uses a cotton or silk ribbon that becomes lighter with use, be sure to change the ribbon before the resulting type impression becomes too light. Typewriters that use a cotton ribbon also need frequent cleaning of the typewriter keys.

COPIER If you are composing with a typewriter, you are probably using a copier for making any necessary copies of the original. Here, too, maintain the copier so that copies are crisp and clear.

STATIONERY

QUALITY The quality of paper unquestionably affects the reader's total impression of the communication. Your stationer or printing company is qualified to advise on the selection of paper, which can range from all-sulfite (a wood pulp) to all-cotton fiber (sometimes called *rag*). Letterhead paper is usually on bond with a 25% or higher cotton fiber content.

The weight of paper is described by a *substance number*. This number is based on the weight of a ream consisting of 500 sheets of 17 × 22-inch paper. The larger the substance number, the heavier the paper. If the ream weighs 24 pounds, the paper is referred to as Sub 24 or 24-pound weight. Letterhead stationery and matching envelopes are usually 16-, 20-, or 24-pound weight.

SIZES Letterhead paper is available in three basic sizes:

- Standard   8½ × 11 inches
- Monarch or executive 7¼ × 10½ inches
- Baronial   5½ × 8½ inches

Standard letterhead is used for general business and professional correspondence. *Monarch* is often used by professional persons for informal business and social correspondence. *Baronial,* which is a half-sheet of Standard, is used for very short letters or memoranda. Each size letterhead should have its matching envelope.

CONTINUATION PAGES The second and continuing pages of a letter or report are placed on plain bond that matches the letterhead in weight and fiber content.

Bond paper has a *felt* side and a *wire* side. Printing and typing are done on the felt side. Pick up a sheet of letterhead and hold it to the light; you will see a design or letters that can be read from the printed side. This design is called a *watermark* and is an indication of quality. The side from which you can read the watermark is the felt side of the paper and is the side on which typing should be done. Always have the watermark read across the page in the same direction as the typing.

Memory Jogger

1 *You may see the notation Sub 24 on a package of paper. What does this tell you?*

Your Personal Tools

Competent handling of written communications requires a basic knowledge of composition (i.e., sentence structure, spelling, and punctuation; see Chapter 12). You will also need a personal reference library that includes an up-to-date standard dictionary, a medical dictionary, and a secretary's manual. Some suggestions are included in the reference list at the end of this chapter.

If you have difficulty with spelling (many people do), you may wish to keep a small looseleaf indexed notebook or card index of words that are troublesome. Whenever it is necessary to look up a word in the dictionary for spelling, record it in the notebook or card index for quick reference.

Your physician or a medical assistant who is familiar with the practice might compile a basic list of frequently used medical terms and abbreviations as a reference for the trainee.

Table 11–1 lists 150 frequently misspelled or misused English words. Table 11–2 lists 100 frequently misspelled medical terms. Your list may be entirely different, depending on your capabilities and the branch of medicine in which you are involved.

Memory Jogger

2 *One of the most frequently misspelled medical words describes the study of the eye. Can you spell this word?*

Composing Tips

WRITING SKILLS

If your only experience in letter writing has been social correspondence, you will have a new set of rules to learn. Social letters tend to be long and chatty, "I" oriented, and do not necessarily follow any organized plan. Most business letters should be less than one page in length, "you" oriented, and carefully organized. This takes practice and preparation.

TABLE 11-1 150 Frequently Misspelled or Misused English Words

absence	corroborate	inimitable	persistent	ridiculous
accede	definitely	inoculate	personal	sacrilegious
accessible	description	insistent	personnel	seize
accommodate	desirable	irrelevant	possession	separate
achieve	despair	irresistible	precede	siege
affect	development	irritable	precedent	similar
agglutinate	dilemma	judgment	predictable	sizable
all right	disappear	labeled	predominant	stationary
altogether	disappoint	led	predominate	stationery
analyses (pl.)	disastrous	leisure	prerogative	subpoena
analysis (s.)	discreet	license	prevalent	succeed
analyze	discrete	liquefy	principal	suddenness
anoint	discriminate	maintenance	principle	superintendent
argument	dissatisfaction	maneuver	privilege	supersede
assistant	dissipate	miscellaneous	procedure	surprise
auxiliary	drunkenness	mischievous	proceed	tariff
balloon	ecstasy	misspell	professor	technique
believe	effect	necessary	pronunciation	thorough
benefited	eligible	newsstand	psychiatry	tranquility
brochure	embarrass	noticeable	psychology	transferred
bulletin	exceed	occasion	pursue	truly
category	exhilaration	occurrence	questionnaire	tyrannize
changeable	existence	oscillate	rearrange	unnecessary
clientele	February	paid	recede	until
committee	forty	pamphlet	receive	vacillate
comparative	grammar	panicky	recommend	vacuum
concede	grievous	parallel	referring	vicious
conscientious	height	paralyze	repetition	warrant
conscious	incidentally	pastime	rheumatism	Wednesday
coolly	indispensable	perseverance	rhythmical	weird

TABLE 11-2 Frequently Misspelled Medical Words

abscess	defibrillator	intussusception	parietal	pruritus
additive	desiccate	ischemia	paroxysmal	psoriasis
aerosol	ecchymosis	ischium	pemphigus	pyrexia
agglutination	effusion	larynx	percussion	respiratory
albumin	epididymis	leukemia	perforation	rheumatic
anastomosis	epistaxis	malaise	pericardium	roentgenology
aneurysm	eustachian	malleus	perineum	sagittal
anteflexion	fissure	melena	peristalsis	sciatic
arrhythmia	flexure	mellitus	peritoneum	scirrhous
bilirubin	glaucoma	menstruation	petit mal	serous
bronchial	gonorrhea	metastasis	pharynx	sessile
cachexia	graafian	neurilemma	pituitary	sphincter
calcaneus	hemorrhage	neuron	plantar	sphygmomanometer
capillary	hemorrhoids	occlusion	pleura	squamous
cervical	homeostasis	optic chiasm	pleurisy	staphylococcus
chromosome	humerus	oscilloscope	pneumonia	suppuration
cirrhosis	idiosyncracy	osseous	polyp	trochanter
clavicle	ileum	palliative	prophylaxis	venous
curettage	ilium	parasite	prostate	wheal
cyanosis	infarction	parenteral	prosthesis	xiphoid

SKILLS AND RESPONSIBILITIES

PLANNING BEFORE ANSWERING A LETTER

1 Carefully read the letter you are to answer.
2 Make note of, or underline, any questions asked or materials requested.
3 Decide on the answers to the questions and verify your information. This is called **annotating.**
4 Draft a reply, using the tools you are most comfortable with (e.g., the computer, typewriter, longhand, or shorthand).
5 Rewrite for **clarity.**

Keep most of your sentences short. Put only one idea in each sentence. Eliminate superfluous words. Be careful about using medical terms in correspondence with patients; use only language that the reader will easily understand.

Every person who writes letters develops his or her own personal style. Most physicians conform to a highly professional and formal style in their dictation.

The medical assistant who is given the responsibility of composing correspondence for the medical office should strive for the same degree of formality used by the physician. It would be inappropriate for the assistant to write in a breezy, informal style when acting as the representative of an employer who is more formal in his or her approach.

The principal point to remember is that every letter produced in your office should project the image of the physician regardless of who composes or signs the letter.

Memoranda are usually intended for interoffice correspondence. Larger facilities often have printed forms that merely require filling in the date, the receiver and sender, and the topic. You can easily prepare a memo in an accepted form. If you are using a computer or word processor, you will probably find a preformatted memorandum already prepared for you. When starting with only plain paper, set the side margins for 1-inch. Begin typing the memo heading 2 inches from the top of the page (line 13). Set up the heading with the words: TO, FROM, DATE, and SUBJECT. Setting a tab stop 10 spaces in from the left margin will enable you to tab to each entry, clearing the headings.

You may start the body of your memorandum at the left margin or set your margin 10 spaces in so that your text starts directly beneath the typed headings. No salutation is necessary in a memorandum. The purpose is to expedite the communication of a message in a manner that provides a record without becoming cumbersome (Fig. 11–1).

INTEROFFICE MEMORANDUM

TO   All Staff

FROM   Office Manager

DATE   December 1

SUBJECT   Holiday Schedule

Our entire facility will be closed on December 24, December 25, December 31, and January 1. The office will be on reduced staff during the days of December 26, 27, 28, 29, and 30. Assignments will be based on seniority of staff members. Please submit your preferences as soon as possible.

A

MEMO TO: George Walker

FROM: Stanley Barr

DATE: February 8, 1999

SUBJECT: Office rental

We are experiencing unexpectedly rapid growth in our business office and will soon need additional space for our increased number of employees. Do you have a larger facility available in this building? If so, I would like to hear from you regarding the location, square footage, and anticipated rental costs.

B

FIGURE 11–1 *A* and *B*, examples of memoranda.

DEVELOPING A PORTFOLIO

Letter composition can be sped up by developing a **portfolio** of sample letters to suit the various situations that frequently arise. As the physician approves your letters you can add them to your portfolio. Suppose, for instance, you need to write to a patient to change an appointment. Compose the very best letter you can—one that is clear, concise, and courteous—and make an extra copy to place in your portfolio of letters. Alternatively, if you are using a computer, store the letter on a disk. Do this each time you write a new kind of letter. Soon you will be able to select a letter from your portfolio and change it slightly to suit the current situation. You will have your letters written in no time!

Watch for sample letters that appear from time to time in the physician's business journals and clip them for your portfolio. Scan the textbooks and office manuals on the market or in your public library for additional help.

OTHER WRITTEN FORMS OF COMMUNICATION

Written communications include more than letters and memoranda. For example, consider telephone messages that you record. Are you sure that they are clearly stated and convey to the reader what you intend? You may need to mail a prescription to a patient, with instructions from the physician.

Make sure that the patient will be able to read and understand what you intend to communicate.

Memory Jogger

3 *Describe the difference between a formal letter and a memorandum.*

Letter Styles

A business letter is usually arranged in one of three styles: *block, modified block (standard),* or *modified block indented.* A fourth style, called *simplified,* is occasionally used. The block and modified block (standard) styles are most commonly used in the physician's office.

BLOCK LETTER STYLE All lines start flush with the left margin. This style is considered the most efficient but is less attractive on the page (Fig. 11–2).

MODIFIED-BLOCK LETTER STYLE (STANDARD) The date line, the complimentary closing, and the typewritten signature all begin at the center. All other lines begin at the left margin (Fig. 11–3).

MODIFIED-BLOCK WITH INDENTED PARAGRAPHS This style is identical to the block style except that the first line of each paragraph is indented five spaces (Fig. 11–4).

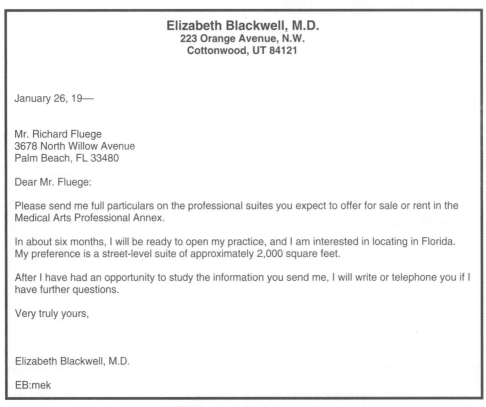

FIGURE 11–2 Block letter style.

MEDICAL ARTS PROFESSIONAL ANNEX
3678 North Willow Avenue
Palm Beach FL 33480

January 29, 19—

Elizabeth Blackwell, M.D.
223 Orange Avenue, N.W.
Cottonwood, UT 84121

Dear Doctor Blackwell:

We have two remaining street-level suites available for occupancy about July 1. These are marked on pages 3 and 4 of the enclosed descriptive brochure. If one of these suites appeals to you, we will be pleased to customize it for your practice.

Please feel free to call me collect at the number on the brochure for further discussion of your needs.

Sincerely yours,

Richard Fluege
Business Manager

RF:ab
Enclosure

FIGURE 11–3   Modified block letter style (standard).

WILLIAM OSLER, M.D.
1000 South West Street
Park Ridge, NJ 07656

January 26, 19—

Robert Koch, M.D.
398 Main Street
Park Ridge, NJ 07656

Dear Doctor Koch:

<u>Mrs. Elaine Norris</u>

Thank you for referring your patient, Mrs. Elaine Norris, for consultation and care. She was examined in my office today.

FINDINGS: The patient complained of pain in the left lower quadrant and some abdominal tenderness. She had a temperature of 100.2 degrees.

RECOMMENDATIONS: The patient was placed on a soft, low-residue, bland diet, antibiotics, and bed rest for a few days. Upper and lower gastrointestinal x-rays will be performed next week.

TENTATIVE DIAGNOSIS: Diverticulitis of large bowel.

Mrs. Norris has been asked to return here for reevaluation in about ten days.

Sincerely yours,

William Osler, M.D.

WO:gm

FIGURE 11–4   Modified block letter style with indented paragraphs.

ROBERT KOCH, M.D.
398 Main Street
Park Ridge, NJ 07656

January 30, 19—

William Osler, M.D.
1000 South West Street
Park Ridge, NJ 07656

ANNABELLE ANDERSON

You will be pleased to know, Bill, that Mrs. Anderson is progressing nicely. Her wound is healing. Her temperature has returned to normal, and she is beginning to resume her usual activities.

Mrs. Anderson has an appointment to return here for one more visit next week. At that time, I will ask her to return to you for any further care.

ROBERT KOCH, M.D.

RK:hb

FIGURE 11–5 Simplified letter style.

SIMPLIFIED LETTER STYLE All lines begin flush with the left margin. The salutation is replaced with an all-capital subject line on the third line below the inside address. The body of the letter begins on the third line below the subject line. The complimentary closing is omitted. An all-capital typewritten signature is entered on the fifth line below the body of the letter (Fig. 11–5).

Punctuation

Traditionally, the punctuation pattern is selected on the basis of letter style. Normal punctuation is always used *within the body* of a business letter. The other parts use either *standard* or *open* punctuation.

STANDARD (MIXED) PUNCTUATION A colon is placed after the salutation, and a comma is placed after the complimentary closing. This is the punctuation pattern most commonly used. It is appropriate with the block or modified-block letter styles.

OPEN PUNCTUATION No punctuation is used at the end of any line outside the body of the letter unless that line ends with an abbreviation. This pattern is always used with the simplified letter style.

Spacing and Margins

Generally, a letter centered on a page is the most attractive. Accomplishing this requires experience, but a few guidelines with which to start are helpful.

SPACING Business letters are almost always single spaced. If a letter consists of only a few lines, you can double-space both the inside address and the message. In this case, you should indent the first line of each paragraph five spaces.

TOP MARGIN The first typed entry (the date) is usually placed on the third line below the letterhead or on line 13 (two inches) if there is no letterhead. Continuation pages begin 1 inch from the top (line 7).

SIDE MARGIN On standard letterhead, the 6½-inch line is common and leaves 1-inch margins on each side. The appearance of a very short letter is improved by increasing the width of all margins.

BOTTOM MARGIN A 1-inch bottom margin is the minimum. This can be increased if the letter is to be carried over to a second page. *Note:* Never use a second page to type only the complimentary closing and signature. Carry over a minimum of two lines of the body of the letter.

Memory Jogger

4 *Why is it important to carry over a minimum of two lines from the body of the letter?*

Parts of Letters

The structure of a letter and its placement on a page have been fairly well standardized into four main parts:

> Heading
> Opening
> Body
> Closing

HEADING

The heading includes the *letterhead* and the *date line.*

The printed letterhead is usually centered at the top of the page and includes the name of the physician or group and the address. It may include the telephone number and the medical specialty (or specialties). In a group or corporate practice, the names of the physicians may also be listed. Occasionally, the heading also includes the name of an office manager.

The date line consists of the name of the month written in full, followed by the day and year. The date should not be abbreviated, nor should ordinal numbers (i.e., 1st, 2nd, and 3rd) be used after the name of the month.

OPENING

The opening consists of the *inside address,* the *salutation,* and the *attention line,* if there is one.

The inside address has two or more lines, starts flush with the left margin, and contains at least the name of the individual or firm to whom the letter is addressed and the mailing address. When the letter is addressed to an individual, the name is preceded by a courtesy title, such as Dr., Mr., Mrs., Miss, or Ms. When addressing a letter to a physician, omit the courtesy title and type the physician's name followed by his or her **academic degree.** (Herbert H. Long, MD). Do not use both a courtesy title and a degree that mean the same thing (e.g., Dr. Herbert H. Long, MD).

The salutation is the letter writer's introductory greeting to the person being addressed. It is typed flush with the left margin on the second line below the last line of the address and is followed by a colon unless open punctuation is used. The words in the salutation vary depending on the degree of formality of the letter.

The attention line, if used, is placed on the second line below the inside address. If you know the name of the person for whom the letter is intended, use that person's name in the inside address and address him or her personally. If the letter is being addressed to a company or organization and directed to a division or department within the company, place the division or department name on the attention line.

BODY

The body of a letter includes the *subject line,* if one is used, and the *message.*

Frequently in medical office correspondence, the subject of a letter is a patient. The patient's name is used as the *subject line.* Because the subject line is considered to be a part of the body of the letter, it is placed on the second line below the salutation. It may start flush with the left margin or at the point of indentation of indented paragraphs, or it may be centered. The word *subject,* followed by a colon, may be used or omitted entirely.

Begin typing the *message* on the second line below the subject line, or on the second line below the salutation if there is no subject line. The first line of each paragraph may be indented five spaces or may start flush with the left margin, depending on the chosen letter style.

CLOSING

The closing includes the *complimentary closing,* the *typewritten signature,* the *reference initials,* and any *special notations.*

The complimentary closing is the writer's way of saying good-bye. It is placed on the second line below the last line of the body of the letter and is followed by a comma unless open punctuation is used. Only the first word is capitalized. The words used are determined by the degree of formality in the salutation. For example, if the salutation is "Dear Herb:" the closing might be "Cordially" or "Sincerely yours" with consistent punctuation. If the letter is addressed to a business, the complimentary closing most used is "Very truly yours."

A typewritten signature is a courtesy to the reader, especially if the name does not appear on the printed letterhead or when the personal signature is difficult or impossible to decipher. Place the typewritten signature on the fourth line directly below the complimentary closing.

Reference initials that identify the typist are placed flush with the left margin on the second line below the typewritten signature. If the writer's name is included on the signature line, the writer's initials need not be included in the reference block unless desired. The writer's initials, if used, should precede the typist's initials and be separated by a colon or diagonal: mek or GB:mek or GB/mek

Special notations are sometimes needed to indicate that enclosures are included with the letter or that copies of the letter are being distributed to others. If the letter indicates an enclosure, type the word *Enclosure* or *Enc.* on the first line below the reference initials. If there is more than one enclosure, specify the number (e.g., Enclosures 3). If copies are to be sent to others, type this notation in the same manner as the enclosure notation or following it if both notations are needed. The copy notation is usually written as cc: or c: or copy to: followed by the name or names of those to whom a copy will be sent. If the person to whom the letter is addressed is not to know that copies are being distributed to others, use the notation bcc: for *blind carbon copy,* on all copies *except* the original. Place this notation either in the upper left of the letter at the margin or below the last notation at the lower left margin.

POSTSCRIPTS

Although a postscript may sometimes be used to express an afterthought, it is more often used to *place emphasis* on an idea or statement.

Begin the postscript on the second line below the last special notation. Follow the style of the letter, indenting the first line if paragraphs were indented in the body of the letter or starting at the margin if indentation was not used in the letter.

Memory Jogger

5 *List the parts of a letter and describe what is included in each part.*

Continuation Pages

If the letter requires one or more **continuation pages,** the heading of the second and subsequent pages must contain three items of information: (1) the name of the addressee, (2) the page number, and (3) the date.

The heading should begin on the 7th line (1 inch) from the top of the page. Continuation of the body of the letter begins on the 10th line or the 3rd line below the heading. There are three accepted forms for the continuation page heading.

Elizabeth Blackwell, M.D.	-2-	July 4, 2000

William Osler, M.D.
Page 2
July 4, 2000

William S. Halsted, M.D.
Page 2
July 4, 2000
Subject: Susan Barstow

Signing the Letter

Some physicians prefer to compose and sign all letters that leave their offices. The majority are more than pleased to delegate to a competent assistant the responsibility of composing and signing letters of a business nature.

Although not all authorities agree on the form to be followed, most recommend that a woman's typewritten signature include a courtesy title (Miss, Mrs., or Ms.) and that the title not be enclosed in parentheses. It is not necessary to include the courtesy title in the handwritten signature.

How will you know which letters to sign? In general, the physician signs all of the following:

- Letters that deal with medical advice to patients
- Letters to officers or committees of the medical society
- Referral and consultation reports to colleagues
- Medical reports to insurance companies
- Personal letters

The medical assistant usually composes and signs letters dealing with the following matters:

- Routine matters such as arranging or rescheduling appointments
- Ordering office supplies
- Notifying patients of surgery or hospital arrangements
- Collecting for delinquent accounts
- Letters of solicitation

The steps in composing business correspondence and an example using composing and writing instructions are given in Procedures 11–1 and 11–2.

PROCEDURE 11–1
Composing Business Correspondence

GOAL

To compose and type a letter ordering medical and office supplies using tabular placement of items and following the guidelines of a commonly used business letter style.

EQUIPMENT AND SUPPLIES

Typewriter or computer
Draft paper
Letterhead paper
Pen or pencil

"Want" list of supplies needed
Medical and office supply catalog
Correction tape (optional)

PROCEDURAL STEPS

1 Locate items from "want" list in catalog.

2 Note the catalog number of each item; the unit price, size, and color; and any special information requirements.
  EXPLANATION: Compare this information with the "want" list to confirm the correctness of the order.

3 Prepare a draft of the letter by hand or machine, tabulating the items ordered.
  PURPOSE: To provide practice in composing a letter and the use of tabulation. (With sufficient experience, preparation of a draft can be eliminated.)

4 Edit the draft carefully for correct information, grammar, spelling, and punctuation.

5 Set line and margins for attractive placement of the letter.

6 Prepare final letter from the corrected draft.

7 Type your signature and identification initials.
  EXPLANATION: The medical assistant signs letters ordering supplies.

8 Proofread the letter for composition errors and accuracy of the order before removing it from typewriter or sending to print.

9 Sign letter in preparation for mailing.

PROCEDURE 11-2

Composing and Writing Instructions

GOAL

To inform new patient of most desirable automobile route to physician's office, including any known landmarks, and description of parking facilities at destination.

EQUIPMENT AND SUPPLIES

Local map
Name and address of patient
Typewriter or word processor
Draft paper
Pen or pencil

Bond paper
Envelope
Dictionary
Correction tape (optional)

PROCEDURAL STEPS

1 Locate the physician's office on the map.

2 Locate the patient's address on the map.
   PURPOSE: To determine the most desirable route between these two points.

3 On draft paper, using a pencil or typewriter, compose directions, using street names and including any prominent intersections, right or left turns, landmarks just preceding the destination, and means of identifying the destination.
   PURPOSE: To create a mental picture of a route and directions that can easily be followed.

4 Read your copy for clarity and recheck with the map for accuracy.
   PURPOSE: Note the spelling of street names and check for the accuracy of direction turns.

5 Describe parking facilities and their utilization.
   EXPLANATION: Include information about meters, validation, time limit, and so forth.

6 Describe route to physician's office entrance from the parking facility.
   PURPOSE: To provide peace of mind to patients who feel apprehensive about traveling to an unfamiliar location.

7 Check the complete draft for clarity and detail.
   PURPOSE: It is very important that directions be accurate, clear, and complete.

8 Prepare directions in narrative form on bond paper.

9 Proofread and make any necessary corrections.

10 Prepare an envelope using the format for optical scanning.

Preparing the Outgoing Mail

ADDRESSING THE ENVELOPE

Mailing Address

The U.S. Postal Service attempts to have all mail (in No. 10 and No. 6¾ envelopes) read, coded, sorted, and canceled automatically at regional sorting stations where mail can be processed at a rate of 30,000 letters per hour. The success of automatic sorting depends on the cooperation of mailers in preparing envelopes in a format that can be read by automatic equipment. Key points are as follows:

- Use dark type on a light background; black on white is best.
- Do not use script or italic type; these cannot be read by an electronic scanner.
- Type all addresses in block format and in the area on the envelope that the scanner is programmed to read.
- Capitalize everything in the address.
- Eliminate all punctuation in the address.
- Use the standard two-letter state code instead of the spelled out name of the state (Table 11–3).
- The last line of the address must contain the city, state code, and ZIP code, and it must not exceed 27 characters in length.

TABLE 11–3 Two-Letter Abbreviations to Be Used with Zip Codes

United States and Territories			
Alabama	AL	Montana	MT
Alaska	AK	Nebraska	NE
Arizona	AZ	Nevada	NV
Arkansas	AR	New Hampshire	NH
California	CA	New Jersey	NJ
Canal Zone	CZ	New Mexico	NM
Colorado	CO	New York	NY
Connecticut	CT	North Carolina	NC
Delaware	DE	North Dakota	ND
District of Columbia	DC	Ohio	OH
Florida	FL	Oklahoma	OK
Georgia	GA	Oregon	OR
Guam	GU	Pennsylvania	PA
Hawaii	HI	Puerto Rico	PR
Idaho	ID	Rhode Island	RI
Illinois	IL	South Carolina	SC
Indiana	IN	South Dakota	SD
Iowa	IA	Tennessee	TN
Kansas	KS	Texas	TX
Kentucky	KY	Utah	UT
Louisiana	LA	Vermont	VT
Maine	ME	Virgin Islands	VI
Maryland	MD	Virginia	VA
Massachusetts	MA	Washington	WA
Michigan	MI	West Virginia	WV
Minnesota	MN	Wisconsin	WI
Mississippi	MS	Wyoming	WY
Missouri	MO		

Canadian Provinces and Territories			
Alberta	AB	Nova Scotia	NS
British Columbia	BC	Ontario	ON
Manitoba	MB	Prince Edward Island	PE
New Brunswick	NB	Quebec	PQ
Newfoundland	NF	Saskatchewan	SK
Northwest Territories	NT	Yukon Territory	YT

The characters should be distributed so that they will not exceed the following limits:

Allowance for city name	13
Space between city name and state code	1
Allowance for state code	2
Space between state code and ZIP code	1
Space for basic ZIP code	5
Space for hyphen and four additional characters	5
	27

If a city name contains more than 13 characters, you must use the approved code for that city as shown in the Abbreviations Section of the National Zip Code Directory.

The Postal Service provides three special sets of abbreviations: (1) state names; (2) long names of cities, towns, and places; and (3) names of streets and roads and general terms, such as University or Institute. You can obtain this information from the Postal Service or purchase a program for the computer. By using these abbreviations, it is possible to limit the last line of any domestic address to 27 strokes. The next-to-last line in the address block

should contain a street address or post office box number.

MEDICAL ASSOCIATES INCORPORATED
4444 AVENIDA WILSHIRE
SAN CLEMENTE CA 92672-1500

HENRY B TURNER MD
PO BOX 845
JACKSONVILLE FL 32232-9950

The address block should start no higher than 2¾ inches from the bottom. Leave a bottom margin of at least ⅝ inch and left and right margins of at least 1 inch. Nothing should be written or printed below the address block or to the right of it.

The regulations for addressing envelopes were developed mainly for volume mailers with computerized mailing lists. Some exceptions are acceptable to the Postal Service and its scanning equipment. For example, the traditional style of typing an address in lower case with initial capital letters is readable by the optical scanners. Also, if you cannot fit the ZIP code on the line with the city and state, you can place it on the line immediately below.

Memory Jogger

6 *What information should appear on the next-to-last line of an address block on the envelope?*

Return Address

Always place a complete return address on your envelope. The US Postal Service will not deliver mail without postage; and if you should forget to stamp the envelope or if the stamp should fall off and there is no return address, it will go to the dead letter office. There the postal employees will open the mail in an attempt to identify the sender.

If they find an address for the sender, they will return the mail in an official envelope with a notice of postage due. If they do not find an address for the sender, the mail is destroyed and you may never know what happened to it. At best, it causes a great delay.

Notations

Any notations on the envelope directed toward the addressee, such as *Personal* or *Confidential*, should be typed and underlined on line 9 or on the third line below the return address, whichever is lower. Align it with the return address on the left edge of the envelope.

Any notations directed toward the postal service, such as SPECIAL DELIVERY or CERTIFIED MAIL,

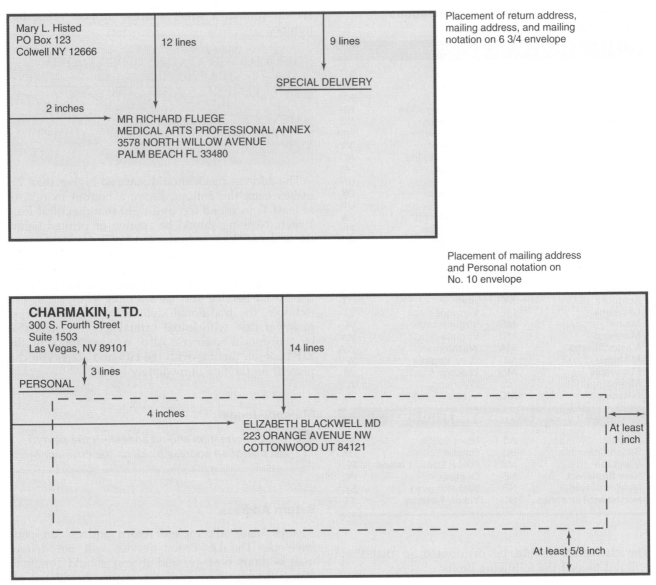

Placement of return address, mailing address, and mailing notation on 6 3/4 envelope

Mary L. Histed
PO Box 123
Colwell NY 12666

12 lines

9 lines

SPECIAL DELIVERY

2 inches

MR RICHARD FLUEGE
MEDICAL ARTS PROFESSIONAL ANNEX
3578 NORTH WILLOW AVENUE
PALM BEACH FL 33480

Placement of mailing address and Personal notation on No. 10 envelope

CHARMAKIN, LTD.
300 S. Fourth Street
Suite 1503
Las Vegas, NV 89101

14 lines

3 lines

PERSONAL

4 inches

ELIZABETH BLACKWELL MD
223 ORANGE AVENUE NW
COTTONWOOD UT 84121

At least 1 inch

At least 5/8 inch

FIGURE 11–6 Addressing envelopes.

should be typed in all capital letters on the upper right side of the envelope immediately below the stamp area. If an address contains an attention line, it should be typed above the organization line, or on the line immediately above the street address or post office box number (Fig. 11–6).

Folding and Inserting Letters

Standard ways of folding and inserting letters are used so that the letter fits properly into the envelope and so that it an be easily removed without damage (Fig. 11–7).

NO. 10 ENVELOPE For a standard-size letter, bring the bottom third of the letter up and make a crease. Fold the top of the letter down to within

about ⅜ inch of the creased edge and make a second crease. The second crease goes into the envelope first.

NO. 6¾ ENVELOPE For a standard-size letter, bring the bottom edge up to within about ⅜ inch of the top edge and make a crease. Then, folding from the right edge, make a fold a little less than one third of the width of the sheet and crease it. Folding from the left edge, bring the edge to within about ⅜ inch of the previous crease. Insert the left creased edge into the envelope first.

WINDOW ENVELOPE To fold a letter for insertion into a window envelope, bring the bottom third of the letter up and make a crease, then fold the top of the letter back to the crease you made before. (The inside address should now be facing you.) This method is often followed for mailing statements.

Sealing and Stamping Hints

Here's a suggestion for speeding up the sealing of a number of envelopes; at statement time, for example, many envelopes go into the mail at one time:

- Fan out unsealed envelopes, address side down, in groups of 6 to 10.
- Draw a damp sponge over the flaps and, starting with the lower piece, turn down the flaps and seal each one.

Do not use too much moisture because this may cause the glue to spread and several envelopes to stick together. A similar process simplifies stamping several letters at one time if you are not using a postage meter. If possible, purchase your stamps by the roll.

- Tear off about 10 stamps from the roll.
- Fanfold the stamps on the perforations so that they separate easily.
- Fan the envelopes address side up.
- Wet a strip of stamps with the sponge and, starting at one end of the fanned envelopes, attach the stamp at the end of the strip, tear it off, and proceed to the next envelope.

Automated sealer/stampers are also available.

Cost-Saving Mailing Procedures

USING ZIP CODES

The ZIP code is a very important part of an address, just as the area code is a very important part of a

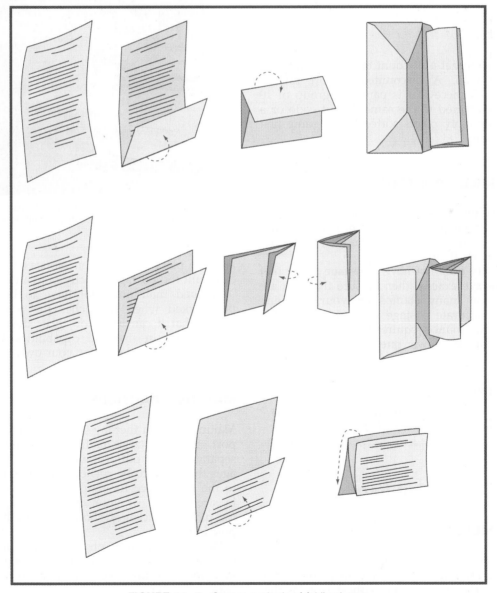

FIGURE 11–7   Correct methods of folding letters.

telephone number. ZIP codes start with the number 0 on the East Coast and gradually increase to number 9 on the West Coast and Hawaii.

The 5-digit ZIP code was introduced in 1961. The first three digits identify a major city or distribution point, and all five digits identify an individual post office, zone of a city, or other delivery unit. Later on the Postal Service added the 9-digit ZIP code, consisting of the original five digits followed by a hyphen and four additional digits that further identify the addressee's street location. The ZIP code is electronically transformed into a bar code. Your office computer may have this capability. The Postal Code claims that the ZIP-plus-4, when used with the automated letter-sorting machinery, can eliminate 20 mail handling steps and result in considerable savings. This saving is passed on to large mailers on mailings of 250 or more pieces of mail that have typewritten addresses in machine-readable format along with the 9-digit ZIP code.

PRESORTING

Large mailers can get a discount on postage for presorting their mail. A discounted presort rate is charged on each piece that is part of a group of 10 or more pieces sorted to the same 5-digit code or a group of 50 or more pieces sorted to the same first 3-digit ZIP code.

USING CORRECT POSTAGE

Although mailing fees are still one of our better bargains, the mailing costs for even a small office are a sizable item in the annual budget, and carelessness can cause them to soar.

If your facility does not have a postage meter that dispenses postage exactly, then be sure that you are not putting too many stamps on your outgoing mail. Use an accurate postage scale and remember that only the first ounce requires the base rate; additional ounces are at a lower rate.

Memory Jogger

7 *At the current rate, how much postage would be needed on a letter that weighs 2¼ ounces?*

Getting Faster Mail Service

POSTAGE METER

The postage meter is the most efficient way of stamping the mail in a large business office (Fig. 11–8). It can print postage onto adhesive strips that

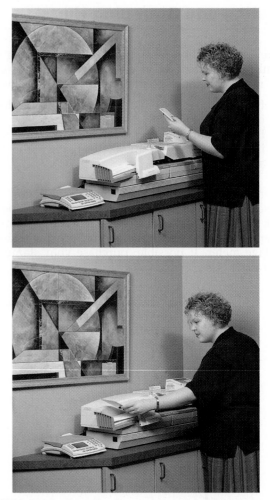

FIGURE 11–8 Example of one type of postage meter-mailing machine and photograph of medical assistant using the machine.

are then placed onto the envelopes or packages, or it can print the postage directly onto an envelope.

Metered mail does not have to be canceled or postmarked when it reaches the post office. This means that it can move on to its destination faster. Meters vary in size and capabilities. Consult your office equipment dealer for your own needs.

MAILING PRACTICES

Mailing early in the day is appreciated by your local post office. For large mailings, local letters should be separated from out-of-town letters. Letters or packages that need to be rushed should be taken directly to the post office for mailing. Others can be placed in street boxes or your own building's mail chute for pickup. Packages should always be taken to a post office.

Place a letter tray on your desk or some other convenient place so that you can keep all outgoing mail together until you are able to send it on its way.

Classifications of Mail

Mail is classified according to *type, weight,* and *destination.* The ounce and pound are the units of measurement.

EXPRESS MAIL NEXT-DAY SERVICE

Express Mail is available 7 days per week, 365 days per year for mailable items weighing up to 70 pounds and measuring 108 inches in combined length and girth. Service features include

- Noon delivery between major business markets
- Merchandise and document reconstruction insurance
- Express mail shipping containers
- Shipment receipt
- Optional return receipt service
- Optional COD service
- Waiver of signature option
- Collection boxes
- Optional pickup service

FIRST CLASS MAIL

This includes sealed or unsealed handwritten or typed material, such as letters, postal cards, postcards, and business reply mail. Postage for letters weighing 11 ounces or less is based on weight, in 1-ounce increments.

Envelopes larger than the standard No. 10 business envelope should have the green diamond border to expedite First Class delivery.

PRIORITY MAIL

First class mail weighing over 11 ounces is classified as priority mail, and the postage is calculated on the basis of weight and destination, with the maximum weight being 70 pounds. Flat-rate envelopes (9½ × 12¼) that can be packed with mailable materials and mailed at a 2-pound postage rate regardless of weight are available from the post office. The amount of postage is predetermined, and the filled envelope can be mailed without having to be weighed.

SECOND CLASS MAIL

Regular and preferred second class rates are available only to newspapers and periodicals that have been authorized to receive Second Class mail privileges. Copies mailed by the public are charged at the applicable express mail, priority mail, or single piece first, third, or fourth class rate.

THIRD CLASS MAIL

Third Class includes such items as catalogs, circulars, books, photographs, and other printed matter. Pieces should be sealed or secured so that they can be handled by machine but must be clearly marked with the words "Third Class."

FOURTH CLASS MAIL

Fourth Class consists of merchandise, books and printed matter that are not included in first or second class and that weigh 16 ounces or more but do not exceed 70 pounds. There are size limitations on fourth class mail; check with your post office regarding regulations on very large parcels. Rates are determined on the basis of *weight* and *destination.* Such mail may be sealed or unsealed.

Domestic Mail

MINIMUM SIZE STANDARDS

All mail must be at least 0.007-inch thick. Mail that is ¼ inch or less in thickness must be rectangular and at least 3½ inches in height and 5 inches long.

NONSTANDARD MAIL

It is important to use a standard size envelope. For each piece of nonstandard mail, the Postal Service assesses a surcharge in addition to the applicable postage and fees. Envelope sizes were standardized when the Postal Service began sorting mail by machine. The following material is considered nonstandard mail: first class mail (except presort first class and carrier route first class) weighing 1 ounce or less and all single-piece rate third class mail weighing 1 ounce or less if

1. Any of these dimensions are exceeded:

   Length—11½ inches
   Height—6½ inches
   Thickness—¼ inch

2. The length divided by the height is not between 1.3 and 2.5.

SPECIAL SERVICES

INSURANCE   Insurance for coverage against loss or damage is available in amounts up to $600 for priority mail, first class, or parcel post.

REGISTRY   Mail of all classes, particularly that of unusually high value, can be additionally protected by registering it. Evidence of its delivery may be requested by the sender. Registering a piece of mail also helps to trace delivery, if necessary.

When sending a registered letter, it is necessary to go to the post office and fill in the required forms. All articles to be registered must be thoroughly sealed with U.S. Postal Service tape (do not use cellophane tape) and have postage paid at first class rates.

On receipt of the item, the recipient is required to sign a form that acknowledges delivery. A registered letter may be released to the person to whom it is addressed or to his or her agent. For an additional fee, a personal receipt may be requested. This ensures that the letter will be released only to the individual to whom it is addressed. Such pieces bear the label *To Addressee Only*.

Registered mail is accounted for by number from the time of mailing until delivery and is transported separately from other mail under a special lock. In case of loss or damage, the customer may be reimbursed up to $25,000, provided that the value of the registered article has been declared at the time of mailing and that the appropriate fee has been paid.

POSTAL MONEY ORDERS Postal money orders are a convenient way of mailing money, especially for the individual who does not have a personal checking account. They may be purchased in amounts as high as $700. If a sum greater than $700 is needed, additional money orders must be purchased in amounts of $700 or less.

SPECIAL DELIVERY Mail of any class that has been marked SPECIAL DELIVERY is charged at the Special Delivery rate. Such pieces may be regular First or Second Class mail, registered, insured, or COD (Collect on Delivery) pieces. The Special Delivery designation generally does not speed up the normal travel time between two cities but does ensure immediate delivery of the item when it arrives at the designated post office.

Special delivery stamps may be purchased at the post office. Alternatively, the equivalent value in regular stamps may be affixed to the envelope, which should always be clearly marked Special Delivery. Use Special Delivery when you need delivery of an item the same day as it is received at the addressee's post office (including weekend delivery that is not available with regular mail). A fee based on the weight of the item is required in addition to the required postage. *Do not* use Special Delivery for mail addressed to a post office box or military installation.

SPECIAL HANDLING Third and Fourth Class mail sent by Special Handling receives the fastest service and ground transportation practicable—about the same as that for First Class mail. The Special Handling fee is in addition to required postage and is determined according to weight. This fee does not include insurance or Special Delivery at the destination, but Special Delivery, if desired, is available at an added cost. If a parcel is sent by Priority Mail, Special Handling is of no additional advantage because it is already traveling at the greatest possible speed.

CERTIFIED MAIL Any piece of mail without **intrinsic value** and on which postage is paid at the First Class rate will be accepted as Certified Mail. Such items as contracts, deeds, mortgages, bank books, checks, passports, insurance policies, money orders, and birth certificates that are not themselves valuable but that would be difficult to duplicate if lost should be certified. Certified Mail is also often used as an aid in collections.

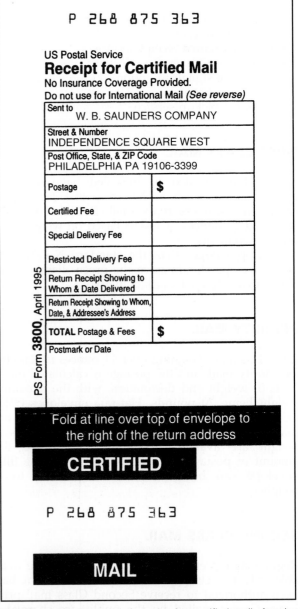

FIGURE 11–9 Example of receipt for certified mail. Attach at top of envelope to the right of return address.

Regular postage in addition to a Certified Mail fee must be affixed. For an additional fee, a receipt verifying delivery can be requested. Certified Mail can be sent Special Delivery if the prescribed Special Delivery fees are paid. A record of delivery of Certified Mail is kept for 2 years at the post office of delivery; however, no record is kept at the post office of origin. Furthermore, this type of mail does not provide insurance coverage.

The medical assistant should keep a supply of Certified Mail forms and return receipts on hand (Figs. 11–9 and 11–10). These may be obtained at any post office. Full instructions are included on the forms. Fees and postage may be paid using ordinary postage stamps, meter stamps, or permit imprint. Certified Mail can be mailed at any post office, station, or branch or can be deposited in mail drops or in street letter boxes if specific instructions are followed.

CERTIFICATE OF MAILING If a sender needs proof of mailing but is not especially concerned with proof of receipt of an item, the most economic method is to obtain a Certificate of Mailing. Obtain this form at your post office and fill in the required information. Attach a stamp for the current fee and hand the form to the postal clerk along with the piece of mail. The clerk will postmark the receipt, initial it, and hand it back as acknowledgment of having received the piece of mail at the post office. This is sometimes used when mailing tax reports or other items that must be postmarked by a certain date.

Memory Jogger

8 *Explain the basic differences between Certified Mail and Certificate of Mailing.*

International Mail

Letters to distant points of the globe are in almost all cases sent by air and can be expected to reach their destination within a very few days. The rates for international mail are based on increments of one-half ounce. A table of rates can be obtained from your post office. If you wish to supply a foreign correspondent with reply postage, international reply coupons may be purchased at the post office and sent to other countries.

Private Delivery Services

Not all mail is delivered by the U.S. Postal Service. Many private services pick up and deliver mail overnight. Among these are Federal Express, United Parcel Service, Emery, and DHL. These services are highly advertised and competitive. All large cities and many smaller communities have centralized points where packages can be dropped off for the service of the sender's choice. Pickup service is also available in many communities.

Handling Special Situations

FORWARDING MAIL

First Class mail only may be forwarded from one address to another without payment of additional postage. Simply cross out the printed address and write in the address to which it should be delivered.

OBTAINING CHANGE OF ADDRESS

If the mailer wants to know an addressee's new address, this service can be obtained from the post office by placing the words *Address Correction Requested* beneath the return address on the envelope. This can be handwritten, stamped, typewritten, or printed. The post office charges a postage-due fee for this service. For First Class mail, the post office will forward the piece of mail and return a card to the sender showing the forwarding address of the addressee. The card will have a postage due stamp on it for the amount of the required fee.

RECALLING MAIL

If you have dropped a letter in the mailbox and want it back, do not ask the mail collector to give it to you; he or she is not permitted to do this. However, mail can be recalled by making written application at the post office, together with an envelope addressed identically to the one being recalled. If your letter has already left the local post office, the postmaster, at the sender's expense, can notify the postmaster at the destination post office to return the letter.

RETURNED MAIL

If a letter is returned to the sender after an attempt has been made to deliver it, it cannot be remailed without new postage. It is best simply to prepare a new envelope with the correct address, affix the proper postage, and remail.

TRACING LOST MAIL

Receipts issued by the post office, whether for money orders, registered mail, certified mail, or in-

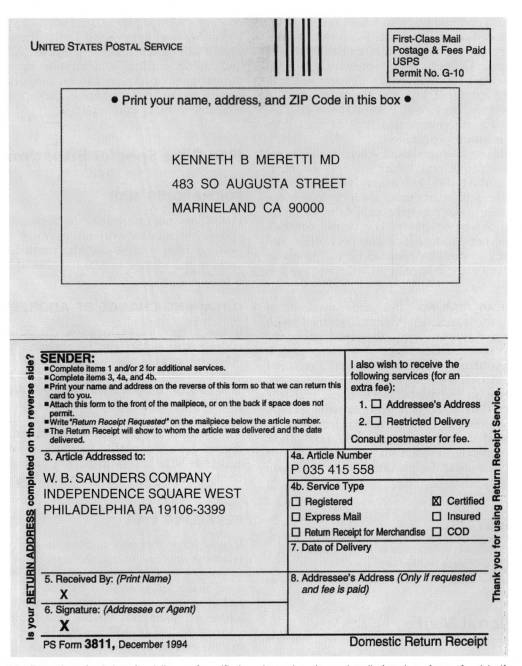

UNITED STATES POSTAL SERVICE

First-Class Mail
Postage & Fees Paid
USPS
Permit No. G-10

● Print your name, address, and ZIP Code in this box ●

KENNETH B MERETTI MD

483 SO AUGUSTA STREET

MARINELAND CA 90000

SENDER:
- Complete items 1 and/or 2 for additional services.
- Complete items 3, 4a, and 4b.
- Print your name and address on the reverse of this form so that we can return this card to you.
- Attach this form to the front of the mailpiece, or on the back if space does not permit.
- Write *"Return Receipt Requested"* on the mailpiece below the article number.
- The Return Receipt will show to whom the article was delivered and the date delivered.

I also wish to receive the following services (for an extra fee):

1. ☐ Addressee's Address
2. ☐ Restricted Delivery

Consult postmaster for fee.

3. Article Addressed to:

W. B. SAUNDERS COMPANY
INDEPENDENCE SQUARE WEST
PHILADELPHIA PA 19106-3399

4a. Article Number
P 035 415 558

4b. Service Type
☐ Registered   ☒ Certified
☐ Express Mail   ☐ Insured
☐ Return Receipt for Merchandise ☐ COD

7. Date of Delivery

5. Received By: *(Print Name)*
X

6. Signature: *(Addressee or Agent)*
X

8. Addressee's Address *(Only if requested and fee is paid)*

Is your RETURN ADDRESS completed on the reverse side?

Thank you for using Return Receipt Service.

PS Form **3811**, December 1994   **Domestic Return Receipt**

FIGURE 11–10 Examples of receipts for delivery of certified, registered, or insured mail. Attach to front of article if space permits. Otherwise, attach to back of article and endorse front of article with "return receipt requested" adjacent to the number.

sured mail, should be retained until receipt of the item has been acknowledged. If, after an adequate time elapses, no acknowledgment of receipt for such mailing arrives, notify the post office to trace the letter or package. Regular First Class mail is not easily traced, but the post office will make every attempt to find it for you. In tracing a lost letter or package, the post office requires that a special form be filled out; data from any original receipt should be written along with any other identifying information on this form.

Incoming Mail

Each day, a great variety of mail comes into the professional office and must be processed. There may be

- General correspondence
- Payments for services
- Bills for office purchases
- Insurance claim forms to be completed
- Laboratory reports

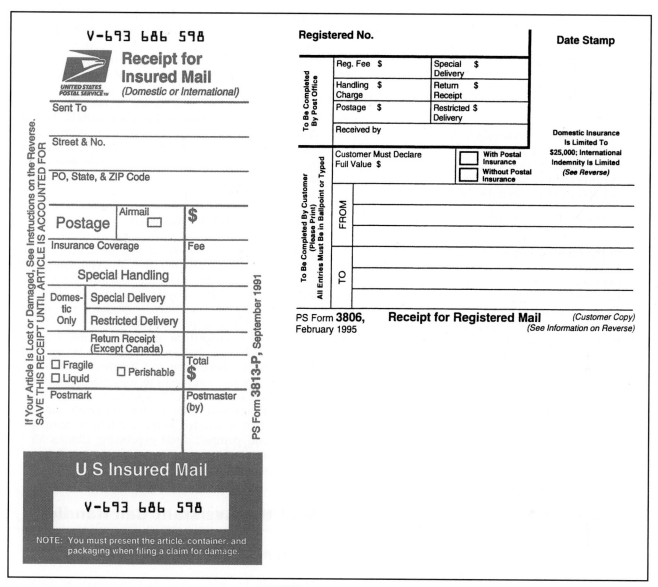

FIGURE 11–10 *Continued*

- Hospital reports
- Medical society mailings
- Professional journals
- Promotional literature and samples from pharmaceutical houses
- Advertisements

In large clinics and medical centers, the mail is opened by specially designated persons in a central department to speed up this daily task. But in the average professional office, a medical assistant opens the mail using the ordinary letter-opener method.

MAIL PROCESSING

Before opening any mail, the medical assistant should have an agreement with the physician as to what procedure to follow regarding incoming mail—in other words, what letters should be opened and what pieces, if any, the physician prefers to open personally. For example, the physician may prefer to open any communications from an attorney or accountant, even when they are not marked *Personal*. If there is any doubt in regard to opening an envelope, the best rule to follow is, "Don't." Treat your physician's mail with the same consideration that you expect others to exercise toward your own. Even a simple procedure such as opening the daily mail can be done with more efficiency if a good system is followed. Have a clear working space on your desk or countertop, and proceed as follows:

Assemble the equipment and supplies you will need:

1. Letter opener
2. Paper clips
3. Stapler
4. Transparent tape
5. Date stamp

Sort the mail according to importance and urgency:

1. Physician's personal mail
2. Ordinary First Class mail
3. Checks from patients
4. Periodicals and newspapers
5. All other pieces, including drug samples

Open the mail neatly and in an organized manner:

1. Stack the envelopes so that they are all facing in the same direction.
2. Pick up the top one and tap the envelope so that when you open it you will not cut the contents.
3. Open all envelopes along the top edge for easiest removal of contents.
4. Remove the contents of each envelope and hold the envelope to the light to see that nothing remains inside.
5. Make a note of the postmark when this is important.
6. Discard the envelope after you have checked to see that there is a return address on the message contained inside. Some offices make it a policy to attach the envelope to each piece of correspondence until it has received attention.
7. Date stamp the letter and attach any enclosures.
8. If there is an enclosure notation at the bottom of the letter, check to be certain that the enclosure was included. Should it be missing, indicate this on the notation by writing the word *no* and circling it. This may be as far as your employer will want you to proceed with handling the correspondence.

ANNOTATING

If you have to **annotate** the mail, you can perform an additional service by reading each letter through, underlining the significant words and phrases, and noting in the margin any action required. If it is a letter that needs no reply, you can code it for filing at this time. A nonprint pencil that does not photocopy may be used for the annotating, if desired.

When mail refers to previous correspondence, obtain this from the file and attach it. Or if the patient's chart is needed in replying to an inquiry, pull the chart and place it with the letter.

A specific place should be agreed on for placing the opened and annotated mail. This will probably be some area on the physician's desk. When you have completed the sorting, opening, and annotating of the mail, place those items that the physician will wish to see in the established place, with the most important mail on top.

Personal mail, of course, is to remain unopened. Should you in error open a piece of personal mail addressed to your employer, fold and replace it inside the envelope, and write across the outside *Opened in Error*, followed by your initials. Use the same procedure with a piece of mail addressed to another office that may have been opened in error. In such cases, reseal the envelope with transparent tape and hand it to your carrier.

RESPONDING TO THE MAIL

In some offices, the physician and the medical assistant go over the mail together. As you gain confidence, you will find that you can draft a reply to some inquiries. Most physicians are very pleased to delegate this responsibility, especially on matters that do not relate to patient care.

Letters of referral from other physicians should be carefully noted so that an answer may be sent after the patient has been seen and the physician can give a report. If considerable time may pass before such information can be sent, it is a courteous gesture to write a thank-you note to the referring physician advising that a detailed letter will follow. Some physicians send printed cards expressing thanks for referrals; others prefer to write thank-you letters to professional colleagues.

Mail the Assistant Can Handle

CASH RECEIPTS

There will be some mail that the medical assistant can handle alone, for instance, payments from patients and insurance forms to be completed. All cash and checks should be separated and recorded immediately in the day's receipts.

INSURANCE FORMS

Insurance forms for completion should be put in a predetermined place for handling at the appropriate time. If there is an insurance clerk or other individual who processes the claims, they should be passed along to that person immediately.

DRUG SAMPLES

Sample drugs and related literature may arrive in the mail. Determine from the physician what types of literature and samples should be saved. Most physicians keep pertinent new samples in their desks, along with the accompanying literature for immediate reference. Other drug samples are **categorically** stored. Drugs should never be tossed into the trash.

Vacation Mail

When the physician is away from the office, it is generally the responsibility of a medical assistant to handle all mail. In this event, all pieces should be examined carefully. The medical assistant can then make a decision in regard to handling each piece on the basis of the following questions:

- Is this important enough that I should phone or FAX the physician?
- Shall I forward this for immediate attention?
- Shall I answer this myself or send a brief note to the correspondent, explaining that there will be a slight delay because the physician is out of the office?
- Can this wait for attention until the physician returns without appearing negligent?

If you are unable to contact the physician or to forward important mail, always answer the sender immediately, explaining the delay and requesting cooperation. Most offices have a copy machine as part of the office equipment. Instead of forwarding an original piece of mail and risking possible loss, make a copy for forwarding. Then, if the physician wishes you to answer the letter, notations can be made on the copy and returned to you without defacing the original letter.

When your employer is traveling from place to place, the envelope on each communication should be numbered consecutively. Doing this enables the physician to easily determine whether any mail has been lost or delayed. By keeping your own record of each piece of mail sent out, with its corresponding number, anything that might be lost can be identified and remailed if necessary.

Correspondence not requiring immediate action that the medical assistant is unable to answer until the physician returns should be placed in a special folder marked *Requires Attention* and placed on top of other accumulated mail. Mail that the medical assistant can compose but that requires the physician's approval before mailing, should be put into another special folder marked *For Approval*. When the physician returns, these letters can be rapidly checked and signed.

Any letters marked *Personal* that you hesitate to open and are unable to forward may be acknowledged to the return address on the envelope. The brief acknowledgment should state that the physician is out of town for a certain length of time and will attend to the letter immediately on returning.

Your acknowledgment should also offer your help in any way possible in the meantime.

Discard any mail that you would ordinarily not bring to the physician's attention. Some promotional literature falls into this category. (Make certain that mailings from professional organizations, whether they are First, Second, Third, or Fourth Class, are saved.)

There may be rare periods when the entire facility is closed. In such cases, the local post office should be notified to forward all First Class mail to an address supplied by the physician, if possible. Your postal carrier cannot accept an oral request to leave the mail with another person or at another address. A formal request must be made. If forwarding is out of the question, place a request with the post office to hold the mail until a specified date when someone will again be on duty. Never leave mail unattended to gather outside a mailbox or clutter up a doorway in a hall. Even mail slots may become filled or magazines may become stuck in them, causing important mail to pile up outside the slot. Far too much money and mail of a confidential nature is sent to physicians' offices to take chances on mail theft or destruction.

Systematizing your routine for processing all incoming and outgoing mail can put you in control of the paper blizzard!

LEGAL AND ETHICAL ISSUES

Every letter sent out from your facility should project a professional image.

The U.S. Postal Service requires that all volume mailers follow a special format in addressing envelopes so that they can be read, coded, sorted, and canceled automatically. Private mailers are requested to follow the same format.

The Postal Service will not deliver mail without postage attached. If there is no return address the mail goes to the dead letter office, where postal employees will open the mail in an attempt to identify the sender.

CRITICAL THINKING

1 What could be a negative effect of poorly written communications?

2 Visit a store that sells office stationery and observe the quality of the various offerings.

3 Examine a few of the promotional letters that arrive in your mail. Think about what is pleasing or not pleasing about their look and content.

4 Can you suggest the reason that volume mailers

would need special regulations for addressing envelopes?

HOW DID I DO? Answers to Memory Joggers

1 Sub 24 is an abbreviation for substance number or weight of a ream of 17×22-inch paper. Heavier weight paper has a higher substance number.

2 Ophthalmology

3 Memorandum is less formal. No salutation or complimentary closing is used.

4 The pages could become separated and difficult to identify.

5 *Heading*—letterhead and date line
Opening—inside address, salutation, and attention line, if used.
Body—subject line and message
Closing—complimentary closing, typed signature, reference initials, special notations.

6 Either the street address or the post office box number.

7 At this writing the postage would be 32¢ + 23¢ + 23¢, a total of 78¢. Rates are periodically changed.

8 The post office keeps a record of delivery of Certified Mail, and the sender may request a receipt verifying delivery. A Certificate of Mailing provides only proof of mailing.

REFERENCES

Sabin W: The Gregg Reference Manual, 7th ed. New York, Glencoe/McGraw-Hill, 1994.
Schwager E: Medical English Usage and Abusage. Phoenix, AZ, The Oryx Press, 1991.
Taber's Cyclopedic Medical Dictionary, 18th ed. Philadelphia, FA Davis, 1997.
The Postal Manual. Washington, DC, US Government Printing Office.

Dictation and Transcription

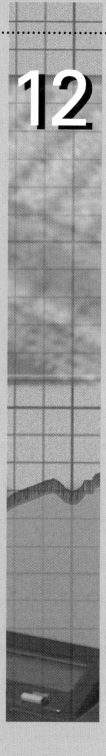

12

LEARNING OBJECTIVES

Cognitive: On successful completion of this chapter, you should be able to:
1 Define and spell the terms listed in the Vocabulary.
2 List six basic educational requirements for the medical transcriptionist.
3 Name two primary requisites for the independently practicing transcriptionist.
4 List the three steps of activity in the machine transcription process.
5 List five functional features of a typical transcribing unit.
6 State the principal differences between a *dedicated word processor* and a *computer.*
7 Name three kinds of frequently dictated reports in the average physician's office.

Performance: On successful completion of this chapter, and given the necessary equipment, you should be able to:
1 Estimate the length of a finished document before transcribing it.
2 Make any necessary corrections in keyboarding before removing the document from the machine.
3 Correctly utilize basic rules of capitalization.
4 Follow the rules for word division.
5 Determine when to use figures for numbers.
6 Correctly format medical reports.
7 Proofread and edit a transcribed document.

VOCABULARY

alignment The state of being in the correct relative position

cassette A magnetic tape wound on two reels and encased in a plastic or metal container; *microcassette* A very small cassette tape that may be used in a hand-held dictating unit

consultation report A report of the findings of the consulting physician to be sent to the referring physician

CPT manual *Current Procedural Terminology* manual

daisy wheel A printing element made of plastic or metal used on some typewriters and impact printers that derives its name from its shape, which is like that of a daisy

dictation The process of recording the spoken word onto a storage medium from which a printed copy will be produced

editing The process of examining text to determine accuracy and clarity

flagging A way of bringing attention to a blank space for possible correction in a transcribed page (also called tagging, carding, or marking)

fonts Sets of printing type that are of one size and style

HCPCS Acronym for HCFA's Common Procedure Coding System, used in determining Medicare fees

ICD manual International Classification of Diseases manual

indicator strip A charted strip that is inserted into the dictation unit and on which the dictator marks the beginning and end point of each document and any corrections to be made

keyboarding The process of entering characters into the memory of a word processor

progress notes Records of patient visits, telephone calls, progress, and treatment that are inserted into the patient's chart

proofreading Checking a document for spelling, sentence structure, punctuation, capitalization, style, and format

subscripts Symbols or numbers written immediately below another character

superscripts Symbols or numbers written immediately above another character

transcription Listening to recorded dictation and translating it into written form

---

A medical transcriptionist is a highly skilled professional whose educational background is similar in some respects to that of the administrative medical assistant. The medical transcriptionist must demonstrate many skills and qualities.

SKILLS AND RESPONSIBILITIES

ESSENTIAL SKILLS OF THE MEDICAL TRANSCRIPTIONIST

- Above-average typing and word processing skills
- Understanding of human anatomy and physiology and of the pathologic conditions that affect the human body
- Knowledge of medical terminology used in medical records, medical and surgical procedures, and laboratory tests
- Superior command of grammar, sentence structure and style, and spelling
- **Editing** and **proofreading** skills
- Ability to use a medical dictionary and other standard reference materials

Administrative medical assistants may find that transcribing **dictation** is one of their job requirements. Transcribing can be performed from handwritten notes, such as those in shorthand, or from machine dictation. In the health care facility the medical transcriptionist is a part of the team. Smooth operation of the facility may depend on the timely and accurate performance of assigned responsibilities, such as record documentation and the preparation of special reports.

Many professional medical transcriptionists practice independently and may affiliate with the American Association for Medical Transcription and become certified (see Chapter 3). The independent transcriptionist will find that *accuracy* and *speed* are primary requisites. Income depends on the transcriptionist's productivity, which may be measured by the number of pages, characters, or lines typed. The person who intends to do transcribing exclusively would do well to take a special course in transcription techniques.

Machine Transcription

Three stages of activity are involved in the process of dictation and transcription:

- Dictating into a dictation unit
- Listening to what has been dictated
- **Keyboarding** the dictated text to a printed document using correct format and required punctuation

Memory Jogger

1 *It is understood that accuracy is essential in preparing medical reports. Why is speed also important to the independent transcriptionist?*

DICTATION UNIT

The dictation unit is used by the physician to record material to be typed. Dictation units vary in design and capabilities. The desktop dictation unit is common in an office setting. This may be a combination unit used for both dictation and transcription. Alternatively, a machine used only for dictation may remain at the physician's desk; a separate **transcription** unit, including headphones and a foot pedal, remains at the transcriptionist's station. A lightweight portable hand-held dictation unit may be used for times when the physician (dictator) wishes to dictate while traveling or attending meetings away from the office. Physicians in a larger setting may install transcribing equipment that they can access by telephone wherever they may be. Many hospitals have this arrangement. All produce a recording that the transcriptionist listens to while keyboarding the text.

TRANSCRIBER UNIT

The unit operated by the transcriptionist may use magnetic tape, a **cassette,** or a disk. A desk-top unit using mini-, micro-, or standard cassettes is typical in the physician's office (Fig. 12–1).

There are many types and manufacturers of transcribing equipment, but most units contain certain standard features. Before using any equipment, the medical assistant should study the manufacturer's instruction manual. Most transcription units have a minimum of the following features:

- Stop and start control, with back-up and fast-forward ability
- Speed control
- Volume control
- Tone control
- Indicator for locating special instructions and determining the document length

STOP AND START CONTROL A foot pedal allows the transcriptionist to start, stop, back up, or fast forward the unit. He or she may wish to stop the unit while catching up with the typing, back up to replay a portion that was not understood, pause to insert additional matter from another source, or stop to check spelling. Most have an optional adjustment so that a slight rewind of the tape occurs when the machine is stopped and restarted. This prevents the loss of any dictated material in the process.

SPEED CONTROL The speed control feature can be used to slow down the recording of a fast dictator or speed up that of a slow dictator to match the speed of the transcriptionist.

VOLUME CONTROL The volume control in the headset can be adjusted to suit each unit of transcription. The headset also serves as a sound barrier by shutting out extraneous office sounds and preserving the confidentiality of the dictation.

TONE CONTROL The tone control feature allows the transcriptionist to increase or decrease the bass or treble to the pitch most understandable and pleasing to the ear.

INDICATOR STRIP For many years, dictating and transcribing machines have had **indicator strips** that could be inserted into the machine to allow the dictator to mark the point at which each item begins and ends and where corrections, if any, are needed. These strips are then attached to the transcribing machine to aid the typist. All too often the dictator refuses or neglects to use these indicators. When this happens, the transcriptionist should courteously remind the dictator of the importance of using this device.

Instead of an indicator strip, the machine may have a display window or cue-tone indexing capability that provides this same information. All of these features assist the transcriptionist in planning his or her transcribing duties.

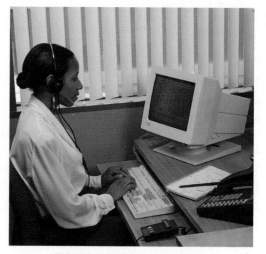

FIGURE 12–1 Transcriptionist.

The beginning transcriptionist tends to listen to a few words, stop the machine, type those words, and then restart the transcriber unit. Through practice, the transcriptionist learns to coordinate keyboarding activity with listening skills and listen ahead, thereby retaining in memory more and more of the dictated material so that it becomes unnecessary to stop and start the machine for this purpose.

Memory Jogger

 What feature of a transcribing unit prevents the loss of dictated material when the machine is stopped and restarted?

KEYBOARDING UNIT

The most important piece of equipment for the transcriptionist is the typewriter or computer on which the printed text will be produced. Many improvements have occurred within the past few years.

The manual typewriter is now virtually a museum piece. The electric typewriter appears to be on its way out as well, having been replaced by the electronic typewriter. The machines of choice in the modern office are the electronic typewriter, with or without memory; the dedicated word processor (display text editor); and the desk-top computer with word processing software.

ELECTRONIC TYPEWRITER

The electronic typewriter improves on the features of the electric typewriter by having the ability to automatically perform many tasks that save time and produce a more pleasing result. It is sometimes referred to as the *intelligent typewriter.* Instead of noisy keys, it has a single element, which is most likely a **daisy wheel.** With a daisy wheel, the typist may choose from among many kinds of type styles and sizes by simply removing one wheel and substituting the one of choice. Automatic features, such as number **alignment,** automatic centering, underlining, indenting, caps lock, and carrier return, are accomplished with the stroke of a key. Most have the capability of storing a limited amount of text and may have a display screen and spell-check capability (see Procedure 12–1).

PROCEDURE 12–1
Transcribing a Machine-Dictated Letter Using a Typewriter

GOAL

To transcribe a machine-dictated letter into a mailable document without error or detectable corrections, using a typewriter.

EQUIPMENT AND SUPPLIES

Transcribing machine
Typewriter
Draft paper

Letterhead Paper
Correcting Supplies
Reference Manual

PROCEDURAL STEPS

1 Assemble supplies

2 Turn on the transcription equipment

3 Set *line* for double spacing
  PURPOSE: To allow room for making changes or corrections

4 Type a draft of the letter

5 Edit the draft for spelling, insertions, and sentence structure

6 Note any necessary corrections

7 Set *line* and *margins* for attractive placement of the letter

8 Retype the draft on letterhead paper

9 Proofread the letter for content and errors before removing it from the typewriter

PROCEDURE 12–2

Transcribing a Machine-Dictated Letter Using a Computer or Word Processor

GOAL

To transcribe a machine-dictated letter into a mailable document without error or detectable corrections, using a computer or word processor.

EQUIPMENT AND SUPPLIES

Transcribing machine
Word processor or computer with
  appropriate software

Stationery
Reference Manual

PROCEDURAL STEPS

1 Assemble supplies
2 Set up the format for selected letter style
3 Keyboard the text while listening to the dictated letter
4 Edit the letter on the monitor
  PURPOSE: The letter should be in mailable form before printing
5 Execute a spell check
6 Direct the letter to the printer

DEDICATED WORD PROCESSOR

The term *word processing* was coined by IBM in the 1960s to describe its innovative Magnetic Tape Selectric Typewriter (MT/ST). The MT/ST was costly and met with some resistance because it required special training. Word processors today are much simpler. The word processor is a computer that is especially designed to perform one function only—word processing. It is more expensive than the electronic typewriter, but in situations that require a great amount of word processing it is a good investment.

COMPUTER

A desk-top computer with word processing software is a third type of keyboarding equipment (Fig. 12–2). The principal difference between it and the dedicated word processor is that other tasks can be performed on the computer.

The person who uses a word processor or computer can throw away the eraser and correcting fluid because the entire text can be edited on the monitor, any necessary corrections or changes made, and a perfect copy obtained before any printing is done (see Procedure 12–2). Revisions can be made easily without retyping a whole document. Blocks of text can be moved from one section of the document to another with just a few keystrokes. Even whole sections of text can be inserted into a document easily and quickly. Paragraphs or statements that are used frequently in letters or reports can be saved as *macros* and with a stroke or two on the keyboard can be retrieved and inserted in the appropriate place without retyping.

Most word processing programs can instruct the printer to print in boldface or in alternate type **fonts.** Some can create **subscripts** and **superscripts.**

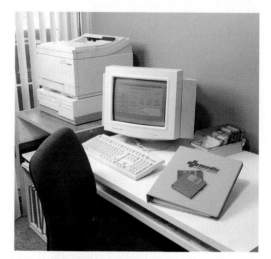

FIGURE 12–2 Desk-top computer.

HISTORY AND PHYSICAL EXAMINATION

CHIEF COMPLAINT:	Severe pain, left hip area, duration for the past couple of years.
PRESENT ILLNESS:	The patient in 1950 was involved in a severe auto accident, at which time he sustained injury to his back and leg as well as to his right shoulder and left hip. He subsequently had back surgery performed as well as a fusion, which was performed at St. Francis Hospital in Yourtown. The patient, however, has had continue sciatica and has been seen by Dr. Thomas Brown. Appropriate studies have been done. It was felt that there is nothing from the neurosurgical standpoint which could be of benefit to his left leg sciatic-type pain.
	In June 1990, the patient underwent insertion of a total right shoulder because of severe progressive degenerative osteoarthritis of the right shoulder. He has done quite well with that, has improved his range of motion, and has minimal to no pain. The patient, however, has had progressive pain about his left hip that has not responded to anti-inflammatory medications. X-rays reveal a progressive degenerative osteoarthritis with cystic formation.
FORMER SURGERIES:	1. Removal of right kidney in 8/85. 2. Former back surgeries in the 1940s. 3. Right total shoulder in 7/90.
SERIOUS ILLNESSES:	None.
MEDICATIONS:	Occasional Darvocet for pain.
HABITS:	Patient does not smoke.
REVIEW OF SYSTEMS:	
HEENT:	Patient denies any recent URIs or chronic sore throat.
CV:	Patient denies history of chest pain or heart disease.
GI:	Patient denies nausea, vomiting, diarrhea.
GU:	Patient denies dysuria or frequency.
MS:	See Present Illness.
HEM:	Patient denies any bleeding tendencies.
VITAL SIGNS:	Blood pressure 132/72.
GENERAL APPEARANCE:	Patient appears to be in good health for his stated age.
HEENT:	PERRL. Funduscopic examination within normal limits. Ears are clear, mouth negative.
NECK:	Supple, Thyroid is not enlarged.
LYMPHADENOPATHY:	None.
HEART:	Regular rate, no murmurs. Patient has good bilateral carotid pulsations.
PHYSICAL EXAMINATION:	
ADBOMEN:	Soft, no abnormal masses.
GENITALIA:	Normal male.
RECTAL:	Prostate is somewhat firm; however, there are no changes from 1992 exam.
EXTREMITIES:	Patient has 0 internal rotation of the left hip. He has abduction approximately 10 degrees, flexion marked pain about 70 degrees. Patient has a very mild left hip flexion contracture.
IMPRESSION:	1. Severe degenerative osteoarthritis, left hip. 2. Postoperative right total shoulder replacement. 3. Residual sciatica, left leg.

xxxx, M.D.

FIGURE 12–3 History and physical examination report.

A *spell-check* feature can proofread a lengthy document in minutes with complete accuracy. One disadvantage of the spell checker is that it can determine only whether a word is spelled correctly. If an incorrect word that is correctly spelled is typed, the checker will not pick it up (e.g., the use of *ilium* instead of *ileum*). With the text stored in memory or on a diskette, additional editing can be done and a corrected copy printed out almost effortlessly at any future time.

Preparation of Reports

The scope of a transcriptionist's duties is determined by each specific employer. In most instances, the preparation of medical reports is a large part of the professional assignment. The reports most frequently dictated in the physician's office are

- History and Physical
- Progress Notes
- Consultation Reports
- Correspondence

TURN-AROUND TIME

Specific time limits may be established for the completion of a variety of reports, with a designation of STAT (abbreviation for the Latin *statim*, meaning *immediate*), CURRENT, or OLD.

> **EXAMPLES OF HOW TO USE TIME LIMITS**
>
> STAT: Radiology, Pathology, and Laboratory Reports, which should be reported in 12 hours or less
> CURRENT: History and Physical, Consultation, and Operation Reports due within 24 hours
> OLD: Discharge Summaries and Emergency Department notes due within 72 hours

Memory Jogger

3 *What reports are most frequently dictated in a physician's office?*

HISTORY AND PHYSICAL

The History and Physical (H & P) may be dictated as the basis for the new patient's chart. When a patient is to be admitted to a hospital for treatment or observation, the physician will dictate an H & P before admitting the patient, and this becomes a part of the patient's hospital chart. No universal standard form exists for the H & P, but Figure 12–3 is a typical example.

Many sections of this report have a standard response that occurs over and over, depending on the patient's complaint and condition. These responses can be stored in memory as macros and used as needed with one or two strokes of the keyboard.

PROGRESS NOTES

The physician who sees many patients during a day does not have the time to handwrite **progress notes** on the medical chart after each patient visit. The physician will either dictate notes in the presence of the patient or immediately after the visit. The transcriptionist will then prepare these notes as an addition to the chart (Fig. 12–4).

By using continuous pages of pressure-sensitive paper, a great deal of time and motion can be saved. The paper is inserted only once and is later separated for the appropriate charts. Some papers have interval perforations that expedite the separation of entries. When typing these progress notes, space is left at the end for the physician's signature. The notes should never be entered into the chart without the physician's approval and signature.

PROGRESS NOTES

1. Brought back to ofc. regarding wart, left dorsal hand, of about 6 mo duration.
   EXAM: 5-mm diameter raised, round, sharply marginated, gray-pink, finely papillomatous and keratotic lesion, left dorsal hand.
   IMP: Verruca vulgaris.
   DISP: 1) Discussed treatment by electrosurgery vs. cryotherapy with father, including scarring with electrosurgery.
   2) Lesion removed by D & C under local anesth with Xyl. + Epi.
   3) Monsels, DSD, H_2O_2 t.i.d.
   4) See prn

2. Has been treating superficial multicentric BCCA, distal left mandible, with Efudex 5% cream b.i.d. for 3 wks. See inflammation with central erosion and peripheral crusting in involved area. Response appears appropriate.
   DISP: 1) Cont Efudex 5% cream b.i.d.
   2) See in 3 wks.

3. Pt. points out very small, quiescent-appearing actinic keratosis—inferior right lateral arm x 1 and proximal left extensor forearm x 1. Discussed nature of lesions with pt. L N2 about 10 sec. each. Re/ck prn persistence.

4. Pt. inquires about lesion, medial right leg. Possibly present since birth. No change in size or color over time. No tmt to date.
   EXAM: Inferior right medial leg: 17 x 15-mm diameter round, sharply marginated, macular, uniformly medium-brown lesions; a few terminal hairs penetrate surface of lesion.
   IMP: Benign pigmented macule.
   DISP: 1) Discussed benign appearance of lesion with pt.
   2) No tmt at this time.
   3) Re/ck prn change.

FIGURE 12–4 Progress reports.

CONSULTATION REPORTS

Physicians who act as consultants are expected to prepare a detailed report of their findings and recommendations and send it to the referring physician. The **consultation report** is dictated by the consulting physician to be transcribed within the office or by an independent transcriptionist if outside services are used. The report may have the same general form as the H & P or may be in correspondence form as the one in Figure 12–5.

OPERATION REPORT

The operation report is dictated by the surgeon immediately after surgery. The heading will show the patient's name, date, hospital code number and room number, plus names of the surgeon, any assistants, and the anesthetist. The report includes a preoperative diagnosis, postoperative diagnosis (these may be identical), the name of the procedure done, and a detailed narrative of the procedure accomplished. The surgeon must sign the report before it

---

December 2, 200x

Thomas Brown, M.D.
234 Maine Avenue
Yourtown, USA

Dear Doctor Brown:

Re: Rebecca Bloom

Rebecca Bloom is a 79-year-old, right-handed lady with known asthma who was seen in neurological consultation for progressive weakness in her legs.

She has had a prior neurological consultation, which suggested motor neuron disease. A muscle biopsy was consistent with neurogenic atrophy, and an EMG revealed positive sharp waves and fibrillation potentials in the quadriceps bilaterally and, to a lesser degree, in the distal groups of both legs below the knees. EMG of the upper extremities was normal.

Chemistry studies were unremarkable.

She denies any exposure to heavy metals or other neurotoxins. She has noted weakness in her legs for the past two years, initially above the knees, left greater than right. The problem has been slowly progressive, but she does not experience any weakness below the knees. She feels that her arms are strong, and she has experienced no difficulty with speech, swallowing, or eye movements. She has lost approximately 20 pounds in the last two years, which she attributes to nausea and poor dentures. She denies any significant muscle wasting or muscle twitching in the thigh muscles. She notes that her feet feel "abnormal," but she does not describe true numbness or tingling. Bowel/bladder function is intact. She has had a vertebral compression fracture due to osteoporosis because of her chronic prednisone therapy for asthma.

Her past medical history is significant for right hip surgery; ectopic pregnancy; status post bladder repair; history of asthma-COPD; status post muscle biopsy; history of mild enlargement of her heart with a valvular dysfunction.

Her medications include prednisone, 7.5 mg q.d. for several years; Brethine; TheoDur, 150 mg p.o. bid; Lanoxin, 0.125 mg p.o. every day; supplemental folic acid; daily Coumadin therapy; Premarin; vitamin D, 50,000 units two times per week; as well as an Alupent Inhalor and Intal; Dyazide, 1 p.o. qd.

Allergies: None known.

The patient denies tobacco or ethanol use. In the past six months, she has required the use of a cane to ambulate.

On physical exam, she is a well-developed, well-nourished female in no acute distress. She is oriented x three with an intact mental status exam. Speech is normal. Blood pressure is 120/80. Neck is supple. Carotids are 2+ bilaterally without bruits over the carotids or the supraclavicular region. Spine is nontender to percussion, HEENT: Normocephalic; atraumatic. Chest is clear to auscultation. Heart has a regular rate and rhythm; S1 and S2 without murmur. Cranial nerves: Olfactory sense is intact. Right disc is sharp with an intraocular lens present; left disc is nonvisible secondary to the presence of a cataract. The right pupil is greater than the left pupil by 0.5 mm; both are round and reactive to light. Visual fields are full. Extraocular movements are intact without nystagmus. Corneal reflexes are intact bilaterally, and there is normal facial symmetry and expression. Hearing is intact bilaterally, and the uvula is midline and upgoing. Sternocleidomastoid function is symmetric, and the tongue is midline.

Motor exam displays strength to be intact in the upper extremities bilaterally. The lower extremities display 3 4/5 strength in the iliopsoas and quadriceps bilaterally. There is trace weakness in the adductors and abductors, as well as hip extensors bilaterally. There is trace weakness of the hamstrings. There is no notable atrophy or fasciculation. The patient is unable to squat and has difficulty arising from a chair. Strength in the musculature distal to the knees is intact. There are no notable fasciculations. Thigh diameter is 33 mm on the right and 34 mm on the left, and the calves are both 30 mm in diameter. Sensory exam displays diminished vibratory and pinprick response in the feet, with position and soft touch intact. Finger-to-nose and heel-to-shin are intact. Fine motor movements and rapid alternating hand movements are normal. Deep tendon reflexes for the bicep, tricep, brachioradialis are 1-2+ bilaterally, with absent knee and ankle jerks; and the toes are downgoing. Gait and tandem are fair. Straight leg raise testing is unremarkable, as is bilateral hip rotation. Pedal pulses are 2+; the feet are cool in temperature, slightly erythematous, and swollen, with evidence of venous stasis.

FIGURE 12–5   Consultation report.

Thomas Brown, M.D.   -2-   December 2, 200x

Data Base: Nerve conduction studies of the lower extremities suggested a peripheral polyneuropathy, and an EMG of the upper extremities was normal. EMG of the left lower extremity revealed denervation to a greater extent in the left quadriceps and, to a minimal extent, in the left gastrocnemius. Some polyphasic small amplitude motor unit potentials were noted in the quadriceps that can be seen in myopathies.

Impression: Rebecca Bloom has evidence of proximal muscle weakness in her lower extremities with associated sensory deficits, including diminished vibratory and pinprick response in her feet and has been on chronic steroid therapy for her asthma-COPD. Her clinical picture, correlating with the electrical studies, suggests a peripheral polyneuropathy and possibly a proximal myopathy from chronic steroid use, rather than a motor neuron disorder, considering the lack of development of symptoms in the bulbar musculature or the upper extremities and the slow rate of progression.

Chemistry studies were unremarkable other than an elevated calcium of 11.3, and this will be further evaluated with the appropriate ionized calcium and PTH level.

I have recommended that we observe her over a period of time to document any evolution of her illness. I have referred her to physical therapy and pointed out that any reduction in her steroid use would be of value.

Further recommendations include a pelvic examination in view of the proximal muscle weakness in the lower extremities.

Her prior records will be reviewed, and the appropriate chemistry studies will be ordered.

Thank you for referring this pleasant lady for neurological evaluation.

Very truly yours,

Oliver South, M.D.

FIGURE 12–5 *Continued*

REGIONAL MEDICAL CENTER
YOURTOWN, USA

REPORT OF OPERATION

DATE: 12/05/99

PREOPERATIVE DIAGNOSIS: MASS, LEFT CALF

POSTOPERATIVE DIAGNOSIS: SAME, PROBABLY DEGENERATIVE MUSCLE DISEASE, LEFT CALF

PROCEDURE: OPEN BIOPSY LEFT CALF MUSCLE

SURGEON: XXXX, M.D.
ASST. SURGEON: XXXX, M.D.
ANESTHESIA: XXXX, M.D. General endotracheal anesthesia

FINDINGS: Under general anesthetic, the patient's left lower extremity was prepped and draped in the usual manner. The left leg was isolated in a sterile field, a well-padded thigh tourniquet was inflated to 300 mm of mercury after elevating and exsanguinating the leg with an Esmarch bandage. Linear incision was made over the posterior medial aspect of the calf, and dissection was carried out through the skin and subcutaneous tissue and superficial fascia. The gastrocnemius muscle was opened posteromedially. It was obvious that the muscle appeared to be rather firm and woody in consistency with infiltrating lighter tissue consistent with fatty tissue throughout the muscle fibers. The muscle fibers also appeared to be essentially relatively avascular and did not contract with direct stimulation. Samples of tissue were sent for frozen section, which indicated both degenerative and reparative process within the muscle without evidence of any tumor infiltration or evidence of infection. The specimens were sent for permanent section. At this point, the wound was thoroughly irrigated with normal saline solution containing bacitracin and neomycin. Previously, the wound was cultured, aerobic and anaerobically. The tourniquet was deflated at 10 minutes of tourniquet time. The wound was closed in layers with 0 and 2-0 Dexon followed by closure of the skin with subcuticular 4-0 Dexon followed by Steri-Strips and dry sterile compression dressings. The patient tolerated the procedure well; she was awakened from the anesthetic and went to the recovery room in good condition. EBL less than 20 mL.

_____ M.D.

NAME: XXXX
HOSPITAL NO.   XXXX
ROOM NO.   OP
ATTENDING: XXXX, M.D.

mek

FIGURE 12–6 Operation report.

is placed in the permanent record. It is important that this report be completed and filed currently, because there may be other physicians attending the patient who were not present during the surgery (Fig. 12–6).

PATHOLOGY REPORT

When tissue or fluid is removed by the surgeon it is examined by the pathologist, who reports on the findings. If a malignancy is suspected, the comple-

tion of the surgery may be delayed pending the pathologist's findings. The pathology report will include the usual heading, followed by a notation of the tissue submitted, with a gross description (meaning as seen by the naked eye), the microscopic description, and the pathologic diagnosis. The pathologist usually dictates the report simultaneously with the examination. As you will note in Figure 12–7, the narrative is dictated in the present tense. The report is signed by the pathologist and becomes a permanent part of the patient's record.

REGIONAL MEDICAL CENTER

PATHOLOGY REPORT

Name: _____ Pathology No. _____

Hospital No.: _____ Sex: _____ Age: _____ Room No.: _____ Date Received: _____

Physicians: _____

Preoperative Diagnosis: _____ Mass of left calf

Postoperative Diagnosis: _____ Pending

Procedure: _____ Open biopsy, left calf muscle

Specimens: (1) _____ Left calf mass-f/s

(2) _____ Left calf mass-f/s

(3) _____ Left calf mass

GROSS:

1. The specimen consists of 3 irregularly shaped fragments of dark maroon-brown muscle tissue measuring in aggregate 1.5 x 1 x 0.3 cm. No discrete lesions are identified. A minimal amount of adipose tissue is present in the largest fragment. The entire specimen is submitted for frozen section diagnosis.

FROZEN SECTION DIAGNOSIS: Benign muscle tissue showing degenerative and regenerative changes.

After frozen section, the tissue submitted is resubmitted and labeled F/S.

2. The specimen consists of 2 fragments of maroon-brown muscle tissue measuring in aggregate 1 x 0.7 x 3 cm. One of the fragments is submitted for frozen section diagnosis.

FROZEN SECTION DIAGNOSIS: Benign muscle tissue showing degenerative and regenerative changes.

After frozen section, the tissue submitted is resubmitted and labeled F/S.

3. Received is a wedge of grossly recognizable muscle tissue, brown-tan, and measuring 2.1 x 1.2 x 0.8 cm in size. On sectioning, this is moderately firm and focally only slightly discolored. All processed.

MICROSCOPIC:

Sections from all three parts show skeletal muscle. There is variable fiber morphology ranging from severely atrophic to markedly hypertrophic. There are abnormal numbers of central nucleoli, and some muscle fibers are vacuolated. In the interstitium there is fatty infiltration but no significant inflammatory infiltrate. No vasculitis is noted.

DIAGNOSIS:

NONSPECIFIC DEGENERATIVE AND HYPERTROPHIC CHANGES CONSISTENT WITH SEQUELA OR PREVIOUS TRAUMATIC INJURY, LEFT LEG MUSCLE BIOPSY.

NOTE: The morphology is somewhat similar to a muscular dystrophy, but the clinical presentation is incompatible. Denervation myopathy could account for some of the features seen. An inflammatory myopathy such as polymyositis is excluded based on the hypertrophic fibers present.

_____

Pathologist

mek

FIGURE 12–7 Pathology report.

RADIOLOGY MEDICAL GROUP, INC.

Name: _____ Age: _____ X-ray No. _____
Doctor: _____ Date _____

DOUBLE-CONTRAST ARTHROGRAM OF THE RIGHT KNEE:

Double-contrast arthrography of the right knee was performed under local anesthesia following intra-articular injection of Conray contrast medium and air.

Multiple views of the medial meniscus in various degrees of internal and external rotation demonstrate a faintly outlined vertically directed linear tear involving primarily the posterior horn and mid segment of the medial meniscus.

The lateral meniscus is intact with no evidence of tear or disruption. Overhead views show normal smooth synovial lining and articular surfaces. No popliteal cyst is demonstrated.

OPINION:

Faintly outlined vertically directed linear tear involving primarily the posterior horn and mid segment of the medial meniscus.

Normal lateral meniscus.

_____
Radiologist

mek

FIGURE 12–8 Radiology report.

RADIOLOGY REPORT

A radiology report contains the usual heading, including the date, name, and age of the patient, and the name of the referring physician. It will describe the radiographic findings and the resulting impression by the radiologist who signs the report (Fig. 12–8).

DISCHARGE SUMMARY

The final progress report for a hospital patient is the discharge summary, which will include the admission date and the date of discharge; admitting diagnosis and principal or discharge diagnosis; history of present illness; hospital course; and disposition and condition at time of discharge. The summary is dictated and signed by the attending physician (Fig. 12–9).

OTHER APPLICATIONS

The office that regularly sends out identical letters, such as recall notices or collection letters, will find word processing very helpful. Form letters can be stored in memory and personalized as needed.

A physician who does academic writing will want a program that can create footnotes, bibliographies, indexes, and so forth.

Transcribing: The Process

In most cases, the transcriptionist aims for finished copy and takes certain preliminary steps toward reaching this goal.

HOW TO PLAN FOR FINISHED COPY

1. Estimate the length of the finished document by first checking the indicator slip or electronic cuing. This makes it possible to decide what margins and spacing to use to produce the desired end product.
2. Look for any special instructions or corrections from the dictator.
3. Try to listen ahead so as to sense the meaning of a sentence and determine the punctuation necessary (some dictators include the punctuation marks).
4. When keyboarding directly on paper, as with a typewriter, it is important to type correctly the first time, whereas with a computer or word processor it is possible to go back and change punctuation, paragraphing, and so forth.
5. Before removing a page from the typewriter or before printing out the document, check the document for any errors.

Hospital No.: _____
Patient Name: _____
Physician: _____
Date of Discharge: _____

YOURTOWN
HOSPITAL

DISCHARGE SUMMARY

DATE OF ADMISSION:	12/15/200X
DATE OF DISCHARGE:	12/19/200X
ADMITTING DIAGNOSIS:	1. TEAR OF THE RIGHT ROTATOR CUFF
PRINCIPAL DIAGNOSIS:	1. TEAR OF THE RIGHT ROTATOR CUFF 2. HYPERTENSION 3. ALLERGIC REACTION
OPERATION:	
BRIEF HISTORY:	Patient came in for an elective surgery on the right rotator cuff. He had injured his shoulder while playing football; and because of continuing pain, an ultrasound vasogram was performed, which revealed a tear of the right rotator cuff.
HOSPITAL COURSE:	Approximately 24 hours following surgery, the patient was provided with patient-controlled anesthesia with intravenous morphine and also received 1 g Ancef every eight hours. Patient developed rather severe itching and subsequent facial flush and mild rash. Both medications were discontinued. It is unknown which medication was the cause of his apparent allergic reaction. Patient also had a very mild hypertension upon admission. During his admission, at times, blood pressure was as high as 190/116, and he ran a rather consistently elevated blood pressure for systolic and diastolic. Dr. Tom Brown was called for consultation because of both the allergic reaction and the hypertension, and initial studies were started concerning the hypertension. Patient was placed on Benadryl and responded rather appropriately to this treatment as far as allergic reaction was concerned.
DISPOSITION:	Patient was discharged home in a sling and strap. He is to remain in this until I see him in approximately two weeks. He will also be followed up with Dr. Tom Brown concerning his hypertension in approximately two weeks, when all studies have been completed.

_____
Signature

mek

FIGURE 12–9 Discharge summary.

ABBREVIATIONS

If transcribing for a hospital, use only abbreviations approved by the hospital for which the reports are intended. The Joint Commission on Accreditation of Healthcare Organizations requires that any abbreviations or symbols used in its medical records be from a list approved by that specific hospital. Progress notes done in the physician's office are less formal, and the physician's personally approved abbreviations are used to conserve space. There are entire books published on abbreviations, and most terminology books contain a list of frequently used abbreviations (see References at the end of this chapter).

CAPITALIZATION

Capitalize the first word of

- Every sentence
- An expression used as a sentence
- Each item in a list or outline
- The salutation and complimentary closing of a letter
- A drug brand name, such as Bufferin. The first letter of a generic name, such as aspirin, is not capitalized.
- The official name of a specific person, place, or thing, for example:

Andrew Jackson
New York City
World Trade Center

- A common noun when it is part of a proper name:

Give the paper to Professor Claudia Lane.
But Give the paper to the professor.
The parade traveled along Madison Avenue.
But: The parade traveled along the avenue.

TABLE 12–1   Basic Rules of Forming Plurals

Nouns ending in	Singular	Plural
	a	ae
	is	es
	um	a
	us	i
	ix, ex	ces

TABLE 12–2   Proper Aligning in Number Systems

Arabic	Decimal	Roman
1	1.23	I
5	3.25	II
13	8.05	III

WORD DIVISION

Avoid excessive division of words at the end of a line. Word divisions clutter a page and may even confuse a reader. Basic rules of word division include

- Dividing words only between syllables
- Never dividing a one-syllable word
- Never setting off a one-letter syllable at the end or beginning of a word
- Never dividing abbreviations or contractions
- Never dividing a word unless you can leave a syllable of at least three characters (including the hyphen) on the upper line and carry a syllable of at least three characters (may include a punctuation mark) to the next line

PLURALS

Some basic rules for forming plurals are

- Plurals of nouns are usually formed by adding *s* or *es* to the singular form.
- Plurals of abbreviations are formed by adding *s* (e.g., ECGs and CVAs); some use an apostrophe before the *s*, but this is unnecessary and losing popularity.
- Medical terms: Many medical terms have Latin roots; the plural of a Latin noun is determined by its gender (masculine, feminine, or neuter) (Table 12–1).

APOSTROPHE

The apostrophe is used to

- Form contractions—It's a sunny day (it is a sunny day).
- Form possessives—the patient's chart (*Exception:* The apostrophe is *omitted* in the possessive form of *it*—its color; not it's color)
- Show omissions in dates—the year '99

NUMBERS

Spell out numbers from 1 to 10. Use figures for numbers greater than 10 except at the beginning of a sentence.

- Use only figures (including 1 through 10) in tables and statistical matter and in expressing dates, money, clock time, and percentages.
- Express related numbers the same way.
- Express measurements in figures.
- Always use figures with AM and PM.
- Do not use zeros with on-the-hour time (e.g., 9 AM, *not* 9:00 AM).
- Always write decimals in figures, without commas in the decimal part of the number.
- Write percentages in figures and spell out *percent* (e.g., 10 percent).
- When typing figures in columns, Arabic numbers (e.g., 1, 2, and 3) are aligned on the right, decimal amounts (e.g., 1.23) are aligned on the decimal, and Roman numerals (e.g., I, II, and III) are aligned on the left (Table 12–2).

Proofreading and Editing

As a final step, the finished printed page should be checked twice—once for typing accuracy and once to be sure that the text makes sense. Never present material for signature unless it makes sense to you and is free of errors.

Proofreading is the process by which you determine whether the copy is exactly what was intended by the dictator and that all words are correctly interpreted and accurately spelled. Be especially careful to watch for sound-alike words, such as site/cite, ilium/ileum, right/write, and anti-/ante- (Table 12–3). Proofreading usually includes checking for sentence structure, correct punctuation, capitalization, style, and format (Table 12–4). Watch for repeated words, substitutions that might change the meaning, the transposition of numbers, and inconsistencies of any kind.

Because you do not have another document with which you can compare the current document, it is your responsibility to make any necessary corrections or, if you are unsure, to mark any questionable area for checking by the dictator. A reliable office worker's reference manual can be your guide in these matters. If you plan to specialize in transcription, a proofreading class is essential.

Editing is the process of questioning the transcribed material for accuracy and clarity. Medical reports generally do not require extensive editing, but as you check for typing accuracy, you should

TABLE 12–3   Sound-Alike Words

addiction	diaphysis	mastitis
adduction	diastasis	mastoiditis
abduction	diathesis	
		menorrhea
alveolus	epigastric	menorrhagia
alveus	epispastic	metrorrhagia
alvus		
	embolus	mucous
amenorrhea	thrombus	mucus
dysmenorrhea		
	endemic	nephrosis
antidiarrheic	epidemic	neurosis
antidiuretic	pandemic	
		palpation
antiseptic	facial	palpitation
aseptic	fascial	
asepsis		precardiac
	foci	pericardium
arteritis	fossae	
arthritis		perineal
	gavage	peroneal
aural	lavage	
oral		perineum
	hypertension	peritoneum
bradycardia	hypotension	
tachycardia		perivascular
	hypocalcemia	perivesical
callus	hypokalemia	
callous		stasis
	ileum	staxis
carbuncle	ilium	
caruncle		sycosis
furuncle	infection	psychosis
	infestation	
carpus		tenia
corpus	insulin	tinea
	inulin	
chronic		trachelotomy
chromic	keratosis	tracheotomy
	ketosis	
contusion		ureter
concussion	larynx	urethra
convulsion	pharynx	
		vesical
corneal	lymphangitis	vesicle
cranial	lymphadenitis	
		xerosis
cocci	maco	cirrhosis
coxa	micro	
cystostomy		
cystotomy		
cystoscopy		

also check the clarity of the text. In making corrections, be careful not to change the meaning. Always check with the dictator when making any changes in what was dictated. Questions to the dictator are done by **flagging** the place in question. Leave a blank space sufficient for insertion of correction. Attach a memo on a Post-it or other adhesive backed note. Include the page number, subject's name, the paragraph and line of the word or sentence in question, and your name if there is more than one transcriptionist in the facility.

Memory Jogger

4 In editing the final copy of a report, certain parts are unclear to the transcriptionist. What action should be taken?

Reference Sources

OFFICE WORKERS' REFERENCE MANUAL

A good reference manual can serve as a ready source of information when you are transcribing. In it, you will find in-depth information on punctuation, capitalization, writing numbers, the use of abbreviations, and plurals and possessives as well as spelling guides. It is also a source of information on typing manuscripts, reports, and bibliographies as well as other information that you may use only occasionally.

ENGLISH LANGUAGE DICTIONARY

Keep a good dictionary near your desk for those times when you are unsure of your spelling or of the meaning of a word (especially one that sounds like another).

MEDICAL DICTIONARY

Not all medical dictionaries have the same arrangement of entries. No matter which one you have available, you will soon become accustomed to finding what you need. In one popular dictionary, terms consisting of two words are primarily defined under the second word—usually the noun. For example, to find *acetic acid,* you would look under the noun *acid* and then for the subheading *acetic;* to find *splenic vein,* you would first find the noun *vein,* and then the subentry *splenic. Syndrome* is a main entry; the many names of syndromes are shown as subentries. Other examples are *tests, disease, culture,* and *method.* Just remember that whenever you must find a two-word entry, you will probably find it under the second word.

A specialized dictionary is available for almost every medical specialty. The transcriptionist in a specialty practice will find it worthwhile to invest in a reference for that specialty.

PHYSICIANS' DESK REFERENCE (PDR)

An unknown drug is difficult to spell, and the spelling must be verified by the transcriptionist. A drug

TABLE 12-4 Proofreader's Marks

Proofreader's Mark	Draft Copy	Finished Copy
⌐⌐ [Single space	⌐⌐ [Read a good book / every day	Read a good book / every day
ds [Double space	*ds* [Where will you go / on your vacation?	Where will you go / on your vacation?
⬚ Indent two spaces	His address is / ⬚ 450 Newport Avenue	His address is / 450 Newport Avenue
⊙ Insert period	Mr⊙ Herbert Hoover	Mr. Herbert Hoover
⋀ Insert comma	Marysville⋀ Indiana	Marysville, Indiana
⊙ Insert colon	Dear Mr. Adams⋀	Dear Mr. Adams:
;/ Insert semicolon	letter of March 6⋀ your question	letter of March 6; your question
?/ Insert question mark	Will he come⋀	Will he come?
⌵ Insert apostrophe	the captains ship	the captain's ship
⌵⌵ Insert quotation marks	his remark,⋀ don't be late⋀	his remark, "don't be late"
=/ Insert hyphen	a one⋀ time thing	a one-time thing
# Insert space	town⋀house	town house
⋀ Caret—to mark exact position of error	Insert caret to # show error	Insert caret to show error
⌐ Delete	⌐ It may ~~not~~ be yours	It may be yours
◡ Close up	Cl◡ose	Close
◡⌐ Delete and close up	Me◡erry Christmas	Merry Christmas
¶ Begin new paragraph	¶ At the time	At the time
no ¶ No paragraph	*no* ¶ This is correct	This is correct
// Align vertically	‖ Ellen Peters / Alice Brown	Ellen Peters / Alice Brown
= Align horizontally	Dear Doctor Roberts	Dear Doctor Roberts
⌐ Move right	$10,000	$10,000
⌐ Move left	⌐ Read a book	Read a book
⊓ Move up	⌐Mo⌐ve	Move
⊔ Move down	⌐Mo⌐ve	Move
⌐⌐ Center	⌐ $10,000 ⌐	$10,000
◠◡ Transpose	resil[ei]nt	resilient
(sp) Spell out	③ years ago	three years ago
stet Let it stand	They were ~~very~~ sad	They were very sad
lc Lower case	It is a Big house	It is a big house
≡ Upper case	Robert birch	Robert Birch
sc Set in small capitals	Regional	REGIONAL
ital Set in italic	special	*special*
bf Set in bold	federal government	**federal government**
wf Wrong font	invest𝐦ent	investment
⌵ Superscript	reference number 3	reference number[3]
⋀ Subscript	reference number 7	reference number[7]
◠ Ligature Æ	aesop	æsop

may have three types of names: chemical, generic, and trade. The chemical name of a drug represents its exact formula, the generic name is the common name of the chemical or drug, and the trade name is the name by which a manufacturer identifies the drug.

The *PDR* is the reference of choice for checking the names and spelling of drugs. It is published each year; and during the year, supplements are published to keep the reference up-to-date. The PDR contains seven different color-coded indexes:

- Alphabetical by Manufacturer
- Alphabetical by Brand Name
- Product (Drug) Category
- Generic and Chemical Name
- Product Identification
- Product Information
- Diagnostic Information

If the dictation contains an unfamiliar drug name, look in the Alphabetical Index for the correct spelling. If this search is unsuccessful, try the Generic and Chemical Name index. In typing the names of drugs, it is important to know whether it is a brand name or a generic name, because brand names are capitalized whereas generic names are not. In addition to being helpful as a source for the spelling and capitalization of drug names, the *PDR* contains a vast amount of information about drugs and their specific uses.

Names of over-the-counter drugs can be found in the *Physicians' Desk Reference for Nonprescription Drugs,* issued annually by the same publisher.

STANDARD ABBREVIATIONS

Except for the physician's own records, any abbreviations used in transcription should be standard and not subject to interpretation. If in doubt, it is always best to check. In some cases there is a difference in meaning if the letters are capitalized or in lower case. Many good books are available for checking abbreviations and should be consulted when the meaning of an abbreviation is in doubt.

CODING BOOKS

If your transcription involves procedural or diagnostic coding, you should have copies of the most recent editions of *Current Procedural Terminology* (**CPT Manual**), the Health Care Financing Administration's Common Procedure Coding System (**HCPCS**), and the *International Classification of Diseases* (**ICD Manual**) in your reference library. Internet sites and CD-ROM databases are available for information about medications and medical terms. Medical spellers can be installed to check spelling of medical terms before a document is printed.

LEGAL AND ETHICAL ISSUES

If you are transcribing for a hospital, remember that the Joint Commission on Accreditation of Healthcare Organizations requires that any abbreviations or symbols used must be from a list approved by that specific hospital.

CRITICAL THINKING

1 Discuss the educational requirements for a medical transcriptionist.

2 Explore some of the published volumes of medical abbreviations and note the similarities/differences of many. How might the use of an incorrect abbreviation affect the patient's care?

3 Discuss the legal aspects of medical reports and the need to be aware of the importance of confidentiality.

4 Can you suggest reasons that a STAT report would be expected for radiology, pathology, and laboratory results?

HOW DID I DO? Answers to Memory Joggers

1 Independent transcriptionists are usually paid on the basis of productivity, and their income depends on the number of pages, characters, or lines typed.

2 A slight rewind of the tape occurs when the machine is stopped and restarted.

3 History and Physical (H & P), Progress Notes, Consultation Reports, Correspondence.

4 Answer depends somewhat on the nature and extent of the lack of clarity. If it is a grammatical error, correct it. If a specific word is in question, consult the dictator before changing it.

REFERENCES

Diehl MO, Fordney MT: Medical Keyboarding, Typing and Transcribing: Techniques and Procedures, 4th ed. Philadelphia, WB Saunders, 1997.

Fordney MT, Diehl MO: Medical Transcription Guide: Do's and Don'ts. Philadelphia, WB Saunders, 1990.

Sabin WA: The Gregg Reference Manual, 7th ed., Lake Forest, IL, Gregg/McGraw-Hill, 1994.

Schwager E: Medical English Usage and Abusage. Phoenix, AZ, The Oryx Press, 1991.

Sloane SB: Medical Abbreviations and Eponyms, 2nd ed. Philadelphia, WB Saunders, 1997.

Strunk W Jr, White EB: The Elements of Style, 3rd ed. New York, Macmillan, 1979.

Tessier C: The AAMT Book of Style for Medical Transcription. Modesto, CA, American Association for Medical Transcription, 1995.

The Computer in Medical Practice

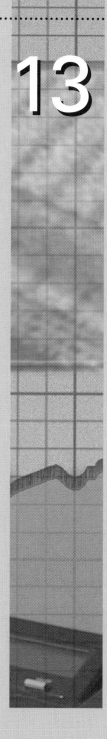

13

LEARNING OBJECTIVES

Cognitive: On successful completion of this chapter you should be able to:

1 Define and spell the terms listed in the Vocabulary.
2 Distinguish between the three types of computers.
3 List the four general categories of computer hardware devices.
4 Name and state the functions of the most important computer hardware devices.
5 Name the pointing device that controls the cursor.
6 Explain the function of the *Enter* key.
7 Describe the cursor-control keys.
8 Name the output devices.
9 Explain the purpose of diskettes.
10 List 10 administrative tasks in a medical practice that might utilize a computer.

Performance: On successful completion of this chapter, and given the necessary equipment, you should be able to:

1 Start the computer
2 Load a program
3 Format a disk
4 Make a back-up copy of a document
5 Generate a patient record
6 Prepare a billing statement
7 Complete a patient insurance form
8 Personalize a computerized form letter
9 Access, add, correct, and delete information on the computer
10 Shut down the computer

VOCABULARY

applications Software programs designed to perform specific tasks

back-space key Key at upper right of keyboard with left arrow that deletes characters as it is struck

back-up A tape or floppy disk for storage of files to prevent their loss in the event of hard disk failure

CD-ROM Compact disk—read-only memory command; an instruction telling the computer to do something with a program

computer A machine that is designed to accept, store, process, and give out information

CPU Central processing unit; the part of a computer system that processes information

cursor A symbol appearing on the monitor that shows where the next character to be typed will appear

cursor-control keys Keys that have an arrow pointing up, down, left, or right that are used to move a cursor

database A collection of related files that serves as a foundation for retrieving information

demographics Relating to the statistical characteristics of populations, such as births, marriages, mortality, and health

disk A magnetic surface that is capable of storing computer programs that sometimes is flexible (*floppy disks*) and sometimes is hard (*hard disks*)

disk drives Devices that load a program or data stored on a disk into a computer

dot matrix printer An impact printer that forms characters using patterns of dots

electronic mail (E-mail) Communications transmitted via computer using a telephone modem

Enter key Key that performs same function as the Return key on a typewriter

floppy disk (diskette) A thin disk (diskette) of magnetic material capable of storing a large amount of information

format To magnetically create tracks on a disk where information will be stored; to initialize

hard copy The readable paper copy or printout of information

hardware Computer components that perform the four main functions

input Information entered into and used by the computer

letter-quality printer A printer that resembles a typewriter and which may be either mechanical or electronic

main memory Section of the computer where information and instructions are stored

modem Acronym for modulator demodulator; a device that enables data to be transmitted over telephone lines

monitor A device used to display computer-generated information; a video screen; a CRT

mouse Pointing device that controls the cursor

output Information that is processed by the computer and transmitted to a monitor, printer, or other device

printout The output from a printer, also called *hard copy*

provider One who provides medical service (e.g., a physician)

random access memory (RAM) The computer's temporary memory that stores data and programs that are input

read-only memory (ROM) Memory that can be altered only by changing the physical structure of the computer chip and that is used to store information essential to the operation of the computer

scanner An input device that converts printed matter into a computer-readable format

software The programming necessary to direct the hardware of a computer system; computer programs

telecommunication The science and technology of communication by transmission of information from one location to another via telephone, television, or telegraph

word processing System used to process written communications

Little more than 50 years ago, in 1946, the first electronic computer (ENIAC) was completed after 2½ years in the making. It weighed 30 tons, required a space of 15,000 square feet, and cost over 1 million dollars. Since that time, a computer explosion has taken place, brought about at first by the application of the transistor, then integrated circuits, and now silicon chips. A compact personal computer in the home and a desk-top monitor in the office are now commonplace.

For many years, the computer has been used in hospitals and large group practices, but the proliferation of software, the decrease in cost of hardware, and the sharp increase in paperwork that must be done in the medical marketplace have brought computerization into private medical practices. The computer is now standard equipment in all health care facilities. Consequently, it is now essential that any person looking toward a medical assisting career must become computer literate.

The development of computers, their programming, and internal operation is extremely complicated. Entire volumes have been written on the minute technical details of the computer. Fortunately, this technical knowledge is not necessary to use the computer, just as it is not necessary to be a mechanic to drive an automobile or to be an electrician to operate a light switch. But a knowledge of the functions that a computer can perform, how it influences our lives, and how it is used to perform tasks in the workplace has become a necessary part of the general education of all students. This chapter is intended to deal only with the use of the computer by the medical assistant as a tool in a medical facility. We will first examine the equipment, and then discuss its applications.

What Is a Computer?

A **computer** is a machine that is designed to accept, store, process, and give out information (Fig. 13–1). The general categories of microcomputer hardware units serve the following functions:

- Processing
- Input
- Output
- Storage

CENTRAL PROCESSING UNIT

The **CPU** is the most important piece of hardware. Acting as the brain of the computer, it interprets the instructions from a program. Although you cannot see it, within the CPU is the memory consisting of electronic and magnetic cells, each of which contains information.

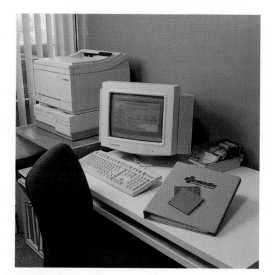

FIGURE 13–1 Microcomputer with software package.

There are two kinds of memory: **read-only memory (ROM)** and **random access memory (RAM).** ROM is internal memory that contains the entire operating system and a computer language. It is also known as the **main memory.** With this permanent memory, much less information has to be transferred from a disk to start the computing process. The ROM cannot be overwritten and is not erased when the power is shut off. RAM can be thought of as the internal scratch pad of the computer. It contains the program instructions and the data that it is currently processing. RAM is normally erased automatically when the power is shut off.

INPUT DEVICES

Information input to the computer is accomplished by means of a keyboard or other input device such as a mouse, scanner, or voice-activated device. The computer keyboard looks very much like an ordinary typewriter keyboard but has a few extra keys, which are called *special function keys*. These special function keys are numbered F1 to F12 and are used to perform specific **word processing** or computer-related operations. Used alone, a function key may create bold print, underline, indent, or call up a HELP screen, as well as other functions. Used in conjunction with the *Ctrl, Alt, or Shift* keys, function keys can produce other desired results, such as activating the printer, inserting the current date into a document, retrieving a file, and moving a designated block of text. A **mouse** is a pointing device with a ball on the bottom that is moved by rolling on a flat table top or mouse pad. Some computers, especially laptops, have a built-in mouse called a trackball that is moved by rotating the ball with the thumb. Others may have a touchpad, which is stroked by the thumb to move the cursor, or a track-point that is manipulated like a joy stick. The mouse controls the **cursor,** which is a flat bar or pointer appearing on the monitor that shows where the next character will appear.

At the right end of the keyboard is a numeric keypad, which has keys that resemble the keypad of a calculator. The numeric keypad is normally not in use during word processing. The *NumLock* key must be pressed to activate this feature.

The *Enter* key performs the same function as the *Return* key on the typewriter but is not used at the end of a line. The computer senses when the next word will not fit on the line and performs a *soft return.* The *Enter* key is used to start a new paragraph or an intentional (or hard) return. The left arrow key at the upper right of the keyboard is the **backspace key** and deletes characters as you move it to the left.

Cursor-control keys have an arrow that points up, down, left, right, and in some cases diagonally.

Memory Jogger

1 *What is ROM, and why is it important?*

OUTPUT DEVICES

Monitor

The monitor, which looks very much like a television screen, is a device used to display computer-generated information. Some monitors are black and white only but may be adjusted for screen brightness and contrast. Color monitors allow the operator to choose the background color that is most pleasing to the eye and easiest to read (Fig. 13–2). A blinking marker on the screen, called the cursor, indicates the position where the next information can be added or inserted. By watching the monitor you have instant feedback on your entries.

Printer

Printers are also **output** devices. Documents appearing on the monitor may be directed to a printer to produce what is called a **printout** or **hard copy** (paper). Four types of printers are commonly used with computers:

* Dot matrix
* Letter-quality or print wheel
* Ink jet
* Laser

Many printers print bidirectionally (i.e., they print both from left to right and from right to left). Some are capable of both draft-quality and correspondence-quality printing. Dot matrix and letter-quality printers are impact printers, using an inked ribbon; ink jet and laser printers are nonimpact and use an ink cartridge.

A **dot matrix printer** is the least expensive of the four types of printer. They are used in many classrooms. Dot matrix printers form the letters or shapes that they are directed to print by arranging patterns of dots on the paper. They operate more quickly than do letter-quality machines, but their print lacks the clarity generally desired for a professional look.

A **letter quality printer** may be either mechanical or electronic. The electronic letter-quality printer generally uses a print wheel, or daisy wheel, that is interchangeable for variations in print style or size. Many printers have 10-, 12-, and 15-pitch typing capability as well as proportional spacing capability.

Ink jet printers use an ink cartridge that feeds an array of nearly microscopic tubes, each of which has a heating element that is energized during the printing process. The ink cartridge may be black-and-white or color. Ink jet printers cost less than laser printers, but the ink cartridges they use are fairly expensive and bring up the operating cost.

Laser printers use xerographic technology similar to that in photocopiers, so the laser printer is able to produce an almost limitless variety of type forms

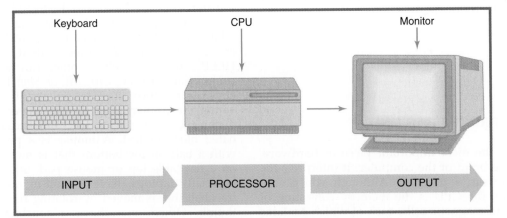

FIGURE 13–2 Input device (keyboard), central processing unit (CPU), and output device (monitor).

and sizes as well as complex graphics. One disadvantage of ink jet and laser printers is that they are incapable of producing multiple copies with carbon sets or multicopy forms, such as many types of insurance forms.

STORAGE

Information may be saved (stored) on a disk for future reference or printing. The amount of information that can be stored depends on the type of **disk** the system uses. Storage is achieved on either a hard disk or **floppy disk (diskette)** or both. The hard disk is inside the computer and you do not see it. The hard disk contains the operating system and the information on all the programs you use. Hard disks store much more information than do diskettes and make possible faster information access. There is a wide variation in the space capacity of hard disks. The disk must be large enough to hold all the programs you use as well as the information that you will store. Diskettes are used principally as an auxiliary storage medium and **back up** for the hard disk. They can also be used for transmitting information between computers. The size of the disk needed depends on the type of drive being used. Older computers used the 5¼-inch floppy, but most computers being sold today accommodate only the 3½-inch floppy. The term *floppy* is misleading, because the disk is quite firm and does not "flop."

A computer may have four or more **disk drives.** There may be two drives for diskettes. Drive A is used for the smaller 3½-inch diskette and drive B for the 5¼-inch diskette. Drive C is the hard disk and Drive D accommodates the CD-ROM. There may also be a ZIP or back-up drive.

Memory Jogger

2 *If your computer is intended principally for insurance billing, what kind of printer would you need? Why?*

Diskette Files

Before information can be stored on a diskette, the diskette must be initialized, or formatted. When correctly instructed your computer will **format** the diskette by creating magnetic tracks (recording bands) on the diskette where information is to be stored. Diskettes that are preformatted are also available at slightly higher cost than nonformatted diskettes. After a diskette has been formatted, the disk operating system (DOS) can both read data from the diskette and write data onto the diskette. When information is stored only on diskettes, it is always wise to make back-up or duplicate diskettes

in case the original diskettes are lost or damaged. These back-up diskettes must be kept in a secure location for protection against fire or theft. Floppy diskettes are more easily damaged than are hard disks (a type of floppy disk different in texture, size, and capacity) and must be carefully stored, always in a jacket, and filed for easy reference. For tips on the proper care of diskettes, see the Care of Diskettes chart. A more dependable system for backing up files is by subscribing to an online backup service on the Internet. The service keeps a copy of your files in two separate locations. For privacy protection your files are encrypted before being transmitted, and a password is needed to retrieve them.

CD-ROM

The **CD-ROM** (compact disk–read-only memory) at this writing is becoming standard equipment on all computers and is increasingly popular as a means of providing programs for installation on computers. The CD-ROM requires a separate disk drive and is able to store much more information than an ordinary diskette. In the medical office it might be used to store a medical dictionary or a medical reference library. It is not used for storing information created on your computer.

CARE OF DISKETTES

- Avoid exposing the diskette to extremes of temperature.
- When the diskette is not in use always return it to its storage envelope, where it will not collect dust.
- Avoid placing a diskette on top of the monitor because this could scramble information on the diskette.
- Keep your fingers off the surface of the diskette, especially around the window in the jacket. Body oils can permanently destroy data.
- Hold the diskette with your thumb on the label.
- Write or type on the label before attaching it to the diskette, if possible, or write with a soft felt-tipped pen. Never write with a ballpoint pen or pencil on a label that is on a diskette. Also, do not erase on a diskette label. All of these can cause impressions in the diskette, and the ink can run.
- Do not force a diskette into a disk drive or its storage envelope. If there is resistance, pull it out and try again. Bending or folding a diskette will render it useless.
- Store the diskettes vertically in dust-tight containers.
- Keep smoke, food, and drink away from the area of use.

Hard Disk Management

The hard disk is the filing cabinet of the computer. Thousands of files can be placed on a hard disk and retrieved with a few specific keystrokes. A hard disk system usually comprises two or more rigid metal plates enclosed in a sealed case. It stores data by magnetic encoding similar to that when using a floppy disk or cassette tape. Hard disks provide much greater storage capacity than do floppy diskettes.

For efficiency in retrieving a given piece of information, a directory is established for each main topic; subdirectories can be set up within directories. Computer files are organized in much the same fashion as ordinary files that contain paper records (Fig. 13–3). When a disk becomes overcrowded, more time is required for the system to retrieve a specific file. The hard disk needs to be periodically purged of files that are outdated or no longer useful just as does any other filing system.

Software

Software consists of sets of instruction placed on magnetic disks. Software is necessary for a computer to function. The operating system, which is preinstalled on your computer, is one kind of software. In operating the computer you will be selecting and using **applications.** Application programs are designed to perform specific tasks such as word processing, patient billing, accounting, appointment scheduling, insurance form preparation and processing, payroll, and database management. Many software applications are available for complete medical practice management. Some health care facilities have software designed specifically for their practices, but this is usually unnecessary in today's market.

Getting Started

Even with some basic knowledge of computer components and of what computers can do, if you have not had any hands-on experience with a computer, you may feel some initial fear—fear of the unknown, fear of machines, or fear of being unable to master the computer. You will soon overcome any such fears if you will remember that you really are smarter than the computer. It is only a machine. All it can do is perform the tasks that you tell it to do. It cannot think. It cannot make decisions, and it will wait for your commands. What it can do is

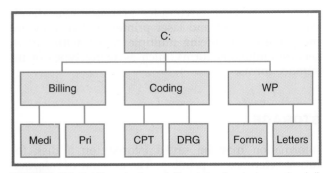

FIGURE 13–3 Organization of files into directories and subdirectories.

- Relieve you of repetitive clerical tasks
- Reduce errors
- Speed up production
- Recall information on command
- Save time
- Reduce paperwork
- Allow more creative use of your time

As you begin your familiarization with the computer, you may key in some wrong information. As a result, the computer will become confused and will respond with a question mark or a comment such as

FILE NOT FOUND or INVALID DRIVE
SPECIFICATION or SYNTAX ERROR

The computer will allow you the opportunity and time to figure out the correct information and input it. Look at the monitor screen. Most of the time it will indicate what to do next. If the answer is not readily available on the monitor, pull down the *Help* menu. Your next resort will be the program instruction manual.

You cannot break the computer simply by hitting the wrong keys. It is unlikely that you will destroy records accidentally; a specific command is necessary. However, if you shut off the computer without saving the information on disk or tape you will lose what you have put in. By using a computer in the classroom, you will gain familiarity with computer operation and confidence that you can master it. Mastery is accomplished only through practice.

The computer that you will encounter on the job is likely to be different from the one on which you will learn in the classroom. The programs and tasks performed may also be different, but you will be given training with that specific system, either by the vendor or by a member of the staff. It is important to keep an open mind while learning to operate any system.

With a knowledge of computer terms, the ability to follow step-by-step instructions, and reasonable expertise with a typewriter keyboard, you should have no problem with learning and using any computer system. In fact, many computer users consider the computer to be their best friend. You probably will, too.

Memory Jogger

 Explain the meaning of application program *and give an example.*

Common Computer Applications

PROCESSING INSURANCE CLAIMS

Claims information can be sent from the physician's office directly to the computer of an insurance company using a **modem,** which transmits information over telephone lines. Electronic processing of insurance claims not only saves transit time but also provides immediate information as to whether a given claim will be accepted. Errors in coding or procedure are immediately evident, and such errors result in the rejection of the claim by the insurance company's computer. Corrections can then be made instantly using the computer.

The codes that are most commonly used for claims processing can be stored on the computer disk and retrieved when needed (Fig. 13–4).

Many insurance companies give preferential treatment to providers who file claims electronically (Fig. 13–5; see p. 188). By the year 2000 all providers of

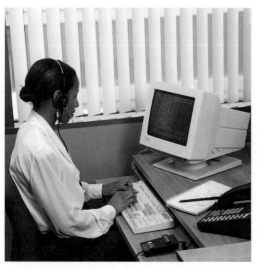

FIGURE 13–4 Computer operator.

care under *Medicare* and *Medicaid* will be required to file their claims electronically.

In medical offices that do not file insurance claims for patients, a computer can generate a *superbill* for the patient to attach to his or her own insurance form. The superbill gives information about diagnosis and procedures that is needed to file a claim.

PATIENT LEDGER

The **demographics** about a patient (e.g., his or her name, address, telephone, number, and insurance carrier) will appear on the patient's computerized ledger (Fig. 13–6; see p. 189). As services are rendered, all charges and payments are entered into the computer. This results in the availability of a current balance at all times.

BILLING AND COLLECTION

At the appropriate time, the computer can print a patient's billing statement that shows detailed charges, payments, adjustments, and a balance (Fig. 13–7; see pp. 190–191). Additionally, the computer can be programmed to age the accounts according to any criteria selected and to include this information on the billing statement. A series of collection letters can also be developed and personalized for individual patients as they are needed.

BOOKKEEPING ENTRIES

With the appropriate software, the computer can easily handle all bookkeeping processes.

EXAMPLES OF SOFTWARE BOOKKEEPING PROCEDURES

- Recording payables and receivables
- Computing the payroll
- Keeping track of bills to be paid
- Generating checks
- Producing a deposit slip for the bank
- Reconciling bank statements
- Preparing daily, monthly, and annual financial and statistical reports

---

DATABASE MANAGEMENT

Database software makes it possible to organize a large volume of information that can be used in a number of ways. One of the most practical uses is organization of identifying information on each patient, which would include name, address, date of

APPROVED OMB-0938-0008

PLEASE
DO NOT
STAPLE
IN THIS
AREA

CARRIER →

PICA

HEALTH INSURANCE CLAIM FORM

PICA

1. MEDICARE	MEDICAID	CHAMPUS	CHAMPVA	GROUP HEALTH PLAN	FECA BLK LUNG	OTHER	1a. INSURED'S I.D. NUMBER	(FOR PROGRAM IN ITEM 1)
X (Medicare#)	(Medicaid #)	(Sponsor's SSN)	(VA File #)	(SSN or ID)	(SSN)	(ID)		

2. PATIENT'S NAME (Last Name, First Name, Middle Initial)

3. PATIENT'S BIRTH DATE **08 27 25** SEX M ☐ F **X**

4. INSURED'S NAME (Last Name, First Name, Middle Initial)

5. PATIENT'S ADDRESS (No., Street)

6. PATIENT RELATIONSHIP TO INSURED
Self **X** Spouse ☐ Child ☐ Other ☐

7. INSURED'S ADDRESS (No., Street)

CITY
STATE **CA**

8. PATIENT STATUS
Single ☐ Married **X** Other ☐

CITY
STATE

ZIP CODE **92683**
TELEPHONE (Include Area Code) **(714)**

Employed ☐ Full-Time Student ☐ Part-Time Student ☐

ZIP CODE
TELEPHONE (INCLUDE AREA CODE) ( )

9. OTHER INSURED'S NAME (Last Name, First Name, Middle Initial)

10. IS PATIENT'S CONDITION RELATED TO:

11. INSURED'S POLICY GROUP OR FECA NUMBER
NONE

a. OTHER INSURED'S POLICY OR GROUP NUMBER

a. EMPLOYMENT? (CURRENT OR PREVIOUS)
☐ YES **X** NO

a. INSURED'S DATE OF BIRTH **08 27 1925** SEX M ☐ F **X**

b. OTHER INSURED'S DATE OF BIRTH **08 27 1925** M ☐ F **X**

b. AUTO ACCIDENT? PLACE (State)
X YES ☐ NO

b. EMPLOYER'S NAME OR SCHOOL NAME

c. EMPLOYER'S NAME OR SCHOOL NAME
RETIRED

c. OTHER ACCIDENT?
☐ YES **X** NO

c. INSURANCE PLAN NAME OR PROGRAM NAME

d. INSURANCE PLAN NAME OR PROGRAM NAME
METLIFE-IL 5090

10d. RESERVED FOR LOCAL USE

d. IS THERE ANOTHER HEALTH BENEFIT PLAN?
X YES ☐ NO *If yes, return to and complete item 9 a-d.*

READ BACK OF FORM BEFORE COMPLETING & SIGNING THIS FORM.

12. PATIENT'S OR AUTHORIZED PERSON'S SIGNATURE I authorize the release of any medical or other information necessary to process this claim. I also request payment of government benefits either to myself or to the party who accepts assignment below.
SIGNED **Signature on File**
DATE **03/12/98**

13. INSURED'S OR AUTHORIZED PERSON'S SIGNATURE I authorize payment of medical benefits to the undersigned physician or supplier for services described below.
SIGNED **Signature on File**

14. DATE OF CURRENT: ILLNESS (First symptom) OR INJURY (Accident) OR PREGNANCY (LMP)

15. IF PATIENT HAS HAD SAME OR SIMILAR ILLNESS. GIVE FIRST DATE MM DD YY

16. DATES PATIENT UNABLE TO WORK IN CURRENT OCCUPATION
FROM MM DD YY TO MM DD YY

17. NAME OF REFERRING PHYSICIAN OR OTHER SOURCE

17a. I.D. NUMBER OF REFERRING PHYSICIAN

18. HOSPITALIZATION DATES RELATED TO CURRENT SERVICES
FROM MM DD YY TO MM DD YY

19. RESERVED FOR LOCAL USE

20. OUTSIDE LAB? ☐ YES **X** NO $ CHARGES

21. DIAGNOSIS OR NATURE OF ILLNESS OR INJURY. (RELATE ITEMS 1,2,3 OR 4 TO ITEM 24E BY LINE)
1. **362.51**
2. **365.11**
3.
4.

22. MEDICAID RESUBMISSION CODE ORIGINAL REF. NO.

23. PRIOR AUTHORIZATION NUMBER

24. A DATE(S) OF SERVICE From / To MM DD YY MM DD YY	B Place of Service	C Type of Service	D PROCEDURES, SERVICES, OR SUPPLIES (Explain Unusual Circumstances) CPT/HCPCS MODIFIER	E DIAGNOSIS CODE	F $ CHARGES	G DAYS OR UNITS	H EPSDT Family Plan	I EMG	J COB	K RESERVED FOR LOCAL USE
1	03 12 98 03 12 98	11		92012	1	43.30	1				
2											
3											
4											
5											
6											

25. FEDERAL TAX I.D. NUMBER SSN ☐ EIN **X**

26. PATIENT'S ACCOUNT NO.

27. ACCEPT ASSIGNMENT? (For govt. claims, see back) **X** YES ☐ NO

28. TOTAL CHARGE $ **43.30**

29. AMOUNT PAID $ **0.00**

30. BALANCE DUE $ **43.30**

31. SIGNATURE OF PHYSICIAN OR SUPPLIER INCLUDING DEGREES OR CREDENTIALS (I certify that the statements on the reverse apply to this bill and are made a part thereof.)
SIGNED **03/12/98** DATE

32. NAME AND ADDRESS OF FACILITY WHERE SERVICES WERE RENDERED (If other than home or office)

33. PHYSICIAN'S, SUPPLIER'S BILLING NAME, ADDRESS, ZIP CODE & PHONE #
SANTA ANA, CA 92704
PIN# GRP# (

(APPROVED BY AMA COUNCIL ON MEDICAL SERVICE 8/88)
WHCFA-1500-2-90

PLEASE PRINT OR TYPE

FORM HCFA-1500 (12-90)
FORM OWCP-1500
FORM RRB-1500

PATIENT AND INSURED INFORMATION

PHYSICIAN OR SUPPLIER INFORMATION

FIGURE 13-5 Computer-generated insurance claims form.

```
                        SMITH, JANE A                    PAGE   1
                        PATIENT LEDGER
                          03/12/99

CHART         DATE   PROV LOC   BILLING     DIAGNOSIS  PROCEDURE      AMOUNT
----------    ------ ---- ----  ----------- ---------- ----------   ----------
973944-00                                      0
              (INSURANCE ID:             INSURANCE PHONE: (714)261-6700)
              11/11/97 02   11   11564     365.04     92004          105.00
              11/11/97 02   11   11564     365.04     PCP            -10.00
              02/19/98 02        11564                IP             -22.00
              02/19/98 02        11564                WO             -73.00
              (INSURANCE 1 BILLED 11/20/97)
              01/20/98 02   11   11983     365.04     92083          120.00
              01/20/98 02        11983                PCP            -10.00
              (INSURANCE 1 BILLED 01/29/98)
                                                                   ------------
                                          PATIENT DEBITS....          225.00
                                          PATIENT CREDITS...         -115.00
                                                                   ------------
                                          BALANCE..........          110.00
                                                                   ============
SMITH, JANE A                             PROVIDER DEBITS...          225.00
                                          PROVIDER CREDITS..         -115.00
                                                                   ------------
                                          PROVIDER BALANCE..          110.00
                                                                   ------------
                                          REPORT DEBITS.....          225.00
                                          REPORT CREDITS....         -115.00
                                                                   ------------
                                          REPORT BALANCE....          110.00
                                                                   ============
```

FIGURE 13–6 Computerized patient ledger.

birth, Social Security number, daytime telephone number, insurance information, and place of employment. The amount and character of information that can be stored on a computer **database** about patients, procedures, diagnoses, and other topics is limitless. After the data are recorded onto the disk, the information can be sorted into any chosen order and retrieved as desired (Fig. 13–8; see p. 192).

HEALTH INFORMATION RECORDS

Computer systems can store clinical information about patients using much less space and with greater security than can papers in a patient chart. Anyone who has worked in a medical office understands the problems that a lost or misfiled patient chart can cause. The chart stored on the computer can be set up in such fashion that a printout of only the most important information can be reviewed by the physician at the time of the patient's visit; as a result, he or she does not have to thumb through an ever-growing stack of papers. Reports from outside sources can be added to the computer record using a scanner. Access to records can be limited with passwords.

APPOINTMENT SCHEDULING

The computer has replaced the appointment book in many medical practices. Software for appointment scheduling ranges from relatively simple programs that merely display available and scheduled times to sophisticated systems into which the operator may enter information such as the length and type of appointment required and day and time preferences of the patient; the computer then selects the best appointment time based on inputted information.

The computer can also be used to keep track of future appointments. For example, when a patient calls and inquires about an appointment, the system can search by his or her name to find the time and date. The computer can provide printouts of the daily schedule that include the patients' names and telephone numbers and the reason for their visiting. Multiple copies of these schedules can be made according to the needs of the practice.

A big advantage of computer scheduling is that more than one person can access the system at one time, and the information is available to all operators. The medical assistant can generate a hard copy of the next day's appointments before leaving for the day. In some facilities, employees still maintain

```
                                                       PAGE    1

                                          Tax ID
                                          95-2585978




                                 June 10 , 1999


        To:



        Diagnosis:                        Patient  :
        1 4659   UPPER RESPIRATORY INFECTI Acct #   :
        2 4959   ALLERGIC ALVEOLITIS & PNE SS#      :
        3 7856   LYMPHADENOPATHY           D.O.B.   :
                                           Phone    :
                                           Employer :
                                           Claim No.:
                                           Group    :


        #    Date   Dr Pl Svc   Description Bil Charge  Credit    Bal    Prev
        ------------------------------------------------------------------------
        1.  052999           777  COURTESY ADJU B        -30.50   0.00   30.50
        2.  052999           742  DEBIT ADJUSTM B         97.50  30.50  -67.00
        3.  043099  INSURANCE BILLED     B/C PRUDE 0401-0430( 30.50)
        4.  043099  INSURANCE BILLED     RISK MANA 0401-0430( 30.50)
        5.  040699  9  1 8706000  NOSE\THROAT C *  30.50         -67.00 -97.50
        6.  093098           751  COURTESY DISC B        -97.50 -97.50   0.00
                                          2/11-2/14/98
        7.  053098           751  COURTESY DISC B       -235.75   0.00  253.75
                                          4/23/98
        8.  043098  INSURANCE BILLED     B/C PRUDEN 0401-0430  253.75
        9.  043098  INSURANCE BILLED     RISK MANAG 0401-0430  253.75
        10. 042398  9  1 9902301  LABORATORY DR *   5.75         253.75 248.00
        11. 042398  9  1 8444300  TSH           *  35.00         248.00 213.00
        12. 042398  9  1 8425100  T4R           *  21.00         213.00 192.00
        13. 042398  9  1 8425000  T3 RESIN      *  21.00         192.00 171.00
        14. 042398  9  1 8429500  SODIUM        *   9.25         171.00 161.75
        15. 042398  9  1 8413200  POTASSIUM     *   9.25         161.75 152.50
        16. 042398  9  1 8371800  HDL CHOLESTER *  27.50         152.50 125.00
        17. 042398  9  1 8011200  CHEM PANEL 12 *  42.50         125.00  82.50
        18. 042398  9  1 8272800  FERRITIN,EIA  *  47.00          82.50  35.50
        19. 042398  9  1 8565100  WESTERGREN SE *  13.50          35.50  22.00
        20. 042398  9  1 8502400  CBC           *  22.00          22.00   0.00
        21. 041998           751  COURTESY DISC B        -41.00   0.00   41.00
                                          BAL APPLD TO DED
        22. 022898  INSURANCE BILLED    B/C PRUDEN 0201-0228   97.50
        23. 022898  INSURANCE BILLED    RISK MANAG 0201-0228   97.50
        24. 022198           751  COURTESY DISC B        -56.50  41.00   97.50
                                          D.O.S.    11/12/97
        25. 021498  4  1 9006000  OFFICE VISIT- *  48.75          97.50  48.75
        26. 021198  4  1 9006000  OFFICE VISIT- *  48.75          48.75   0.00
        27. 013198           751  COURTESY DISC B        -56.50   0.00   56.50
                                          TO DEDUCTIBLE
```

FIGURE 13–7   Patient's billing statement.

```
                                                        PAGE    2

28.    112397   INSURANCE BILLED         AETNA LIFE 1001-1123  56.50
29.    111297  10  1 8720503  10% KOH PREP  *    10.50           56.50   46.00
30.    111297   6  1 9006000  OFFICE VISIT- *    46.00           46.00    0.00
31.    053197           751  COURTESY DISC B                     0.00  220.25
32.    022897   INSURANCE BILLED         AETNA LIFE 0201-0228  178.00
33.    020297   6  1 9902200  ALLIED CLINIC *     8.00          220.25  212.25
                                          \FERRITIN
34.    020297   6  1 8444300  TSH           *    33.00          212.25  179.25
35.    020297   6  1 8425100  T4R           *    19.75          179.25  159.50
36.    020297   6  1 8425000  T3 RESIN      *    19.75          159.50  139.75
37.    020297   6  1 8371800  HDL CHOLESTER *    26.00          139.75  113.75
38.    020297   6  1 8011200  CHEM PANEL 12 *    38.00          113.75   75.75
39.    020297   6  1 8565100  WESTERGREN SE *    12.75           75.75   63.00
40.    020297   6  1 8502400  CBC           *    20.75           63.00   42.25
41.    093096   INSURANCE BILLED         AETNA LIFE 0901-0930  42.25
42.    091996   3  1 8565100  WESTERGREN SE *    12.00           42.25   30.25
43.    091996   3  1 8503100  Not in ISAM   *    19.50           30.25   10.75
44.    091996   3  1 9902201  ALLIED SPECIM *    10.75           10.75    0.00
                                          /FER,IBC,SE IRON
45.    010096   3  1 9999900  BALANCE FORWA B     0.00            0.00    0.00
                                          COMPRESSED TO BALF


               Current    30-day    60-day    90-day    120 + Balance
Bal Fwd Age:     0.00      0.00      0.00      0.00      0.00     0.00


Treatment Rendered by:

Referring Physician   : NO REFERRAL

Please Make Check Payable to:
```

FIGURE 13–7 *Continued*

an appointment book as a back-up to computer scheduling.

WORD PROCESSING

Word processing software is available for all desktop computers. The latest software is very sophisticated with the capability to create footnotes, bibliographies, indexes, graphics, and much more. Formatting processes are quick and easy, and error detection is continuous. A word processing applications program is used in transcription and preparing written communications such as correspondence and reports, as well as many other tasks.

Styles and formatting of all kinds can be established and stored in the application program for use as needed. Formatting includes setting margins, determining line spacing, justification, setting tabs, pagination, page breaks, and so forth. If the document is to be saved, you must first assign a file name and complete the "save" process before exiting the item or turning off the computer.

NETWORKING

With the exception of the very small facility, the computer system will be set up to communicate with other systems or individuals via networks and telecommunication systems. The network will link one or more computers in the same facility or farther away, such as with a hospital or the home of one or more physicians, via modem and special software.

Clinical Research

Patient information stored in a database can be used by the physician to develop research reports from this source. For example, if a study were being done on the results of a specific treatment, the physician could gather the needed information from the database.

```
DATE : 00/00/00 TIME : 08:37 AM                              PAGE   1

LIST OF PATIENTS


                          R E G I S T R A T I O N
06/10/92
 1.CHART #:                     10.RESP PARTY:
 2.NAME    :                    11.ADDRESS   :
 3.ACCT #  :                    12.CITY/STATE:
 4.DR/PL #: 03/01               13.ZIP       :
 5.SEX     : F                  14.RELATION  :
 6.MARITAL: M                   15.PHONE RES :
 7.BIRTH   : 7/22/57            16.PHONE BUS :
 8.REF DOC:    1  NO REFERRAL   17.EMPLOYER  :
 9.ACC DAY:   /  / 0            18.SSN       :
- - - - - - - - - - - - - I N S U R A N C E - - - - - - - - - - - - - -
 20.CODE   : 851                26.CODE      : 856   B/C PRUDENT BUYER
 21.PRIMARY: RISK MANAGEMENT RESO 27.SECONDARY :
 22.ID #   : 429-27-7469        28.ID #      :
 23.GROUP  : 664-626            29.GROUP     : 336631/101/3
 24.ASSN:1            25.STAT: 0  30.ASSN:0            31.STAT: 0
- - - - - - - - - - - - - - - - - - - - - - - - - - - - - - - - - - - -
 32.NOTE 1: PARENTS     524-8240 34.RECALL DATE:08/18/88 36.RECALL TYPE:  0
 33.NOTE 2: SISTER      -524-6995 35.RECALL DONE:08/30/88 37.PAN:NEW INS 1/91
- - - - - - - - - - - - - - - - - - - - - - - - - - - - - - - - - - - -
 38.ICD #1:4659    39.DESC:UPPER RESPIRATORY INFECTI  44.ADMITTED   :00/00/00
 40.ICD #2:4959    41.DESC:ALLERGIC ALVEOLITIS & PNE  45.DISCHARGED :00/00/00
 42.ICD #3:7856    43.DESC:LYMPHADENOPATHY            46.LAWYER     :   0


SECPAG — Extra Patient Information

 1. Pat Address :              10. Family Planning   :
 2.      Address :             11. Other Accident    :
 3.      City St :             12. Patient Employed   : Y
 4.          Zip :             13. Patient P/T Std.   :
 5. O.I. Emp/Sch:              14. Patient F/T Std.   :
 6. Time of Inj.:              15. Insured's Sex      : F
 7. Active/Ret. :              16. Other Ins. Sex     : M
 8. Date to Clinic        :    17. Insured's D.O.B.  : 07/22/57
 9. Discharge Date        :    18. Other Ins. D.O.B. : 10/21/45

19. Refered Out :             25. Auto Accident   :
20.     Contact :             26. Work Related    :
21.     Address :             27. Return Mod Work:
22.     City St :             28. Return Reg Work:
23.         Zip :             29. Claim #         :
24.       Phone :             30. Examiner        :

31. Extra Info 1:


              Change what # ( 0 for none ) :
```

FIGURE 13–8 Patient registration information stored in a database.

Electronic Mail (E-Mail)

Telecommunication (or **electronic mail**) software allows one computer to communicate with another computer via telephone lines through the use of a modem. Letters and reports travel along telephone lines to your computer, which can provide a printout in a manner not unlike that previously discussed concerning the electronic transmission of insurance claims.

Electronic Signature

Physicians are sometimes negligent about signing clinical reports generated in the hospital as well as those reports originating in the private office. Recently introduced on the market is the electronic signature option. Electronic signature programs are offered both as stand-alone products and as part of a computerized medical record system. After the dictated report is transcribed, the physician by using a password and personal identification number (PIN) can log on to the patient record system by computer. The physician accesses and reviews a report, makes any necessary changes or additions, then "signs" the report by clicking on an icon. Once the record has been signed it cannot be altered; only addenda are allowed.

Ergonomic Work Areas

The increase in utilization of computers in the workplace has emphasized the need to choose and arrange furniture and equipment that employees use to maintain comfort and safety. Repetitive strain injury (RSI) accounts for a majority of job-related injuries. RSI includes a number of conditions that are caused by repeatedly straining certain nerves, muscles, or tendons. Carpal tunnel syndrome is one example of RSI.

To avoid such injuries it is very important that posture chairs support the lumbar section of the back with correct angle of the knee and the feet resting on the floor. Many designs for keyboards are available and every effort should be made to choose a keyboard height that allows a right angle at the elbow with the wrist being held in a neutral position. Extensive studies have been done to ensure the comfort and safety of employees. Prevention of RSI is possible; a cure is sometimes not possible.

Eyestrain is another danger arising from continuous use of a computer. The monitor should be just below eye level and at an arm's length away. At least once each hour take a break from looking at the monitor to rest your eyes.

Security Guidelines for Computerized Data

As we learned in an earlier chapter, the patient is entitled to utmost confidentiality with respect to his or her medical records and the release of any information of a personal nature. Computer technology allows the accumulation and storage of a vast amount of data that may be accessible to a variety of individuals, making it imperative that guidelines be set up for the protection of that data. Security guidelines have been established by the Council on Ethical and Judicial Affairs of the American Medical Association and are included in the 1996–1997 edition of the *AMA Code of Ethics* (see Chapter 5).

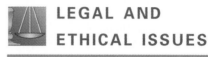

LEGAL AND ETHICAL ISSUES

The patient is entitled to complete confidentiality of his or her records. Follow the security guidelines that have been established by the Council on Ethical and Judicial Affairs of the American Medical Association.

CRITICAL THINKING

1 Why are security guidelines so important for computerized data?

2 Is security more important for medical records than it is for other kinds of data?

HOW DID I DO? Answers to Memory Joggers

1 ROM (read-only memory) is the internal memory of the computer that contains the entire operating system and computer language. It remains stored in the computer when the power is off and is present to start the computer process when the power is turned on.

2 Dot matrix and letter-quality printers are impact printers and can generate multiple form copies.

3 Application program is software designed to perform specific tasks (e.g., Word Perfect, a word processing program).

REFERENCES

American Medical Association: Code of Medical Ethics, 1996–1997 edition. Chicago, AMA 1996.

Gylys BA: Computer Applications for the Medical Office. Philadelphia, FA Davis, 1997.

Filing Methods and Record Keeping

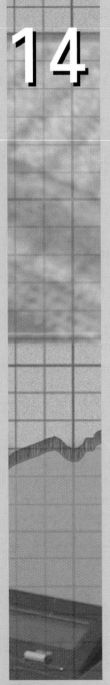

14

LEARNING OBJECTIVES

Cognitive: *On successful completion of this chapter, you should be able to:*

1 Define and spell the terms listed in the Vocabulary.
2 List and discuss the basic equipment and supplies in a filing system.
3 Describe the seven sequential steps in filing a document.
4 List and discuss application of the four basic filing systems.
5 Explain how color coding of files can be advantageous in a health care facility.

Performance: *On successful completion of this chapter, you should be able to:*

1 Type a list of names in indexing order and arrange them alphabetically for filing.
2 Arrange a group of patient numbers in filing sequence for a terminal digit filing system.
3 Using the color key in this chapter, state the tab color to be used for a given list of names.

VOCABULARY

alphabetic filing Any system that arranges names or topics according to the sequence of letters in the alphabet

alphanumeric Systems made up of combinations of letters and numbers

caption A heading, title, or subtitle under which records are filed

direct filing system A filing system in which materials can be located without consulting an intermediary source of reference

indirect filing system A filing system in which an intermediary source of reference, such as a card file, must be consulted to locate specific files

numeric filing The filing of records, correspondence, or cards by number

OUTfolder A folder used to provide space for the temporary filing of materials

OUTguide A heavy guide that is used to replace a folder that has been temporarily moved from the filing space

shelf filing A system that uses open shelves (rather than cabinets) for storing records

subject filing Arranging records alphabetically by names of topics or things rather than by names of individuals

tab The projection on a file folder or guide on which the caption is written

tickler file A chronologic file used as a reminder that something must be taken care of on a certain date

transfer Removing inactive records from the active file

unit Each part of a name that is used in indexing

A filing system is only as good as the ease of retrieval of everything in the files. A modern filing system should have three key components: (1) a symbol on the outside of the jacket or folder indicating the active or inactive status of the record, (2) safeguards to prevent misfiling, and (3) a filing technique that allows quick, accurate retrieval and refiling. Files may be kept as hard copy (on paper) or on the computer disk. Most medical facilities use a combination, with the patients' notes as hard copy.

Filing Equipment

The vertical four-drawer steel filing cabinet, used with manila folders with the patient's name on the tab, was the traditional system of choice for years. The most popular system today is color coding on open shelves. There are also rotary, lateral, compactable, and automated files. Some records are kept in card or tray files. Regardless of the type or style of equipment, the best quality is always an economy.

Some of the considerations in selecting filing equipment are

- Office space availability
- Structural considerations
- Cost of space and equipment
- Size, type, and volume of records
- Confidentiality requirements
- Retrieval speed
- Fire protection

DRAWER FILES

Drawer files should be full suspension; they should roll easily, close securely, and be equipped with a locking device. The best cabinets have a center trough at the bottom of each drawer with a rod for holding divider guides. Floor space of twice the depth of the drawer must be allowed so that the drawer can be pulled out to its full extent. A drawback of the vertical four-drawer files is that only one person can use a file cabinet at any given time. Filing is also slower because the drawer must be opened and closed each time a file is pulled or filed. Drawer files are relatively easy to move, but for safety reasons they should be bolted to the wall or to each other.

 Safety Alert: File drawers are heavy and can tip over, causing serious damage or injury unless reasonable care is observed. Open only one file drawer at a time and close it when the filing has been completed. A drawer left even slightly open can cause injury to a passerby.

SHELF FILES

Shelf files should have doors to protect the contents. A popular type of shelf file has doors that slide back

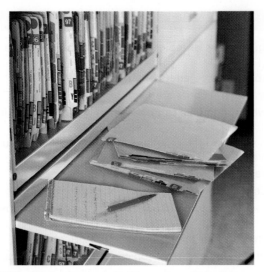

FIGURE 14–1 Open shelf filing using shelf door as work space.

into the cabinet; the door from a lower shelf may be pulled out and used for work space (Fig. 14–1). About 50% more material per square foot of floor space may be filed in shelf files as compared with the four-drawer file. Open shelf units hold files sideways and can go higher on the wall because there is no drawer to pull out. File retrieval is faster because several individuals can work simultaneously.

Open shelf units without doors are the most economical but offer little protection or confidentiality to the records. They are susceptible to water and fire damage. Shelf files are available in many attractive colors and can add a decorative note to the business office.

Special storage or shelf space should be provided for x-ray films if many films are stored.

ROTARY CIRCULAR FILES

Rotary circular files can hold a large volume of records. They save space and clerical motion. The files revolve easily; some come with push-button controls. Several persons can work at one rotary file and use records at the same time. One disadvantage is that they afford less privacy and protection than files that can be closed and locked.

LATERAL FILES

Lateral files are good for personal files and are especially attractive for the physician's private office. They use more wall space than the vertical file but do not extend out into the room so far. The folders are filed sideways in the lateral file, left to right, instead of front to back as in a vertical file. Some have a pull-out drawer, as the vertical file does;

others have doors that slide into the cabinet, exposing the filing space.

COMPACTABLE FILES

The office with little space and a great volume of records might use compactable files, which are a variation of open shelf files. The files are mounted on tracks in the floor, and the units slide along the tracks so that access is gained to the needed records. They may be either automated or manual. One drawback is that not all records are available at the same time.

AUTOMATED FILES

Automated files are very expensive initially and require more maintenance than do the other types of filing equipment. They will probably be found only in very large installations such as clinics or hospitals. These files bring the record to the operator instead of the operator going to the record. When the operator presses a button indicating the appropriate shelf, the shelf automatically moves into position in front of the operator for record retrieval. The automated or power file is fast and can store large amounts of records in a small amount of space. Only one person can use the unit at one time.

CARD FILES

Almost every office has some occasion to use a card file. This may be for patient ledgers, a patient index, library index, index of surgical tray setups, telephone numbers, or numerous other records. A good-quality steel box or tray is a sound investment.

SPECIAL ITEMS

Metal framework is available that can convert a regular drawer file into suspension-folder equipment. The assistant with a great deal of filing may wish to purchase a portable filing shelf that fits on the side of an opened drawer and can be moved from place to place as needed. Another special filing item is a sorting file, which can be a great time saver. A portable file cart for the temporary filing of unbilled insurance claims may be quite useful. It may also be used for the preliminary sorting of charts to be refiled. This is sometimes called a suspense file.

Memory Jogger

1 *Discuss the various styles of file storage, noting their advantages and disadvantages.*

Supplies

DIVIDER GUIDES

Each file drawer or shelf should be equipped with plenty of dividers or guides. Some authorities recommend one guide for approximately each inch and a half of material, or every 8 to 10 folders. Guides should be of good-quality pressboard. Economy guides will soon become bent and frayed and have to be replaced. Divider guides have a protruding tab, which may be either an integral part of the card or may be made of metal or plastic. The guides reduce the area of search and serve as supports for the folders. They are available in single, third, or fifth cut (one, three, or five different positions). The guide may have a projection at the bottom edge with a ring or hole through which a rod may go. This type of guide card is used in drawers that have a trough for the projection and a rod to hold the guides in place.

OUTGUIDES

An **OUTguide** is a heavy guide that is used to replace a folder that has been temporarily removed. It should be of a distinctive color for quick detection. This makes refiling simpler and alerts the file clerk that a file is missing. Several colors may be used, each color designating the temporary location of the file. The OUTguide may have lines for recording information, or it may have a plastic pocket for inserting an information card (Fig. 14–2).

CHART COVERS OR FOLDERS

Most records to be filed are placed in covers or tabbed folders. The most commonly used is a general-purpose third-cut manila folder that may be expanded to ¾ inch. These are available with a double-thickness reinforced tab that will greatly lengthen the life of the folder. Folders kept in drawers have tabs at the top; those kept on shelves have tabs at the side. There are many variations of folder styles obtainable for special purposes:

- A classification folder separates the papers in one file into six categories yet keeps them all together.
- An **OUTfolder** is used like the OUTguide and provides space for temporary filing of materials.
- The vertical pocket, which is heavier weight than the general purpose folder, has a front that folds down for easy access to contents and is available with up to 3½ inch expansion. These are used for bulky histories or correspondence.
- Hanging or suspension folders are made of heavy stock and hang on metal rods from side to side of a drawer. They can be used only with files equipped with suspension equipment.
- Binder folders have fasteners with which to bind papers within the folder. These offer some security for the papers but are time consuming in filing the materials.

The number of papers that will fit in one folder depends on the thickness of the papers. Near the bottom edge of most folders are one or more score marks, which should be used as the contents of the folders expand. If folders are refolded at these score marks, the danger of their bending and sliding under other folders is reduced, and a neater file results. Papers should never protrude from the folder edges, and they should always be inserted with their tops to the left. When papers start to ride up in any folder, the folder is overloaded.

Memory Jogger

2 *Describe an OUTguide and its uses.*

LABELS

The label is a necessary filing and finding device. Use labels to identify each shelf, drawer, divider guide, and folder.

A label on the drawer or shelf identifies the nature of its contents. It should also indicate the range (alphabetic, numeric, or chronologic) of the material filed in that space.

> **EXAMPLES OF TYPES OF LABELS**
>
> PATIENT HISTORIES (ACTIVE)
> A–F
>
> OR
>
> GENERAL CORRESPONDENCE
> 1997–1998

The label on the divider guide identifies the range of folder headings following that divider guide up to the next divider, for example, Ba–Bo.

The label on the folder identifies the content of that folder only. This may be the name of the patient, subject matter of correspondence, a business topic, or anything at all that needs to be filed. You will need to label a folder when a new patient is seen or existing folders are full or when you need to **transfer** materials within the filing system.

Paper labels may be purchased in rolls of gummed tape or have adhesive backs that are peeled from a protective sheet. They are available in

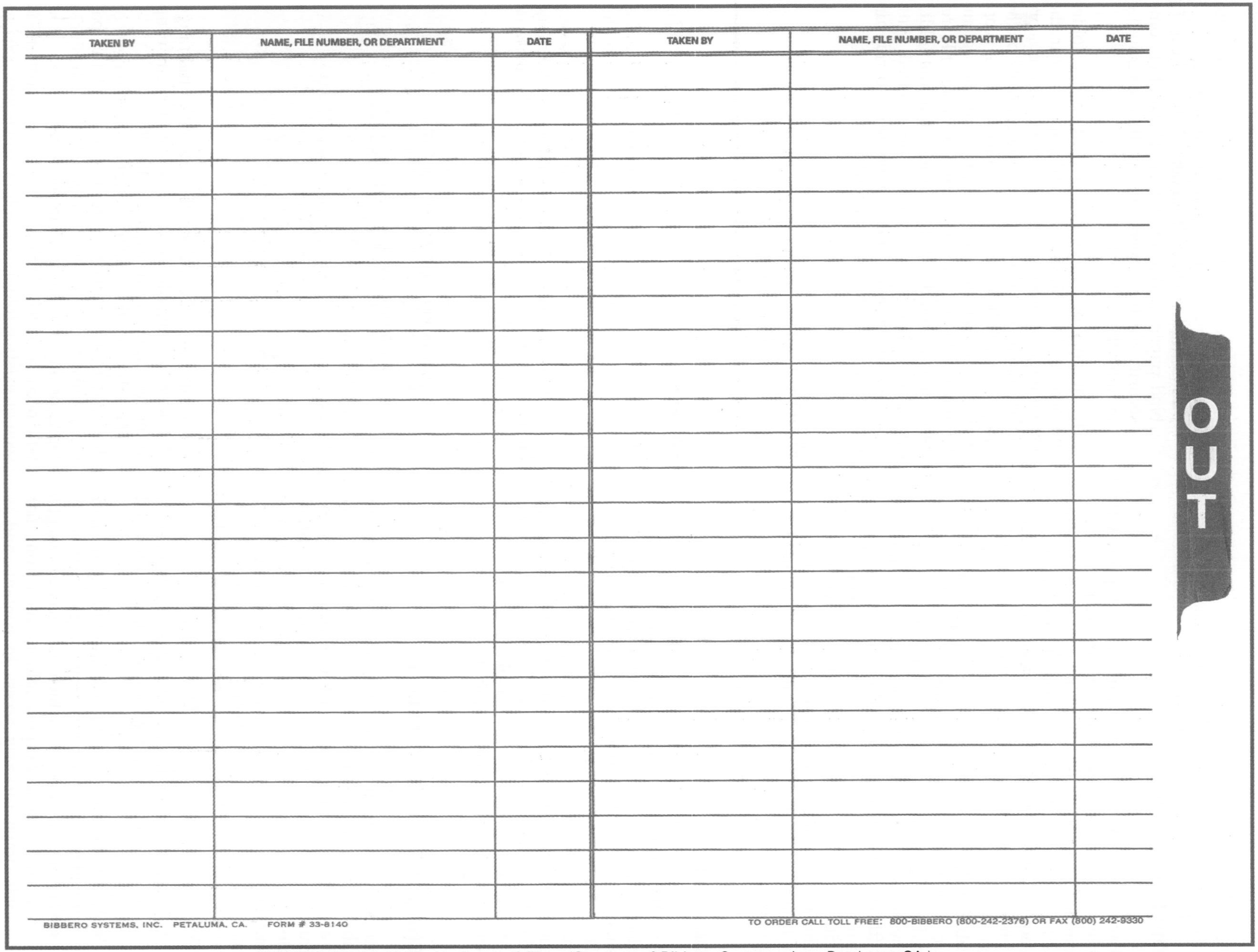

TAKEN BY	NAME, FILE NUMBER, OR DEPARTMENT	DATE	TAKEN BY	NAME, FILE NUMBER, OR DEPARTMENT	DATE

FIGURE 14–2 OUTguide for shelf filing. (Courtesy of Bibbero Systems, Inc., Petaluma, CA.)

TABLE 14–1 Application of Indexing Rules

Indexing Rule	Name	Unit 1	Unit 2	Unit 3
1	Robert F. Grinch	Grinch	Robert	F.
	R. Frank Grumman	Grumman	R.	Frank
2	J. Orville Smith	Smith	J.	Orville
	Jason O. Smith	Smith	Jason	O.
3	M. L. Saint-Vickery	Saint-Vickery	M.	L.
	Marie-Louise Taylor	Taylor	Marielouise	
4	Charles S. Anderson	Anderson	Charles	S.
	Anderson's Surgical Supply	Andersons	Surgical	Supply
5	Ah Hop Akee	Akee	Ah	Hop
6	Alice Delaney	Delaney	Alice	
	Chester K. DeLong	Delong	Chester	K.
7	Michael St. John	Stjohn	Michael	
8	Helen M. Maag	Maag	Helen	M.
	Frederick Mabry	Mabry	Frederick	
	James E. MacDonald	Macdonald	James	E.
9	Mrs. John L. Doe (Mary Jones)	Doe	Mary	Jones (Mrs John L.)
10	Prof. John J. Breck	Breck	John	J. (Prof.)
	Madame Sylvia	Madame	Sylvia	
	Sister Mary Catherine	Sister	Mary	Catherine
	Theodore Wilson, M.D.	Wilson	Theodore (M.D.)	
11	Lawrence W. Sloan, Jr.	Sloan	Lawrence	W. (Jr.)
	Lawrence W. Sloan, Sr.	Sloan	Lawrence	W. (Sr.)
12	The Moore Clinic	Moore	Clinic (The)	

almost any size, shape, or color to meet the individual needs of any facility. Visit your stationer and study the catalogs to find the best product for you.

A narrow label applied to the front of the folder tab is the easiest to use and is satisfactory for folders kept in a drawer file. Labels for shelf filing should be identifiable from both front and back. Always type the label before separating it from the roll or protective sheet. Type the **caption** on the label in indexing order (see Indexing Rules and Table 14–1).

Filing Procedures

Filing of all materials involves five basic steps: conditioning, releasing, indexing and coding, sorting, and storing and filing.

CONDITIONING

Conditioning of papers involves (1) removing all pins, brads, and paper clips, (2) stapling related papers together, (3) attaching clippings or items smaller than page size to a regular sheet of paper with rubber cement or tape, and (4) mending damaged records.

RELEASING

The term *releasing* simply means that some mark is placed on the paper indicating that it is now ready for filing. This will usually be either the medical assistant's initials or a FILE stamp placed in the upper left corner.

INDEXING AND CODING

Indexing means deciding where to file the letter or paper, and coding means placing some indication of this decision on the paper. This may be done by underlining the name or subject, if it appears on the paper, or writing in some conspicuous place the indexing subject or name. If there is more than one logical place to file the paper, the original is coded for the main location and a cross-reference sheet prepared, indicating this location and coded for the second location. Every paper placed in a patient's chart should have the date and name of the patient on it, usually in the upper right corner.

SORTING

Sorting is arranging the papers in filing sequence. Sort papers before going to the file cabinet or shelf. Do any necessary stapling of papers at your desk or filing table. Invest in a desktop sorter with a series of dividers between which papers are placed in filing sequence. One general-purpose sorter has six means of classification: alphabetic sections, numbers 1 to 31, days of the week, months of the year, numbers in groups of five, and space on the tabs for special captions to be taped when desired. In the preliminary sorting you place the papers in the appropriate division in the sorter. Then it is comparatively simple to arrange these groups into the proper sequence for filing.

PROCEDURE 14–1

Initiating a Medical File for a New Patient

GOAL

To initiate a medical file for a new patient that will contain all the personal data necessary for a complete record and any other information required by the agency.

EQUIPMENT AND SUPPLIES

Computer or Typewriter
Clerical supplies (pen, clipboard)
Information on agency's filing
  system
Registration form
File folder
Label for folder

ID card if using numeric system
Cross-reference card
Financial card
Routing slip
Private conference area

PROCEDURAL STEPS

1 Determine that the patient is new to the office.

2 Obtain and record the required personal data.
  PURPOSE: Complete information is necessary for credit and insurance claim processing.

3 Type the information onto the patient history form.

4 Review the entire form.
  PURPOSE: To confirm that the information is complete and correct.

5 Select a label and folder for the record.
  EXPLANATION: If color coding is used, a decision must be made regarding the appropriate color for the patient name.

6 Type the caption on the label and apply to the folder.
  EXPLANATION: Use patient's name for alphabetic filing or appropriate number for numeric filing.

7 For numeric filing system, prepare a cross-reference card and a patient ID.
  PURPOSE: Numeric filing is an indirect system and requires a cross-reference to a patient's name for locating a chart. The patient will use the number of the ID card when arranging appointments or making inquiries.

8 Prepare the financial card, or place the patient's name in the computerized ledger.

9 Place the patient's history form and all other forms required by the agency into the prepared folder.

10 Clip a routing slip on the outside of the patient's folder.

STORING AND FILING

In storing or filing papers in the folder, items should be placed face up, top edge to the left, with the most recent date to the front of the folder. Lift the folder 1 or 2 inches out of the drawer before inserting new material, so that the sheets can drop down completely into the folder.

If you are refiling completed folders, arrange them in indexing order before going to the file cabinets. Procedure 14–1 provides the steps for initiating a new patient file.

Memory Jogger

3 *List and describe the five steps in filing.*

Locating Misplaced Files

Unless files are promptly replaced after use, they may become lost. Papers may be misfiled, requiring a thorough search to find them. After you have made a methodical and complete search through the proper folder, there are several places you may look for a misplaced paper: (1) in the folder in front of and behind the correct folder; (2) between the folders; (3) on the bottom of the file under all the folders; (4) in a folder of a patient with a similar name; or (5) in the sorter.

Indexing Rules

Indexing rules are fairly well standardized, based on current business practices. The Association of Records Managers and Administrators takes an active part in updating the rules. Some establishments adopt variations of these basic rules to accommodate their needs. In any case the practices need to be consistent within the system.

1. Last names of persons are considered first in filing; given name (first name), second; and middle name or initial, third. Compare the names beginning with the first letter of the name. When you find a letter that is different in the two names, that letter determines the order of filing. Example:

> ab*e*
> ab*i*
> ab*x*
> ac*l*
> ac*m*
> a*d*a
> ad*e*
> ad*i*

2. *Initials* precede a *name* beginning with the same letter. This illustrates the librarian's rule, "Nothing comes before something." Example:

> Smith, J.
> Smith, Jason

3. *Hyphenated personal names.* The hyphenated elements of a name, whether first name, middle name, or surname, are considered to be one **unit.** Example:

> Carlotta Freeman-Duque is filed as
> Freemanduque, Carlotta
> Cindy-Jean Green is filed as
> Green, Cindyjean

4. The apostrophe is disregarded in filing. Example:

> Andersons' Surgical Supply
> Andersons Surgical Supply

5. When you are indexing a foreign name and *cannot* distinguish the first and last name, you should index each part of the name in the order in which it is written:

> Cau Liu
> Talluri Devi

If you *can* make the distinction, you should use the last name as the first indexing unit:

> Liu, Jason

6. Names with prefixes are filed in the usual alphabetic order with the prefix being considered as part of the name. Example:

> DeLong is filed as Delong
> LaFrance is filed as Lafrance
> von Schmidt is filed as Vonschmidt

7. Abbreviated parts of a name are indexed as written if that is the form generally used by that person. Example:

> Ste. Marie is filed as Stemarie
> St. John is filed as Stjohn
> Wm. is filed as Wm
> Edw. is filed as Edw
> Jas. is filed as Jas

8. Mac and Mc are filed in their regular place in the alphabet:

> Maag
> Mabry
> *Mac*Donald
> Machado
> *Mac*Hale
> Maville
> *Mc*Aulay
> *Mc*Williams
> Meacham

If your files contain a great many names beginning with Mac or Mc, you may, for convenience, wish to file them as a separate letter of the alphabet.

9. The name of a married woman is indexed by her legal name (her husband's surname, her given name, and her middle name or maiden surname). Example:

> Doe, Mary Jones (Mrs. John L.)
> *not* Doe, Mrs. John L. (unless first name is unknown)

10. Titles, when followed by a complete name, may be used as the *last* filing unit if needed to distinguish from another identical name. Example:

Dr. James D. Conley	Conley James D Dr.
Mr. James D. Conley	Conley James D Mr.

Titles without complete names are considered the *first* indexing unit:

Madame Sylvia
Sister Theresa

11. Terms of seniority, or professional or academic degree, are used only to distinguish from an identical name. Example:

Theodore Wilson, Sr.
Theodore Wilson, Jr.
Theodore Wilson, MD
Theodore Wilson, PhD

would be filed in the following order

Theodore Wilson, Jr.
Theodore Wilson, MD
Theodore Wilson, PhD
Theodore Wilson, Sr.

12. Articles such as *The* or *A* are disregarded in indexing:

Moore Clinic (The)

Filing Methods

The three basic methods of filing used in health care facilities are

- Alphabetic by name
- Numeric
- Subject

Patient charts are filed either alphabetically by name or by one of several numeric methods. Subject filing is used for business records, correspondence, and topical materials.

ALPHABETIC FILING

Alphabetic filing by name is the oldest, simplest, and most commonly used system. It is the system of choice for filing patient records in the majority of physicians' offices. If you can find a word in the dictionary or a name in the telephone directory, you already know some of the rules.

The alphabetic system of filing is traditional and simple to set up, requiring only a file cabinet or shelf, folders, and some divider guides. It is a **direct filing system** in that you need only know the name in order to find the desired file.

Alphabetic filing does have some drawbacks:

- You must know the correct spelling of the name
- As the number of files increases, more space is needed for each section of the alphabet. This results in periodic shifting of folders from drawer to drawer or shelf to shelf to allow for expansion.
- As the files expand, more time is required for filing or retrieving each folder because of the greater number of folders involved in the search. The time can be greatly reduced by color coding, which is discussed in detail later in this chapter. Procedure 14–2 explains how to add material to existing patient files.

NUMERIC FILING

Some form of **numeric filing** combined with color and **shelf filing** is used by practically every large clinic or hospital. Management consultants differ in their recommendations; some recommend numeric filing only if there are more than 5,000 charts, more than 10,000 charts, or in some cases more than 15,000 charts. Others recommend nothing but numeric filing. Numeric filing is an **indirect filing system**, requiring the use of an alphabetic cross-reference in order to find a given file. Some people object to this added step and overlook the advantages, which are that it

- Allows unlimited expansion without periodic shifting of folders, and shelves are usually filled evenly
- Provides additional confidentiality to the chart
- Saves time in retrieving and refiling records quickly. One knows immediately that the number 978 falls between 977 and 979. By contrast, an alphabetic system, even with color coding, requires a longer search for the exact spot.

There are several types of numeric filing systems. In the *straight* or *consecutive* numeric system, patients are given consecutive numbers as they visit the practice. This is the simplest of the numeric systems and works well for files of up to 10,000 records. It is time consuming, and there is a greater chance for error when filing documents with five or more digits. Filing activity is greatest at the end of the numeric series (Table 14–2).

In the *terminal digit* system, patients are also assigned consecutive numbers, but the digits in the number are usually separated into groups of twos or

PROCEDURE 14-2
Adding Supplementary Items to Established Patient File

GOAL

To add supplemental documents and progress notes to patient histories, observing standard steps in filing, while creating an orderly file that will facilitate ready reference to any item of information.

EQUIPMENT AND SUPPLIES

Assorted correspondence, diagnostic reports, and progress notes
Patient files
Computer or typewriter
Mending tape
FILE stamp or pen
Sorter
Stapler

PROCEDURAL STEPS

1 Group all papers according to patients' names.
   PURPOSE: Some related papers may require stapling.

2 Remove any pins or paper clips.
   PURPOSE: Pins in file folders are hazardous; paper clips are bulky and may become inadvertently attached to other materials.

3 Mend any damaged or torn records.

4 Attach any small items to standard-size paper.
   PURPOSE: Small items are easily lost or misplaced in files.

5 Staple any related papers together.

6 Place your initials or FILE stamp in the upper left corner.
   PURPOSE: To indicate that the document is released for filing.

7 Code the document by underlining or writing the patient's name in the upper right corner.
   PURPOSE: To indicate where the document is to be filed.

8 Continue steps 2 through 7 until all documents have been conditioned, released, indexed, and coded.

9 Place all documents in the sorter in filing sequence.
   EXPLANATION: Sorter can be taken to file cabinet or shelf for placing documents in patient folders.

threes and are read in groups from right to left instead of from left to right. The records are filed backward in groups. For example, all files ending in 00 are grouped together first, then those ending in 01, etc. Next the files are grouped by their middle digits so that the 00 22s come before the 01 22s. Finally the files are arranged by their first digits, so that 01 00 22 precedes 02 00 22 (Table 14–3).

Middle digit filing begins with the middle digits, followed by the first digit and finally by the terminal digits.

Some practices use the last four digits of each patient's Social Security number to file patient records. However, there is no legal requirement that every United States resident have a Social Security

TABLE 14-2 Consecutive Sequencing

Morales, Maria	012479
Rees, Charles	012480
Dreis, Patrick	012481

TABLE 14-3 Terminal Digit Sequence

Carter, John	01 99 00
Delgado, Juan	00 73 01
Geiselmann, Troy	05 55 11
Herr, Leonard	01 68 21
Julian, Bruce	01 68 22
Grissom, Randal	88 34 23
Cook, Robert	90 34 23

number, in which cases a "pseudo number" would have to be issued.

Numeric filing requires more training, but once the system is mastered, fewer errors occur than with alphabetic filing.

SUBJECT FILING

Subject filing can be either alphabetic or **alphanumeric** (A 1-3, B 1-1, B1-2, etc.) and is used for general correspondence. The main difficulty with subject filing is indexing, or classifying—deciding where to file a document. Many papers require cross-referencing. All correspondence dealing with a particular subject is filed together. The papers within the folders are filed chronologically, the most recent on top. The subject headings are placed on the tabs of the folders and filed alphabetically.

Memory Jogger

4 a. Name the three most commonly used systems of filing.
b. Which of the three is the simplest?
c. Which is an indirect system?

Color Coding

When a color coding system is used, both filing and finding are easier, and misfiled folders are kept to a minimum. The use of color visually restricts the area of search for a specific record. A misfiled chart is easily spotted even from a distance of several feet. In color coding, a specific color is selected to identify each letter of the alphabet. The application of the principle may be through using colored folders, adhesive colored identification labels, or various combinations of these (Fig. 14–3; Procedure 14–3). Any selection of colors may be used, and the division of the alphabet is determined by one's own needs. However, studies have shown that there is wide variation in the frequency with which different letters occur. One division that has been used successfully is shown in Table 14–4. Experience has proved that this breakdown results in almost equal representation of the five colors.

TABLE 14-4 Division of Letters in Color Coding

Color of Label	Letters of Alphabet
Red	A B C D
Yellow	E F G H
Green	I J K L M N
Blue	O P Q
Purple	R S T U V W X Y Z

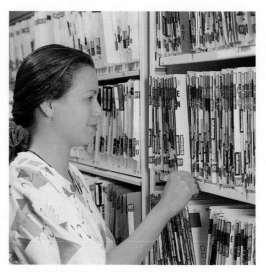

FIGURE 14–3 Application of color coding.

ALPHABETIC COLOR CODING

There are several ways of color coding files. One alphabetic system utilizes five different colored folders, with each color representing a segment of the alphabet. The *second* letter of the patient's last name determines the color, as shown in Table 14–5.

As medicine continues to consolidate into larger facilities, with more patients under one management, the filing of patient charts becomes more complicated and color coding becomes more useful. Sev-

TABLE 14-5 Division of Alphabet in 5-Color System

RED FOLDER (second letters a, b, c, d)	Canfield Eberhart Ackerman Adams
YELLOW FOLDER (second letters e, f, g, h)	Venable Effron Igawa Thill
GREEN FOLDER (second letters i, j, k, l, m, n	Histed Bjork Ak Ullman Imhoff Anderson
BLUE FOLDER (second letters o, p, q)	Gordon Epperley Aquino
PURPLE FOLDER (second letters r, s, t, u, v, w, x, y, z)	Trout Osterberg Atherton Auer Uvena Owsley Oxford Nye Azzaro

PROCEDURE 14–3
Color Coding Patient Charts

GOAL
To color code patient charts using the agency's established coding system to effectively facilitate filing and finding.

EQUIPMENT AND SUPPLIES

20 patient charts
Information on agency's coding
  system

20 file folders
Full range of color labels

PROCEDURAL STEPS

1 Assemble patient charts.

2 Arrange charts in indexing order.
   PURPOSE: When charts have been color coded, they will be in filing order.

3 Pick up the first chart and note the second letter of the patient's surname.
   EXPLANATION: For purpose of this activity, the color coding system in the text will be used.

4 Choose a folder and/or caption label of the appropriate color.

5 Type patient's name on label in indexing order and apply to folder tab.
   PURPOSE: To identify sequence of folder in filing system.

6 Repeat steps 4 and 5 until all charts have been coded.

7 Check entire group for any isolated color.
   PURPOSE: If the order and color of the folders is correct, all charts of the same color within each letter of the alphabet will be grouped together.

---

eral color-coding systems use two sets of 13 colors—one set for letters A–M, and a second set of the same colors on a different background for the letters N–Z.

There are many ready-made systems available (e.g., Bibbero, Colwell, Kardex, Remington Rand, Smead, TAB, VisiRecord). Self-adhesive colored letter blocks with either two or three letters in the specific colors are supplied in rolls. The color blocks with the appropriate letter are placed on the index tab of the folder, along with the patient's full name. The letters are in pairs so that they can be seen from either side of the chart. Strong, easily differentiated colors are used, creating a band of color in the files that makes it easy to spot out-of-place folders.

NUMERIC COLOR CODING

Color coding is also used in numeric filing. Numbers 0 through 9 are each assigned a different color. In a terminal digit filing system, the colors for the last two numbers would be affixed to the tab. If the number 1 is red and 5 is yellow, all files with numbers ending in 15 form a red and yellow band. Usu-

ally a predetermined section of the number is color coded.

OTHER COLOR CODING APPLICATIONS

There are many other ways to make color work for you. Small pressure-sensitive tabs in a variety of colors may be used to identify certain types of insured patients and other specific information. For example, a red tab over the edge of the folder may identify a patient on Medicaid, a blue tab may identify a CHAMPUS patient; a green tab may identify a Workers' Compensation patient; matching tabs may be attached to the insured's ledger card; research cases may be identified by a special color tab; and brightly colored labels on the outside of a patient chart can indicate certain health conditions, such as drug allergies. In a partnership practice, a different color folder or label may identify each physician's patients. Color can also be used to differentiate dates—one color for each month or year.

Business records may also utilize color coding. Main divider guide headings may be of one color, subheadings in a second color, and subdivisions in a

TABLE 14–6 Color Coding for Business Records

Main Heading:	DISBURSEMENTS	Red label
Subheading:	Equipment	Blue label
Subdivisions:	Typewriter	Yellow label
	Copier	Yellow label
	Calculator	Yellow label

third color (Table 14–6). A fourth color might be used for personal items.

The use of color in filing is limited only by the imagination. One word of caution: Every person in the facility who uses the files must know the key to the coding, and the key should also be written in the facility's procedures manual.

Organization of Files

PATIENT HEALTH INFORMATION

It is very difficult for a physician to study a disorganized history. Some systematic method must be followed in placing items in the patient folder. The content of the patient record has already been discussed. From the filing standpoint, it should be emphasized that when a patient record is not in actual use, there is only one place it should be—in the filing cabinet or shelf. Many precious hours can be lost in searching for misplaced or lost records that were carelessly left unfiled.

The patient's full name, in indexing order, should be typed on a label and attached to the folder tab. A strip of transparent tape can be placed on the label to prevent smudging if this is a problem. The patient's full name should also be typed on each sheet within the folder.

HEALTH-RELATED CORRESPONDENCE

Correspondence pertaining to patients' medical records should be filed with the case history. Other medical correspondence should probably be filed in a subject file.

GENERAL CORRESPONDENCE

The physician's office operates as a business as well as a professional service. There will be correspondence of a general nature pertaining to the operation of the office. In all likelihood, a special drawer or shelf is set aside for the general correspondence. The correspondence is indexed according to subject matter or names of correspondents. The guides in a subject file may appear in one, two, or three posi-

tions, depending on the number of headings, subheadings, and subdivisions. Examples are shown in Table 14–6.

PRACTICE MANAGEMENT FILES

The most active financial record is, of course, the patient ledger. In facilities that still use a manual system, this will be a card or vertical tray file, and the accounts will be arranged alphabetically by name. There will be at least two divisions:

- Active accounts
- Paid accounts

MISCELLANEOUS FOLDER

Papers that do not warrant an individual folder are placed in a miscellaneous folder. Within the folder, all papers relating to one subject, or with one correspondent, are kept together in chronologic order, the most recent on top, and then filed alphabetically with other miscellaneous material. Related materials may be stapled together. Never use paper clips for this purpose. When as many as five papers accumulate with one correspondent or subject, a separate folder should be prepared.

> **EXAMPLES OF SPECIAL CATEGORIES THAT MAY BE SET UP**
> Government-sponsored insurance
> Workers' Compensation
> Delinquent accounts
> Collection accounts

Other business files include records of income and expense, financial statements, income and payroll tax records, canceled checks, and insurance policies. These papers may be filed chronologically.

TICKLER OR FOLLOW-UP FILE

The most frequently used follow-up method is that of a **tickler file,** so called because it tickles the memory that something needs to be done or followed up on a particular date. The tickler file is always a chronologic arrangement. In its simplest form, it consists of notations on the daily calendar. If information, such as an x-ray report or laboratory report, is expected concerning a patient who has an appointment to come in, the medical assistant might make a note on the calendar or tickler file a day ahead to check on whether the report has arrived.

The tickler file is often a card file with 12 guides for the names of the months and 31 guides printed with numbers 1 through 31 for the days of the month. The guide for the current month, followed by the 31 day guides, is placed at the front of the file. Notations of actions to be taken are placed behind the guides for specific days of the current month. Notations for future months are placed behind the guide for that month. To be effective, the tickler file must be checked the first thing each day.

There are many ways to use the tickler file. It is a useful reminder for recurring events such as payments, meetings, and so forth. On the last day in each month, all the notations from behind the next month's guide are distributed among the daily numbered guides, and the guide for the month just completed is placed at the back of the file.

TRANSITORY OR TEMPORARY FILE

Many papers are kept longer than necessary because no provision is made for segregating those that have a limited usefulness. This situation is avoided by having a *transitory* or *temporary* file. For example, if the medical assistant writes a letter requesting a reprint, the file copy is placed in the transitory folder. When the reprint is received, the file copy is destroyed. The transitory file is used for materials having no permanent value. The paper may be marked with a T and destroyed when the action is completed.

LEGAL AND ETHICAL ISSUES

Shelf units with doors afford the best protection of confidentiality of patient records. Make certain that every paper placed in a patient's chart carries the date and name of the patient.

CRITICAL THINKING

1 Explain why the number of patient records might determine the method of filing.

2 Discuss the difference between a direct filing system and an indirect system. What is the determining factor?

3 Explain how color coding can speed up filing and retrieval.

HOW DID I DO? Answers to Memory Joggers

1 Answers will vary but should include six styles.

2 An OUTguide is used to indicate the place of a file that has been temporarily removed. It also avoids unnecessary search for a missing file.

3 Conditioning, releasing, indexing and coding, sorting, storing, and filing

4 a. alphabetic, numeric, subject
   b. alphabetic
   c. numeric

REFERENCES

Huffman EK: Health Information Management, 10th ed. Berwyn, IL, Physicians' Record Company, 1994.
Sabin WA: The Gregg Reference Manual, 7th ed. New York, Glencoe Division, McGraw-Hill, 1994.

Health Information Management

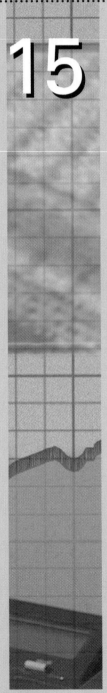

15

LEARNING OBJECTIVES

Cognitive: On successful completion of this chapter, you should be able to:

1 Define and spell the terms listed in the Vocabulary.

2 State five important reasons for keeping good medical records.

3 Explain ownership of the record.

4 List three advantages of the POMR.

5 Explain the basic differences between a traditional medical record and a problem-oriented record.

6 Illustrate the meaning of *subjective* and *objective* information in a medical record.

7 List four categories each of *subjective* and *objective* information contained in a complete case history.

8 List 15 items of personal data needed on a patient history.

9 Discuss changing an entry in the medical record and the importance of following correct procedure.

10 List and describe the three classifications of patient files.

Performance: On successful completion of this chapter, you should be able to:

1 Initiate a medical record for a new patient.

2 Add reports and correspondence into the patient's file in the correct manner and sequence.

3 Make a correction in a patient's chart in a manner affording legal protection.

VOCABULARY

augment To make larger or more intense

chronologic order In the order of time

continuity The quality or state of being continuous

correlation To show a mutual relationship

demographic Relating to the statistical characteristics of populations, such as births, marriages, mortality, health, and so forth

litigation Contest in a court of justice for the purpose of enforcing a right

microfilming Photographic records in reduced size on film.

objective information Perceptible to the external senses (e.g., conclusions reached by a physician after listening to body sounds with a stethoscope)

obliteration To remove from existence; destroy

OUTfolder A folder used to provide space for the temporary filing of materials

parlance Manner or mode of speech

pejorative Having negative connotations; a deprecatory word

POMR Problem-oriented medical record

procrastination The intentional putting off of doing something that should be done

retention schedule A listing of dates until which records are to be kept, based on statutes of limitation, tax regulations, and other factors

sequential Succeeding or following in order or as a result

statute of limitations The time limit within which an action may legally be brought upon a contract

subjective information Findings perceptible only by the affected person (the patient) (e.g., pain experienced in a specific area under certain circumstances)

Complete and accurate records are essential to a well-managed medical practice. They provide a continuous story of a patient's progress from the first visit to the last. The treatment and therapy prescribed are noted, along with regular reports on the patient's condition. When a patient is discharged, the degree of improvement is noted in the record. Health information management includes not only the assembling of the medical record for each patient but also having an efficient system for the saving, retrieval, transferring, protection, retention, storage, and destruction of these records.

SKILLS AND RESPONSIBILITIES

OBJECTIVES OF GOOD INFORMATION MANAGEMENT

- Save space
- Reduce the creation of unnecessary records
- Retrieve information fast
- Comply with legal safeguards
- Save time for the physician and the patient

Ownership of the Record

The information in a medical record is private and confidential. The medical record should be kept away from patient care areas. Its contents should not be made public. Authority to release information from the medical record lies solely with the patient unless required by law. The *record* belongs to the physician; the *information* belongs to the patient.

Reasons for Health Information Records

The three traditionally important reasons for careful recording of health information are to

- Provide the best medical care
- Supply statistical information
- Provide legal protection

PROVIDE THE BEST MEDICAL CARE

The physician examines the patient and enters the findings on the patient's medical record. These findings are the clues to diagnosis. The physician may order many types of tests to confirm or **augment** the clinical findings. As the reports of these tests come in, the findings fall into place like the pieces of a jigsaw puzzle. Now, with the confirmation data to support the diagnosis, the physician can prescribe treatment and form an opinion about the patient's chances of recovery, assured that every resource has been used to arrive at a correct judgment.

Keeping good medical records helps a physician provide **continuity** in a patient's care. Earlier illnesses and difficulties that appear on the patient's record may supply the key to current medical problems. For example, information that the patient was treated for rheumatic fever as a child can be extremely important in determining the course of treatment the physician prescribes for that patient when an illness develops a number of years later.

SUPPLY STATISTICAL INFORMATION

Medical records may be used to evaluate the effectiveness of certain kinds of treatment or to determine the incidence of a given disease. **Correlation** of such statistical information may result in a new outlook on some phases of medicine and can lead to revised techniques and treatments. The statistical data from medical records are also valuable in the preparation of scientific papers, books, and lectures.

PROVIDE LEGAL PROTECTION

Sometimes a physician must produce case histories and medical records in court. For example, a patient may wish to substantiate claims made to an insurance company for damages resulting from an accident in which he or she was injured and required medical treatment. The physician's record can be a help or a hindrance, depending on the care with which the record is kept.

In recent years other increasingly important reasons for keeping adequate health information records have affected the practice of medicine: financial reimbursement and participation in managed care.

FINANCIAL REIMBURSEMENT

Those who pay the bills require complete data to evaluate the necessity for care and the level and quality of that care before reimbursing the provider. Services must be carefully documented to justify insurance billing. The motto is "If it is not documented, it was not done (even if it was done)."

PARTICIPATION IN MANAGED CARE

Managed care organizations randomly conduct chart reviews and judge the physician on the quality of his or her documentation. The managed care organization must be able to assure its members that the physician is providing appropriate care.

Memory Joggers

1 Discuss the statement "If it is not documented, it was not done."

2 How would you answer the question "Who owns the medical record?"

Form and Quality of the Record

A record is any form of documented information. It may be kept on paper, film, or magnetic medium, such as computer tapes or disks.

FACTORS IN CREATING A USEFUL RECORD

- Easily retrievable
- Orderly
- Timely
- Legible
- Complete
- Understandable by anyone who needs to use it

Using shortened forms of words in records may be a timesaver, but any such system should be clearly understandable by anyone who needs to consult the chart. If the short forms vary from standard abbreviations (e.g., inf. could mean *infirm, inform,* or *information*), an explanation should be prepared and placed in the front of the files for immediate reference (Table 15–1).

If a record is to be *helpful*, it must be completely accurate. To be *good*, the record must be brief.

Style of the Record

NATURE OF PRACTICE

The style selected by a physician for recording case histories depends partly on the nature of the practice. General practitioners and some specialists keep

TABLE 15–1 Abbreviations Commonly Used in Patient History and Physical Examination

Abbreviation	Meaning
A&W	Alive and well
CC	Chief complaint
CNS	Central nervous system
CR	Cardiorespiratory
CV	Cardiovascular
Dx	Diagnosis
FH	Family history
GI	Gastrointestinal
GU	Genitourinary
GYN	Gynecology
HEENT	Head, ears, eyes, nose, throat
MM	Mucous membrane
PH	Past history
PI	Present illness
prn	As necessary *(pro re nata)*
ROS/SR	Review of systems/Systems review
TPR	Temperature, pulse, respirations
UCHD	Usual childhood diseases
VS	Vital signs
w/d	Well developed
w/n	Well nourished
WNL	Within normal limits

very detailed records. A specialist who sees patients only on a consultant basis, or a specialist who is likely to see a patient only once, such as a radiologist or an anesthesiologist, need not keep complex records.

NATURE OF PATIENT'S COMPLAINT

The nature of the patient's complaint is also a factor in determining how detailed a record should be. If a patient comes into a physician's office to have a foreign body removed from an eye or to have some minor injury such as a cut finger treated, a less detailed past medical history or family history is required. In contrast, the patient who is being treated for cardiac, hypertensive, or diabetic symptoms requires a complete examination and a detailed history.

USE OF SIMPLIFIED FORM

In some health care facilities where detailed histories are less common, a simple patient registration form (Fig. 15–1) can be used to record personal data and a plain sheet of paper used to record the complaint and treatment rendered. The physician who uses a

plain sheet of paper for the patient record generally develops an outline that serves as a guide to taking down the information required for a history. The physician then dictates the history, and the medical assistant types it according to an established format and places it in the patient's folder after having it read and initialed by the physician. In every medical facility certain technical terms are used frequently in the physician's reports. The medical assistant who types the reports should become familiar with the correct spelling and meaning of the medical terms. Because of the close similarity in sound and spelling of some medical terms it is also wise to check the definition to verify that the word fits the context in which it is used.

STRUCTURED FORMAT

For the physician who wishes to use a more structured format, there are many different types of forms available from professional suppliers: forms for general practice, obstetrics, surgery, pediatrics, internal medicine, or any other of the established specialties. Some physicians design their own forms to suit their particular practice and have them printed to order.

Suppliers that specialize in medical forms sometimes provide a planning kit for the physician to use. Local printers, too, often can be very helpful with form design. The record may be **sequential,** or it may be separated into problems, as described later in the section on the problem-oriented medical record. Regardless of the form used, the record will contain certain basic information (see Legal Considerations of the Patient Record).

LEGAL CONSIDERATIONS OF THE PATIENT RECORD

For adequate legal protection, the patient record should include the following:

* Patient's name and the date on every page
* Patient's medical history
* Specific quotes of comments made by the patient about symptoms or reasons for consultation
* Physician's response to any such comments
* Results of examinations
* All notations of vital signs, dated and initialed
* Records of treatment, including all possible complications that might arise
* Any failed appointments, dated and initialed by receiver
* Copies of laboratory reports
* Notations of all instructions given

Thank you for selecting our health care team!
To help us meet all your health care needs, please
fill out this form completely in ink. If you have any questions
or need assistance, please ask us - we will be happy to help.

Welcome

Patient # _____

Soc. Sec. # _____

Date _____

Patient Information (CONFIDENTIAL)

Name_____ Birth date _____ Home phone _____

Address_____ City _____ State_____ Zip _____

Check appropriate box: ☐ Minor ☐ Single ☐ Married ☐ Divorced ☐ Widowed ☐ Separated

If student, name of school/college _____ City _____ State__ ☐ Full time ☐ Part time

Patient's or parent's employer _____ Work phone _____

Business address _____ City _____ State_____ Zip _____

Spouse or parent's name _____ Employer _____ Work phone _____

Whom may we thank for referring you?_____

Person to contact in case of emergency_____ Phone _____

Responsible Party

Name of person responsible for this account _____ Relationship to patient _____

Address _____ Home phone _____

Driver's license # _____ Birth date _____ Financial institution _____

Employer_____ Work phone _____ SSN# _____

Is this person currently a patient in our office? ☐ Yes ☐ No

Insurance Information

Name of insured _____ Relationship to patient _____

Birth date _____ Social Security # _____ Date employed _____

Name of employer_____ Union or local # _____ Work phone _____

Address of employer _____ City _____ State_____ Zip _____

Insurance company_____ Group # _____ Policy/ID # _____

Ins. co. address_____ City _____ State _____ Zip _____

How much is your deductible? _____How much have you used?_____ Max. annual benefit _____

DO YOU HAVE ANY ADDITIONAL INSURANCE? ☐ Yes ☐ No   IF YES, COMPLETE THE FOLLOWING:

Name of insured _____ Relationship to patient _____

Birth date _____ Social Security # _____ Date employed _____

Name of employer_____ Union or local # _____ Work phone _____

Address of employer _____ City _____ State_____ Zip _____

Insurance company_____ Group # _____ Policy/ID # _____

Ins. co. address_____ City _____ State _____ Zip _____

How much is your deductible? _____How much have you used?_____ Max. annual benefit _____

I authorize release of any information concerning my (or my child's) health care, advice and treatment provided for the purpose of evaluating and administering claims for insurance benefits. I also hereby authorize payment of insurance benefits otherwise payable to me directly to the doctor.

X_____

Signature of patient or parent if minor _____ Date _____

FIGURE 15–1 Patient registration form.

- Documentation of information disclosed during the informed consent process when applicable
- Any correspondence that relates to the patient's diagnosis or treatment
- Any other data pertinent to the patient's health

When a patient fails to follow instructions or refuses recommended treatment, a letter to this effect should be sent to the patient by certified, return-receipt mail and a copy retained in the patient record. A similar type of letter should be sent if the patient leaves the physician's care or if the physician feels it is necessary to withdraw from the case (Fig. 15–2).

EXAMPLES OF ITEMS TO EXCLUDE FROM THE RECORD

- Reports from consulting physicians *should not* be placed in the record until they have been carefully reviewed to ensure that the overall diagnostic and treatment plan is consistent or that any inconsistencies have been identified and justified. If the report contains confidential data from another source, release of such data without authorization can lead to legal difficulties.
- Transferred records from the patient's previous physicians should never be added to the patient's new record until the physician has reviewed them. The same advice would apply to records received from any outside source (e.g., hospital emergency departments or free-standing urgent-care clinics).
- **Pejorative** or flippant comments should never be entered in the record. For example, after seeing a patient who tended toward hypochondria, a physician might be tempted to enter only one note, such as "new verse, same refrain." This comment would reflect negatively on the physician in court. In some states, patients or their representatives have the legal right to a copy of their medical records.

Organization of the Record

SOURCE-ORIENTED RECORD

The traditional patient record is *source oriented;* that is, observations and data are catalogued according to their source—physician, laboratory, x-ray, nurse, technician—with no recording of a logical relation-

Date

Dear (Patient):

I find it necessary to inform you that I am withdrawing from providing you medical care for the reason that _____ .

Because your condition requires medical attention, I suggest that you promptly seek the care of another physician. If you do not know of another physician, you may wish to contact the county medical society for a referral.

If you so desire, I shall be available to provide care to you for a reasonable time after you have received this letter, but in no event for more than 15 days.

When you have selected a new physician, I would be pleased to make available to him or her a copy of your medical chart or a summary of your treatment.

Very truly yours,

FIGURE 15–2 Letter of withdrawal from a case.

ship between them. Forms and progress notes are filed in reverse **chronologic order** (most recent on top) and filed in separate sections of the record by the type of form or service rendered—all laboratory reports together, all x-ray reports together, and so forth.

PROBLEM-ORIENTED RECORD

The problem-oriented medical record (**POMR**) is a radical departure from the traditional system of keeping patient records. It is sometimes referred to as the Weed system because it was originated by Dr. Lawrence L. Weed, a professor of medicine at the University of Vermont's College of Medicine. The POMR is a record of clinical practice that divides medical action into four bases:

- The *database* includes chief complaint, present illness, and patient profile and also a review of systems, physical examination, and laboratory reports.
- The *problem list* is a numbered and titled list of every problem the patient has that requires management or workup. This may include social and **demographic** troubles as well as strictly medical or surgical ones.
- The *treatment plan* includes management, additional workups needed, and therapy. Each plan is titled and numbered with respect to the problem.
- The *progress notes* include structured notes that are numbered to correspond with each problem number.

One company, which designed the Andrus/Clini-Rec Charting System, has developed a file folder for

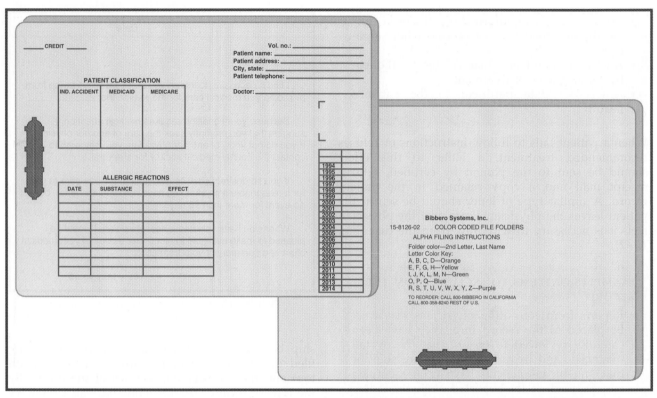

FIGURE 15–3   File folder for organization of patient data. (Courtesy of Bibbero Systems, Inc., Petaluma, CA.)

its recommended organization of patient data. The folder is preprinted on the front for age dating and easy access to basic information. With the calendar years printed on the cover, it is simple to keep track of when the patient was last seen. On the initial visit, the year, say 1998, is checked on the cover. If the patient appears again in 2000, and the year 1999 is not checked, it is immediately evident that more than a year has elapsed since the last visit (Fig. 15–3). The system includes dividers for laboratory reports, consultations, hospital reports, and radiologic and electrocardiograph reports (all scientific information) on the left side and database and progress notes (communication and supervision) on the right side.

The chart is begun by obtaining a patient-completed database system record, which contains family and past medical history together with many carefully selected screening questions (Fig. 15–4). There are also questionnaires designed for screening problems in specialty practices.

The problem list is entered on the divider cover for laboratory reports. Special sections are provided for current major and chronic problems and for inactive major or chronic problems. The divider cover for progress notes is a chart for listing medications and other therapeutic modalities. Progress notes follow the SOAP approach (Fig. 15–5).

SOAP APPROACH

- *Subjective impressions*
- *Objective clinical evidence*
- *Assessment or diagnosis*
- *Plans for further studies, treatment, or management*

The POMR has the advantage of imposing order and organization on the information added to a patient's medical record. The records are more easily reviewed, and the likelihood of overlooking a problem is greatly reduced. The SOAP approach essentially forces a rational approach to patient problems and assists in formulating a logical and orderly plan of patient care.

Popularity of the POMR has continued to grow since its introduction in the 1960s, and it is especially advantageous in clinics, group practices, and hospitals, where more than one person must be able to find essential information in the chart.

Memory Jogger

3 *Explain the SOAP approach.*

PART A — PRESENT HEALTH HISTORY (continued)

IV. GENERAL HEALTH, ATTITUDE AND HABITS (continued)

Have you recently had any changes in your: If yes, please explain:
Marital status?   No ____ Yes ____ _____
Job or work?   No ____ Yes ____ _____
Residence?   No ____ Yes ____ _____
Financial status?   No ____ Yes ____ _____
Are you having any legal problems
or trouble with the law?   No ____ Yes ____ _____

PART B — PAST HISTORY

I. FAMILY HEALTH

Please give the following information about your immediate family:

Relationship	Age, If Living	Age At Death	State of Health Or Cause of Death
Father			
Mother			
Brothers and Sisters			
Spouse			
Children			

Have any **blood relatives** had any of the following illnesses?
If so, indicate relationship (mother, brother, etc.)

Illness	Family Members
Asthma	
Diabetes	
Cancer	
Blood Disease	
Glaucoma	
Epilepsy	
Rheumatoid Arthritis	
Tuberculosis	
Gout	
High Blood Pressure	
Heart Disease	
Mental Problems	
Suicide	

PART C — BODY SYSTEMS REVIEW

MEN: Please answer questions 1 through 12, then skip to question 18.
WOMEN: Please start on question 6.

MEN ONLY
Have you had or do you have
prostate trouble? .... No____ Yes____
Do you have any sexual problems
or with impotency? .... No____ Yes____
Have you ever had sores or
lesions on your penis? .... No____ Yes____
Have you ever had any discharge
from your penis? .... No____ Yes____
Do you ever have pain, lumps
or swelling in your testicles? .... No____ Yes____
Check here if you wish to discuss any special problems with the doctor.

Is it sometimes hard to start your urine flow?

	Rarely/ Never	Occasionally	Frequently

II. HOSPITALIZATIONS, SURGERIES

Please list all times you have been hospitalized

Year	Operation

III. ILLNESS AND MEDICAL PROBLEMS

Please mark with an (X) any of the following
If you are not certain when an illness started,

Illness	(X)
Eye or eye lid infection	
Glaucoma	
Other eye problems	
Ear Trouble	
Deafness or decreased hearing	
Thyroid trouble	
Strep throat	
Bronchitis	
Emphysema	
Pneumonia	
Allergies, asthma or hay fever	
Tuberculosis	
Other lung problems	
High blood pressure	
Heart attack	
High cholesterol	
Arteriosclerosis	
(Hardening of arteries)	
Heart murmur	
Other heart condition	
Stomach/duodenal ulcer	
Diverticulosis	
Colitis	
Other bowel problem	
Hepatitis	
Liver trouble	
Gallbladder trouble	

Page 2   © 1979, 1983 Bibbero Systems International
(REV. 6/92)

Chart No. _____

ANDRUS/CLINI-REC® HEALTH HISTORY QUESTIONNAIRE

Identification Information   Today's Date _____

Name _____   Date of Birth _____

Occupation _____   Marital Status _____

PART A — PRESENT HEALTH HISTORY

I. CURRENT MEDICAL PROBLEMS

Please list the medical problems for which you came to see the doctor. About when did they begin?

Problems	Date Began

What concerns you most about these problems?

If you are being treated for any other illnesses or medical problems by another physician, please describe the problems and write the name of the physician or medical facility treating you.

Illness or Medical Problem	Physician or Medical Facility	City

II. MEDICATIONS

Please list all medications you are now taking, including those you buy without a doctor's prescription (such as aspirin, cold tablets or vitamin supplements)

III. ALLERGIES AND SENSITIVITIES

List anything that you are allergic to such as certain foods, medications, dust, chemicals, or soaps, household items, pollens, bee stings, etc., and indicate how each affects you.

Allergic To:	Effect	Allergic To:	Effect

IV. GENERAL HEALTH, ATTITUDE AND HABITS

How is your overall health now? .... Health now: Poor ____ Fair ____ Good ____ Excellent ____
How has it been most of your life? .... Health has been Poor ____ Fair ____ Good ____ Excellent ____
In the past year:
Has your appetite changed? .... Appetite: Decreased ____ Increased ____ Stayed same ____
Has your weight changed? .... Weight: Lost ____ lbs. Gained ____ lbs. No change ____
Are you thirsty much of the time? .... Thirsty: No ____ Yes ____
Has your overall 'pep' changed? .... Pep: Decreased ____ Increased ____ Stayed same ____
Do you usually have trouble sleeping? .... Trouble sleeping: No ____ Yes ____
How much do you exercise? .... Exercise: Little or none ____ Less than I need ____ All I need ____
Do you smoke? .... Smokes: No ____ Yes ____ If yes, how many years? ____
How many each day? ....   Cigarettes ____ Cigars ____ Pipesfull ____
Have you ever smoked? .... Smoked No ____ Yes ____ If yes, how many years? ____
How many each day? ....   Cigarettes ____ Cigars ____ Pipesfull ____
Do you drink alcoholic beverages? .... Alcohol: No ____ Yes ____ I drink ____ Beers ____ Glasses of Wine ____
                                                          Drinks of hard liquor - per day
Have you ever had a problem with alcohol? ..... Prior problem: No ____ Yes ____
How much coffee or tea do you usually drink? .. Coffee/Tea: ____ cups of coffee or tea a day.
Do you regularly wear seatbelts? .... Seatbelts: No ____ Yes ____

DO YOU:	Rarely/ Never	Occasionally	Frequently	DO YOU:	Rarely/ Never	Occasionally	Frequently
Feel nervous?				Ever feel like committing suicide?			
Feel depressed?							
Find it hard to make decisions?				Feel bored with your life?			
Lose your temper?				Use marijuana?			
Worry a lot?				Use "hard drugs"?			
Tire easily?				Do you want to talk to the			
Have trouble relaxing?				doctor about a personal matter? No ____ Yes ____			
Have any sexual problems?							

Created and Developed by "Medical Economics" Professional Systems
Copyright © 1979, 1983 Bibbero Systems International, Inc.   STOCK NO. 19-711-4 5/83

Page 1

19-711-4 5/83   Page 3

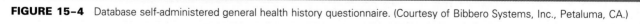

FIGURE 15–4 Database self-administered general health history questionnaire. (Courtesy of Bibbero Systems, Inc., Petaluma, CA.)

OUTLINE FORMAT PROGRESS NOTES

Patient Name ___Fletcher, LeRoy___

Prob. No. or Letter	DATE	**S** Subjective	**O** Objective	**A** Assess	**P** Plans	Page___1___
2	01/26/00	Patient complains of two days of severe high epigastric pain and burning, radiating through to the back. Pain accentuated after eating.				
			On examination there is extreme guarding and tenderness, high epigastric region. No rebound. Bowel sounds normal. BP 110/70			
				R/O gastric ulcer, pylorospasm.		
					To have upper gastrointestinal series. Start on Cimetidine, 300 mg. q.i.d. Eliminate coffee, alcohol, and aspirin. Return in two days.	

Start each Progress Note (Subjective, Objective, through the intervening columns to the right   Assessment and Plans) at the appropriate margin of the page.   shaded column to create an outline form. Write

ANDRUS/CLINI-REC® PRIMARY CARE CHARTING SYSTEM FORM NO. 26-7115, ©1976 BIBBERO SYSTEMS, INC., PETALUMA, CA.

FIGURE 15–5 SOAP progress note form. (Courtesy of Bibbero Systems, Inc., Petaluma, California (800) 242-2376, Fax (800) 242-9330.)

Contents of the Complete Case History

The medical case history is the most important record in a physician's practice. For completeness, each patient's record should contain **subjective information** provided by the patient and **objective information** provided by the physician. If all entries are completed, the case history will stand the test of time. No branch of medicine is exempt from the necessity of keeping records. Records aid the physician in the practice of medicine, as well as provide legal protection.

SUBJECTIVE INFORMATION

Routine Personal Data

The patient's case history begins with routine personal data, which the patient usually supplies on the first visit. The basic facts needed are

- Patient's full name, spelled correctly
- Names of parents if patient is a child
- Patient's sex
- Date of birth
- Marital status
- Name of spouse, if married
- Number of children, if any
- Home address and telephone number
- Occupation
- Name of employer
- Business address and telephone number
- Employment information for spouse
- Health care insurance information
- Source of referral
- Social Security number

Personal and Medical History

This portion of the medical record, which is often obtained by having the patient complete a questionnaire, provides information about any past illnesses or surgical operations that the patient may have had and includes data about injuries or physical defects, whether congenital or acquired. It also includes information about the patient's daily health habits.

Patient's Family History

The family history comprises the physical condition of the various members of the patient's family, any past illnesses or diseases that individual members may have suffered, and a record of the causes of death. This information is important, because a hereditary pattern may be present in the case of certain diseases.

Patient's Chief Complaint

This is a concise account of the patient's symptoms, explained in the patient's own words. It should include

- Nature and duration of pain, if any
- Time when the patient first noticed symptoms
- Patient's opinion as to the possible causes for the difficulties
- Remedies that the patient may have applied before seeing the physician
- Other medical treatment received for the same condition in the past

OBJECTIVE INFORMATION

Objective findings, sometimes referred to as signs, become evident from the physician's examination of the patient.

Physical Examination and Findings and Laboratory and Radiology Reports

This section of the case history varies greatly with the specialty of the physician and the complaint of the patient. After the physician has examined the patient, the physical findings are recorded on the history. Results of other tests or requests for these tests are then recorded or, if they appear on separate sheets, attached to the history.

Diagnosis

The physician, on the basis of all evidence provided in the patient's past history, the physician's examination, and any supplementary tests, places the diagnosis of the patient's condition on the medical record. If there is some doubt, it may be termed *provisional diagnosis.*

Treatment Prescribed and Progress Notes

The physician's suggested treatment is listed after the diagnosis. Generally, instructions to the patient to return for follow-up treatment in a specific period of time are noted here as well.

On each subsequent visit, the date must be entered on the chart and information about the patient's condition and the results of treatment added to the history, on the basis of the physician's observations. Notations of all medications prescribed or instructions given, as well as the patient's own progress report, should be placed in the record. Any home visits are noted. If the patient is hospitalized, the name of the hospital, the reason for the admission, and the dates of admission and discharge are recorded. Much of this information may be obtained from the hospital discharge summary.

Condition at Time of Termination of Treatment

When the treatment is terminated, the physician will record that information, for example, *August 18, 1999. Wound completely healed. Patient discharged.*

Memory Joggers

 Explain the difference between subjective *and* objective *information.*

Obtaining the History

The medical assistant usually secures the routine personal data. The personal and medical history and the patient's family history may be secured by asking the patient to complete a questionnaire, with the physician **augmenting** the information provided during the patient interview.

BY THE MEDICAL ASSISTANT

When the medical assistant is responsible for recording the patient's history, care must be exercised to ensure that the patient's answers are not heard by others in the reception room. If privacy is not possible, it is better to give the patient a form to fill out and then transfer this information to permanent records later. When privacy is available, the medical assistant may ask the patient questions and at the same time type the answers directly on the record. This method offers an opportunity to become better acquainted with the patient while completing the necessary records. In facilities where lengthy questionnaires are to be completed by the new patient, the questionnaire is mailed to the patient with a request that it be completed and returned to the physician before the appointment. If the record is to be computerized, requesting the information ahead of time gives the office staff the opportunity to transfer information to the computer before the new patient's visit.

BY THE PHYSICIAN

The patient's chief complaint may have been indicated to the medical assistant, but the physician will question the patient in more detail. Many practitioners write their own entries on the chart in longhand. Some may keyboard the findings direct into the computer. Others may dictate the material, either directly to the medical assistant or by using a recording device. If the material is dictated and typed, the physician should check each entry and then initial the entry to verify accuracy. Although the physician may find this a "bother," it should be encouraged. For a chart to be admissible as evidence in court, the person dictating or writing the entries must be able to attest that they were true and correct at the time they were written. The best indication of that is the physician's signature or initials on the typed entry.

Making Additions

As long as the patient is under the physician's care, the medical history is building. Each laboratory report, radiology report, and progress note is added to the record with the latest information always on top. Although each item is important, the most recent is usually of greatest significance to the patient's care. Again, the physician should read and initial each of these reports before it is placed in the record.

LABORATORY REPORTS

Different colors of paper are often used for reporting different procedures. For example, urinalysis report forms may be yellow, blood count forms pink, and so forth. When laboratory slips are smaller than the history form, they should be placed on a standard 8½ × 11-inch sheet of colored paper. Type the patient's name in the upper right corner, and then, with transparent tape, fasten the first report even with the bottom of the page. The second laboratory report will be taped or glued in place on top of and about ½ inch above the first slip, allowing the date to show on the first report. By this method, called shingling, the latest report always appears on top. When checking previous reports, it is necessary only to run your finger down the slips until you find the desired date; then flip up the slips above. Laboratory report carrier forms with adhesive strips may be purchased (Fig. 15–6).

RADIOLOGY REPORTS

Radiology reports are usually typed on standard letter-size stationery. They are placed in the patient's history folder, with the most recent report on top. All radiology reports may be stapled together or kept behind a special divider in the chart.

PROGRESS NOTES

Reports on the patient's progress are continually being added to the case history. Each visit of the patient should be entered on the chart, with the date preceding any notations about the visit. The medical

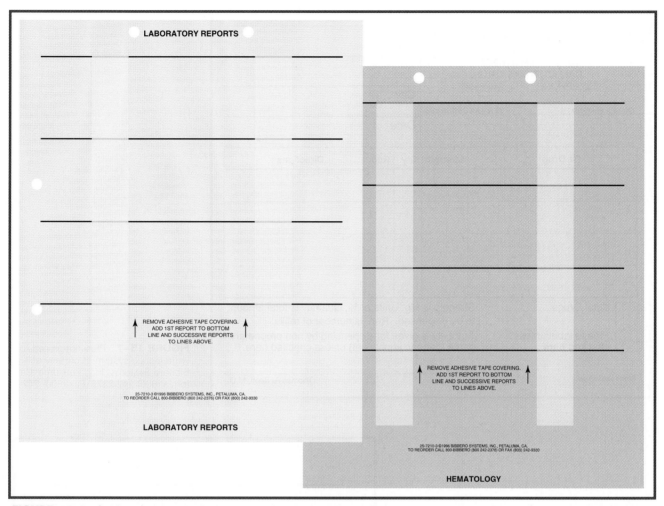

FIGURE 15–6   Quick-stick color-coded lab carriers. (Courtesy of Bibbero Systems, Inc., Petaluma, California (800) 242-2376, Fax (800) 242-9330.)

assistant can type or stamp the date on the chart when readying the charts for the patient's visits. Every instruction, prescription, or telephone call for advice should be entered with the correct date. If several persons are handling and making entries on a patient's record, it is advisable to initial each entry. This aids in tracing entries about which there may be some question.

Making Corrections

Sometimes it is necessary to make corrections on medical records. Erasing and **obliteration** must be avoided. To correct a handwritten entry, follow these three steps:

1. Draw a line through the error
2. Insert the correction above or immediately after the error.
3. In the margin, write correction or *Corr.,* your initials, and the date.

Errors made while typing are corrected in the usual way. However, an error discovered in a typed entry at a later date is corrected in the same manner as described for a handwritten entry.

Keeping Records Current

One of the greatest dangers to good record keeping is **procrastination.** The record must be methodically kept current. It is the medical assistant's responsibility to see that this is done.

The case histories and reports may accumulate on the physician's or the medical assistant's desk during the day. After the last patient has gone, check each history to make certain that all necessary information has been recorded and that each entry is sufficiently clear for future understanding. Give the physician all extra reports, such as laboratory and radiology reports, to read and initial so that they may be filed in the patient's case history folder.

While the physician is reviewing these reports,

THOMAS A. SCOTT
General Practice
135 SO. ELM STREET
DALLAS, TEXAS 75019
TELEPHONE: (214) 340-9999

TX. LIC. #6099914   DEA #AK08888888

Name

Address

City

Date

Rx Drug	Strength	Qty.	Rep.	Directions

☐ Total Drugs

☐ Please label unless checked here

Strength is Mg. Units or %; Quantity is total amount to be dispensed. Rep. is number of refills.

Authority is given for dispensing by non proprietary name (generic equivalent) unless checked here. ☐

FORM #25-8298

Thomas A. Scott, M.D.

FIGURE 15–7 Prescription pad for write-it-once system. (Courtesy of Bibbero Systems, Inc., Petaluma, California (800) 242-2376, Fax (800) 242-9330.)

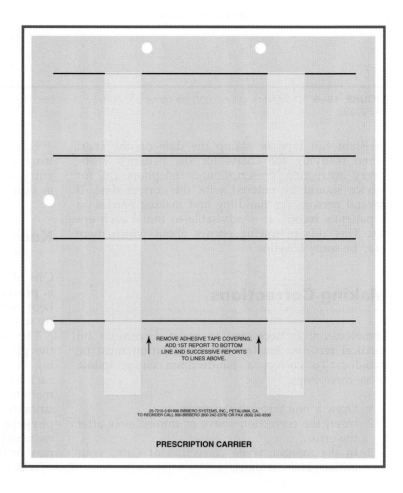

REMOVE ADHESIVE TAPE COVERING. ADD 1ST REPORT TO BOTTOM LINE AND SUCCESSIVE REPORTS TO LINES ABOVE.

25-7210-3 ©1996 BIBBERO SYSTEMS, INC., PETALUMA, CA. TO REORDER CALL 800-BIBBERO (800 242-2376) OR FAX (800) 242-9330

PRESCRIPTION CARRIER

FIGURE 15–8 Quick-stick prescription carrier. (Courtesy of Bibbero Systems, Inc., Petaluma, California (800) 242-2376, Fax (800) 242-9330.)

you can pull the histories of any patients seen outside the office that day, as well as those of patients who have been given special instructions by telephone or for whom prescriptions were ordered. These entries are made in the same manner as for an office visit, but the type of call is explained in parentheses after the date.

> **EXAMPLE OF A HOME VISIT ENTRY**
>
> May 23, 1998 (Res.). Routine PX. Temp 98.6. Chest clear.
> Cont. Rx. May now eat semi-bland diet.

> **EXAMPLE OF A TELEPHONE CALL TO PHYSICIAN**
>
> June 26, 1998 (Tel.). To change Rx (Vit. B Comp) to one b.i.d.
> Force fluids. Feeling much better.

> **EXAMPLE OF CHARTING TESTS ORDERED FOR PATIENT**
>
> April 10, 1999. Consultation. Bil. mammograms scheduled at SJH on April 17. Scheduled with Dr. Abbot for office consultation on April 26.

> **EXAMPLE OF CHARTING PRESCRIPTIONS**
>
> April 25, 1999. Refill Tylenol c Cod. #25

A prescription pad, printed on no-smear, spot carbon paper, is available for a timesaving, write-it-once system. By placing the prescription blank over the patient's record, the prescription is automatically copied on the record as it is written (Fig. 15–7). Prescription carriers with adhesive strips are also available for the physician who uses duplicate prescription blanks (Fig. 15–8).

The patient record should not leave the office. A physician's pocket call record, as shown in Figure 15–9, can be used for outside calls, and the information can be transferred to the chart in the office.

Notations should be made of any unkept appointments or of refusals to cooperate with instructions as they occur.

After all records have been reviewed, they should be placed in a file tray and locked away for the night, if there is insufficient time to file them the same day. Do not leave histories out in view at night, especially if the facility has a night cleaning service.

On arrival the next morning, the medical assistant can index the histories for filing. Attach extra reports and information sheets (do not simply drop them into the folders). When this has been done, the records are ready for filing.

The physician may prefer to dictate progress notes rather than write them in longhand. At appropriate times during the day, everything is dictated: patient histories, physical examination findings, medications prescribed, follow-up findings, summaries of telephone conversations. At the end of the day the recorded information is given to the medical assistant for transcribing onto the records.

A great deal of time may be saved in transcribing these notes by using a continuous roll or pages of

PHYSICIANS POCKET CALL RECORD DATE______

NAME	ADDRESS OR REMARKS	SYMBOL	MONEY RECEIVED	HOME CHARGES	HOSPITAL CHARGES
	Post these TOTALS to office book daily. ☛				

FIGURE 15–9 Physician's pocket call record.

self-adhesive strips (Fig. 15–10). When the transcription has been completed, the physician may wish to check the notes, underline important points, and initial each entry before returning the notes to the medical assistant for insertion into the charts to verify that they are correct in the event of audit or **litigation.** The use of self-adhesive strips saves removing the sheet from a chart that may be bound with metal fasteners, inserting the sheet into the typewriter, and putting the sheet back into the

J. Barton
4-17-99   Examination: 5 mm diameter raised, round, sharply marginated, gray-pink, finely
          papillomatous and keratotic lesion, left dorsal hand.
          Impression: Verruca vulgaris
Disp: 1) Discussed treatment by electrosurgery vs. cryotherapy, with father, including
             scarring with electrosurgery.
          2) Lesion removed by D & C under local anesth with Xyl. + Epi.
          3) Monsels, DSD, T.I.D.
          4) See prn

B. Kolo
4-17-99   Has been treating superficial multicentric BCCA, distal left mandible, with Efudex 5%
          cream b.i.d. for 3 wks. See inflammation with central erosion and peripheral crusting in
          involved area. Response appears appropriate.
Disp: 1) Cont Efudex 5% cream b.i.d.
          2) See in 3 wks

F. Schroeder
4-17-99   Pt. points out very small, quiescent-appearing actinic keratosis—inferior right lateral
          arm x 1 and proximal left extensor forearm x 1. Discussed nature of lesions with pt. L
          N2 about 10 sec. each.
          Re/ck p.r.n. persistence.

N. Mywea
4-17-99   Pt. inquires about lesion, medial right left. Possibly present since birth. No change in
          size or color over time. No trmt to date.
Exam: Inferior right medial left: 17 x 15 mm diameter round, sharply marginated, macular,
          uniformly medium-brown lesion; a few terminal hairs penetrate surface of lesion.
Imp: 1) Discussed benign appearance of lesion with pt.
          2) No treatment at this time
          3) Re/ck prn change

A

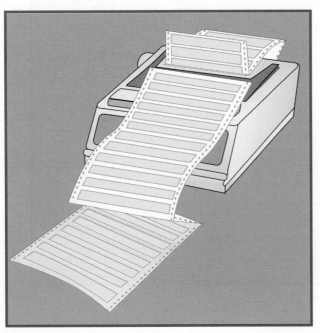

B

FIGURE 15–10 *A* and *B,* Self-adhesive strip and continuous roll used to transcribe notes.

folder. It also simplifies the physician's part in checking and initialing the notes, because only the transcribed material is handled, not the bulky charts.

Memory Jogger

 Why is it important for the physician to sign or initial typewritten progress notes?

Regular Transfer of Files

In most medical offices, records are filed according to three classifications:

- *Active files* are those of patients currently receiving treatment.
- *Inactive files* generally are those of patients whom the doctor has not seen for 6 months or longer. When such individuals return for care, their folders are replaced in the active file.
- *Closed files* are records of patients who have died, moved away, or otherwise terminated their relationship with the physician.

Some system must be established for regular transfer of files from active to inactive status or possibly destruction. The yearly expansion of charts and the file space available can influence the transfer period. Charts for patients who are currently hospitalized may be kept in a special section for quick reference, then placed in the regular active file when the patient is discharged from the hospital. In a surgical practice, there frequently is a specific date on which the patient is discharged from the physician's care and the notation made on the chart "Return prn" (for the Latin *pro re nata:* as the occasion arises). This record may safely be placed in the inactive file. In a general practice office, the outside of the folder may be stamped with the date of the visit each time the patient is seen. It will then be a simple matter to determine when the chart should be transferred to the inactive status. In the **parlance** of filing, this is called the *perpetual transfer method.*

Retention and Destruction

Physicians have an obligation to retain patient records that may reasonably be of value to a patient, according to the AMA Council on Ethical and Judicial Affairs. There is no standard rule to follow in establishing a records **retention schedule**.

- Medical considerations are the primary basis for deciding how long to retain medical records. For example, operative notes and chemotherapy records should always be part of the patient's chart.

- If a particular record no longer needs to be kept for medical reasons, the physician should check state law to see if there is a requirement that records be kept for a minimum length of time (most states do not have such a provision). The time is measured from the last professional contact with the patient.
- In all cases, medical records should be kept for at least as long as the length of time of the **statute of limitations** for medical malpractice claims, which may be 3 or more years, depending on the state law. In the case of a minor, the statute of limitations may not apply until the patient reaches the age of majority.
- The records of any patient covered by Medicare or Medicaid must be kept at least 5 years.
- Before discarding old records, patients should be given an opportunity to claim the records or have them sent to another physician, if it is feasible to give the patient that opportunity.
- To preserve confidentiality when discarding old records, the documents should be destroyed.

Protection of Records

Releasing original case histories to anyone outside the health care facility should be avoided if possible. Instead, prepare a summary or photocopy the materials needed for reference and retain the original in the physician's office. With the facsimile machine becoming standard equipment in business facilities, as well as in many of our homes, the transfer of information is simplified and the records remain in safekeeping. Often only certain aspects of the record are requested by colleagues or others, and these can easily be supplied by faxing the required pages, observing precautions for confidentiality.

Occasions may arise when records are temporarily out of the office. Some physicians release case histories to their colleagues, or an original record may be subpoenaed by the court. In such instances, a colored **OUTfolder** should be inserted in the file in place of the regular folder and a notation made of the name, date, and to whom the record was released. Interim papers may be placed in the OUTfolder until the original is returned.

Long-Term Storage

Large health care facilities may find it advisable to microfilm records for storage. Another option is the transfer of paper records by laser beam onto optical disks. **Microfilming** and optical disk technology are both very expensive and probably are not practical for any but the very large group practice or health maintenance organization.

Facilities that have computerized the patient records will be able to keep those records indefinitely on disk. Scanners can convert a paper record into an image on the computer screen resulting in an electronic medical record. The bulky paper files can then be put in storage or eliminated. There is no longer a need to fill hundreds of square feet of storage space or search through stack upon stack of storage file boxes for an inactive or closed file.

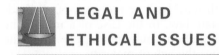

LEGAL AND ETHICAL ISSUES

Authority to release information from the medical record lies solely with the patient unless required by law.

Ownership of the record is often a subject of controversy. The record belongs to the physician; the information belongs to the patient.

When the physician withdraws from the care of a patient, or if the patient leaves the physician's care, a letter acknowledging this situation should be sent by the physician to the patient by certified, return-receipt mail.

When a medical chart is used as evidence in a court case, the person dictating or writing the entries must be able to attest to their authenticity.

The person making corrections to a medical record always must follow the steps as outlined in this chapter.

The records of any patient covered by Medicare or Medicaid must be kept at least 5 years. All records should be kept until the statute of limitations for medical malpractice claims has expired.

CRITICAL THINKING

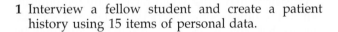

1 Interview a fellow student and create a patient history using 15 items of personal data.

2 Using the Discharge Summary in Chapter 12, demonstrate the correct method of making an alteration in the record.

HOW DID I DO? Answers to Memory Joggers

1 Example: In performing a physical examination, the physician may actually examine every body system but may record information about only those systems that are abnormal. This record would not stand up in court.

2 The answer should explain the ownership of both the physician and the patient.

3 *Subjective* impressions
Objective clinical evidence
Assessment or diagnosis
Plans for further studies, treatment, or management.

4 Subjective information is supplied by the patient and includes personal data, past medical history, family medical history, and the patient's current complaint (symptoms). Objective information is what the physician notes on examination of the patient (signs).

5 It is important for the physician to initial typewritten notes to verify that they are correct, in the event of audit or litigation.

REFERENCES

American Medical Association: Current Opinions with Annotations of the Council on Ethical and Judicial Affairs, 1996–97 edition. Chicago, AMA, 1997.
Huffman EK: Health Information Management, 10th ed. Berwyn, IL, Physician Record Company, 1994 (revised by American Health Information Management Association).

Notes

SECTION 5

Financial Management

Professional Fees and Credit Arrangements

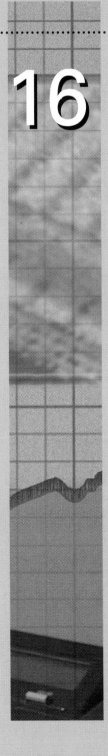

16

LEARNING OBJECTIVES

Cognitive: On successful completion of this chapter you should be able to:
1 Define and spell the terms listed in the Vocabulary.
2 Discuss how fees are determined.
3 List three values that are considered in determining professional fees.
4 Give an example of usual and customary fee.
5 Explain how a physician's fee profile is determined.
6 List three reasons for giving patients an estimate slip.
7 Discuss the concept of professional courtesy.
8 List four kinds of charges that should be avoided.
9 List the items to be included on a credit form.
10 Explain what is meant by third-party liability.
11 Identify the three items of information that can be released in response to a request for credit information.
12 State three items that should be *excluded* in replying to a request for credit information.
13 Discuss the Truth in Lending Regulation.
14 Discuss how confidentiality relates to credit.

Performance: On successful completion of this chapter you should be able to:
1 Make financial arrangements with a patient requesting credit.
2 Prepare a Truth in Lending form.
3 Respond to patient's request for explanation of the physician's fee.

VOCABULARY

assignment of benefits Statement authorizing the insurance company to pay benefits directly to physician

capitation System of payment in which providers are paid a fixed per capita fee for each enrolled patient, not dependent on the services rendered

fee profile Compilation of a physician's fees over a given period of time

fee schedule Compilation of preestablished fee allowances for given services or procedures.

fiscal agent An organization under contract to the government as well as some private plans to act as financial representative in handling insurance claims from providers of health care; also referred to as fiscal intermediary

medically indigent Able to take care of ordinary living expenses but cannot afford medical care

professional courtesy Reduction or absence of fee to professional associates

third-party payer Someone other than the patient, spouse, or parent who is responsible for paying all or part of the patient's medical costs

usual, customary, and reasonable A formula for determining medical insurance benefits payable

The practice of medicine is a business as well as a profession, and the details of conducting the business aspects are often the responsibility of the medical assistant. While service to the patient is the primary concern of the medical profession, a physician must charge and collect a fee for such services to continue providing medical care. The physician is one of many contributors in determining the amount of the fees. The medical assistant usually has the responsibility of informing the patient on financial matters, collecting the payment, and, in some cases, making arrangements for deferred payment.

How Fees Are Determined

Setting fees is no simple matter. The physician has three commodities to sell—time, judgment, and services. Yet the value of these commodities is never exactly the same to any two individuals. Medical care has little value except to the patient, and the value to the patient may not be consistent with the ability to pay. In every case, the physician must place an estimate on the value of the services. Such an arrangement is known as fee for service. This value may then be modified by other considerations.

THE EFFECTS OF MANAGED CARE

An important consideration in today's atmosphere of managed care is the preponderance of patients who are enrolled in health maintenance organization (HMO)-type insurance contracts. Under managed care the physician agrees to accept predetermined fees for specific procedures and services instead of

the fee-for-service arrangement described in the preceding paragraph. The patient may be subject to a copay that is determined by the insurance contract and is collected at the time of service. When payment is made on a **capitation** basis the records of all patients in each plan are kept together and billed collectively.

- In 1993 only about half the Americans insured through employers were in managed care.
- In 1995 three of four insured U.S. workers had health coverage through managed care.
- In 1997 fewer than one fourth of U.S. workers had fee-for-service plans.

PREVAILING RATE IN THE COMMUNITY

One of the bases for determining charges on the fee-for-service basis is the economic level of the community. Different communities reflect different living scales, and this situation is reflected in medical fees as well. Consequently, the prevailing rate in the community—the average composite fee—must be taken into consideration by each individual physician. Strangely enough, fees that are too low drive patients away just as quickly as do fees that are too high because the average person tends to judge worth of a product on its cost—low cost translates as low value.

USUAL, CUSTOMARY, AND REASONABLE FEE

Most insurance plans base their payments on what has become known as a usual and customary fee for a given procedure. Some include the word "reasonable," that is, **usual, customary, and reasonable:**

- **usual**—The physician's usual fee for a given service is the fee that that an individual physician most frequently charges for the service.
- **customary**—The customary fee is a range of the usual fees charged for the same service by physicians with similar training and experience practicing in the same geographic and socioeconomic area. There is now a growing tendency for fees to be determined by national trends rather than by local custom.
- **reasonable**—The term *reasonable* usually applies to a service or procedure that is exceptionally difficult or complicated, requiring extraordinary time or effort on the part of the physician.

It should be noted that under Medicare Part B, *customary and prevailing* corresponds to *usual and customary* as defined here.

To illustrate, let us suppose that Dr. Wallace usually charges private patients $100 for a first office visit. The usual fees charged for a first visit by other physicians in the same community with similar training and experience range from $75 to $125. Dr. Wallace's fee of $100 is within the customary range and would therefore be paid by an insurance plan that pays on a usual and customary basis. If, on the other hand, the range of usual fees in the community is from $60 to $85, the insurance plan would allow only the maximum within the range, or $85, to Dr. Wallace.

FEE SETTING BY THIRD-PARTY PAYERS

The physician does not act alone in determining fees. A **third-party payer** may provide the physician with a predetermined **fee schedule** that it will approve for payment. Some require preapproval of the fee before service is rendered. A third-party payer may require precertification before it will pay for a specific service. Government programs such as Medicare and Medicaid (see Chapter 20) have strict guidelines regarding reimbursement for fees and the raising of fees.

PHYSICIAN'S FEE PROFILE

The **fiscal agent,** or **fiscal intermediary,** for government-sponsored insurance programs as well as some private plans keeps a continuous record of the usual charges submitted for specific services by each individual physician. By compiling and averaging these fees over a given period, usually a year, the physician's **fee profile** is established. This fee profile is then used in determining the amount of third-party liability for services under the program. One of the

objections voiced by physicians is the lag between the time of a private fee increase and the time it is reflected in payments by an insurance carrier. It may be as long as 2 to 3 years.

INSURANCE ALLOWANCE

In some individual cases, the physician may not wish to charge the patient in addition to what will be allowed by the patient's insurance. This is often a professional courtesy for other health care professionals. The full fee should be quoted to the patient and charged to the account, with the understanding that after the insurance allowance has been received, the balance may be discounted. If a smaller fee is quoted and charged, several problems may arise:

- The lower fee will alter the physician's fee profile.
- If it should become necessary to bring suit for payment of the fee, only the reduced fee can be recovered.
- If the insurance allowance is paid on the basis of a certain percentage of the physician's fee and a lower fee is charged, the insurance allowance will be correspondingly lower. Also, if the physician does this with many patients, the insurance company may take the position that the reduced fee is the physician's usual fee and base its payments accordingly. It may even be considered fraudulent in some instances.

Explaining Costs to Patient

It is natural for the patient, particularly one new to the practice, to wonder, "How much is this going to cost?" However, some patients may be reluctant to voice this concern.

RESPONSIBILITY TO DISCUSS FEES

It is the responsibility of the physician or the medical assistant to raise the discussion of fees if the patient does not do so (see Procedure 16–1). Be prepared to discuss fees with any patient who is interested, but do not assume that you must do so with everyone. You might open the discussion of fees with something like this: "Mr. Willardson, do you have any questions about the costs of your operation? If you do, I'll be glad to review them." On the other hand, in this preliminary discussion of fees, the physician must not sidestep the issue by saying, "Don't worry about the bill, let's just get you well first." Avoid attempting to calm a worried patient about to undergo surgery by saying, "There's

PROCEDURE 16 – 1
Explaining Professional Fees

GOAL

To explain the physician's fees so that the patient understands his or her obligations and rights for privacy.

EQUIPMENT AND SUPPLIES

Patient's statement
Copy of physician's fee schedule

Quiet private area where the patient
feels free to ask questions

PROCEDURAL STEPS

1 Determine that the patient has the correct bill.
  PURPOSE: To make certain that the bill belongs to this patient and that the insurance numbers, the address, and the telephone number are correct.

2 Examine the bill for possible errors.
  PURPOSE: To demonstrate that the patient's concerns are important and that you are willing to make any necessary adjustments.

3 Refer to the fee schedule for the services rendered.
  PURPOSE: To explain how physicians determine their fees. If an error has occurred, correct it immediately with a sincere apology.

4 Explain itemized billing:
  • Date of each service
  • Type of service rendered
  • Fee
  PURPOSE: To make certain that the patient realizes the number and extent of services rendered.

5 Display professional attitude toward the patient.
  PURPOSE: To reassure the patient that you have a thorough understanding of the fee schedule and show willingness to answer questions politely and completely.

6 Determine whether the patient has specific concerns that may hinder payment.
  PURPOSE: To provide an opportunity for making special arrangements if needed.

7 Make appropriate arrangements for a discussion between the physician and patient if further explanation is necessary for resolution of the problem.

---

really nothing to it." The patient may later complain loudly about the bill because he or she misunderstood the complexity of the service.

Even in those cases in which the physician quotes a fee, the medical assistant often has the responsibility of explaining the physician's fees to the patient. The medical assistant must know how fees are determined and why charges vary, as well as have a thorough knowledge of the physician's practice and policies to handle perplexing situations involving fees.

As the medical assistant's understanding of the practice increases, he or she can build respect for the physician's services by educating patients that money spent for medical care is an excellent investment in the future. It is a rare patient who understands the intricate procedures involved in diagnosis and treatment.

ADVANCE DISCUSSION OF FEES

Advance fee discussions help the patient to plan ahead for medical expenditures. Most patients want to pay their financial obligations but rightly insist on an accurate estimate of those obligations before they contract for purchase of goods or services. When a physician frankly discusses fees in advance with patients, even to the point of describing how a fee is established, misconceptions and complaints about overcharging and fee discrepancies are usually eliminated.

Memory Jogger

1 *List and explain six factors that may affect the determination of the fee for a given service.*

EXPLAINING ADDITIONAL COSTS

Explanations of medical costs should extend beyond the physician's own charges. For example, if a patient is to undergo surgery, the physician should also explain the costs of the operation, the anesthesiologist's and radiologist's charges, the laboratory fees, and the approximate hospital bill. The importance of calling in another physician for consultation should be explained to patients when consultation becomes necessary. It should be made clear, in advance, that there will be a separate bill submitted by the consulting physician. Patients do not always understand that the consultation is for the benefit of the patient, not the physician.

ESTIMATE SLIPS

Some physicians give patients an estimate of medical expenses before hospitalization (Fig. 16–1). A few medical societies cooperatively develop such estimate sheets with local hospitals. Individual physicians occasionally work up their own estimate forms when a patient is embarking on long-term treatment. The physician should, however, emphasize that it is an estimate only and that the actual cost may vary somewhat.

Estimate slips should be prepared in duplicate so that the patient may have a copy and the original is retained in the patient's file. Duplicate estimate slips may help to

- Avoid your forgetting that a fee was quoted
- Eliminate the possibility of later misquoting the fee
- Simplify collection by preventing misunderstanding and confusion over charges

Adjusting or Canceling Fees

CARE FOR THOSE WHO CANNOT PAY

The medical profession has traditionally accepted the responsibility of providing medical care for individuals unable to pay for these services. In spite of the increased scope of government-sponsored care for the **medically indigent,** physicians still donate thousands of dollars' worth of such medical services each year.

In many instances, medical care of the indigent is available through social service agencies. The medical assistant should learn about any local organizations and agencies that can aid the patient in obtaining the necessary assistance. The physician can provide only medical services. Other agencies must provide hospitalization, for example, or arrange for

SURGICAL COST ESTIMATE

Name of Patient: ______________________ Date: ______________
Procedure: ______________________
Your surgery has been scheduled at ______________ Hospital on ______________.
You should report to the Admitting Office between the hours of ______ (AM) (PM) and ______ (AM) (PM).

Although medical and hospital expenses are seldom welcome, knowing in advance what expenses to expect and how to plan for them can lessen the burden. This estimate is prepared to assist you in budgeting your surgical costs.

PROFESSIONAL FEES

When you have major surgery, the surgical team includes the operating surgeon, the assistant surgeon, and the anesthetist. Each has an important part in your care, and each will render a separate statement for services. While each doctor will independently set his/her own fee, it is usually possible to estimate in advance an approximate range of fees. Assuming an uncomplicated course for your surgery, the charges are estimated as follows:

Operating Surgeon	$ ________	to $ ________
Assistant Surgeon	________	to ________
Anesthetist	________	to ________

The assistant surgeon and the anesthetist usually base their fees on the operating time; consequently, if a surgical procedure turns out to be more complicated than was expected, their fees may be correspondingly increased.

The estimated duration of your hospital stay is ______ days at $______ per day for a (semi-private) (private) room. During your hospital stay there will be charges for laboratory tests, medications as required, and other services. It is impossible to estimate in advance what these charges will be; they will be itemized on your hospital bill. If you have health insurance, please take the appropriate forms and I.D. information with you on the day of your admittance.

PLEASE KEEP IN MIND THIS IS ONLY AN ESTIMATE

FIGURE 16–1 Form for surgical cost estimate.

paying the costs of special therapy, rehabilitation, or medications. Unfortunately, there is still another segment of the population that consists of uninsured employees who are not eligible for public assistance, are not covered under a group policy, and cannot afford the high premiums for private medical insurance. Special attention must be given to helping these persons arrange to pay their medical bills.

If a physician accepts a case for which a fee will not be paid, complete records must still be kept on the patient. The only deviation in procedure is that the financial record indicates no charge (n/c) in the debit column.

FEES IN HARDSHIP CASES

Sometimes a physician is faced with the problem of deciding whether to reduce or cancel a fee in a hardship case. Before adjusting or canceling a fee, the physician or the medical assistant should engage in a frank discussion of the patient's financial situation. Find out whether the patient is entitled to an insurance settlement of some kind. Circumstances may qualify the patient for local or state public assistance. If so, the assistant may direct the patient to the appropriate agency.

If the circumstances of hardship are known before the services are rendered, thorough discussion of what the fee will be and how it will be paid should take place at that time. In most cases, it is far better to adjust a fee before rather than after treatment. The physician may suggest that a medically indigent patient seek care at a county hospital with public assistance. A physician should be free to choose his or her form of charity and not feel obligated to substantially reduce or cancel a fee when the circumstances are known in advance.

After the physician and patient have agreed on a fee, special circumstances may arise that create a hardship. If the physician then agrees to reduce the fee, the patient should be told that the reduction will be effective only after the adjusted amount is paid in full. For instance, if a fee of $500 is reduced to $350, the full amount of the $500 charge should appear on the ledger and when $350 has been received the remainder can be written off as an adjustment.

PITFALLS OF FEE ADJUSTMENTS

Great care should be taken in reducing the fee for care of a patient who dies. The physician's sympathy is with the family in such instances, but the physician's generosity in reducing a fee could be misinterpreted and result in a suit for malpractice.

If the physician agrees to settle for a reduced fee in a situation in which the patient is disputing the fee, care should be taken to make certain the negotiations are *without prejudice*. By taking this precau-

tion, the physician protects the right to collect the original sum should the patient refuse to pay the lowered fee. The offer of a discount, therefore, should be made in writing, with the insertion of the words "without prejudice" and a definite time limit for making payment stated. Prepare two copies of the agreement and have the signatures witnessed. Keep the original for the physician and give a copy to the patient.

A fee should never be reduced on the basis of a poor result or as a means of obtaining payment to avoid the use of a collection agency. A reduction for these reasons degrades the physician and the practice of medicine.

PROFESSIONAL COURTESY

Traditionally, physicians do not charge professional colleagues or their immediate dependents for medical care. Although the concept of **professional courtesy** is often attributed to Hippocrates, the foundations of professional courtesy today are derived from Thomas Percival's Code of 1803.

In some cases, the giving of professional courtesy represents the loss of a large amount of potential income. If there is a substantial outlay in the cost of materials, the professional colleague will probably wish to reimburse the physician for the materials used. Most physicians today subscribe to a health insurance plan. If the care they receive is covered by insurance, it is entirely ethical for the attending physician to accept the insurance benefits in payment for services.

If the services are frequent enough to involve a significant portion of the physician's professional time, or extend over a long period of time, the physician may wish to charge on an adjusted basis.

When professional courtesy has been offered and the recipient still insists on paying, the physician need not hesitate on ethical grounds to accept a fee for service.

Professional courtesy is often extended beyond fellow physicians and their dependents. Most physicians treat their own medical assistants without charge and grant discounts to nurses and medical assistants not in their direct employ. Professional courtesy is sometimes extended to others in the health care field, for instance pharmacists and dentists. There is a growing sentiment that professional courtesy has outlived its usefulness and should be abandoned.

Charges to Avoid

TELEPHONE CALLS

It is generally considered inadvisable to charge for telephone calls. Some physicians, especially pediatricians, find they must give considerable advice over the telephone. However, many of these calls are fairly routine to the office—although not to the worried mother or patient—and an able medical assistant can be trained to answer many of the questions or a special time can be set aside for telephone calls.

LATE PAYMENTS

Levying late charges on fees for professional services not paid within a prescribed time is usually not in the best interest of the public or the profession. However, the physician who has experienced problems with delinquent accounts may properly choose to request that payment be made at the time of treatment or add interest or other reasonable charges to delinquent accounts. The physician must comply with state and federal regulations applicable to the imposition of such charges (see Truth in Lending Act).

MISSED APPOINTMENTS

Most physicians believe that charging for a missed appointment or for one not canceled 24 hours in advance, although not unethical if the patient is fully advised, is nevertheless not in the best interest of their patients or their practices.

FIRST INSURANCE FORM

If the patient has multiple insurance forms to be completed, the physician is justified in making a charge but should be willing to complete the first standard form without charge. Exceptions are Medicare and Medicaid, which prohibit charging for completing forms.

Credit Arrangements

EXTENDING CREDIT

Whenever a service is rendered before payment is received, an extension of credit has been made. If payment is collected on completion of the service, no problem exists. But if payment is deferred, credit arrangements are best made during the patient's initial visit (see Procedure 16–2). Successful collection of an account may depend on the skill and tact with which the medical assistant conducts the first interview.

Under the Federal Equal Credit Opportunity Act of 1975, once you agree to extend credit to one patient, you must offer the same arrangement to any other patient who requests it. You can refuse to do so only on the basis of ability or inability to pay. One way to avoid involvement with the credit laws is to accept bank credit cards. The Equal Credit Opportunity Act bars discrimination in all areas of credit, with the purpose of ensuring that credit is made available fairly and impartially, and specifies prohibited bases under the law. The law prohibits discrimination against any applicant for credit because (1) of race, color, religion, national origin, sex, marital status, or age; (2) the applicant receives income from any public assistance program, and (3) he or she has exercised rights under consumer credit laws.

Many medical assistants inform a patient who is telephoning for a first appointment that new patients are expected to pay cash for their first visit, at which time credit arrangements can be established if further care is needed. For example:

> Mr. Barrington, your appointment is scheduled for 9:30 AM, Tuesday, September 25, with Dr. Newhouse. The usual charge for a first office visit is about XX dollars, and we ask that payment for a first visit be made at the time of service. If you wish to establish credit arrangements in case further care is needed, please plan to be here 15 minutes early so that the necessary papers can be completed.

This approach informs the patient in advance that he or she will be expected to complete a credit application.

Information from the Patient

Maintaining records is essential to the follow-up of collections. It is extremely important that the medical assistant get adequate information about the patient's ability to pay—on the first visit, if possible. It is neither unprofessional nor time consuming to get full credit information from patients. The public is conditioned to supplying such information and respects a business-like approach if it is done tactfully and without apology. Although a patient needing medical care is rarely turned away because of a credit risk, the information provided on the initial visit may alert the medical assistant to be cautious about allowing an account to fall in arrears.

The medical assistant should check the completed form carefully, to make certain that nothing was overlooked. The new patient will view these questions as reasonable, but the established patient may resent such an inquiry. Consequently, it is important that the form be completed on the first visit.

Although the registration form the patient completes in the physician's office is usually not as detailed as an application for credit in, for example, a department store, it must establish an information base, should future collection steps become necessary.

Many printed forms are available, but some physicians design their own to include specific information desired in their practices. Whatever form is used, it should include certain basic information and

PROCEDURE 16–2
Making Credit Arrangements with a Patient

GOAL
To assist the patient in paying for services by making mutually beneficial credit arrangements according to established office policy.

EQUIPMENT AND SUPPLIES
Patient's ledger
Calendar
Truth in Lending form
Assignment of Benefits form

Patient's insurance form
Typewriter
Private area for interview

PROCEDURAL STEPS

1 Answer thoroughly and kindly all questions about credit.

2 Inform the patient of office policy regarding credit:
- Payment at the time of first visit
- Payment by bank card
- Credit application

PURPOSE: To ensure complete understanding of mutual responsibilities.

3 Have the patient complete the credit application.
PURPOSE: To comply with office practices on the extension of credit.

4 Check the completed credit application.
PURPOSE: To confirm that all necessary information is included.

5 Discuss with the patient the possible arrangements and ask the patient to decide which of those arrangements is most suitable.
PURPOSE: Better compliance can be expected when the patient makes the choice.

6 Prepare the Truth in Lending form and have the patient sign it if the agreement requires more than four installments.
PURPOSE: To comply with Regulation Z.

7 Have the patient execute an assignment of insurance benefits.
PURPOSE: To comply with credit policy.

8 Make a copy of the patient's insurance ID and have the patient sign a consent for release of the information to insurance company.
PURPOSE: Consent for the release of information is necessary on most insurance forms before a claim can be processed

9 Keep credit information confidential.

---

not ask for information that is disallowed under the 1977 Federal Equal Credit Opportunity Act (ECOA). For instance, under the ECOA "marital status" can be requested only as *married, unmarried,* or *separated.* Terms such as *divorced, single,* or *widow/er* are illegal. *Age* is also forbidden, but *date of birth* is acceptable.

INFORMATION FROM PATIENT

Patient's full name. The patient's first, middle, and last names, correctly spelled, should be at the top of the form.

Patient's birth date. With this information, the patient's age can be calculated at any time.
Telephone number
Social Security number
Responsible person's full name. Relationship to the patient, his or her address, telephone number, Social Security number, and driver's license number should be included.
Responsible person's employer. Name, address, and telephone number of the employer and the responsible person's occupation or department

Insurance information

Spouse of responsible person. Same information as for responsible person. (Community property laws in some states make each and both responsible.)

Nearest relative. Name, relationship to patient, address, and telephone number

Referral. Name of physician or other person who referred the patient (see Fig. 8–3)

An individualized form can ask for further specific information appropriate for a particular practice. When a patient applies for credit you may *not* ask for the patient's race, color, religion, or national origin. It is also illegal to gather information on the patient's birth control practices or plans to have children. Those questions may be asked when it is part of a medical history but not when it is related to granting credit.

Third-Party Liability

If financial responsibility is attributed to an individual other than the patient, spouse, or parent, be sure to obtain full name, address, employment data, and other credit information about that person. Also, contact the named individual for verification of the obligation. If a third-party payer's agreement to pay is contingent on the patient's failure to pay, such an agreement must be in writing to be enforceable and must be made before treatment. Any agreement made after completion of treatment could be considered as a moral obligation only. The guarantee of a person to pay the account of another may be very simple. It may be typewritten or handwritten, stating:

I, the undersigned, do promise to pay for the medical services rendered by Theodore Wilson, MD, to my nephew, Robert L. Smith.
Date:
Signed: _____

or

I, the undersigned, promise to pay the medical bill of Robert L. Smith, if his mother, Mrs. Lydia Smith, does not pay by the 15th of July, 19xx.
Date:
Signed: _____

Accounts for services rendered to a spouse or child should always carry full data about the party responsible, which in most cases is the other spouse or the parent. Generally, a responsible spouse or parent pays the account without any follow-up col-

lection procedures. In the case of a minor, it is generally held that the parent accompanying the child to the medical facility is responsible for paying. Any agreement between divorced or separated parents is solely between them and does not affect the obligation to the physician.

If you foresee legal difficulties in collecting an account in which divorce, legal guardianship, or the involvement of an emancipated minor complicates the matter, it is best to contact the physician's attorney for advice. The laws governing such matters vary according to each state. One regulation is that you must always have the signature of the third party responsible for the debt if he or she is not otherwise obligated by law. An oral agreement in this case is not binding.

Memory Jogger

2 *What is the purpose of the Equal Credit Opportunity Act of 1977? What are its restrictions?*

Health Insurance Information

The initial interview is the best time to get full information on the patient's insurance coverage. The patient registration form usually provides a place for the name of the insurance company. Ask to see the patient's identification card and make a photocopy for your records. The card usually shows the name of the subscriber and the group and member number and often includes a service code indicating the patient's coverage. Also obtain information on any supplementary coverage—for instance, a plan in which the spouse is the subscriber and the patient is covered as a dependent. There may also be major medical or supplementary benefits to the patient's policy. Verify this information on each visit.

Assignment of Benefits

Many physicians ask the patient to execute an **assignment of benefits** at this time. The assignment, authorizing the insurance company to pay benefits directly to the physician, may be stamped on the insurance form or may be subsequently attached to a completed insurance form.

Consent for Release of Information

Use a standard claim form or the form the patient has brought to the office. Have the patient sign the consent for release of the information that is on the claim form. In this way, the insurance billing can be processed without delay as services are performed. Some states require a special form for release of information separate and apart from the insurance claim form itself. The medical assistant should check local regulations.

INSTALLMENT BUYING OF MEDICAL SERVICES

Because installment buying is so much a part of our economic system today, the physician's office must be prepared to help patients budget for their medical care. Patients expect to use their credit resources and appreciate business-like assistance in establishing a payment plan. The medical profession has too long suffered a poor collection record because of its fear of appearing too commercial. The physician should be ready to arrange credit when medical bills will be high or when a patient for some reason is unable to pay at the time of service. In general, fees for routine office calls and small medical bills should be kept on a pay-as-you-go basis.

Credit Cards

The acceptance of credit cards, sometimes called bank cards, has become commonplace in medical practice. Patients appreciate the convenience, and paying by credit card may help to improve collections. The signed credit card voucher is deposited to the physician's bank account. The card company deducts a percentage (from 1% to 5% depending on volume) for the collection service. The patient may pay the full amount when billed by the card company or may pay a portion and be charged interest on the balance.

Special Budget Plans

If a patient appears concerned about the ability to meet his financial obligations, the physician or the medical assistant can suggest in a tactful way:

> Mr. Elwood, if you think you will have difficulty paying for your treatments at one time, we can work out some special arrangement.

This allows the patient to ask what sort of plan you have in mind, and the discussion progresses very easily into various payment plans. Generally, it is better to let the patient decide what arrangements are best rather than to suggest a plan. However, if the patient has no suggestion, the medical assistant can say:

> Mr. Elwood, would you be able to pay $50 each month until the account is paid in full?

or

> Usually an account of this size can be settled in 3 to 4 months. Would you be able to pay $100 now, then $50 a month until the account is paid in full?

When the amount of each installment has been agreed on, it is then wise to establish definite dates on which the payments will be expected. Strive for an arrangement that will result in the balance being paid within a reasonable time, generally within 6 months.

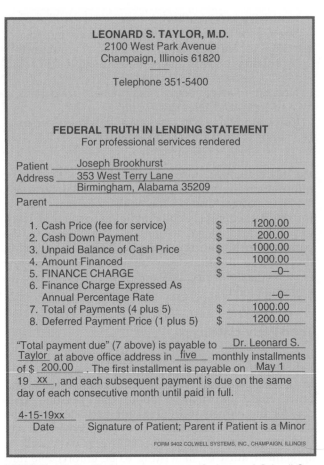

FIGURE 16–2 Disclosure statement. (Courtesy of Colwell Systems, Inc., Champaign, IL.)

Truth in Lending Act

Regulation Z of the Truth in Lending Act, which is enforced by the Federal Trade Commission, requires that when there is a bilateral agreement between physician and patient to accept payment in more than four installments, the physician is required to provide disclosure of information regarding finance charges. Even if there are no finance charges involved, the form must be completed stating this fact. A copy of the form is retained by the physician, and the original is given to the patient. Specific wording is required in the disclosure. The form in Figure 16–2 meets the requirements. Have the patient sign the agreement in your presence, because you must have proof of signing. The disclosure statement must be kept on file for 2 years. Although the disclosure statement is designed as protection for the debtor, it can be a good collection tool for the creditor.

It is recognized that physicians generally permit their patients to pay in installments, and as long as there is no specific agreement on the part of the physician for payment to be made in more than four installments, and no finance charge is made, the account is not subject to the regulation. If the patient chooses to pay in installments instead of the full amount, this is considered a unilateral action. The physician, in accepting such payments, probably would not be subject to the provisions of the regulation. The physician's office, however, must be certain to bill for the full balance each time. If the statement is for only a partial payment, it then becomes a bilateral agreement and as such is subject to Regulation Z.

Helping patients budget their medical expenses is a rather new aspect of the business side of medical practice. However, it is a real service to patients and demonstrates that the physician and the office staff are sincerely anxious to help patients pay their own way. It may also prevent many collection problems.

Memory Jogger

3 *What is the purpose of Regulation Z of the Truth in Lending Act and when is it applied?*

CONFIDENTIALITY

Obtaining Credit Information

Credit information is confidential. It should be guarded as carefully as a confidential medical history and should be disclosed to no one. When you ask for credit information from patients in the office, do so in a private area where others cannot overhear the conversation. A desk or table away from the reception area where a patient can sit in total privacy and complete a credit application is a great asset. Credit information is personal—it should be kept that way.

Credit Bureaus

Some physicians join a credit bureau, particularly in large cities where it is more difficult to gauge informally the patients' ability to pay. Credit bureaus gather credit information from many sources, pool it, and make it available to dues-paying bureau members. If you receive a request for credit information about one of your patients, it is permissible to furnish it because the debtor, by giving the physician's name as a reference, has given implied consent; otherwise, the credit bureau would not have contacted you. According to the Fair Credit Practices Act Amendments of 1975, you can reply by giving ledger information only, including

- When the account was opened
- How much the patient now owes
- The highest amount of the account at any time

You should avoid any reference to

- Character
- Paying habits
- Credit rating

Medical-Dental-Hospital Bureaus

The Medical-Dental-Hospital Bureaus of America (MDHBA), with headquarters in Chicago, is a national organization of agencies serving physicians, dentists, and hospitals. It seeks to maintain the highest standards among its members and is committed to following the collection methods most acceptable to physicians. Members who use their collection services have access to credit information on accounts assigned by other clients. Member bureaus of the MDHBA frequently assist the medical assistant by sponsoring collection seminars as well as by providing speakers for medical assistant society meetings.

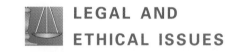

LEGAL AND ETHICAL ISSUES

Government plans such as Medicare and Medicaid have strict guidelines regarding setting fees and reimbursement.

If a physician allows or suggests to a patient that the insurance payment will be considered payment in full, discounting the deductible, the physician may be judged guilty of fraud.

The tradition of not charging professional colleagues (professional courtesy) is diminishing because most physicians today carry health insurance, and it is entirely ethical for the attending physician to accept the insurance in payment of services.

The Federal Equal Credit Opportunity Act of 1977 bars discrimination in all areas of credit. If the physician agrees to extend credit to one patient, then the same arrangement must be offered to any other patient who requests it.

If both the physician and the patient agree that payment for services may be made in more than four installments, the physician must complete a Federal Truth in Lending Statement and have it signed by the patient.

CRITICAL THINKING

1 Explain the meaning of "bilateral agreement."

2 When does the matter of third-party liability become an issue?

3 How would the medical assistant know when it is ethical to release credit information about a patient? What information can be released?

HOW DID I DO? Answers to Memory Joggers

1 a. Managed care participation
b. Prevailing rate in the community

c. Usual, customary, and reasonable fee
d. Third-party fee schedule
e. Physician's fee profile
f. Insurance allowance

2 The purpose of the Equal Credit Opportunity Act is to bar discrimination in all areas of credit, ensuring that credit is available fairly and impartially. It prohibits discrimination because of race, color, religion, national origin, sex, marital status, or age or because applicant receives public assistance or has exercised rights under consumer credit laws.

3 Regulation Z requires the physician to provide disclosure regarding finance charges and becomes effective when there is a bilateral agreement between physician and patient to accept payment in more than four installments.

REFERENCES

Federal Reserve Board: Equal Credit Opportunity Act, October 28, 1977.
Truth in Lending Act, 1968.

Managing Practice Finances

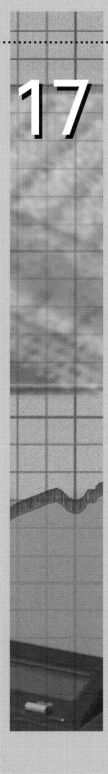

17

LEARNING OBJECTIVES

Cognitive: On successful completion of this chapter you should be able to:

1 Define and spell the terms listed in the Vocabulary.
2 Name the two bases of accounting and explain their differences.
3 State the four kinds of information that the financial records of any business should show at all times.
4 Differentiate between a debit balance and a credit balance.
5 Describe and demonstrate the entry for a credit balance.
6 List six kinds of bookkeeping records.
7 Compare the three most common systems used in the professional office.
8 State the basic accounting equation.
9 Discuss the importance of a trial balance.
10 Describe how to maintain a petty cash fund.
11 List and state the purpose of the five common periodic accounting reports.

Performance: On successful completion of this chapter you should be able to:

1 Prepare a ledger account for a new patient.

2 Prepare a patient charge slip.

3 Journalize service charges and payments using a single-entry system.

4 Post the entries from the daily journal to patient ledger cards.

5 Prepare a daily proof of posting.

6 Prepare a daily proof of cash control.

7 Prepare a monthly trial balance.

8 Establish and maintain a petty cash fund.

9 Post service charges and payments using a pegboard.

VOCABULARY

account A single financial record.

account balance The debit or credit balance remaining in the account

accounting equation Assets = Liabilities + Proprietorship (Capital)

accounts payable Debts incurred and not yet paid

accounts receivable Amounts owed to the physician

accounts receivable control A summary of unpaid accounts

accounts receivable ledger The combined record of all patient accounts

accounts receivable trial balance A method of determining that the journal and the ledger are in balance

accrual basis of accounting Income is recorded when earned, and expenses are recorded when incurred

adjustment column An account column, sometimes included to the left of the balance column, that is used for entering discounts

balance The difference between the debit and credit totals

balance column The account column on the far right that is used for recording the difference between the debit and credit columns

balance sheet A financial statement for a specific date that shows the total assets, liabilities, and capital of the business

bookkeeping The recording part of the accounting process

cash basis of accounting Income is recorded when received, and expenses are recorded when paid

cash flow statement A financial summary for a specific period that shows the beginning balance on hand, the receipts and disbursements during the period, and the balance on hand at the end of the period

cash payment journal A record of all cash paid out

credit The record of a payment received

credit balance The amount of advance payment or overpayment on an account (amount of receipts exceeding amount chargeed)

credit column The account column to the right of the debit column that is used for entering funds received

daily journal The book in which all transactions are first recorded; the book of original entry, or general journal

debit The record of a charge or debt incurred

debit column The account column on the left that is used for entering charges

disbursements Money paid out

disbursements journal A summary of amounts paid out

discounts Subtractions from the patient's balance

general journal The book of original entry in bookkeeping

in balance Total ending balances of patient ledgers equal total of accounts receivable control

invoice A paper describing a purchase and the amount due

packing slip An itemized list of objects in a package

payables Amounts owed to others

petty cash fund A fund maintained to pay small unpredictable cash expenditures

posting The act of transferring information from one record to another

receipts Money received

receivables Amounts owing from others

statement A request for payment

statement of income and expense A summary of all income and expenses for a given period

superbill A combination charge slip, statement, and insurance reporting form

transaction The occurrence of a financial event or condition that must be recorded

trial balance A method of checking the accuracy of accounts

A physician's business records are the key to good management practice. The medical assistant who can keep accurate financial records and who will conduct the nonclinical side of the practice in a business-like fashion is genuinely needed and appreciated.

Financial records that are complete, correct, and current are essential for

- Prompt billing and collection procedures
- Professional financial planning
- Accurate reporting of income to federal and state agencies

What Is Accounting?

Accounting is a system of recording, classifying, and summarizing financial transactions.

Bookkeeping is mainly the recording part of the accounting process. The bookkeeping must be done daily and is the responsibility of the administrative medical assistant in a small practice. In a larger practice, the office manager or financial manager assumes this responsibility.

ACCOUNT BASES

There are two general bases for accounting: the cash basis and the accrual basis (Table 17–1). Most physicians use the **cash basis of accounting.** Expressed simply, this means that (1) charges for services are entered as income when payment is received and (2) expenses are recorded when they are paid. Merchants, on the other hand, generally use an **accrual basis of accounting.** Income is considered earned when services have been performed or goods have been sold, even though payment may not have been received. Expenses are recognized and recorded when incurred, even though they have not been paid.

FINANCIAL SUMMARIES

The financial records of any business should at all times show

- How much was earned in a given period
- How much was collected
- How much is owed
- The distribution of expenses incurred

From the daily entries, the accountant can prepare monthly and annual summaries that provide a basis for comparing any given period with another similar period.

Periodic analyses of the financial records can result in improved business practices, better management of time, curtailment or elimination of unprofitable services, and better budgeting of expenses. With the appropriate software these analyses can be accomplished using the computer.

Bookkeeping

A willingness to pay attention to detail, good organizational skills, and the ability to concentrate and maintain consistency in working patterns and procedures are all necessary qualifications for the person who has the responsibility of keeping financial records.

TABLE 17–1 Accounting Bases

	Cash Basis	Accrual Basis
Income is recorded	When received	When service is performed or goods are sold
Expense is recorded	When paid	When incurred (even if not paid)

SKILLS AND RESPONSIBILITIES

BOOKKEEPING PROCEDURES

- Use good penmanship.
- Use the same pen style and ink consistently.
- Keep columns of figures straight.
- Write well-formed figures (a careless 9 may look like a 7; an open 0 may resemble a 6).
- Carry decimal points correctly.
- Do not erase, write over, or blot out figures. If an error is made, a straight line should be drawn through the incorrect figure and the correct figure written above it.

Bookkeeping procedures are not difficult or complicated, but they do require concentration to avoid errors. There is no such thing as *almost* correct financial records. The books either balance, or they do not balance. The bookkeeping is either right or wrong. This is not the place to be creative or take shortcuts.

The medical assistant should set aside a certain time each day for bookkeeping tasks, if possible. Do not attempt to work on financial records when you are busy attending patients or when there are other distractions.

CARDINAL RULES OF BOOKKEEPING

- Enter all charges and receipts immediately in the daily record or journal.
- Write a receipt in duplicate for any currency received. Writing receipts for checks is optional, but a consistent pattern should be followed.
- Post all charges and receipts to the patient ledger daily.
- Endorse checks for deposit as soon as received.
- Deposit all receipts in the bank.
- Verify that the total of the deposit plus the amount on hand equals the total to be accounted for in the daily journal.
- Use a petty cash fund to pay for small unpredictable expenses. Pay all other expenses by check (a cancelled check is the best proof of payment).
- Pay all bills before their due dates, after checking them for accuracy. Place date of payment and number of check on paid bills.

Memory Jogger

1 *What four items of information must be available from the financial records of a business at all times?*

Terminology of Accounts

To understand and perform bookkeeping procedures, it is first necessary to learn some of the terminology of accounts.

A business **transaction** is the occurrence of an event or of a condition that must be recorded.

EXAMPLES OF BUSINESS TRANSACTIONS

- A service is performed for which a charge is made.
- A debtor makes a payment on account.
- A piece of equipment is purchased.
- The monthly rent is paid.

Each example is a transaction that must be recorded within the accounting system. You will very likely encounter various other business transactions as you become more familiar with the individual needs of your employer's practice.

The **daily journal** is called the book of original entry because this is where all transactions are first recorded (Fig. 17–1).

A patient's financial record is called an **account.** All of the patients' accounts together constitute the **accounts receivable ledger.**

Account cards vary in design, but all will have at least three columns for entering figures. In the manual system these are

- **Debit** (abbreviation: Dr) **column** on the left is used for entering charges and is sometimes called the charge column
- **Credit** (abbreviation: Cr) **column** to the right, sometimes headed Paid, is used for entering payments received
- **Balance column** on the far right is used for recording the difference between the debit and credit columns

An **adjustment column** is available in some systems and is used for entering professional discounts, write-offs, disallowances by insurance companies, and any other adjustments (Fig 17–2).

In a computer system, when you call up a patient by name or ID you will get the patient's balance. This is the individual patient's ledger.

Posting means the transfer of information from one record to another. Transactions are posted from the journal to the ledger (this is accomplished in one writing on the pegboard system).

The **account balance** is normally a debit balance (charges exceed payments). A **debit** balance is entered by simply writing the correct figure in the balance column.

A **credit balance** exists when payments exceed charges; for example, when a patient pays in advance. This is common in obstetric practices. To

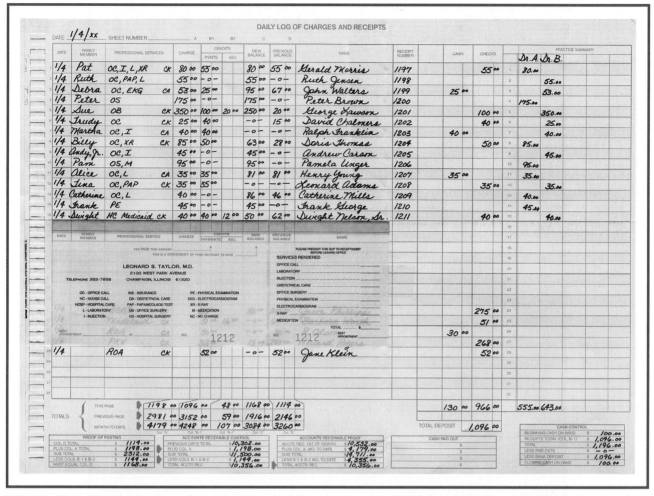

FIGURE 17–1 Sample day sheet for pegboard bookkeeping system, with deposit list of checks and optional business analysis summaries. (Courtesy of Colwell Systems, Inc., Champaign, IL.)

show a credit balance, record the figures in one of the following two ways:

- Write the credit balance on the card in regular ink and enclose the figure in parentheses or circle it.
- Write the credit balance in red ink (this cannot be done on the pegboard system).

Discounts are also credit entries and are entered in the adjustment column, or, if there is no adjustment column, the discount is entered in the debit column in red ink or enclosed in parentheses. By making the entry this way, it is recognized as a subtraction from the charges. When totaling columns, any figure in red or in parentheses is always *subtracted.*

Receipts are cash and checks taken in payment for professional services. **Receivables** are charges for which payment has not been received—amounts that are owing. **Disbursements** are cash amounts paid out. **Payables** are amounts owed to others but not yet paid.

Kinds of Financial Records

DAILY JOURNAL

The daily journal day sheet is the chronologic record of the practice—the financial diary. All information regarding services rendered, charges, and receipts is first recorded in the general journal. It is important that every transaction be recorded.

In addition to professional services rendered in and out of the office, there may be income from other sources, such as rentals, royalties, interest, and so forth. Usually a special place is provided in the journal for such income. Any income that is not practice related should be recorded separately from patient receipts.

LEDGER

The accounts receivable ledger comprises all the individual patients' financial accounts on which there is a balance.

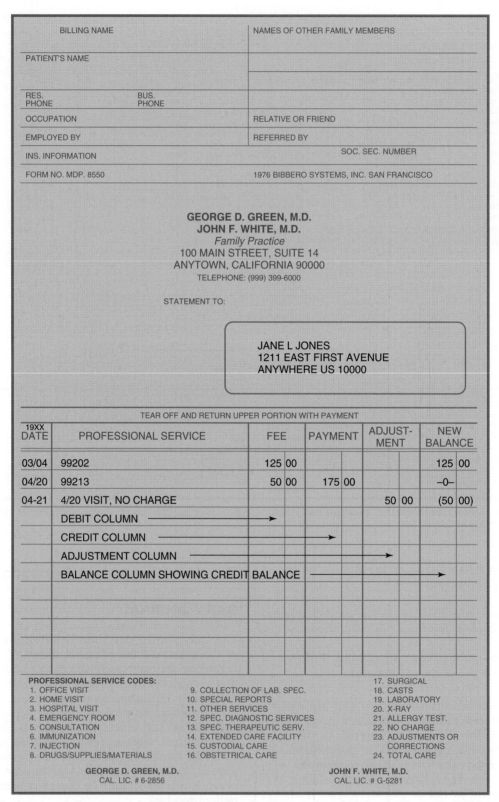

BILLING NAME		NAMES OF OTHER FAMILY MEMBERS	
PATIENT'S NAME			
RES. PHONE	BUS. PHONE		
OCCUPATION		RELATIVE OR FRIEND	
EMPLOYED BY		REFERRED BY	
INS. INFORMATION		SOC. SEC. NUMBER	
FORM NO. MDP. 8550		1976 BIBBERO SYSTEMS, INC. SAN FRANCISCO	

GEORGE D. GREEN, M.D.
JOHN F. WHITE, M.D.
Family Practice
100 MAIN STREET, SUITE 14
ANYTOWN, CALIFORNIA 90000
TELEPHONE: (999) 399-6000

STATEMENT TO:

JANE L JONES
1211 EAST FIRST AVENUE
ANYWHERE US 10000

TEAR OFF AND RETURN UPPER PORTION WITH PAYMENT

19XX DATE	PROFESSIONAL SERVICE	FEE		PAYMENT		ADJUST-MENT		NEW BALANCE	
03/04	99202	125	00					125	00
04/20	99213	50	00	175	00			–0–	
04-21	4/20 VISIT, NO CHARGE					50	00	(50	00)
	DEBIT COLUMN ⟶								
	CREDIT COLUMN ⟶								
	ADJUSTMENT COLUMN ⟶								
	BALANCE COLUMN SHOWING CREDIT BALANCE ⟶								

PROFESSIONAL SERVICE CODES:

1. OFFICE VISIT
2. HOME VISIT
3. HOSPITAL VISIT
4. EMERGENCY ROOM
5. CONSULTATION
6. IMMUNIZATION
7. INJECTION
8. DRUGS/SUPPLIES/MATERIALS

9. COLLECTION OF LAB. SPEC.
10. SPECIAL REPORTS
11. OTHER SERVICES
12. SPEC. DIAGNOSTIC SERVICES
13. SPEC. THERAPEUTIC SERV.
14. EXTENDED CARE FACILITY
15. CUSTODIAL CARE
16. OBSTETRICAL CARE

17. SURGICAL
18. CASTS
19. LABORATORY
20. X-RAY
21. ALLERGY TEST.
22. NO CHARGE
23. ADJUSTMENTS OR CORRECTIONS
24. TOTAL CARE

GEORGE D. GREEN, M.D.
CAL. LIC. # 6-2856

JOHN F. WHITE, M.D.
CAL. LIC. # G-5281

FIGURE 17–2   Account card/statement showing debit, credit, adjustment, and credit balance. (Courtesy of Bibbero Systems, Inc., Petaluma, California (800) 242-2376, Fax (800) 242-9330.)

Manual Posting

All charges and payments for professional services are posted to the ledger daily. The ledger then becomes a reliable source of information for answering all inquiries from patients about their accounts.

A separate account card or page is prepared for each patient (or each family) at the time of the first visit or service (Fig. 17–3). The heading of the account should include all information pertinent to collecting the account:

- Name and address of person responsible for payment
- Insurance identification

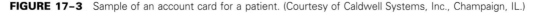

STATEMENT

LEONARD S. TAYLOR, M.D.
2100 WEST PARK AVENUE
CHAMPAIGN, ILLINOIS 61820

TELEPHONE 351-5400

DATE	FAMILY MEMBER	PROFESSIONAL SERVICE	CHARGE	PAYMENTS	ADJ.	BALANCE
		BALANCE FORWARD ▷				
5/13/00		Office consult 99203	60 –	60 –		0

Form 1625

PAY LAST AMOUNT IN THIS COLUMN

OC - OFFICE CALL	INS - INSURANCE	PE - PHYSICAL EXAMINATION
HC - HOUSE CALL	OB - OBSTETRICAL CARE	EKG - ELECTROCARDIOGRAM
HOSP - HOSPITAL CARE	PAP - PAPANICOLAOU TEST	XR - X-RAY
L - LABORATORY	OS - OFFICE SURGERY	M - MEDICATION
I - INJECTION	HS - HOSPITAL SURGERY	NC - NO CHARGE

FIGURE 17–3 Sample of an account card for a patient. (Courtesy of Caldwell Systems, Inc., Champaign, IL.)

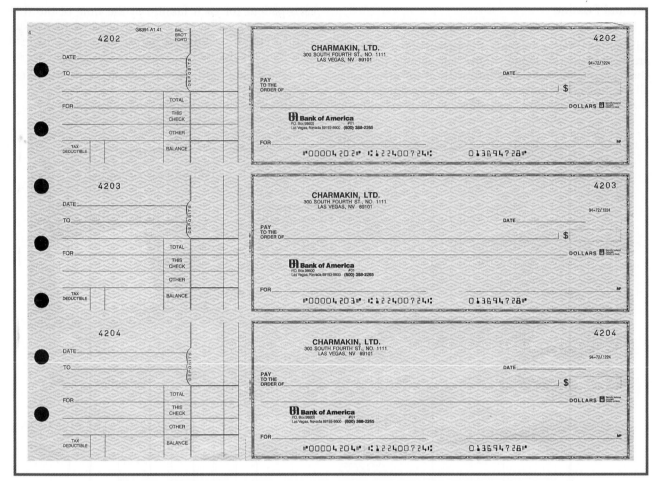

FIGURE 17–4 Page from a commercial checkbook with end stubs.

- Social Security number
- Home and business telephone numbers
- Name of employer
- Any special instructions for billing

Billing statements to the patient and the patient's insurance carrier are prepared from the ledger.

Computer Posting

The patient's name, date, diagnosis, and procedures are posted when the patient leaves the office. The database will retrieve the correct charges and post the charges on the computerized patient record and the accounts receivable ledger.

CHECKBOOK

All receipts are deposited in the checking account, and a record of the deposit is entered in the journal and on the check stub. A copy of each deposit slip should be kept with the financial records. All bills are paid by check, and a record of the payment is entered on the check stub and in the disbursements section of the general journal (Fig. 17–4).

DISBURSEMENTS JOURNAL

Manual Posting

In simplified accounting systems, the **disbursements journal** usually consists of a section at the bottom of each day sheet and a check register page at the end of each month, plus monthly and annual summaries. It must show

- Every amount paid out
- Date and check number
- Purpose of payment

Disbursements that are not practice related should be recorded separately.

Computer Posting

Use cash or check payments screen. Enter payment information and the computer can print the check, *or* enter information after the check has been manually prepared.

PETTY CASH RECORD

A **petty cash fund** and voucher system should be established to take care of minor unpredictable expenditures such as postage due, parking fees, small contributions, emergency supplies, and miscellaneous small items. In the average facility, $25 to $50 is sufficient for the petty cash fund. If a larger sum is available, there is a tendency to pay too many bills out of petty cash instead of writing a check.

When the check for this fund is exchanged at the bank for small bills and coins, the money is placed in a cashbox or drawer that can be locked or kept in the safe at night. One person only should be in charge of the petty cash fund. This person must be able to account for the full amount of the fund at any time.

PAYROLL RECORD

The payroll record is an auxiliary disbursement record. A separate page or card for each employee, as well as a summary record, should be kept. This procedure is discussed in more detail in Chapter 24 as a management responsibility.

Memory Jogger

2 *Briefly explain the difference between a* debit *balance and a* credit *balance.*

Comparison of Common Bookkeeping Systems

Success in bookkeeping requires a thorough understanding of the system and what it is expected to accomplish. There are many variations in bookkeeping systems, from simple to complex, no one of which can meet the needs of every physician. The basic principles are the same for all; only the system of recording varies.

The three most common systems found in the professional office are

- Single-entry
- Double-entry
- Pegboard or write-it-once

An overview of the three systems is presented here (Table 17–2), followed later in the chapter by more detailed instruction for the pegboard system,

TABLE 17–2 Accounting Systems

	Advantages	Disadvantages
Single-entry	Inexpensive Requires little training Simple to use	Provides only simple summaries Errors difficult to locate No built-in controls
Double-entry	Provides comprehensive financial picture Built-in accuracy controls	Requires special training, more time, and greater skill
Pegboard	Generates all records with one writing Daily control on accounts receivable Daily record of bank deposits and cash on hand	Cost of supplies greater than single-entry system Some training required (usually included in medical assistant programs)

which is currently the most widely used manual system in medical practices.

SINGLE-ENTRY SYSTEM

Single-entry bookkeeping is inexpensive, is simple to use, and requires very little training. It is the oldest and simplest of bookkeeping systems and includes at least three basic records:

- A **general journal,** which may also be called a daily log, daybook, daysheet, daily journal, or charge journal
- A **cash payment journal,** which in its simplest form is a checkbook
- An accounts receivable ledger, which is a record of the amounts owed by all the patients. The accounts receivable ledger may be a bound book, a loose-leaf binder, a card file, or loose pages in a ledger tray.
- There may also be auxiliary records for petty cash and payroll records.

The records of charges and receipts are usually entered into a bound journal with a page for each day of the year, monthly summary pages, and an annual summary. Daily pages have columns for entering each transaction that show the patient's name, the service performed and the charge, any payments received, and the totals for charges and receipts. The daily totals are entered on the monthly summary, and the monthly totals are carried forward to the annual summary (Figure 17–5).

The same bound book may also have space for recording cash payments, or the checkbook may be the only cash payment journal. Monthly and annual summaries would be done from the checkbook.

The accounts receivable ledger usually consists of an account card for each patient on which are entered the charges and payments from the general

FIGURE 17–5   Page from a daily log used in single-entry bookkeeping. (Courtesy of Bibbero Systems, Inc., Petaluma, California (800) 242-2376, Fax (800) 242-9330.)

journal. The patients' statements are prepared from these cards (Fig. 17–6).

In a single-entry system, each entry is made separately.

SKILLS AND RESPONSIBILITIES

RECORDING AN ENTRY

1 Record the entry on the daily journal or log.
2 Write a patient receipt if payment was made.
3 Post the transaction to the ledger.
4 Generate a monthly statement from the ledger.

Although the single-entry system may satisfy the requirements for reporting to government agencies, it does have some drawbacks:

• Errors are not easily detected.
• There are no built-in controls.
• Periodic analyses are inadequate for financial planning.

The single-entry system was at one time widely used in health care facilities but has been mostly replaced in favor of more complete accounting systems.

DOUBLE-ENTRY SYSTEM

Double-entry bookkeeping is also inexpensive but requires a trained and experienced bookkeeper or the regular services of an accountant. The transactions may be recorded manually or by computer. In addition to the basic journals used in a single-entry system, there may be numerous subsidiary journals. The system is based on the **accounting equation:**

Assets = Liabilities + Proprietorship (Capital)

Every transaction requires an entry on each side of the accounting equation, and the two sides must always be in balance. For this reason the system is called *double-entry.* It is the most complete of the three systems. An understanding of the basics of double-entry bookkeeping will help to clarify the principles of all systems.

	BILLING NAME		NAMES OF OTHER FAMILY MEMBERS	

PATIENT'S NAME

RES. PHONE	BUS. PHONE	

OCCUPATION | RELATIVE OR FRIEND

EMPLOYED BY | REFERRED BY

INS. INFORMATION | SOC. SEC. NUMBER

THE BIBBERO SYSTEM FORM NO. MDP. 8510   ©1965 BIBBERO SYSTEMS, INC. - SAN FRANCISCO

GEORGE D. GREEN, M.D.
JOHN F. WHITE, M.D.
Family Practice
100 MAIN STREET, SUITE 14
ANYTOWN, CALIFORNIA 90000
TELEPHONE: (999) 399-6000

STATEMENT TO:

— — — — — — — — — TEAR OFF AND RETURN UPPER PORTION WITH PAYMENT — — — — — — — — —

DATE	PAYMENTS			PROFESSIONAL SERVICE	FEE	LAST AMOUNT IN THIS COLUMN IS BALANCE DUE
	BANK NUMBER	BY CHECK OR P.M.O.	BY COIN OR CURRENCY			

PROFESSIONAL SERVICE CODES:

1. OFFICE VISIT	9. COLLECTION OF LAB. SPEC.	17. SURGICAL
2. HOME VISIT	10. SPECIAL REPORTS	18. CASTS
3. HOSPITAL VISIT	11. OTHER SERVICES	19. LABORATORY
4. EMERGENCY ROOM	12. SPEC. DIAGNOSTIC SERVICES	20. X-RAY
5. CONSULTATION	13. SPEC. THERAPEUTIC SERV.	21. ALLERGY TEST.
6. IMMUNIZATION	14. EXTENDED CARE FACILITY	22. NO CHARGE
7. INJECTION	15. CUSTODIAL CARE	23. ADJUSTMENTS OR CORRECTIONS
8. DRUGS/SUPPLIES/MATERIALS	16. OBSTETRICAL CARE	24. TOTAL CARE

GEORGE D. GREEN, M.D.
CAL. LIC. # 6-2856

JOHN F. WHITE, M.D.
CAL. LIC. # G-5281

FIGURE 17–6 Combination account card/statement from accounts receivable ledger. (Courtesy of Bibbero Systems, Inc., Petaluma, California (800) 242-2376, Fax (800) 242-9330.)

Assets are the properties owned by a business, such as bank accounts, accounts receivable, buildings, equipment, and furniture. The rights to these assets are called *equities*. The equity of the owner is called *capital, proprietorship,* or *owner's equity.* The equities of the creditors (those to whom money is owed) are called *liabilities.* The owner's equity (capital) is what remains of the value of the assets after the creditor's equities (liabilities) have been subtracted.

For example, if the physician purchased equipment for $1000, paid $250 down, and gave a promissory note for $750, the accounting equation would be:

$$\text{Assets} \quad \$1000 = \text{Liabilities} \quad \$\ 750$$
$$+$$
$$\text{Capital} \qquad 250$$
$$\overline{\$1000} \qquad \overline{\$1000}$$

The total value of the asset is $1000. The owner's equity is $250, and the creditor's equity is $750. The accounting terms *capital, proprietorship, owner's equity,* and *net worth* are used interchangeably.

Few medical assistants are trained in accounting. If a double-entry system is used, it is usually set up by a practice management consultant or the accountant who does most of the actual bookwork and reports. The medical assistant in this instance generally maintains only the daily journal, from which the accountant takes the figures once a month.

The double-entry system provides a more comprehensive picture of the practice and its effect on the physician's net worth. Errors show up readily, and there are many built-in accuracy controls; but because of the time and skill required, it is not frequently used in the small practice.

PEGBOARD OR WRITE-IT-ONCE SYSTEM

The initial cost of materials for the pegboard system is slightly more than that for a single- or double-entry system but is still moderate. The system is simple to operate, and training is included in most medical assisting programs.

The system gets its name from the lightweight aluminum or masonite board with a row of pegs along the side or top that hold the forms in place. The accounting forms are perforated for alignment on the pegs. All of the forms used in any system must be compatible so that they may be aligned perfectly on the board.

The pegboard system generates all the necessary financial records for each transaction with one writing:

- Charge slip and receipt
- Ledger card
- Journal entry

It may also include a statement and bank deposit slip.

The system provides current accounts receivable totals and a daily record of bank deposits and cash on hand, in addition to the record of income and expenses. The need for separate posting to patient accounts is eliminated, and the chance for error is decreased.

Memory Jogger

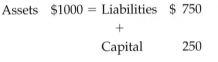 *Compare the advantages and disadvantages of the three bookkeeping systems. Why would pegboard be the most popular of the three?*

Using the Pegboard System

The pegboard system provides positive control over cash, collections, and receivables and ensures that every cent is accounted for and properly entered (see Procedure 17–1). It provides a record of every patient, every charge, and every payment, plus a daily recap of earnings—a running record of receivables and an audited summary of cash. The system requires a minimum of time. One writing allows one to

- Enter a transaction on the daysheet.
- Give the patient a receipt for payment.
- Bring the patient's account up to date.
- Provide a current statement of account for the patient.
- Give the patient a notation of the next appointment.

All of these features communicate the money message to patients effectively and courteously and generate good financial records.

MATERIALS REQUIRED

The pegboard may be of inexpensive masonite construction with pegs down the left side, or it may be a more sophisticated aluminum sliding board that allows flexible positioning of materials. The basic forms are

- Day sheet
- Patient ledger
- Patient charge slip/receipt or superbill

All of the forms must be compatible and are available from medical office supply companies. They are customized to the practice, incorporating the usual services and procedure codes of the practice.

PREPARING THE BOARD

At the beginning of each day, place a new daysheet on the accounting board. Some systems have a sheet of clean carbon attached to the daysheet; others use

> Ruling and column headings to match your current system.
> Please enclose sample of daysheet for an exact match.

LEONARD S. TAYLOR, M.D.
Internal Medicine
2100 WEST PARK AVENUE
CHAMPAIGN, IL 61820
Telephone: (217) 352-5400
Fax: (217) 351-5413

Tax I.D. # 123456
S.S. No. 000-00-0000
UPIN #E00000

IL LIC. #00-00000
MC #TA 000000
BCBS 123-45678-00

OFFICE VISIT - NEW PATIENT	CPT-4
Focused	☐ 99201
Expanded	☐ 99202
Detailed	☐ 99203
Comprehensive	☐ 99204
Complex	☐ 99205

OFFICE VISIT - ESTABLISHED PATIENT	
Minimal	☐ 99211
Focused	☐ 99212
Expanded	☐ 99213
Detailed	☐ 99214
Comprehensive	☐ 99215
Comprehensive Service	☐ 90080

CONSULTATIONS - INITIAL	
Limited	☐ 90600
Intermediate	☐ 90610

IMMUNIZATION INJECTIONS	
Diphtheria and Tetanus Toxoids	☐ 90718
Influenza Virus Vaccine	☐ 90724
Pneumococcal Vaccine. Polyvalent	☐ 90732
Therapeutic Injection	☐ 90782
Specify Material: _____	
Therapeutic IV	☐ 90784
Specify Material: _____	
Inj., B - 12	☐ J3420
Inj. Ampicillin, 500 mg	☐ J0290

GENERAL SERVICES	
Allergen Immunotherapy,	☐ 95115
Single Injection	☐
Removal Impacted Cerumen	☐ 69210

GENERAL SERVICES (Cont.)	CPT-4
Sigmoidoscopy, Flexible Fiberoptic	☐ 45330
Cardiovascular Stress Test	☐ 93015
Spirometry	☐ 94010
Spirometry with BD	☐ 94060
ECG, with Interpre. and Report	☐ 93000
Handing and / or	☐ 99000
Conveyance Specimen	
Tuberculosis, Intradermal	☐ 86580
LABORATORY	
Routine Venipuncture	☐ 36415*
Florescent Antibody, Screen	☐ 86255
Hemogram (CBC) Manual Differential	☐ 85022
General Health Screen Panel	☐ 80050
Digoxin, RIA	☐ 82643
Glucose, Blood	☐ 82948
Blood; Occult, Feces, Screening	☐ 82270
Hematocrit	☐ 85014
Heterophile Antibodies(Monotype)	☐ 86300
Platelet Count	☐ 85580
Potassium: Blood	☐ 84132
Prothrombin Time	☐ 85610
Quinidine, Blood	☐ 84230
Syphilis Test, Qualitative	☐ 86592
Culture or Direct Bacterial	☐ 87072
Commercial Kit	
Urinalysis, by Reagent Strips	☐ 81002
_____	☐ ___
_____	☐ ___
_____	☐ ___

PATIENT NAME _____

DIAGNOSTIC CODES: ICD-9-CM

☐ 789.0	Abdominal Pain	☐ 401.0	Hypertension, Malignant
☐ 795.0	Abnormal Pap Smear	☐ 402.90	Hypertension, W / O CHF
☐ 706.1	Acne Vulgaris	☐ 244.9	Hypothyroidism, Primary
☐ 477.0	Allergic Rhinitis,	☐ 380.4	Impacted Cerumen
☐ 285.9	Anemia, NOS	☐ 487.1	Influenza
☐ 281.0	Anemia, Pernicious	☐ 564.1	Irritable Bowel Syndrome
☐ 411.1	Angina, Unstable	☐ 464.0	Laryngitis, Acute
☐ 427.9	Arrhythmia, NOS	☐ 454.9	Leg Varicose Veins
☐ 440.9	Arteriosclerosis	☐ 424.0	Mitral Valve Prolapse
☐ 714.0	Arthritis, Rheumatoid	☐ 412	Myocardial Infarction, Old
☐ 414.0	ASHD	☐ 715.90	Osteoarthritis, Unspec. Site
☐ 493.90	Asthma, Bronchial W/O Status. Ast.	☐ 620.2	Ovarian Cyst
☐ 493.91	Asthma, Bronchial W/Status Ast.	☐ 614.9	Pelvic Inflammatory Disease
☐ 466.1	Bronchiolitis, Acute	☐ 685.1	Pilonidal Cyst
☐ 466.0	Bronchitis, Acute	☐ 462	Pharyngitis, Acute
☐ 727.3	Bursitis	☐ 486	Pneumonitis
☐ 786.50	Chest Pain	☐ 627.1	Postmenopausal Bleeding
☐ 574.20	Cholelithiasis	☐ 625.4	Premenstrual Tension
☐ 372.30	Conjunctivitis, Unspecified	☐ 782.1	Rash
☐ 564.0	Constipation	☐ 569.3	Rectal Bleeding
☐ 496	COPD	☐ 398.90	Rheumatic Heart Disease, NOS
☐ 692.9	Dermatitis, Allergic	☐ 461.9	Sinusitis, Acute, NOS
☐ 250.01	Diabetes Mellitus, ID	☐ 782.1	Skin Eruption, Rash
☐ 250.00	Diabetes Mellitus, NID	☐ 845.00	Sprain, Ankle
☐ 558.9	Diarrhea	☐ 848.9	Sprain, Muscle, Unspec. Site
☐ 562.11	Diverticulitis	☐ 785.6	Swollen Glands
☐ 562.10	Diverticulosis	☐ 246.9	Thyroid Disease, Unspecified
☐ 782.3	Edema	☐ 463	Tonsillitis, Acute
☐ 492.8	Emphysema	☐ 474.0	Tonsillitis, Chronic
☐ V18.0	Family History Of Diabetes	☐ 465.9	Upper Respir. Infection, Acute
☐ 780.6	Fever of Undetermined Origin	☐ 599.0	Urinary Tract Infection
☐ 578.9	G. I. Bleeding, Unspecified	☐ V03.9	Vaccination / Bacterial Dis.
☐ 727.41	Ganglion Of Joint	☐ V06.8	Vaccination / Combination
☐ 535.0	Gastritis, Acute	☐ V04.8	Vaccination, Influenza
☐ V72.3	Gynecological Exam	☐ 616.10	Vaginitis, Vulvitis, NOS
☐ 748.0	Headache	☐ 780.4	Vertigo
☐ 785.2	Heart Murmur, Innocent	☐ 787.0	Vomiting, Nausea
☐ 550.90	Hernia, Inguinal, NOS	☐	_____
☐ 054.9	Herpes Simplex	☐	_____
☐ 053.9	Herpes Zoster	☐	_____
☐ 708.9	Hives / Urticaria	☐	_____
☐ 401.1	Hypertension, Benign		

DATE OF SERVICE	CPT CODE	DIAGNOSIS CODE(S)	CHARGE

Place of Service:
( ) Office
( ) Emergency Room
( ) In-Patient Hospital
( ) Out-Patient Hospital
( ) Nursing Home

TOTAL CHARGE	$
AMOUNT PAID	$
PREVIOUS BALANCE	$
BALANCE DUE	$

Doctor's Signature

FORM 7201 COLWELL SYSTEMS, CHAMPAIGN, IL

FIGURE 17-7 Example of a superbill. (CPT only © American Medical Association. All Rights Reserved.)

special carbon with holes for the pegs; some use NCR (no carbon required) paper. The carbon goes on top of the daysheet. Over the carbon, place the charge slip/receipt or **superbill** (Fig. 17-7). The receipt has a carbonized writing line that should align with the first open writing line on the daysheet. If the slips are shingled, lay the entire bank of receipts over the pegs, with the top one aligned as mentioned. The remainder will be automatically in place. Receipts should be used in numerical order.

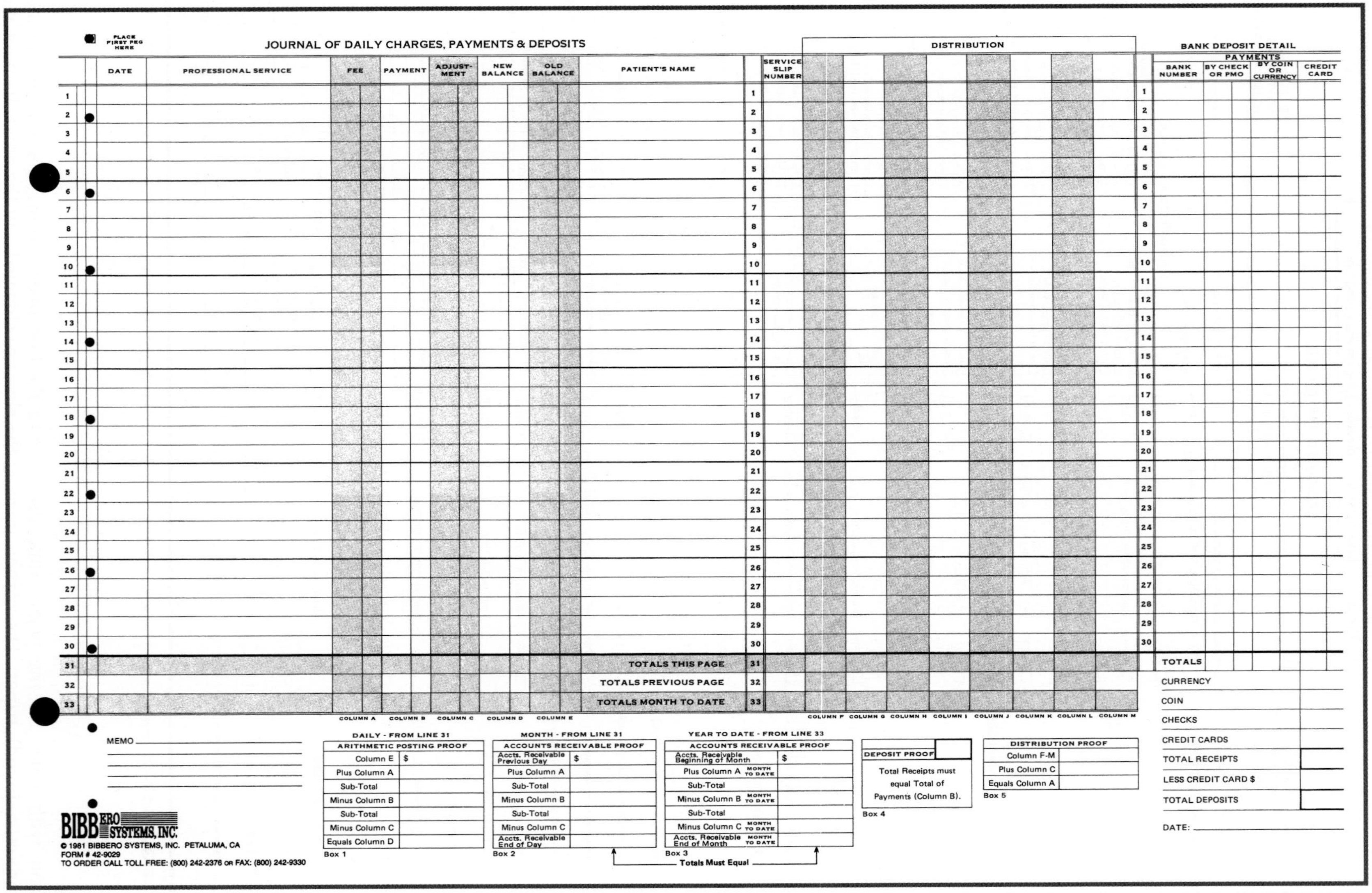

FIGURE 17–8 Sample daily log of charges and receipts. (Courtesy of Bibbero Systems, Inc., Petaluma, California (800) 242-2376, Fax (800) 242-9930.)

PULLING THE LEDGER CARDS

If a great many patients are to be seen in one day, pulling the ledger cards for all the scheduled patients at the beginning of the day will save time. Keep the cards in the order in which the patients are scheduled to be seen.

ENTERING AND POSTING TRANSACTIONS

As each patient arrives, insert the patient's ledger card under the first receipt, aligning the first available writing line of the card with the carbonized strip on the receipt. Enter the receipt number and date, the account balance in the space labeled previous balance, and the patient's name. The information recorded on the receipt is automatically posted to the ledger and the daysheet (Fig. 17–8).

The charge slip is then detached and clipped to the patient chart to be routed to the physician, who now has an opportunity to see how much the patient owes and can discuss the account in privacy, if desired.

After the service has been performed, the physician enters the service on the charge slip and asks the patient or the nurse to return it to the medical assistant. The assistant then has an opportunity to ask the patient whether this is to be a charge or cash transaction before completing the posting.

Again, insert the ledger card under the proper receipt, checking the number that was previously entered to make sure you have the correct card. Record the service by procedure code, post the charge from the fee schedule, enter any payment made, and write in the current balance. If there is no balance, place a zero or straight line in the balance column. If another appointment is required, enter the date and time at the bottom of the receipt.

The transaction has now been posted to the journal and the ledger, and, if payment was made by the patient, a receipt has been generated. The service receipt is given to the patient; no other receipt is necessary. The ledger card is ready for refiling.

File the charge slips in numerical order for your internal audit. At the end of the month, the total of the charge slips should equal the total of the charges recorded on the daysheets for the month.

RECORDING OTHER PAYMENTS AND CHARGES

Payments will be received in the mail and may be brought in by patients some time after a service was performed. These payments are entered on the daysheet and the ledger card in the same manner as previously explained. Payments by mail do not require a receipt.

The physician may have daily charges for visits to patients in a hospital or convalescent facility. Enter these charges on the daysheet and ledger card only. Surgery fees are usually recorded as one entry that includes the surgery and aftercare.

END-OF-DAY SUMMARIZING

At the end of the day, all columns must be totaled and proved. Although all bookkeeping is done in ink, it is a good idea to write the totals in pencil until they have been proved. If an error is discovered, you must correct the entry in which it occurred. Do not attempt to erase or write over the incorrect entry. Simply draw a line through it and make a new entry on the first open writing line. Remember that you must reinsert the ledger card for these corrections. Also, if the entry included a receipt for the patient, you must make a new receipt and notify the patient of the correction.

The pegboard system provides several ways for proving the arithmetic on the day sheet. Two examples are shown.

EXAMPLE OF POSTING PROOF FOR DAY

Old Balance $_____$
  Plus total charges $_____$
                   Subtotal $_____$
  Less payments received $_____$
                   Subtotal $_____$
  Less adjustments $_____$
New Balance *$_____$

*This figure is carried forward to next page for "old balance."

EXAMPLE OF CASH CONTROL PROOF

Cash on hand at beginning of day $_____$
  Cash received $_____$
                   Subtotal $_____$
  Less cash paid out $_____$
  Less bank deposit $_____$
Cash on hand at end of day *$_____$

*This figure is carried forward to next page for "cash on hand at beginning of day."

Special Bookkeeping Entries

The following special entries are necessary occasionally and may be used with pegboard or any other accounting system.

ADJUSTMENTS

At times, it is necessary to enter a credit adjustment. These could be for (1) professional discounts, (2) insurance disallowances, or (3) writeoffs. If the system has an adjustment column, enter them there. Otherwise, because the adjustment is actually a subtraction from the charge, enter it in the charge column with the figure enclosed in parentheses or circled and an explanation of the entry in the description column. When the column of figures is totaled, the circled figure is *subtracted* rather than added. The learner has a tendency to ignore the circled figures. This is incorrect—they must be subtracted.

CREDIT BALANCES

A credit balance occurs when

* A patient has paid in advance
* There has been an overpayment

For example, an overpayment occurs if the patient made a partial payment and later the insurance allowance was more than the remaining **balance.** The difference between the total amount of money received and the amount owed must be entered in the balance column and enclosed within parentheses or circled. This indicates a credit balance.

The credit balance is money owed to the patient. If the patient has paid in advance or wishes to leave the overpayment in the account in anticipation of future charges, care must be taken in figuring the balance on future transactions. Whereas normally a charge increases the balance, it will decrease a credit balance.

REFUNDS

If a patient wishes to have an overpayment refunded, write a check for the amount due and enter the transaction on the daysheet as shown.

SKILLS AND RESPONSIBILITIES

HOW TO GENERATE A REFUND
1 Place the ledger card on the daysheet.
2 Enter an explanation in the description column.
3 Show the existing credit balance within parentheses or circled.
4 Write the amount of the refund in the payment column within parentheses or circled to show that it is a subtraction.
5 Show a zero balance.

NONSUFFICIENT FUNDS (NSF) CHECKS

Sometimes a patient sends in a check without having sufficient funds to cover it; this check is later deposited to the physician's account. The bank will return the check to you marked NSF. You must now perform two accounting functions as shown.

SKILLS AND RESPONSIBILITIES

HOW TO RECORD NSF CHECKS
1 Deduct the amount from your checking account balance.
2 Add the amount back into the patient's account balance by
  * Entering the amount in the paid column in parentheses
  * Increasing the balance by the same amount
3 Write a brief explanation of the transaction in the description column (Fig. 17–9).

ONE-ENTRY CASH TRANSACTIONS

For the transient patient who has no ledger card and pays at the time of service, use a receipt as previously described. Enter the amount of the fee in the charge column and in the paid column and a zero balance. This records the transaction on the journal page and provides a receipt for the patient. There is no need for a ledger card.

COLLECTION AGENCY PAYMENTS

When a collection agency recovers an account for the physician, the agency deducts a commission, usually 40% to 50% of the amount recovered. For example, if the patient had a balance of $100 and pays it in full, the agency will send the physician $50. The patient now has a zero balance and the physician has only $50. This transaction is recorded on the ledger card and the daysheet in the following manner:

SKILLS AND RESPONSIBILITIES

RECORDING A COLLECTION AGENCY PAYMENT
1 $100 appears in the balance column.
2 Enter $50 in the cash received or paid column.

NAME BROWN, JOHN		S.S.# 000 00 0000					

ADDRESS 429 WEST MARKET STREET, LONG DESERT, NV 80056							

TELEPHONE 702-345-6789		INSURANCE METROPOLITAN					REF. BY BAFFLE

DATE	FAMILY MEMBER	PROFESSIONAL SERVICE	CHARGE		CREDITS PAYMENT	ADJ.	BALANCE
2000			BALANCE FORWARD ▷				
10-20	self	99245	200 00		50 –		150 00
11-15		99213	100 00				250 00
11-20		Personal check			100 00		150 00
11-28		Check retd NSF			(100)		250 00

Form 5128 Colwell Systems, Champaign, IL

FIGURE 17–9   Entry for returned NSF (nonsufficient funds) checks.

---

3 Enter $50 in the adjustment column.
4 Enter zero in the new balance column.
5 If there is no adjustment column, the $50 commission is entered in the charge column in parentheses ($50), so that the total charge is reduced by this amount and the transaction is reflected correctly in the accounts receivable control.

Accounts Receivable Control— Pegboard System

The **accounts receivable control** is a daily summary of what remains unpaid on the accounts.

This is an integral part of the pegboard and double-entry systems but is a separate operation in single-entry accounting. A simple form such as the one

---

ACCOUNTS RECEIVABLE CONTROL

Month of ____December____ , 19____   Accounts receivable at end of last day of preceding month: __$37,506__

Day	Value of Services Rendered	Received from Patients	Adjustments	+	−	Accounts Receivable Balance
1	785	1098			313	37,193
2	210	630			420	36,773
3	950	510	33	407		37,180
4						

FIGURE 17–10   Accounts receivable control for a single-entry bookkeeping system.

PROCEDURE 17 – 1

Posting Service Charges and Payments Using Pegboard

GOAL

To post one day's charges and payments and complete the daily bookkeeping cycle using a pegboard.

EQUIPMENT AND SUPPLIES

Pegboard	Carbon
Calculator	Receipts
Pen	Ledger cards
Daysheet	Balances from previous day

PROCEDURAL STEPS

1 Prepare the board:
   * Place a new daysheet on the board.
   * Cover daysheet with carbon.
   * Place bank of receipts over the pegs aligning the top receipt with the first open writing line on the daysheet.

2 Carry forward balances from the previous day.
   PURPOSE: To keep all totals current.

3 Pull ledger cards for patients to be seen today.

4 Insert the ledger card under the first receipt, aligning the first available writing line of the card with the carbonized strip on the receipt.
   PURPOSE: To ensure that one writing will correctly post the entry to receipt, ledger, and daysheet.

5 Enter the patient's name, the date, receipt number, and any existing balance from the ledger card.

6 Detach the charge slip from the receipt and clip it to the patient's chart.
   PURPOSE: The physician will indicate the service performed on the charge slip and return it to you.

7 Accept the returned charge slip at the end of the visit.

8 Enter the appropriate fee from the fee schedule.

9 Locate the receipt on the board with a number matching the charge slip.
   PURPOSE: To make certain it is the correct receipt.

10 Reinsert the patient's ledger card under the receipt.

11 Write the service code number and fee on the receipt.

12 Accept the patient's payment and record the amount of payment and new balance.
   PURPOSE: Brings patient's account up to date and provides current statement for patient.

13 Give the completed receipt to the patient.

14 Follow your agency's procedure for refiling the ledger card.

15 Repeat steps 4 to 14 for each service for the day.

16 Total all columns of the daysheet at the end of the day.
   PURPOSE: To determine total amount of charges, receipts, and resulting balances for the day.

17 Write preliminary totals in pencil.
   PURPOSE: To facilitate any necessary changes.

18 Complete proof of totals and enter totals in ink.

19 Enter figures for accounts receivable control.
   PURPOSE: To complete daily accounting cycle.

illustrated in Figure 17–10 is useful. Using a separate page or card for each month, proceed as listed below:

SKILLS AND RESPONSIBILITIES

PERFORMING AN ACCOUNTS RECEIVABLE CONTROL

1 Total the unpaid balances from the entire ledger on the last day of the preceding month and enter this figure at the top of the card or page.
2 Total the charges and receipts at the end of each day and enter these figures in columns 1 and 2.
3 Determine the **accounts receivable** figure as follows:

• If charges for the day are greater than the receipts, there is an increase in the accounts receivable. Enter this figure in column 4 and add it to the balance in column 6.
• If receipts for the day are greater than the charges, there is a decrease in the accounts receivable. Enter this figure in column 5 and subtract it from the balance in column 6.

Note that the accounts receivable figure changes at the end of any day on which there is financial activity. The balance consists of the accounts receivable figure from the previous day, plus the charges for the day, minus the day's receipts and adjustments.

The total of the entire file of ledger card balances at the end of any given day should equal the accounts receivable balance shown for that day on the control form.

EXAMPLE OF ACCOUNTS RECEIVABLE CONTROL

Total outstanding A/R balance
(from previous day) $_____
  Plus today's charges _____
    Subtotal $_____
  Less today's payments _____
    Subtotal $_____
  Less today's adjustments _____
Balance outstanding *$_____

*This figure is carried forward to next page for "total outstanding A/R balance."

Trial Balance of Accounts Receivable

A trial balance should be done once per month *after* all posting has been completed and *before* preparing the monthly statements.

The purpose of a trial balance is to disclose any discrepancies between the journal and the ledger. It does not prove the accuracy of the accounts.

For example, if a charge or payment were posted to the wrong account, or if the wrong amount were entered in the journal and then posted to the ledger, the totals would still "balance," but the accounts would not be accurate.

To begin, pull all the account cards that have a balance, enter each balance on the adding machine, and total the figures. This should equal the accounts receivable balance figure on your control.

If you have not kept a daily control, you must total all of the charges, all of the payments, and all of the adjustments for the month, and then do the computation illustrated below.

The end-of-month accounts receivable figure must agree with the figure arrived at by adding all the account card balances. The accounts are then said to be **in balance.** If the two totals do not agree, you must locate the error.

EXAMPLE OF BALANCING END-OF-MONTH ACCOUNTS RECEIVABLE

Accounts receivable at first of month $_____
  Plus total charges for month _____
    Subtotal $_____
  Less total payments for month _____
    Subtotal $_____
  Less total adjustments for month _____
Accounts receivable at end of month $_____

LOCATING AND PREVENTING ERRORS

After you have checked your tape and verified that you have not made an error in calculation, the first step in locating an error in your trial balance is to find the difference between the two totals. Then search the daily journal pages and the account cards for an entry of the identical amount. Check each one you find, to verify that it was posted correctly. Of course, there may be more than one error that adds up to this amount.

If there is only one error, and the amount of the error is divisible by 9, you may have transposed a figure. For example, if the difference is $81 (a number divisible by 9), you may find that you wrote $209 instead of $290. If the amount of the error is divisible by 2, you may have posted to the wrong column, reversing a debit and a credit.

A common error is made by entering the wrong amount in the previous balance column or in figuring the new balance. This kind of error will show up on the pegboard daily proof but could easily go undetected in the single-entry system.

Another common error is made by carrying forward a wrong total from one day to the next (e.g., carrying forward the beginning accounts receivable total rather than the ending accounts receivable total).

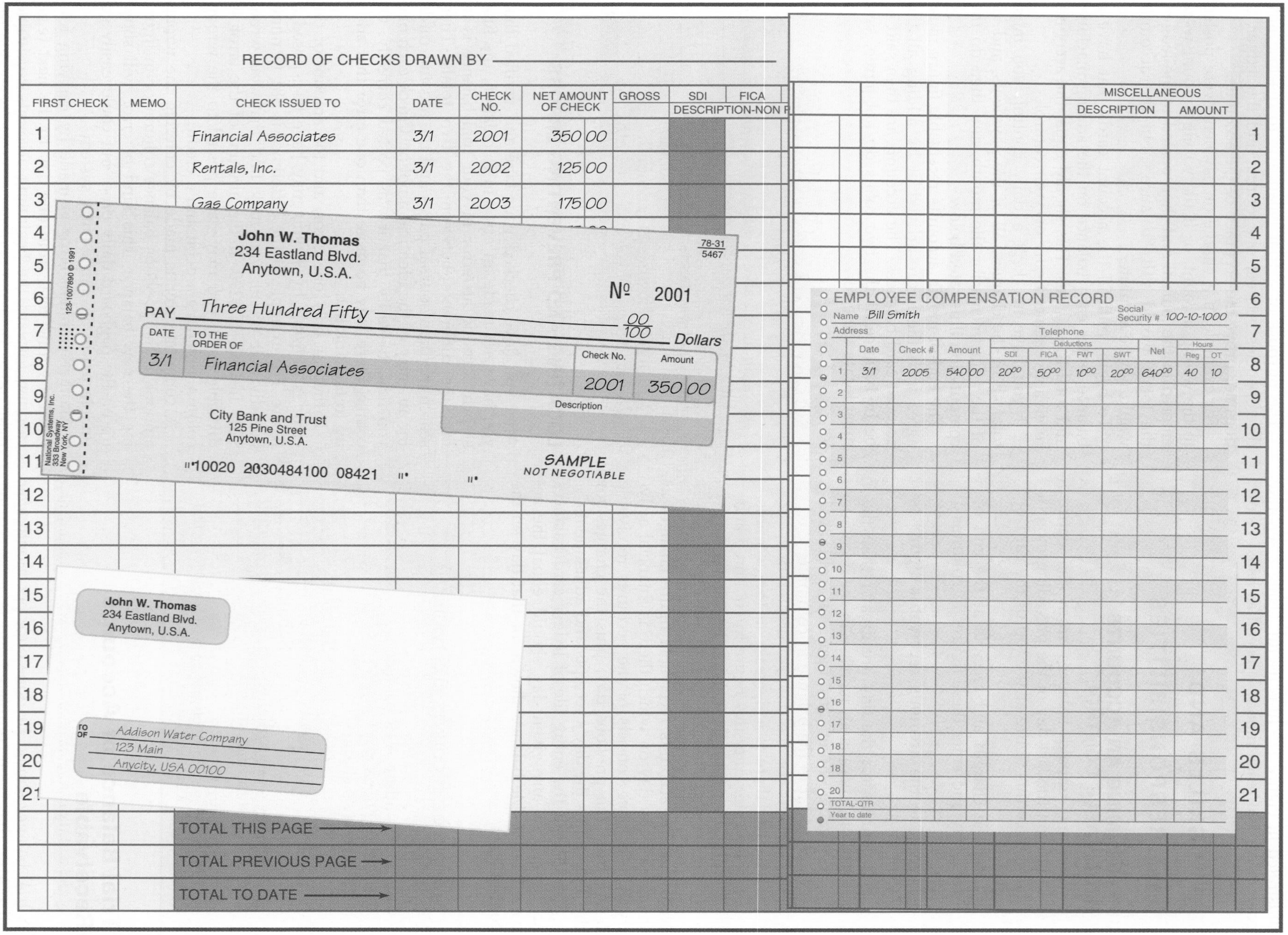

FIGURE 17–11 Payroll and cash disbursement journal showing payroll check that has been prepared for an employee and a window envelope for mailing a check.

There is always a chance of sliding a number, that is, writing the first digit in the wrong column, such as writing 400 for 40 or 60 instead of 600.

Many bookkeepers avoid errors in the cents column by using a line (—) instead of writing two zeros when only even dollars are involved. For example, instead of writing $12.00, the bookkeeper will write $12.—. This eliminates the possibility of misreading zeros as other numbers. It also speeds the adding process when columns must be totaled.

If you are unable to locate any numerical error, there is the possibility that an account card was lost or overlooked or was transferred as paid in full.

Memory Jogger

4 *What is the purpose of preparing a trial balance, and what does it reveal? Does it prove the accuracy of the accounts?*

Accounts Payable Procedures

INVOICES AND STATEMENTS

When time purchases are made, that is, the item is not paid for at the time of purchase, the vendor usually includes a **packing slip** with delivery of the merchandise. A packing slip describes the items enclosed. The vendor may also enclose an **invoice.** An invoice describes the items and shows the amount due. Always check to verify that the items listed on the packing slip and invoice are included in the delivery.

Invoices should be placed in a special folder until paid. You may be making more than one purchase from the same vendor during the month. Some vendors request that payment be made from the invoice; others expect to send a **statement** later. A statement is a request for payment.

PAYING FOR PURCHASES

At the time of payment, compare the statement with the invoice(s) to verify accuracy, fasten the statement and invoices together, write the date and check number on the statement, and place it in the paid file.

RECORDING DISBURSEMENTS

Both the pegboard and the single-entry bookkeeping systems provide pages for recording disbursements. This is sometimes called a *check register* (Fig. 17–11). On these pages, disbursements are distributed to specific expense accounts such as

- Auto expense
- Dues and meetings
- Equipment
- Insurance
- Medical supplies
- Office expenses
- Printing, postage, and stationery
- Rent and maintenance
- Salaries
- Taxes and licenses
- Travel and entertainment
- Utilities
- Miscellaneous
- Personal withdrawals

Each check should be entered on the disbursement page, showing the date, to whom the check was written, the number and amount of the check, and the payment allocated to one or more of the expense accounts. It is important to separate personal expenditures from business expenses. Business expenses are tax deductible and are considered in determining net income from the practice, but personal expenditures are not.

RECORDING PERSONAL EXPENDITURES

Some system must be established for transferring funds from the practice account to the physician's personal account. If the practice is incorporated, the physician is paid a salary. In the unincorporated practice, the transfer is usually accomplished through what is known in accounting terms as a *drawing account.*

The physician establishes a personal checking account and perhaps one or more savings accounts. Each month, or at any specified time, the medical assistant writes a check payable to the physician, which is then endorsed and deposited to the physician's personal account. In the disbursements journal, the amount of the check is posted in a special column headed *Personal* or *Drawing.*

Although personal expenses are not deductible in determining net income from the practice, some qualify as personal deductions in computing personal income tax, so a careful accounting should be kept. Deductible expenses would include property taxes, interest paid out, contributions, and so forth.

ACCOUNTING FOR PETTY CASH

The petty cash fund is a revolving fund. It does not change in amount except to increase or decrease the established fund. To establish the petty cash fund, a check is written payable to Cash or Petty Cash and entered in the disbursements journal under Miscellaneous (see Procedure 17–2). This is the *only* time the petty cash check is charged to Miscellaneous.

No.	Date	Description	Amount	Office Exp.	Automobile	Misc.	Balance
	04-01	Fund established					50.00
1	04-02	Postage due	.55	.55			49.45
2	04-08	Parking fee	6.00		6.00		43.45
3	04-10	Delivery charge	2.32			2.32	41.13
4	04-25	Stationery supplies	3.38	3.38			37.75
		TOTAL	12.25	3.93	6.00	2.32	
	05-01	Balance 37.75					
	Ch #	374 12.25					50.00

FIGURE 17–12 Petty cash record.

Each time the fund is replenished, the amount of the check is spread among the various accounts for which the money was used. This is determined from a record of expenditures such as that shown in Figure 17–12. The headings of the columns should correspond to headings in the disbursements journal to which they will be posted.

A pad of petty cash vouchers is kept in or near the cash box. For every disbursement from the fund, the petty cashier should either have a receipt or prepare a voucher similar to the one in Figure 17–13. The total of the petty cash vouchers and receipts plus the amount of cash in the box must always equal the original amount of the fund.

Receipt and voucher total	$12.25
Cash on hand	37.75
Amount of fund	$50.00

Figure 17–12 shows that $50 was received into the fund on April 1. This is entered in the Description column and in the Balance column. On April 2 postage due was paid out, a voucher prepared, the number of the voucher and the amount of 55 cents entered, and a new balance brought down. On April 8, the physician paid a parking fee. The amount of $6 was entered in the record, $6 taken from petty cash to reimburse the physician, and the new balance of $43.45 brought down.

Amount $ 20.00 No. 17

RECEIVED OF PETTY CASH

For Nurses' Benefit, Mercy Hospital

Charge to Miscellaneous

Approved by Received by

FIGURE 17–13 Petty cash voucher.

At the end of the month, or sooner if the fund is depleted, a check is written to Cash for replenishing the fund, but instead of being charged to Miscellaneous as previously, the amount of the check is divided among the various accounts affected. Our record shows that at the end of April, we have $37.75 remaining in the fund and need $12.25 to bring it back to $50.

When the check is written for $12.25, it is accounted for in the monthly distribution of expenditures by posting $3.93 as office expense, $6 as car expense, and $2.32 as a miscellaneous expense. In this way, the expenditures from petty cash are charged to the specific accounts affected.

The accounted-for vouchers are clipped together and placed with paid invoices, the check for $12.25 is cashed, and the money is placed in the petty cash fund. The amount of the check is entered as being received into the fund, and the new balance of $50 is brought down.

Avoid the habit of borrowing from the petty cash fund. This admonition applies to the physician as well as to the medical assistant. If the physician requests cash from the fund, request a personal check or an office check in exchange for cash from the fund.

It is also poor policy to use the petty cash fund for making change. In facilities where patients frequently pay with currency, a separate change fund should be kept.

Periodic Summaries

Financial summaries are compiled on monthly and annual bases. They may be prepared either by the medical assistant or by the accountant (or by computer). Common summary reports include

- Statement of Income and Expense
- Cash Flow Statement
- Trial Balance

PROCEDURE 17-2
Accounting for Petty Cash

GOAL
To establish a petty cash fund, maintain an accurate record of expenditures for 1 month, and replenish the fund as necessary.

EQUIPMENT AND SUPPLIES
Form for petty cash fund   Two checks
Pad of vouchers   List of petty cash expenditures
Disbursements journal

PROCEDURAL STEPS

1 Determine the amount needed in the petty cash fund.

2 Write a check in the determined amount.
PURPOSE: To establish a fund.

3 Record the beginning balance in the petty cash record.

4 Post the amount to miscellaneous on the disbursement record.
PURPOSE: To account for original amount of fund.

5 Prepare a petty cash voucher for each amount withdrawn from the fund.
PURPOSE: Voucher will be used for internal audit.

6 Record each voucher in the petty cash record and enter the new balance.
PURPOSE: To record current balance and determine the need for replenishing the fund.

7 Write a check to replenish the fund as necessary.
NOTE: The total of the vouchers plus the fund balance must equal the beginning amount.

8 Total the expense columns and post to the appropriate accounts in the disbursement record.
PURPOSE: To record expenditures in the correct expense category.

9 Record the amount added to the fund.

10 Record the new balance in the petty cash fund.

- Accounts Receivable Trial Balance and Aging Analysis
- Balance Sheet

The **statement of income and expense** is also known as the profit and loss statement and covers a specific period. It lists all the income received and all expenses paid during the period. The total income is called *gross income* or *earnings*. The income after deduction of all expenses is the *net income*.

A **cash flow statement** starts with the amount of cash on hand at the beginning of the month (or for any specified period). It then lists the cash income and the cash disbursements made throughout the period and concludes with a statement of the amount of cash remaining on hand at the end of the period.

A **trial balance** is necessary to determine that the books are in balance. All of the columns on the disbursements journal must be totaled at the end of the month. The combined totals of all the expense columns must be equal to the total of the checks written. If the figures do not balance, it is necessary to recheck every entry until an error is found.

The **accounts receivable trial balance** is done before sending out the monthly statements. First, record the total of the accounts receivable ledger at the end of the previous month; then add the charges for the current month and subtract the adjustments and the payments received. The remainder should equal the total of the accounts receivable ledger at the end of the current month.

The **balance sheet,** also known as a statement of financial condition, shows the financial picture of the practice on a specific date. Often, it is done only on an annual basis. The balance sheet is set up using the accounting equation: *Assets = Liabilities + Proprietorship.* The title of the statement had its origin in the equality of the elements—the balance between the sum of the assets and the sum of the liabilities and capital.

At the end of the accounting year, it is very simple to combine the monthly reports to compile the annual summaries. The annual summaries simplify the reporting of income for tax returns.

Bookkeeping with the Aid of the Computer

The office with an in-house computer and the appropriate software can accomplish all the described accounting operations and more in a fraction of the time required to do them manually. The role of the computer in the medical practice was discussed in Chapter 13. The office without a computer can still reap some of the benefits by using an outside computer service.

A computer service can relieve the office staff of the repetitive clerical procedures necessary in the recording of charges and in the preparation and mailing of statements and insurance forms. It can produce weekly and monthly financial reports that would be too time-consuming and perhaps beyond the capabilities of the staff to do manually.

Memory Jogger

5 *Name the five periodic financial summaries.*

Payroll Records

The office accounting system must include records of payroll, federal and state tax deductions, Social Security tax information, and quarterly and annual reports. These topics are discussed in Chapter 24, Management Responsibilities.

 ## LEGAL AND ETHICAL ISSUES

The keeping of the financial records is a position of great trust and responsibility. The records must be accurate and completed on a daily basis. Daily jour-

nal pages should be kept indefinitely in support of tax returns.

CRITICAL THINKING

1 Discuss the statement "There is no such thing as almost correct financial records."

2 In what bookkeeping record is all financial information first recorded?

3 What symbol or mark is used to indicate that a figure must be subtracted rather than added?

4 What are the three most common bookkeeping systems used in a professional office?

HOW DID I DO? Answers to Memory Joggers

1 *a.* How much was earned in a given period
b. How much was collected
c. How much is owed
d. The distribution of expenses incurred

2 A debit balance represents money due to the provider.
A credit balance represents an advance or overpayment.

3 Answers will vary.

4 The purpose of preparing a trial balance is to determine that the journal and ledger are in balance. The trial balance will reveal any discrepancies.

5 *a.* Statement of income and expense.
b. Cash flow statement
c. Trial balance
d. Accounts receivable trial balance
e. Balance sheet

REFERENCES

Colwell Systems: One-Write Pegboard Bookkeeping System. Champaign, IL, Colwell Systems, 1997.
Fess PE, et al: Accounting Principles, 17th ed. Cincinnati, South-Western Publishing Company, 1989.

Banking Services and Procedures

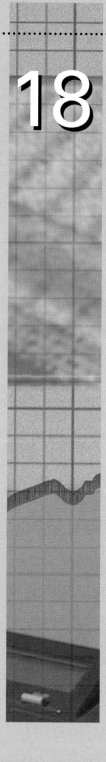

18

LEARNING OBJECTIVES

Cognitive: On successful completion of this chapter you should be able to:

1 Define and spell the terms listed in the Vocabulary.
2 State the four requirements of a negotiable instrument.
3 Discuss six advantages of using checks for the transfer of funds.
4 State why it is important to complete the check stub before writing a check.
5 Explain how you would handle mistakes made in preparing a check.
6 List and discuss eight precautions to observe in accepting checks.
7 State the purpose of a check endorsement.
8 Name and compare four kinds of endorsements.
9 Cite five reasons for depositing checks promptly.
10 Discuss the action necessary when a deposited check is returned.

Performance: On successful completion of this chapter you should be able to:

1 Prepare a bank deposit.
2 Correctly write a check.
3 Pay office bills by checks.
4 Reconcile a bank statement with the checkbook balance.

VOCABULARY

disbursements Funds paid out.

endorser Person who signs his or her name on the back of a check for the purpose of transferring title to another person.

maker (of a check) Any individual, corporation, or legal party who signs a check or any type of negotiable instrument.

negotiable Legally transferable to another party.

payee Person named on a draft or check as the recipient of the amount shown.

payer Person who writes a check in favor of the payee.

power of attorney A legal statement in which a person authorizes another person to act as his or her attorney or agent. The authority may be limited to the handling of certain procedures. The person authorized to act as the agent is known as an *attorney in fact.*

reconciliation (of bank statement) The process of proving that the bank statement and the checkbook balance are in agreement.

teller A bank employee who is assigned the duty of waiting on the bank's customers.

third-party check A check written to the order of the person offering payment and unknown to the payee, who is a third party in the process.

Financial transactions in the professional office nearly always involve banking services and the use of checks. Therefore, the medical assistant must understand the responsibilities involved in accepting payments, in endorsing and depositing checks, in writing checks, and in regularly reconciling bank statements.

- Checks provide a permanent reliable record of disbursements for tax purposes.
- The deposit record provides a summary of receipts.
- Checking accounts protect the money while on deposit.

Checks

A check is a draft or an order on a bank for the payment of a certain sum of money to a certain person therein named, or to the bearer, and is payable on demand. It is considered to be a negotiable instrument. A **negotiable** instrument must

- Be written and signed by **a maker**
- Contain a promise or order to pay a sum of money
- Be payable on demand or at a fixed future date
- Be payable to order or bearer

ADVANTAGES OF USING CHECKS

Using checks for the transfer of funds has many advantages:

- Checks are both safe and convenient, particularly for making payments by mail.
- Expenditures are quickly calculated.
- Specific payments can be easily located from the check record.
- A stop-payment order can protect the payer from loss due to stolen, lost, or incorrectly drawn checks.

TYPES OF CHECKS

You are probably already familiar with the standard personal check, but there are many additional types of checks in use in business transactions. You should be familiar with the following:

BANK DRAFT   A check is drawn by a bank against funds deposited to its account in another bank.

CASHIER'S CHECK   A bank's own check is drawn on itself and signed by the bank cashier or other authorized official. It is also known as an officer's or treasurer's check. A cashier's check is obtained by paying the bank cashier the amount of the check, in cash or by personal check. Some banks charge a fee for this service. Cashier's checks are often issued to accommodate the savings account customer who does not maintain a checking account.

CERTIFIED CHECK   This is the depositor's own check, on the face of which the bank has placed the word *certified* or accepted with the date and a bank official's signature. Because the bank deducts the amount of the check from the depositor's account at the time it certifies the check, the bank can guarantee that the amount is available. A certified check, like a cashier's check, can be used when an ordinary personal check might not be acceptable. If not used,

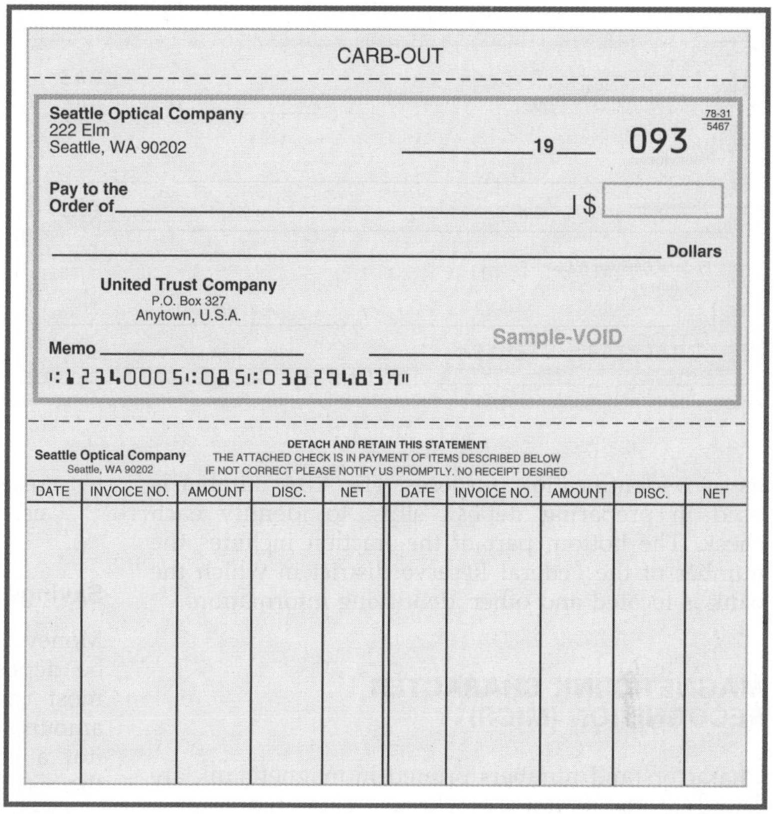
CARB-OUT

Seattle Optical Company
222 Elm
Seattle, WA 90202

78-31 / 5467

______19___ 093

Pay to the Order of ______ $

______ Dollars

United Trust Company
P.O. Box 327
Anytown, U.S.A.

Memo ______

Sample-VOID

⑆1234000 5⑆085⑆038 2948 39⑈

Seattle Optical Company
Seattle, WA 90202

DETACH AND RETAIN THIS STATEMENT
THE ATTACHED CHECK IS IN PAYMENT OF ITEMS DESCRIBED BELOW
IF NOT CORRECT PLEASE NOTIFY US PROMPTLY. NO RECEIPT DESIRED

DATE	INVOICE NO.	AMOUNT	DISC.	NET	DATE	INVOICE NO.	AMOUNT	DISC.	NET

FIGURE 18–1 Page from bank order book showing sample voucher check.

a certified check should be redeposited promptly, so that the funds previously set aside are credited back to the depositor's account.

LIMITED CHECK A check may be limited as to the amount written on it and as to the time during which it may be presented for payment. The limited check is often used for payroll or insurance checks.

MONEY ORDER Domestic money orders are sold by banks, some stores, and the United States Postal Service. The maximum face value varies according to the source. International money orders may be purchased for limited amounts, indicated in U.S. dollars, for use in sending money abroad.

TRAVELER'S CHECK Traveler's checks are designed for persons traveling where personal checks may not be accepted or for use in situations in which it is inadvisable to carry large amounts of cash. Traveler's checks are usually printed in denominations of $10, $20, $50, and $100, and sometimes $500 and $1000. They require two signatures of the purchaser, one at the time of purchase and the other at the time of use. They are available at banks and some travel agencies.

VOUCHER CHECK A voucher check is one with a detachable voucher form. The voucher portion is used to itemize or specify the purpose for which the check is drawn. It is used for the convenience of the **payer** and shows discounts and various other itemizations. This portion of the check is removed before presenting the check for payment and provides a record for the **payee** (Fig. 18–1).

Memory Jogger

1 *a.* Explain the difference between a cashier's check and a certified check.
b. What kind of check needs to be signed twice by the payer?

ABA NUMBER

The ABA number is part of a coding system originated by the American Bankers Association. It appears in the upper right area of a printed check. The number is used as a simple way to identify the area where the bank upon which the check is written is located and the particular bank within the area. The code number is expressed as a fraction, for example, $\frac{90\text{-}1822}{1222}$ (Fig. 18–2). In the top part of the fraction, before the hyphen, the numbers 1 to 49 designate cities in which Federal Reserve banks are located or other key cities; the numbers from 50 to 99 refer to states or territories. The part of the number following the hyphen is a number issued to each bank for

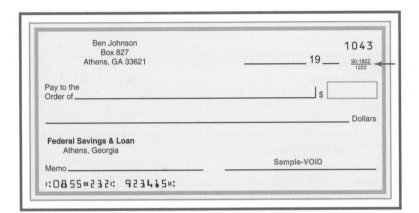

FIGURE 18–2 Sample check. Arrow indicates American Bankers Association number.

its own identification purposes. The ABA number is used in preparing deposit slips, to identify each check. The bottom part of the fraction includes the number of the Federal Reserve district in which the bank is located and other identifying information.

MAGNETIC INK CHARACTER RECOGNITION (MICR)

Characters and numbers printed in magnetic ink are found at the bottom of checks. They represent a common machine language, readable by machines as well as by humans. When a check is deposited, the amount of the check can also be printed in magnetic ink below the signature. MICR identification facilitates processing through a high-speed machine that reads the characters, sorts the checks, and does the bookkeeping.

Bank Accounts

COMMON TYPES OF ACCOUNTS

Checking Accounts

By placing an amount of money on deposit in a bank, a depositor can set up a checking account. Simply stated, a checking account is a bank account against which checks can be written. Many variations in checking accounts have been developed over the years. Instead of a straight non–interest-bearing account, one might have an insured money market checking account, which bears interest at the daily money market rate if a certain minimum balance is retained.

A physician often requires three different checking accounts:

1. An account for personal and family expenses
2. A separate checking account for office expenses
3. A high-yield interest-bearing account for funds reserved for paying insurance premiums, property taxes, and other seasonal expenses

Savings Accounts

Money that is not needed for current expenses can be deposited in a savings account (Fig. 18–3). In most cases, savings accounts earn interest on the amounts deposited; that is, the bank pays the depositor a certain percentage monthly or quarterly for the use of the money in the savings account. The ordinary savings account draws interest at the lowest prevailing rate and has no minimum balance requirement and no check-writing privileges.

Money Market Savings Account

An insured money market savings account requires a minimum balance, frequently $2500, draws interest at money market rates, and allows the writing of a specified number of checks (frequently three) per month. There may be a minimum amount for each transaction. Such checks are usually written for transfer of funds to a checking account.

Memory Jogger

2 *How does an insured money market savings account differ from an ordinary savings account?*

Systematizing Bill Paying

A systematic plan should be established for the writing of checks and the paying of bills. Check writing usually is done on a specific day or days of each month. An exception sometimes arises when it is possible to realize a good discount if payment of a bill is made within a specified time, for instance,

Statement of Account   14700 CT

014143759	R		1	12/20/99
Account Number	Type	Items	Page No.	Statement Date

001

Current Balance	Previous Statement Date	Previous Balance
2896.34	11/21/99	2886.59

ANSWERS TO YOUR BANKING QUESTIONS 24 HOURS A DAY,
7 DAYS A WEEK.   CALL ANSWERLINE TODAY

**** SUPER INSURED MONEY MARKET ACCOUNT ****

YOUR OPENING BALANCE OF: 2,886.59

                        NO   DEPOSITS LISTED TOTALING: .00

- OTHER CREDITS -

12-20 SUPER INSURED MONEY MKT. INT. PAID   9.75

            1   CREDITS LISTED TOTALING: 9.75

       NO   CHECKS LISTED TOTALING: .00

       NO   DEBITS LISTED TOTALING: .00

EQUALS YOUR ENDING BALANCE OF: 2,896.34

DAILY ACCOUNT BALANCES

DATE	BALANCE	DATE	BALANCE	DATE	BALANCE
12-20	2896.34				

- - - - - - - - - - - - - - - - - SUPER INSURED MONEY MARKET STATEMENT - - - - - - - - - - - - - - - - -

DATE	COLLECTED BALANCE	INTEREST RATES	DATE	COLLECTED BALANCE	INTEREST RATES
11-22	2,886.59	04.40	11-25	2,886.59	04.40
11-26	2,886.59	04.40	11-27	2,886.59	04.40
12-02	2,886.59	04.40	12-03	2,886.59	04.40
12-04	2,886.59	04.15	12-05	2,886.59	04.15
12-06	2,886.59	04.15	12-09	2,886.59	04.15
12-10	2,886.59	04.15	12-11	2,886.59	04.15
12-12	2,886.59	04.15	12-13	2,886.59	04.15
12-16	2,886.59	04.15	12-17	2,886.59	04.15
12-18	2,886.59	04.15	12-19	2,886.59	04.15
12-20	2,886.59	04.15			04.15

FIGURE 18–3 Example of a money market account statement. This type of check-writing has limited privileges.

PROCEDURE 18 – 1

Writing Checks in Payment of Bills

GOAL

To correctly write checks for payment of bills

EQUIPMENT AND SUPPLIES

Checkbook   Bills to be paid

PROCEDURAL STEPS

1 Locate the first bill to be paid. Before writing the check, fill out the stub or the place designated for recording expenditures. Include the date, name of payee, amount of check, the new balance to be carried forward, and usually the purpose of the check.
   PURPOSE: To prevent the possibility of delivering or mailing a check without entering the information in the checkbook.

2 Complete both the check and the stub with pen or typewriter.
   PURPOSE: To avoid danger of alteration for any reason.

3 Date the check the day it is written (do not postdate).

4 Write the name of the payee after the printed words, "Pay to the Order of _____" with the necessary information following. Do not use abbreviations unless so instructed.

5 Leave no space before the name, and follow it with three dashes if there is space remaining.

6 Omit personal titles from the names of payees.

7 If a payee is receiving a check as an officer of an organization, the name of the office should follow the name. Example: "John F. Jones, Treasurer."

8 Start writing at the extreme left of each space. Leave no blank spaces. Keep the cents notation close to the dollars figure to prevent alteration.

9 Verify that the amount of the check is recorded correctly on the stub, in the box for the dollar ($) amount, and on the line where the amount is written in words.

10 If a check is written for an amount less than one dollar, the figures by the $ sign may be circled or enclosed in parentheses ($0.65) to emphasize the amount.

---

10 days. Such discounts are usually indicated at the bottom of invoices or billing statements.

When a check is written in payment of a statement or invoice, it is good practice to write on the invoice the number of the check and the date it was paid. Then if any question arises about whether or when the bill was paid, you can readily locate the check stub. The handling and writing of checks must be done with extreme care (see Procedure 18–1).

THE BUSINESS CHECKBOOK

The checkbook most generally used in the professional office has three checks per page with a perforated stub at the left end of the check (Fig. 18–4). The checks may be in a bound soft cover or punched for a ring binder. The check and matching stubs are numbered in sequence and preprinted with the depositor's name and account number and any additional optional information such as address and telephone number. From 100 to 300 checks are usually ordered at one time, and the cost is charged against the account. Numbered deposit slips are also supplied to the depositor.

CHECKBOOK STUBS

The check stub (the part that remains in the book after the check has been written and removed) is the depositor's own record of the checks written, date, amount, payee, and purpose. It is important that the stub be completed before the check is written (Fig. 18–5). This prevents the possibility of writing a

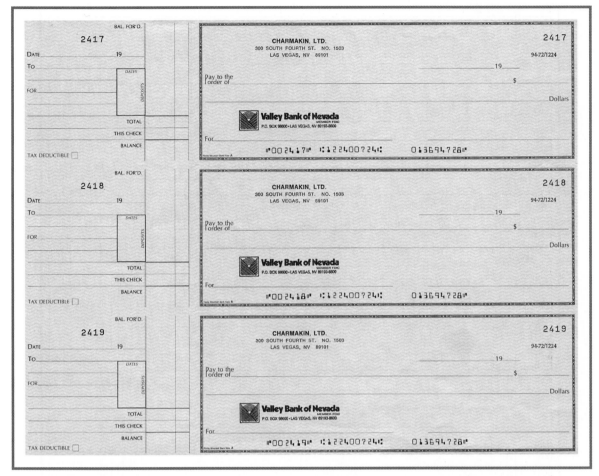

FIGURE 18–4 Example of business check with stub. (Courtesy of Valley Bank of Nevada, Las Vegas, NV.)

check and neglecting to complete the stub. If the stub is not completed and the check is sent out, you will have no record of the payee and the amount taken from the account until the canceled check is returned at a later date. Consequently, you will be unable to balance the account or determine the amount on hand until those canceled checks are returned by the bank. It is possible to get this information from the bank after the check has been cashed. There may be a charge for this service.

Check stub		Deposit record

FIGURE 18–5 Methods of filling out check stubs.

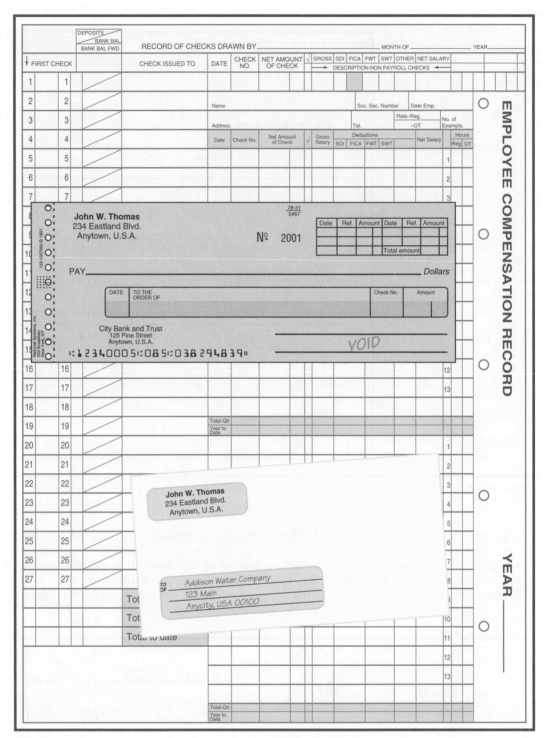

FIGURE 18–6 Pegboard system for check writing. (Courtesy of Bibbero Systems, Inc., Petaluma, California (800) 242-2376, Fax (800) 242-9330.)

COMPUTER-GENERATED CHECKS

Instead of ordering checks to be printed by the bank, personalized checks can be ordered from printing houses to fit your computer financial program (e.g., *Quicken*). Checks can be prepared on the computer in much the same manner as using a typewriter. The checks may have one or more copies that serve as the record of checks written.

ONE-WRITE CHECK WRITING

A one-write system of writing checks can save time and minimize errors in medical office **disbursements.** The office with a pegboard bookkeeping system (see Chapter 17) may wish to include one-write check writing. By using a combination check-writing system, such as the one illustrated in Figure 18–6, one check and one record of checks drawn handle both bill paying and payroll check writing.

When the check is written, a permanent record is created through the carbonized line of the check onto the record of checks drawn and the employee's payroll record, including a record of all deductions. Space is provided for the payee's address so that the check can be mailed in a window envelope. This not only saves time but also ensures that the check goes to the right address. Suppliers of basic pegboard systems can also provide a check-writing system such as the one described.

LOST AND STOLEN CHECKS

If any of the checks are lost, report this to the bank promptly. The bank will place a warning on the account, and signatures on incoming checks will be carefully inspected to detect possible forgeries.

If you suspect that checks have been stolen, first make a report to the police in the city or town where the theft took place. Then notify the bank and relate the time, date, and place the police report was made. A warning will be placed on the account. In some cases, you may be asked to close the account and open a new one under a different number.

As long as the loss of the checks missing or stolen has been reported to the proper authorities, the depositor usually will not be held responsible for losses due to forgery. The bank or merchant who accepts the forged checks will be charged for the loss. For this reason, anyone accepting a check from a person who is not known personally must be very careful about establishing the person's identity.

WRITING CHECKS

HANDLING CORRECTIONS AND MISTAKES Do not cross out, erase, or change any part of a check.

Checks are printed on sensitized paper so that erasures are easily noticeable, and the bank has the right to refuse to pay on any check that has been altered. Figures 18–7 and 18–8 show examples of correct and incorrect check writing.

If a mistake is made, write the word **VOID** on the stub and the check, but do not throw out or destroy the check. It should be filed with the canceled checks so that it is available for auditing purposes.

WRITING CASH CHECKS A cash check is a check made payable to cash or bearer. Such checks are completely negotiable. Because these checks are easily cashed without positive identification, it is poor policy to write cash checks unless they are to be cashed at the time they are written. Banks may require that the person receiving the cash endorse the check.

SIGNING CHECKS After all checks have been written, place them, along with the invoices or other verifying information, on the physician's desk for signature. In some practices, the medical assistant who has charge of the financial matters is also allowed to sign the checks. This is accomplished by filing a **power of attorney** at the depositor's bank. The power of attorney may limit the check-signing authorization to a certain amount or to a limited time period.

Memory Jogger

3 *Why is it important to complete the check stub before writing a check?*

MAILING CHECKS When checks are sent through the mail, the check should not be visible through the envelope. Either place the check within a letter or fold it into a plain sheet of paper. Checks may be folded at the right end to conceal the amount of money written. Make certain the envelopes are sealed before mailing, and mail all checks yourself as soon as possible after writing.

Special Problems with Checks

Special problems may arise when a check is written on nonexistent funds or when a payer wishes, for a legitimate reason, to prevent the payee from cashing a check.

ACCOUNT OVERDRAWN OR OVERDRAFT

When a depositor draws a check for more than the amount on deposit in the account, the account becomes overdrawn. In most states, it is illegal to issue

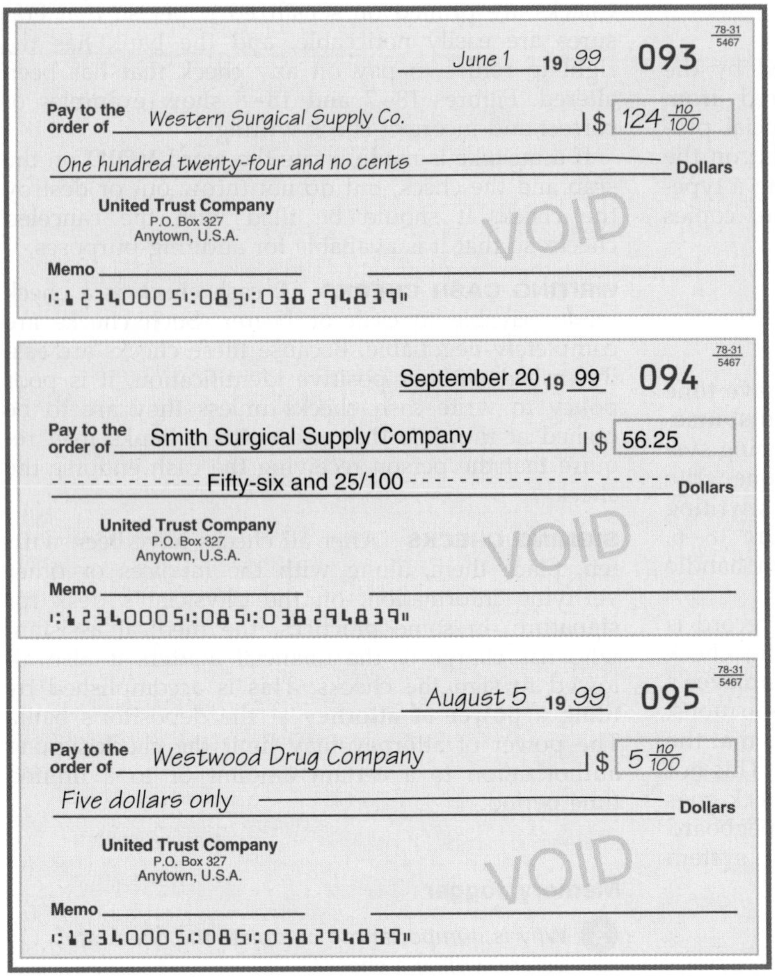

_____June 1_____ 19 _99_ **093**   78-31/5467

Pay to the order of _Western Surgical Supply Co._ | $ 124 $\frac{no}{100}$

One hundred twenty-four and no cents ——————— **Dollars**

United Trust Company
P.O. Box 327
Anytown, U.S.A.

Memo _____   _____

⑈123400051⑉085⑈038294839⑆

VOID

September 20 19 99 **094**   78-31/5467

Pay to the order of _Smith Surgical Supply Company_ | $ 56.25

- - - - - - - - - Fifty-six and 25/100 - - - - - - - - - - - - - **Dollars**

United Trust Company
P.O. Box 327
Anytown, U.S.A.

Memo _____

⑈123400051⑉085⑈038294839⑆

VOID

_____August 5_____ 19 _99_ **095**   78-31/5467

Pay to the order of _Westwood Drug Company_ | $ 5 $\frac{no}{100}$

Five dollars only ——————————— **Dollars**

United Trust Company
P.O. Box 327
Anytown, U.S.A.

Memo _____   _____

⑈123400051⑉085⑈038294839⑆

VOID

FIGURE 18–7 Correct methods of writing checks.

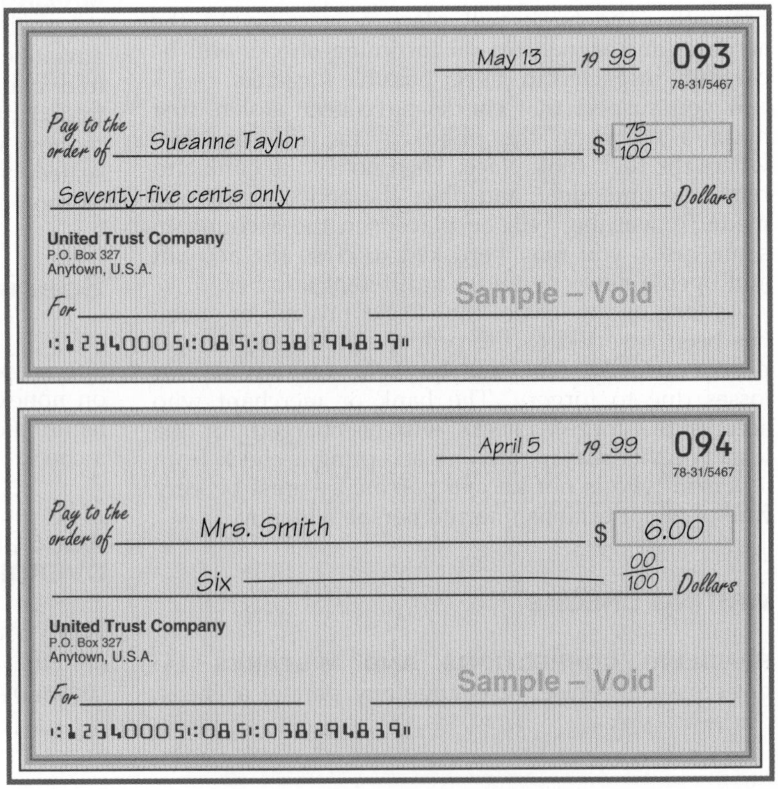

May 13 _19 99_ **093**   78-31/5467

Pay to the order of _Sueanne Taylor_ ——————— $ $\frac{75}{100}$

Seventy-five cents only ——————————— _Dollars_

United Trust Company
P.O. Box 327
Anytown, U.S.A.

For _____   _____

⑈123400051⑉085⑈038294839⑆

Sample – Void

April 5 _19 99_ **094**   78-31/5467

Pay to the order of _Mrs. Smith_ ——————— $ 6.00

Six ——————————— $\frac{00}{100}$ _Dollars_

United Trust Company
P.O. Box 327
Anytown, U.S.A.

For _____   _____

⑈123400051⑉085⑈038294839⑆

Sample – Void

FIGURE 18–8 *Top,* Correct method of writing a check. *Bottom,* Incorrect method of writing a check, with incomplete name and space for altering (e.g., 6.00 could be made into 26.00 or more and 00 could be made into 88).

a check for more than the amount on deposit in the bank. Should this happen through error or oversight, the bank may refuse to honor the check and will return it to the bank that presented it for payment. Such a check is said to "bounce."

If the check is written by an established depositor, the bank may honor the check and notify the depositor that the account is overdrawn. If the bank thus pays or covers the check, it issues an overdraft on the depositor's account.

STOP-PAYMENT ORDER

A depositor or maker of a check who wishes to rescind or stop payment of that check has the right to request the bank to stop payment on it. Stop-payment orders should be used only in emergencies. Reasons for stop-payment requests are

- Loss of a check
- Disagreement about a purchase
- Disagreement about a payment

Payment from Patients

ACKNOWLEDGING PAYMENT IN FULL

If payment in full is to be recognized in regard to a given check, the statement "Payment in Full to Date" must appear *on the back of the check*, above the endorsement, not on the face of the check. Canceled checks are a receipt for the maker of the check, not for the payee.

PRECAUTIONS IN ACCEPTING CHECKS

The medical assistant is frequently presented with checks in payment for the physician's services. In most cases, these are personal checks. See Guidelines for Accepting Checks

GUIDELINES FOR ACCEPTING CHECKS

- Scan the check carefully for the correct date, amount, and signature.
- Do not accept a check with corrections on it.
- If you do not know the person presenting a personal check, ask for identification and compare signatures.
- Accept an out-of-town check, government check, or payroll check only if you are well acquainted with the person presenting it and it does not exceed the amount of the payment.
- Acceptance of a **third-party check** is generally unwise. A third-party check is one made out to your patient by a party unknown to you. A check from the patient's health insurance carrier is an exception.
- When accepting a postal money order for payment, make certain it has only one endorsement. Postal money orders with more than two endorsements will not be honored.
- Do not accept a check marked "Payment in Full" unless it does pay the account in full up to and including the date on which it is received. If a check so marked is less than the amount due, you will be unable to collect the balance on the account once you have accepted and deposited such a check. It is illegal for you to scratch out the words "Payment in Full."
- Accepting checks written for more than the amount due and returning cash for the difference between the amount of the check and the amount owed is poor policy. If the check is not honored by the bank, your office will suffer the loss not only of the amount of the check but also of the amount returned in cash.

Endorsement of Checks

An endorsement is a signature plus any other writing on the back of a check by which the **endorser** transfers all rights in the check to another party. Endorsements are made in ink, with either pen or rubber stamp, on the back of the check across the left (or perforated) end.

NECESSITY FOR ENDORSEMENT

The Uniform Negotiable Instrument Act, applicable in all states, explains the need of an endorsement as follows:

An instrument is negotiated when it is transferred from one person to another in such a manner as to pass title to another party. If payable to bearer, it is negotiated by delivery. If payable to order, it is negotiated by the endorsement of the holder completed by delivery.

The name of the last endorser of the check shows who last received the money. If a check is cashed for someone who did not endorse it and is returned for some reason, the bank will charge the check to the last endorser, not to the last person receiving the money. For this reason, it is not wise to cash a check made payable to another party without having the endorsement of the person who delivered the check to you for cashing.

KINDS OF ENDORSEMENTS

There are four principal kinds of endorsements. Blank and restrictive endorsements are the ones most commonly used.

BLANK ENDORSEMENT The payee signs only his or her name. This makes the check payable to the bearer. It is the simplest and most common type of endorsement on personal checks but should be used only when the check is to be cashed or deposited immediately.

RESTRICTIVE ENDORSEMENT This specifies the purpose of the endorsement. You use a restrictive endorsement in preparing checks for deposit to the physician's checking account. An example is shown in Figure 18–9.

SPECIAL ENDORSEMENT This endorsement includes words specifying the person to whom the endorser makes the check payable. For instance, a check naming Helen Barker as payee may be endorsed to the physician by writing on the back of the check

Pay to the order of
Theodore F. Wilson, M.D.
Helen Barker

The check is still negotiable but requires Dr. Wilson's signature or endorsement.

QUALIFIED ENDORSEMENT The effect of the endorsement is qualified by disclaiming or destroying any future liability of the endorser. Usually the words "without recourse" are written above by an attorney who accepts a check on behalf of a client but who has no personal claim in the transaction.

ENDORSEMENT METHODS

The medical assistant may use a blank endorsement when cashing a check to replenish the petty cash fund. This endorsement should be made only at the time of exchanging the check for cash.

As checks from patients and other sources arrive, they should be recorded on the ledger and immediately stamped with the restrictive endorsement *For Deposit Only*. This is a safeguard against lost or stolen checks.

Any endorsement should agree exactly with the name on the face of the check. If the name of the payee is misspelled, it is usually necessary for the payee to endorse the check the way the name is spelled on the face, followed by the correctly spelled signature. The Uniform Commercial Code, Section 3-203, states

Where an instrument is made payable to a person under a misspelled name or one other than his

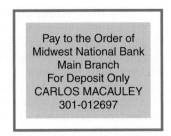

own, he may endorse in that name or his own or both; but signature in both names may be required by a person paying or giving value for the instrument.*

Most banks accept routine stamp endorsement that is restricted to deposit only, if the customer is well known and maintains an established account. Some insurance checks or drafts require a personal signature endorsement; a stamped endorsement is not acceptable. This will be stated on the back of the check. In such cases, ask the payee to endorse the check, then stamp immediately below the signature the restrictive endorsement *For Deposit Only*.

Memory Jogger

4 *Name and describe the endorsement that is usually used in preparing checks for deposits to the physician's checking account.*

Making Deposits

Financial duties of the medical assistant include depositing checks and reconciling the bank statements with the checkbook. Checks should be deposited promptly because

- There is the possibility of a stop-payment order.
- The check may be lost, misplaced, or stolen.
- Delay may cause the check to be returned because of insufficient funds.
- The check may have a restricted time for cashing.
- It is a courtesy to the payer.

PREPARING THE DEPOSIT

Deposit slips are itemized memoranda of cash or other funds that a depositor presents to the bank with the money to be credited to the account. All deposits must be accompanied by a deposit slip. A carbon or photocopy of the deposit slip should be kept on file. (See Procedure 18–2.)

There are several types of deposit slips, sometimes

PROCEDURE 18–2

Preparing a Bank Deposit

GOAL
To prepare a bank deposit for the day's receipts and complete appropriate office records related to the deposit.

EQUIPMENT AND SUPPLIES
Currency
Six checks for deposit
Deposit slip

Endorsement stamp (optional)
Typewriter
Envelope

PROCEDURAL STEPS

1 Organize currency.
   PURPOSE: To arrange currency in the best order for speedy and accurate presentation to the teller.

2 Total the currency and record the amount on the deposit slip.

3 Place restrictive endorsements on the checks, using an endorsement stamp or the typewriter.
   PURPOSE: To transfer the title and protect checks from loss or theft.

4 List each check separately on the deposit slip by ABA number and its amount.

5 Total the amount of currency and checks and enter on the deposit slip.

6 Enter the amount of the deposit in the checkbook.
   PURPOSE: To record the current balance in the account.

7 Prepare a copy of the deposit slip for the office record, including the names of the payers.
   PURPOSE: For verification of checks deposited, if necessary.

8 Place the currency, checks, and deposit slip in an envelope for transporting to the bank.

---

called *deposit tickets*. The commercial slip is used for the office checking account. The deposit slips are printed with the number of the account in magnetic ink characters to correspond with the checks. Preprinted deposit slips are ordered along with the checks.

Some write-it-once accounting systems include a deposit slip that the bank will accept as the itemization if it is attached to the customer's numbered deposit slip. The deposit slip should be prepared before you go to the bank, with the money organized and ready to present to the bank **teller.**

Payment on patient accounts is generally made by check, but some payments are made in currency (paper money). Each type of funds is recorded separately on the deposit slip. The currency is usually listed first. Organize the currency so that all of the bills are facing in the same direction—that is, the black side up with the portrait right-side-up. Place the largest bills on top.

Checks are recorded individually by the ABA number. If the checks are arranged alphabetically by the names of the patient accounts, with these names included on your office copy of the deposit slip, you will have a ready reference of checks deposited

should a question arise regarding a patient's payment. Follow the procedure listed below for preparing a deposit slip (Fig. 18–10):

1. List all checks on the back of the deposit slip.
2. Transfer the total to the front of the slip.
3. Enter the amount of the total deposit on the deposit slip stub.

Money orders, either postal, express, or others, are identified by PO Money Order or Express MO. Remember that money orders cannot have more than two endorsements.

The deposit slip should be carefully totaled and the total entered in the checkbook. Any torn bills should be mended with transparent tape. Clip the currency together, and clip the checks in a separate packet. Then place the entire amount in a heavy envelope for taking to the bank. Deposit the currency and checks daily if possible.

Memory Jogger

4 *How are checks identified when they are listed on a deposit slip?*

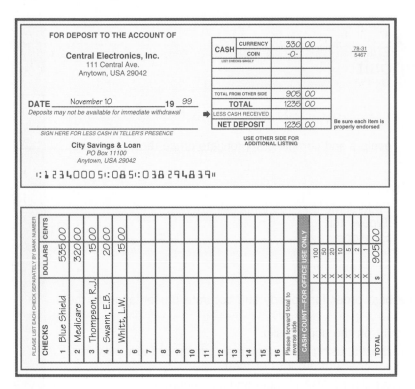

FIGURE 18–10 Front and back of deposit slip.

DEPOSITING BY MAIL

Depositing by mail saves time and is easily accomplished if the deposit consists of checks only. Banks usually supply their customers with special mailing deposit slips and envelopes on request (Fig. 18–11). Some mailing deposit slips have an attached portion that the bank will stamp and return to the customer as a receipt. Others may provide the customer with a receipt card that is sent along with the deposit each time for the bank's notation. The mailer shown in Figure 18–11 has a peel-off receipt for the depositor's records. Mailed deposits are prepared in the same manner as are regular deposits, but certain precautions should be observed.

DEPOSIT BY MAIL PRECAUTIONS

1 Do not send cash or currency by mail. If this is absolutely necessary, then send it by registered mail.
2 Use only a restrictive endorsement; use a deposit stamp or write the notation "For Deposit Only to the account of _____."
3 If you have not obtained mailing deposit slips or your bank does not provide them, make duplicate slips and mail them with your deposit. Ask the bank to stamp one copy and return it to you as a receipt.

RETURNED CHECKS

Occasionally, the bank may return a deposited check because of some irregularity such as a missing signature or missing endorsement. More often, it is because the payer has insufficient funds on deposit to cover the check.

If the check is stamped "NSF," indicating nonsufficient funds, do not delay in contacting the person who gave you the check. If you are unable to contact the maker of a bad check, waste no time in tracking down all leads, such as referrals, numbers you obtained from credit cards, driver's license, and so forth. There are several places to which bad checks may be reported. Credit associations are often a great help when such problems arise. Turn the account over to a qualified collection agency if you do not succeed in collecting on the account yourself within a short time.

If a check is returned to your office marked "No Account," and it is a check that you had deposited promptly, you have obviously been swindled. This check should be given to the police, the local Better Business Bureau, or your collection agency.

Bank Statement

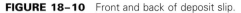

A statement is periodically sent by the bank to the customer; it shows the status of the customer's account on a given date. This statement indicates the

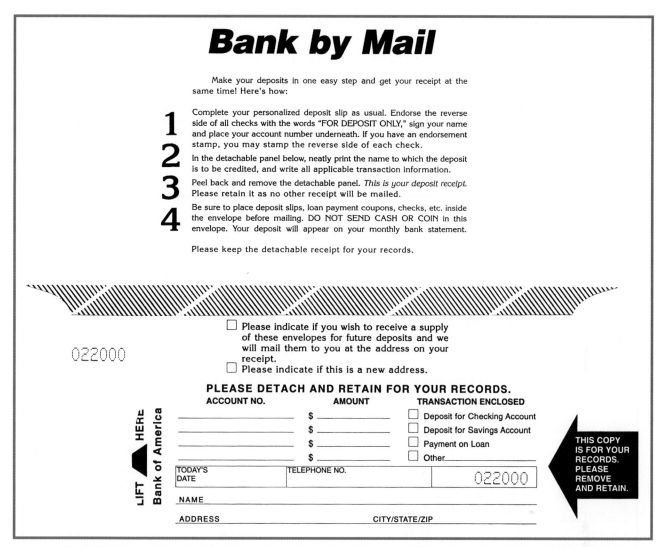

Bank by Mail

Make your deposits in one easy step and get your receipt at the same time! Here's how:

1 Complete your personalized deposit slip as usual. Endorse the reverse side of all checks with the words "FOR DEPOSIT ONLY," sign your name and place your account number underneath. If you have an endorsement stamp, you may stamp the reverse side of each check.

2 In the detachable panel below, neatly print the name to which the deposit is to be credited, and write all applicable transaction information.

3 Peel back and remove the detachable panel. *This is your deposit receipt.* Please retain it as no other receipt will be mailed.

4 Be sure to place deposit slips, loan payment coupons, checks, etc. inside the envelope before mailing. DO NOT SEND CASH OR COIN in this envelope. Your deposit will appear on your monthly bank statement.

Please keep the detachable receipt for your records.

022000

☐ Please indicate if you wish to receive a supply of these envelopes for future deposits and we will mail them to you at the address on your receipt.
☐ Please indicate if this is a new address.

PLEASE DETACH AND RETAIN FOR YOUR RECORDS.

ACCOUNT NO.   AMOUNT   TRANSACTION ENCLOSED

$ _____ ☐ Deposit for Checking Account
$ _____ ☐ Deposit for Savings Account
$ _____ ☐ Payment on Loan
$ _____ ☐ Other_____

TODAY'S DATE   TELEPHONE NO.   022000

NAME

ADDRESS   CITY/STATE/ZIP

LIFT HERE Bank of America

THIS COPY IS FOR YOUR RECORDS. PLEASE REMOVE AND RETAIN.

FIGURE 18–11   Example of bank-by-mail deposit envelope. (Courtesy of Valley Bank of Nevada, Las Vegas, NV.)

- Beginning balance
- Deposits received
- Checks paid
- Bank charges
- Ending balance

The bank statement (Fig. 18–12) is usually accompanied by the customer's canceled checks. Many banks are now microfilming canceled checks and storing the information in the bank's computer. The customer is asked for permission to use this procedure and has the privilege of requesting a copy of any check when needed. Bank statements are prepared at regular intervals, usually once per month.

RECONCILING THE BANK STATEMENT

The bank statement balance and the customer's checkbook balance will usually be different, except in a relatively inactive account. The two balances must be reconciled. The **reconciliation** discloses any errors that may exist in the checkbook or, on rare occasions, in the bank statement (Fig. 18–13).

The bank statement may include an entry for service charges that must be deducted from the checkbook balance. In all types of accounts, the bank may charge a fee for services. Usually in the case of an individual account, it is a flat fee; in a business account, the fee is based on services rendered. If the average or minimum balance is maintained at an established level, the bank may forego a service charge.

Most banks ask to be notified within 10 days of any error found in the statement. The bank statement should be reconciled as soon as it is received. You will usually find a form to follow in carrying out this procedure on the back of the bank statement.

0821-402054

#821

||l|ıını|ıl|l|ıl|ın|ıl|ılıl|ılıııl|||ını||ıını|ılıl|ıınl|ıll

N
2

CALL (888) 555-2932
24 HOURS/DAY, 7 DAYS/WEEK
FOR ASSISTANCE WITH
YOUR ACCOUNT.

PAGE 1 OF 2   THIS STATEMENT COVERS: 6/22/99 THROUGH 7/22/99

INTEREST CHECKING
0821-402054

SUMMARY

PREVIOUS BALANCE	252.10	MINIMUM BALANCE	142.55
DEPOSITS	68.74 +	AVERAGE BALANCE	220.00
INTEREST EARNED	.18 +	ANNUAL PERCENTAGE	
WITHDRAWALS	109.55 −	YIELD EARNED	.96 %
CUSTOMER SERVICE CALLS	.00 −		
INTERLINK/PURCHASE FEE	.00 −	INTEREST EARNED 1994	2.23
MONTHLY CHECKING FEE AND OTHER CHARGES	.00 −		

► **NEW BALANCE**   **211.47**

USE YOUR EXPRESS CARD TO MAKE UNLIMITED PURCHASES AT RETAILERS DISPLAYING
THE INTERLINK SYMBOL. (A $1 MONTHLY FEE MAY APPLY.)

TRY IT TODAY AT ARCO . . . MOBIL . . . LUCKY . . . RALPHS . . . SAFEWAY & MORE!

CHECKS AND WITHDRAWALS	CHECK 202	DATE PAID 7/05	AMOUNT 15.05	CHECK 203	DATE PAID 7/15	AMOUNT 94.50

DEPOSITS			DATE POSTED	AMOUNT
	CUSTOMER DEPOSIT		7/22	68.74
	INTEREST PAYMENT THIS PERIOD		7/22	.18

BALANCE INFORMATION	DATE 6/22	BALANCE 252.10	DATE 7/05	BALANCE 237.05	DATE 7/15	BALANCE 142.55
					7/22	211.47

---

24 HOUR CUSTOMER SERVICE

EACH ACCOUNT COMES WITH 3 COMPLIMENTARY CALLS PER STATEMENT PERIOD.

CALLS TO 24 HOUR CUSTOMER SERVICE THIS STATEMENT PERIOD: 0

INTEREST INFORMATION

FROM	THROUGH	INTEREST RATE	ANNUAL PERCENTAGE YIELD (APY)
6/22	7/22	1.00%	1.01%

INTEREST RATE/APY AS OF 7/22/94 IF YOUR BALANCE IS

$ 0 - 4,999 . . . . .1.00%		1.01%
$ 5,000 - 9,999 . . . . .1.00%		1.01%
$ 10,000 AND OVER. 1.00%		1.01%

CALL 1-800-555-2932 IN CALIFORNIA ANYTIME FOR CURRENT RATES.

MEMBER FDIC

STATEMENT

FIGURE 18–12   Example of regular checking account statement.

THIS WORKSHEET IS PROVIDED TO HELP YOU BALANCE YOUR ACCOUNT

1. Go through your register and mark each check, withdrawal, Express ATM transaction, payment, deposit or other credit listed on this statement. Be sure that your register shows any interest paid into your account, and any service charges, automatic payments, or Express Transfers withdrawn from your account during this statement period.

2. Using the chart below, list any outstanding checks, Express ATM withdrawals, payments or any other withdrawals (including any from previous months) that are listed in your register but are not shown on this statement.

3. Balance your account by filling in the spaces below.

ITEMS OUTSTANDING	
NUMBER	**AMOUNT**
TOTAL	$

ENTER

The NEW BALANCE shown on this statement _ _ _ _ _ _ _ _ _ _ _ _ _ _ _ _ _ _ _ $_____

ADD

Any deposits listed in your register $_____
or transfers into your account $_____
which are not shown on this $_____
statement.   +$_____

TOTAL _ _ _ _ _ _ _ _   +$_____

CALCULATE THE SUBTOTAL _ _ _ _ _ _ _ _ _ $_____

SUBTRACT

The total outstanding checks and withdrawals from the chart at left _ _ _ _ _ _ _ _ _   −$_____

CALCULATE THE ENDING BALANCE

This amount should be the same as the current balance shown in your check register _ _ _ _ _ _ _ _ _ _ _ _ _ _ _ _ _ $_____

IF YOU SUSPECT ERRORS OR HAVE QUESTIONS ABOUT ELECTRONIC TRANSFERS

If you believe there is an error on your statement or Express ATM receipt, or if you need more information about a transaction listed on this statement or an Express ATM receipt, please contact us immediately. We are available 24 hours a day, seven days a week to assist you. Please call the telephone number printed on the front of this statement. Or, you may write to us at United Trust Company, P.O. Box 327, Anytown, USA.

1) Tell us your name and account number or Express card number.

2) As clearly as you can, describe the error or the transfer you are unsure about, and explain why you believe there is an error or why you need more information.

3) Tell us the dollar amount of the suspected error.

You must report the suspected error to us no later than 60 days after we sent you the first statement on which the problem appeared. We will investigate your question and will correct any error promptly. If our investigation takes longer than 10 business days (or 20 days in the case of electronic purchases), we will temporarily credit your account for the amount you believe is in error, so that you may have use of the money until the investigation is completed.

FIGURE 18–13   Reverse side of bank statement to be used for reconciling checking account.

PROCEDURE 18-3
Reconciling a Bank Statement

GOAL
To reconcile a bank statement with the checking account

EQUIPMENT AND SUPPLIES

Ending balance of previous statement
Current bank statement
Canceled checks for current month

Checkbook stubs
Calculator
Pen

PROCEDURAL STEPS

1 Compare the opening balance of the new statement with the closing balance of the previous statement.
   PURPOSE: To determine that the balances are in agreement.

2 Compare the canceled checks with the items on the statement.
   PURPOSE: To verify that they are your checks and that they are listed in the right amount.

3 Arrange the canceled checks in numerical order and compare with the checkbook stubs.

4 Place a checkmark (√) on each stub for which a canceled check has been returned.
   PURPOSE: To locate any outstanding checks.

5 List and total the outstanding checks.

6 Verify that all previous outstanding checks have cleared.

7 Subtract the total of the outstanding checks from the bank statement balance.
   NOTE: Do not include any certified checks as outstanding because their amount has already been deducted from the account.

8 Add to the total in Step 7 any deposits made but not included in the bank statement.
   PURPOSE: To correct the credits in the bank statement balance.

9 Total any bank charges that appear on the bank statement and subtract them from the checkbook balance. Such charges may include service charges, automatic withdrawals or payments, and NSF checks.
   PURPOSE: To correct the checkbook balance.

10 If the checkbook balance and the statement balance do not agree, match the bank statement entries with the checkbook entries.

The reconciliation procedure may be put in a formula, as shown below:

BANK STATEMENT RECONCILIATION FORMULA

Bank statement balance	$_____	
Less outstanding checks	$_____	
Plus deposits not shown	$_____	
Corrected Bank Statement Balance		$_____
Checkbook balance	$_____	
Less any bank charges	$_____	
Corrected Checkbook Balance		$_____

If the two *corrected balances* agree, you may stop there. If they do not agree, *subtract* the lesser figure from the greater figure; the difference will usually give you a clue to locating the error. (See Procedure 18-3.)

QUESTIONS TO ASK IN SEARCHING FOR A POSSIBLE ERROR

- Is your arithmetic correct?
- Did you forget to include one of the outstanding checks?
- Did you fail to record a deposit or did you record it twice?

- Do all stubs and checks agree?
- Have you carried your figures forward correctly?
- Have you transposed a figure? (If the amount of your error is divisible by nine, you probably did.)
- Did someone write a check without your knowledge?
- Did you fail to correct your checkbook balance at the time of the previous statement?

Many persons find the reconciliation process confusing at first, but after a few times it becomes easier and fairly routine.

Medical Assistant's Position of Trust

The medical assistant who manages the financial responsibilities of a medical practice is in a position of great trust. Conscientious and reliable attention to detail in this position can be a great source of job satisfaction and an attribute toward job security.

 LEGAL AND ETHICAL ISSUES

If a mistake is made in preparing a check, do not destroy this check. Rather, write VOID across the check, make a note on the check stub, and file the check with canceled checks for auditing purposes.

A stop-payment order may be placed with the bank in an emergency, such as a check being lost, or a disagreement about a purchase or payment.

Do not accept a check made payable to another party without having the endorsement of the person who gives it to you. If the check is returned by the bank for any reason, the responsibility for the check will be charged to the last endorser, not the last person to receive the money.

CRITICAL THINKING

1 Shortly after you arrive at the office on Monday morning you discover that the office checkbook is missing. What action(s) would you take?

2 What is the simplest type of check endorsement, and when can it safely be used?

3 A patient wishes to pay an outstanding account at the end of an office visit. The balance is $70 and the patient offers a check in the amount of $100 written to the patient by a party unknown to you. How would you handle this situation? Why?

HOW DID I DO? Answers to Memory Joggers

1 *a.* A cashier's check is the bank's own check signed by an authorized officer of the bank. A certified check is a depositor's check that has been certified by a bank officer's signature.
b. A traveler's check requires a signature at the time of purchase and a second signature when it is used.

2 An insured money market savings account usually requires a minimum balance, draws interest at money market rates, and allows the writing of checks (limited number).
The ordinary savings account has no minimum balance, draws interest at the lowest prevailing rate, and has no check-writing privileges.

3 Prevents the possibility of neglecting to complete stub, which would leave you unable to balance checkbook until that check is returned.

4 Restrictive endorsement. Specifies the purpose of the endorsement (e.g., deposit to account).

5 By ABA number.

REFERENCES

American Medical Association: The Business Side of Medical Practice. Chicago, AMA, 1989.
Fess PE, et al: Accounting Principles, 17th ed. Cincinnati, South-Western Publishing, 1993.

Billing and Collection Procedures

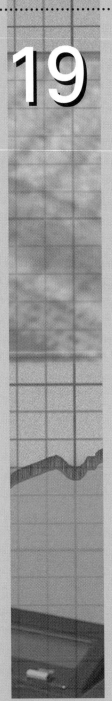

19

LEARNING OBJECTIVES

Cognitive: On successful completion of this chapter you should be able to:

1 Define and spell the terms listed in the Vocabulary.
2 Name the three ways by which payment for medical services is accomplished.
3 List nine items that should be addressed in developing a credit policy.
4 State three reasons for itemizing billing statements.
5 Describe cycle billing and its advantages.
6 Discuss the significance of determining the collection ratio and the accounts receivable ratio.
7 List the three most common reasons for patients' failure to pay accounts.
8 Discuss the do's and don'ts of telephone collection procedures.
9 Name five sources of information in tracing skips.
10 State the procedure to follow on receiving notice of a debtor's bankruptcy.
11 List three advantages of using small claims courts for collecting delinquent accounts.
12 Discuss five appropriate follow-up actions after assigning accounts to a collection agency.

Performance: On successful completion of this chapter you should be able to:

1 Prepare patients' monthly statements.
2 Calculate a collection ratio and an accounts receivable ratio.
3 Prepare an age analysis of accounts receivable.
4 Initiate proceedings to collect delinquent accounts.
5 Demonstrate telephone collection techniques.

VOCABULARY

accounts receivable ratio A formula for measuring how fast outstanding accounts are being paid

age analysis A procedure for classifying accounts receivable by age from the first date of billing

collection ratio A formula for measuring the effectiveness of the billing system

invasion of privacy Unauthorized disclosure of a person's private affairs

statute of limitations The time limit within which an action may legally be brought upon a contract

subsidize To aid or promote something (such as a private enterprise) with public money

superbill A combination charge slip, statement, and insurance reporting form

In Chapter 16 we discussed how fees are determined, the importance of advance discussion of fees, the adjusting or canceling of fees in hardship cases, and the legal aspects of credit arrangements. We also addressed the importance of getting adequate information on the first visit when it appears that an extension of credit will be necessary. Attention to these details helps immeasurably in the collection efforts that follow.

The collection of fees and account management of the medical practice is often entrusted to the medical assistant.

PERSONAL QUALITIES

HOW THE MEDICAL ASSISTANT CAN BE AN EFFECTIVE ACCOUNT MANAGER

- Believe that the physician and the facility have a right to charge for the services provided.
- Do not be embarrassed to ask for payment for the value of the service.
- Possess tact and good judgment.
- Give individual attention and personal consideration to each situation.
- Be courteous and show a sincere desire to help the patient who has financial problems.
- Try to find out the patient's reason for non-payment when this occurs.

The payment for medical services is accomplished in four ways: (1) payment at time of services, (2) billing when extension of credit is necessary, (3) insurance or other third party, and (4) using outside collection assistance.

Payment at Time of Service

A large percentage of patients will have some type of health insurance for at least major items. Every practice in which there are patient visits should encourage time-of-service collection. It is especially important to collect copayments and payment for office visits not covered by insurance. If patients get into the habit of paying their current charges before they leave the office, there are no further billing and bookkeeping expenses. If patients are informed when making an appointment that payment is expected at the time of service, they are not surprised when you say at the end if the visit,

> Your charge for today is $xx. Will that be cash or check?

Many patients are hesitant to ask about charges and are unsure whether to offer to pay or to wait until asked. You will make it easier for the patients by offering to accept their payments, because most people are prepared to pay small bills on a cash basis. Even if a patient requests to be billed, you can say,

> The normal procedure is to pay at the time of service, but we can make an exception this time.

A patient who may have forgotten his or her checkbook should be given a self-addressed envelope with the charge slip and asked to send the payment in the next mail.

Memory Jogger

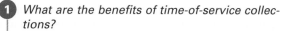

1 *What are the benefits of time-of-service collections?*

Billing After Extension of Credit

In some types of practice, particularly those involving large fees for surgery or long-term care, it becomes necessary to extend credit and establish a regular system of billing. This requires informing the patient of (1) what the charges will be, (2) what professional services these charges cover, and (3) the credit policy of the office.

CREDIT POLICY

Many practices do not have a true credit policy; thus, each account continues to be evaluated individually. It is almost impossible to judge accounts objectively and equitably under such circumstances.

The physician and the staff should think through their situation, decide what they expect of patients with respect to payments, and how they will inform the patient. Although there will always be exceptions to any rule, there must *be* a rule, which should be in writing and conveyed to the patient at the outset of the relationship.

Some medical practices prepare an information booklet that includes the payment policy. New patients are given a copy of the booklet. Any patient who needs special consideration can be counseled by the medical assistant. (See Issues to be Addressed in Credit Policy.) The medical assistant who has the guidance and support of an established credit policy can perform with confidence when handling patient accounts.

ISSUES TO BE ADDRESSED IN CREDIT POLICY

1 When payment is due from patients
2 When the practice requires payment at time of service
3 When or if assignment of insurance benefits is accepted
4 Whether insurance forms will be completed by the office staff
5 Billing procedures
6 Collection protocol
7 How long an account will be carried without payment
8 Telephone collection protocol
9 Sending accounts to a collection agency

INDEPENDENT BILLING SERVICE

Many health care facilities find it advantageous to refer their billing and collections to an independent billing service. The information related to services and fees is sent to the billing service on a daily or weekly basis. The servicing agent then handles all billing and collections, as well as any telephone inquiries. This system frees the regular office staff for more patient-oriented duties. An added advantage is that any dispute that may arise is handled by a person who is not connected with the patient care on a personal basis.

Memory Jogger

2 *How does having a credit policy benefit the collection of fees?*

Internal Billing by the Account Manager

This chapter is directed to billing fee-for-service patients in a private practice. Insurance and managed care billing are addressed in following chapters.

METHODS AND APPEARANCE OF BILLING

In a practice with only a moderate number of accounts, the medical assistant handles the preparation and mailing of statements. This may be accomplished by a (1) computer-generated statement, (2) superbill, (3) typewritten statement, or (4) photocopied statement.

The appearance of the statement carries a visual impact just as a letter does, so the statement heads should be carefully chosen and the typing clean and accurate. Statement heads are usually imprinted with the same information as the physician's letterhead. They should be of good quality and large enough to allow itemization of charges. Envelopes should be imprinted with "Address Correction Requested" under the return address, to maintain up-to-date mailing lists. A self-addressed return envelope included with the statement encourages prompt payment. This is mainly for the convenience of patients who do not always have stationery available for sending a return payment or who are less likely to return a payment immediately if they must address an envelope.

Computer-Generated Statement

Patient accounts are generated and stored in the computer, and a statement can be produced whenever needed. The statement can show the service rendered on each date, the charge for each service, the date on which a claim was submitted to the insurance company, the date of payment, and the balance due from the patient. The computer may also be programmed to print messages on the statement, such as "Balance now 30 days past due," or a selection of other messages.

Superbill

The **superbill** is a combination charge slip, statement, and insurance reporting form. There are variations in style, but they are usually personalized for the practice. Figure 19–1 is an example of a form used in the practice of an endocrinologist. It has space for all the elements required in submitting medical insurance claims:

- Name and address of patient
- Name of insurance carrier
- Insurance identification number
- Brief description of each service by code number

LIC. # 181181
S.S. # 052-56-3472
UPIN # F29065

MARGARET J. NACHTIGALL, M.D.
Reproductive Endocrinology
251 EAST 33RD STREET
NEW YORK, N.Y. 10016

TELEPHONE: (212) 683-0519
FAX: (212) 779-8432

PATIENT INFORMATION

| PATIENT'S LAST NAME | FIRST | | INITIAL | BIRTHDATE / / | SEX ☑FEMALE | TODAY'S DATE / / |
| ADDRESS | CITY | STATE | ZIP | RELATION TO SUBSCRIBER | REFERRING PHYSICIAN | |

SUBSCRIBER OR POLICYHOLDER — INSURANCE CARRIER

ADDRESS CITY STATE ZIP — INS. ID — COVERAGE CODE — GROUP

OTHER HEALTH COVERAGE? ☐ NO ☐ YES IDENTIFY — DISABILITY RELATED TO: ☐ IND. ☐ ACCIDENT ☐ PREGNANCY ☐ OTHER — DATE SYMPTOMS APPEARED, INCEPTION OF PREGNANCY, OR ACCIDENT OCCURRED: / /

ASSIGNMENT & RELEASE: I hereby assign my insurance benefits to be paid directly to the undersigned physician. I am financially responsible for non-covered services. I also authorize the physician to release any information required to process this claim.
SIGNED: (Patient, or Parent, if Minor) — DATE: / /

✔ DESCRIPTION	CODE	FEE	✔ DESCRIPTION	CODE	FEE	✔ DESCRIPTION	CODE	FEE
OFFICE VISIT			**OFFICE PROCEDURES**			**LABORATORY - IN OFFICE**		
New Patient			Sperm Wash	58323		Pregnancy Test	85160	
Consultation	99204		Cauterization of Cervix	57510		Urinalysis	81002	
Comprehensive	99205		Cervical Biopsy	57500		Stool Occult Blood	82270	
OFFICE VISIT			Endocervical Curettage	57505		Lyme Titer	86317	
Established Patient			Endometrial Biopsy	58100		Estradiol	82670	
Limited	99211		Office Endometrial Curettage	58102		Chemistry	80019	
Intermediate	99212		Post Coital Test	89300		CBC, pit., Diff.	85024	
Extended	99213		Artificial Insemination	58310		T3 Uptake	84479	
Comprehensive	99214		Pelvic Sonogram	76856		T4	84435	
Comprehensive	99215		Vulvar Biopsy	56600		TSH	84443	
SURGERY			Bilateral Mammogram	76091		ESR	85650	
D & C	58120		Unilateral Mammogram	76090		Pregnancy Test	84702	
Pregnancy Termination	59840		Breast Ultrasound	76645		FSH	83000	
Laparoscopy	56305		Abdominal Ultrasound	76700		Prolactin	84146	
Hysteroscopy	56351		Polypectomy	57500				
Laporotomy	49000							
Myomectomy	58140							
Hysterectomy	58150							

DIAGNOSIS: ICD-9
☐ Abortion, Incomplete 634.71
☐ Abortion, Spontaneous 634.90
☐ Alopecia 704.09
☐ Amenorrhea 626.0
☐ Anemia 285.9
☐ Anovulation 628.0
☐ Atrophic Vaginitis 627.3
☐ Breast Cyst 610.1
☐ Breast Mass 611.72
☐ Breast Pain 611.71
☐ Cervical Polyp 622.7
☐ Cervicitis 616.0
☐ Condyloma 091.3
☐ Cyclic Adrenal Hyperplasia .255.2
☐ Cystocele 618.0
☐ Cystitis 595.9

☐ Diabetes Mellitus 250.0
☐ Dysmenorrhea 625.3
☐ Dyspareunia 625.0
☐ Dysuria 788.1
☐ Ectopic Pregnancy 633.9
☐ Edema 782.3
☐ Endometrial Hyperplasia .621.3
☐ Endometriosis 617.0
☐ Fatigue 780.7
☐ Fibrocystic Breast Disease .610.1
☐ Galactorrhea 676.6
☐ Headache 784.0
☐ Hemorrhoids 455.6
☐ Herpes 054.1
☐ Hypercholesterolemia 272.0
☐ Hyperprolactinemia 253.1
☐ Hypertension 401.9

☐ Hyperthyroidism 242.9
☐ Hypothyroidism 244.9
☐ Infertility 628.9
☐ Luteal Phase Insufficiency .628.8
☐ Menometrorrhagia 626.2
☐ Menopausal Syndrome ...627.2
☐ Menorrhagia 626.2
☐ Monilial Vaginitis 112.1
☐ Obesity 278.0
☐ Osteoarthritis 715.9
☐ Osteopenia 733.9
☐ Osteoporosis 733.0
☐ Ovarian Cyst 620.2
☐ Ovarian Insufficiency ...256.3
☐ Pelvic Pain 625.9
☐ Polycystic Ovary Syndrome 256.4
☐ Postmenopausal Bleeding .627.1

☐ Pregnancy V22.2
☐ Pregnancy Termination ..V72.4
☐ Premature Ovarian Failure .256.3
☐ Premenopausal Menorrhagia .627.0
☐ Prolactinoma 253
☐ Prolapsed Uterus 618.1
☐ Rectocele 569.1
☐ Thyroiditis 245.2
☐ Trichomonas 131.0
☐ Urinary Tract Infection ...599.0
☐ Uterine Fibroids 218.9
☐ Vasomotor Instability 780.2
☐ Vaginitis 616.1
☐ Vulvitis 616.1

DIAGNOSIS: (IF NOT CHECKED ABOVE) — ADDITIONAL INFORMATION: — DOCTOR'S SIGNATURE

SERVICES PERFORMED AT: ☐ OFFICE ☐ University Hospital ☐ Day Surgery / University Hosp.
560 First Avenue / 530 First Avenue N.Y., N.Y. 10016

ACCEPT ASSIGNMENT? ☐ YES ☐ NO
TOTAL TODAY'S FEE

REFERRING PHYSICIAN: — PREVIOUS BALANCE

INSTRUCTIONS TO PATIENT FOR FILING INSURANCE CLAIMS:
1. COMPLETE UPPER PORTION OF THIS FORM; SIGN AND DATE.
2. MAIL THIS FORM DIRECTLY TO YOUR INSURANCE COMPANY. YOU MAY ATTACH YOUR OWN INSURANCE COMPANY'S FORM IF YOU WISH, ALTHOUGH IT IS NOT NECESSARY.
PLEASE REMEMBER THAT PAYMENT IS YOUR OBLIGATION, REGARDLESS OF INSURANCE OR OTHER THIRD PARTY INVOLVEMENT.

AMT. REC'D. TODAY — NEW BALANCE

INSUR-A-BILL ® BIBBERO SYSTEMS, INC. • PETALUMA, CA • © 5/95 (SB M-N) — (REV. 9/96)

FIGURE 19–1 Superbill. (Courtesy of Bibbero Systems, Inc., Petaluma, California (800) 242-2376, Fax (800) 242-9330.)

- Fee for each service
- Place and date of service
- Diagnosis
- Physician's name and address
- Physician's signature

The superbill can be used as a charge slip for office treatments if the physician checks the services performed at the completion of the visit and asks the patient to hand it to the medical assistant when leaving. Either the physician or the medical assistant may write in the amount of the fee. If a payment is made, it can be so indicated. Instructions to the patient for filing insurance claims are on the bottom left. The physician's office keeps one copy, the patient is given the original, and one copy is for filing with the insurance company.

Statements must be correct and must include the

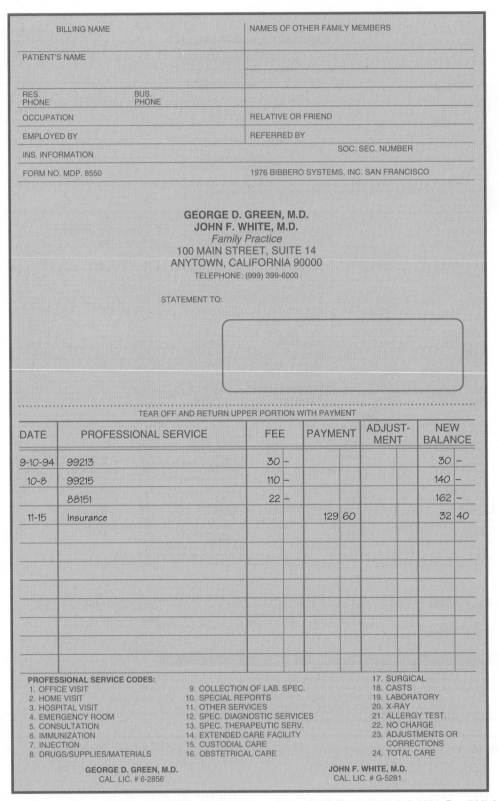

		BILLING NAME		NAMES OF OTHER FAMILY MEMBERS	

PATIENT'S NAME

RES. PHONE   BUS. PHONE

OCCUPATION   RELATIVE OR FRIEND

EMPLOYED BY   REFERRED BY

INS. INFORMATION   SOC. SEC. NUMBER

FORM NO. MDP. 8550   1976 BIBBERO SYSTEMS, INC. SAN FRANCISCO

GEORGE D. GREEN, M.D.
JOHN F. WHITE, M.D.
Family Practice
100 MAIN STREET, SUITE 14
ANYTOWN, CALIFORNIA 90000
TELEPHONE: (999) 399-6000

STATEMENT TO:

TEAR OFF AND RETURN UPPER PORTION WITH PAYMENT

DATE	PROFESSIONAL SERVICE	FEE		PAYMENT		ADJUST-MENT		NEW BALANCE	
9-10-94	99213	30	–					30	–
10-8	99215	110	–					140	–
	88151	22	–					162	–
11-15	Insurance			129	60			32	40

PROFESSIONAL SERVICE CODES:

1. OFFICE VISIT	9. COLLECTION OF LAB. SPEC.	17. SURGICAL
2. HOME VISIT	10. SPECIAL REPORTS	18. CASTS
3. HOSPITAL VISIT	11. OTHER SERVICES	19. LABORATORY
4. EMERGENCY ROOM	12. SPEC. DIAGNOSTIC SERVICES	20. X-RAY
5. CONSULTATION	13. SPEC. THERAPEUTIC SERV.	21. ALLERGY TEST.
6. IMMUNIZATION	14. EXTENDED CARE FACILITY	22. NO CHARGE
7. INJECTION	15. CUSTODIAL CARE	23. ADJUSTMENTS OR CORRECTIONS
8. DRUGS/SUPPLIES/MATERIALS	16. OBSTETRICAL CARE	24. TOTAL CARE

GEORGE D. GREEN, M.D.
CAL. LIC. # 6-2856

JOHN F. WHITE, M.D.
CAL. LIC. # G-5281

FIGURE 19–2 Itemized statement. (Courtesy of Bibbero Systems, Inc., Petaluma, California (800) 242-2376, Fax (800) 242-9330.)

patient's name and address as well as the balance owed. If statements are photocopied or microfilmed, special care must be taken that the ledger card is correct because it will be duplicated in the billing process.

Typewritten Statements

The use of continuous form billing statements is a timesaver. The statements are printed in a roll with perforated edges for separation. The roll is fed into the typewriter for the first statement and remains until the last statement is typed, eliminating the time and energy necessary for inserting and removing each statement form from the typewriter.

Another timesaver is the multiple-copy statement. The Colwell Company calls its version "E-Z Statements." The E-Z Statement features three monthly statements plus one patient's ledger card in each set, all in NCR (no carbon required) paper. Services and payments are posted during the month, and at billing time the top sheet is removed, folded, and mailed in a window envelope. If more than three mailings are required, a new set must be headed and the balance forwarded.

Photocopied Statements

Coordinated ledger cards and copy paper are used in preparing photocopied statements. A perfect statement is ready for mailing in minimum time. Extra care must be used in posting the ledgers. A black pen should be used in making entries on the ledger card, because other ink colors do not reproduce well. Writing must be clear and legible. There should be no personal notes made on the ledger cards unless it is something you wish conveyed to the patient. (It is possible to buy pencils with nonreproducible lead if you believe this is necessary for making collection entries.) Usually a window envelope is used for mailing, which means that the name and address on the ledger must be neat, correct, and in the right position for the envelope window.

PROCEDURE FOR INTERNAL BILLING

Itemizing the First Statement

If the medical fee has been explained in advance, as discussed in Chapter 16, the monthly statement is merely a confirmation of what is owed, and there should be no misunderstanding. However, it is good business practice—and a courtesy to the patient—to itemize the charges. This is essential if the statement is to be used for billing the patient's insurance. Patients are entitled to an understanding of the physician's statement for medical services (Fig. 19–2).

Itemizing statements is not difficult. The simplest method is merely to allow space on the original statement, below the "For Professional Services" line, on which to list the separate charges for office, house, or hospital calls or for treatments or tests performed in the medical facility.

Many physicians have devised their own itemized charge slips; these are given to the patient when payment is made at the time of service or later mailed in a combination statement-reply envelope. Use of such charge slips simplifies the itemization procedure, because filling out the slips is usually just a matter of checking the procedures listed. An itemized charge slip is shown in Figure 19–3. Although the itemization of bills may seem an unnecessary waste of time, if you do itemize you will spend less time in explaining services provided, clearing up misunderstandings with patients, and following up on delinquent accounts.

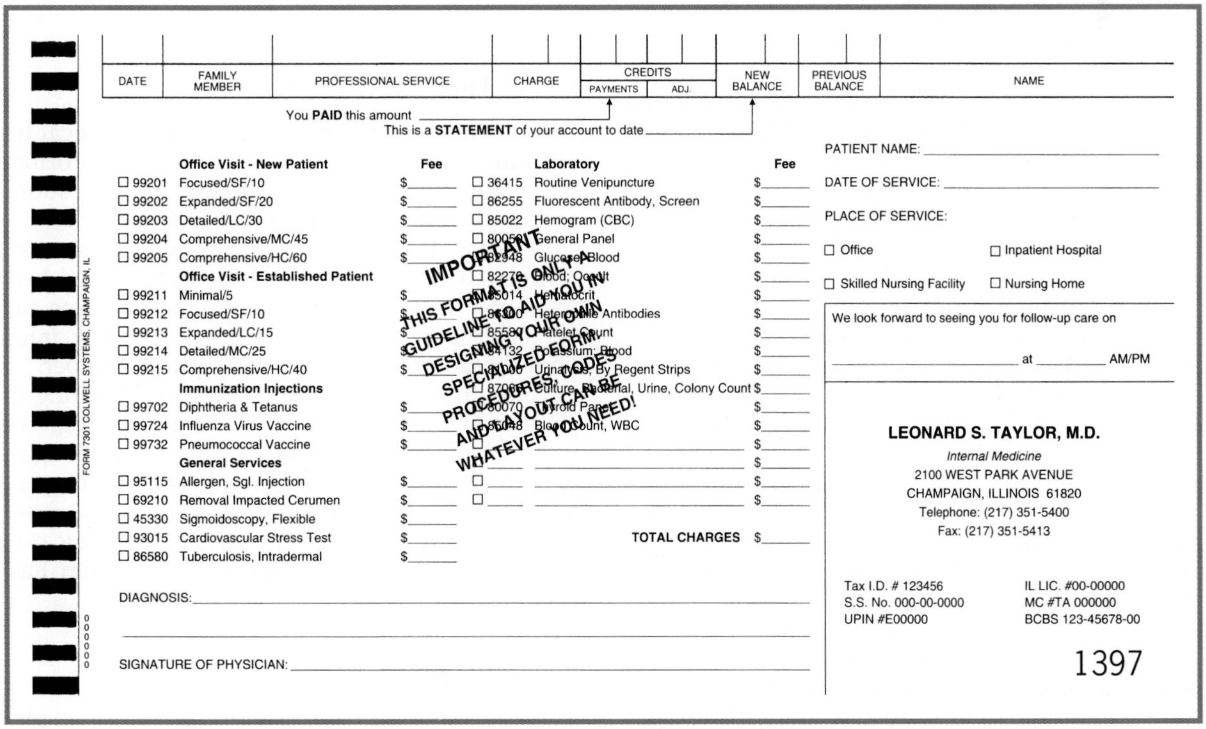

DATE	FAMILY MEMBER	PROFESSIONAL SERVICE	CHARGE	CREDITS PAYMENTS	CREDITS ADJ.	NEW BALANCE	PREVIOUS BALANCE	NAME

You **PAID** this amount ____
This is a **STATEMENT** of your account to date ____

Office Visit - New Patient — Fee
- ☐ 99201 Focused/SF/10 $____
- ☐ 99202 Expanded/SF/20 $____
- ☐ 99203 Detailed/LC/30 $____
- ☐ 99204 Comprehensive/MC/45 $____
- ☐ 99205 Comprehensive/HC/60 $____

Office Visit - Established Patient
- ☐ 99211 Minimal/5 $____
- ☐ 99212 Focused/SF/10 $____
- ☐ 99213 Expanded/LC/15 $____
- ☐ 99214 Detailed/MC/25 $____
- ☐ 99215 Comprehensive/HC/40 $____

Immunization Injections
- ☐ 99702 Diphtheria & Tetanus $____
- ☐ 99724 Influenza Virus Vaccine $____
- ☐ 99732 Pneumococcal Vaccine $____

General Services
- ☐ 95115 Allergen, Sgl. Injection $____
- ☐ 69210 Removal Impacted Cerumen $____
- ☐ 45330 Sigmoidoscopy, Flexible $____
- ☐ 93015 Cardiovascular Stress Test $____
- ☐ 86580 Tuberculosis, Intradermal $____

Laboratory — Fee
- ☐ 36415 Routine Venipuncture $____
- ☐ 86255 Fluorescent Antibody, Screen $____
- ☐ 85022 Hemogram (CBC) $____
- ☐ 80050 General Panel $____
- ☐ 82948 Glucose; Blood $____
- ☐ 82270 Blood; Occult $____
- ☐ 85014 Hematocrit $____
- ☐ 86308 Heterophile Antibodies $____
- ☐ 85580 Platelet Count $____
- ☐ 84132 Potassium; Blood $____
- ☐ 81000 Urinalysis, By Regent Strips $____
- ☐ 87086 Culture, Bacterial, Urine, Colony Count $____
- ☐ 80070 Thyroid Panel $____
- ☐ 85048 Blood Count, WBC $____
- ☐ ____ ____ $____
- ☐ ____ ____ $____
- ☐ ____ ____ $____
- ☐ ____ ____ $____

TOTAL CHARGES $____

IMPORTANT THIS FORMAT IS ONLY A GUIDELINE TO AID YOU IN DESIGNING YOUR OWN SPECIALIZED FORM. PROCEDURES, CODES AND LAYOUT CAN BE WHATEVER YOU NEED!

PATIENT NAME: ____

DATE OF SERVICE: ____

PLACE OF SERVICE:

☐ Office ☐ Inpatient Hospital

☐ Skilled Nursing Facility ☐ Nursing Home

We look forward to seeing you for follow-up care on

____ at ____ AM/PM

LEONARD S. TAYLOR, M.D.
Internal Medicine
2100 WEST PARK AVENUE
CHAMPAIGN, ILLINOIS 61820
Telephone: (217) 351-5400
Fax: (217) 351-5413

Tax I.D. # 123456 — IL LIC. #00-00000
S.S. No. 000-00-0000 — MC #TA 000000
UPIN #E00000 — BCBS 123-45678-00

DIAGNOSIS: ____

SIGNATURE OF PHYSICIAN: ____

1397

FORM 7301 COLWELL SYSTEMS, CHAMPAIGN, IL

FIGURE 19–3 Charge slip. (Courtesy of Colwell Systems, Champaign, IL.)

Time and Frequency of Billing

A regular system of mailing statements should be put into operation. Most people expect to receive statements from their creditors, and they plan their budgets around first-of-the-month bills received. Punctuality in billing encourages prompt payment.

Statements should be sent at least once each month. Some offices send bills immediately after treatment; others bill all patients on the same day each month. Mailing statements twice a month—for example, half of the accounts on the 10th and the remaining half on the 25th—is also common practice.

According to the Fair Credit Billing Act of October 28, 1975, when a billing date for an account has been established, the date of mailing the statement must not vary more than five days without notification to the patient/debtor. If there is a *balance due* or a *credit balance* of one dollar or more, the account must be billed every 30 days.

ONCE-A-MONTH BILLING   If a monthly pattern is followed, bills should leave your office in time to reach the patient no later than the last day of each month and preferably by the 25th of the month. Planning ahead for the preparation of statements can lighten the burden of once-a-month billing. The statement can be prepared at the time of service (or during slack periods), postdated, and mailed at the end of the month.

CYCLE BILLING   Many physicians prefer to use the cycle billing system, which calls for the billing of certain portions of the accounts receivable at given times during the month instead of preparing all statements at the end of each month. Cycle billing is used in large businesses such as department stores, banks, and utility companies. Its many advantages include avoiding once-a-month peak workloads and stabilizing the cash flow. In a small office in which billing is done only once per month, the unexpected illness or absence of the medical assistant for any emergency can leave the physician in a financial bind if the statements do not go out.

The accounts are separated into fairly equal divisions, the number of divisions depending on how many times billing will be done during a month. For example, if you expect to bill twice per month, divide the accounts into two equal sections; for weekly billing, divide into 4 groups; for daily billing, divide into 20 groups.

Small alphabetical groups can be combined to keep the divisions nearly equal in the number of statements to prepare on each billing day. If the files are color coded, you may wish to use the same alphabetical breakdown in billing. Regardless of constant changes in the individual accounts, the mailing dates for accounts in each section remain the same. A schedule for processing and mailing of accounts is thus established, and the workload is apportioned throughout the entire month.

Cycle billing allows the medical assistant to continue all routine duties each day, handling the statements on a day-to-day or weekly schedule rather than in one intensive period at the end of the month. This means that whole days need not be sacrificed from other duties to get statements in the mail. By spacing the billing throughout the month, more time and consideration can be given to each statement, the itemization of bills is less burdensome, and the likelihood of error is decreased.

Patients generally accept the cycle billing system quickly, often with enthusiasm. However, if your office decides to change from a once-a-month billing system to a cycle billing system, patients should be notified in advance, and the new plan should be explained to them. To explain the new system to established patients, enclose a notice in each statement for 2 months preceding the transfer, describing the plan and indicating the future dates on which each patient will receive the bill.

Before a physician adopts the cycle billing system, particularly in a small community, several factors should be taken into consideration, such as

* What is the general income level of the community, and how and when does the average patient get paid?
* Do local companies pay employees at various times during the month, or are most paychecks handed out at the beginning of the month?
* Would cycle billing benefit patients as well as the overall operation of the office?

Memory Jogger

3   *How does the Fair Credit Billing Act affect the frequency or date of mailing statements?*

Billing Third-Party Payers

Collection problems may arise if the medical assistant fails to get the necessary insurance information, particularly Medicare and Medicaid information (see section on Credit Arrangement in Chapter 16).

In some instances, the insurance forms are not completed correctly, and the claim is denied because of minor infractions such as failing to name the responsible party or omitting Social Security information, the policy number, or the group number.

Time limits must also be observed in billing third-party payers. In cases of Medicare patients with a terminal illness, it may be best to accept assignment of benefits. If the physician does not take assignment he or she may receive nothing because the family is not obligated to pay, and Medicare will not pay after a certain time or if the claim has not been correctly filed.

Billing Minors

Minors cannot be held responsible for payment of a bill unless they are emancipated (see Chapter 6).

PROCEDURE 19-1
Preparing Monthly Billing Statements

GOAL
To process monthly statements and evaluate accounts for collection procedures in accordance with the agency's credit policy.

EQUIPMENT AND SUPPLIES
Typewriter or computer
Patient accounts

Agency's credit policy
Statement forms

PROCEDURAL STEPS
1 Assemble all accounts that have outstanding balances

2 Separate accounts that need special attention in accordance with the agency's credit policy.
EXPLANATION: Routine statements should be prepared first, after which special attention can be given to delinquent accounts.

3 Prepare routine statements, including
- Date the statement is prepared
- Name and address of the person responsible for payment
- Name of the patient if different from the person responsible for payment
- Itemization of dates, services, and charges for the month
- Any unpaid balance carried forward (may or may not be itemized, depending on office policy)

4 Determine the action to be taken on accounts separated in step 2.

5 Make a note of the necessary action on the ledger card (telephone call, collection letter series, small claims court, or assignment to collection agency).
PURPOSE: For guidance in executing an action and for later follow-up when necessary.

Bills for minors must be addressed to a parent or legal guardian. If a bill is addressed to a minor, the parent or parents could take the attitude that they are not responsible because they never received the bill.

If the parents are separated or divorced, the parent who brings the child in for treatment is responsible for payment. Whatever financial agreement exists between the parents is strictly their personal business and should not concern the medical office. The responsible parent should be so informed from the beginning.

If an emancipated minor appears in the office and requests treatment and you can ascertain that the person is not living at home, the minor is responsible for the bill. It may be wise to make a determination either with the business manager or with the physician as to whether your office wishes to treat this emancipated minor. (See Procedure 19–1.)

Memory Jogger

 When is a minor responsible for paying the cost of medical care?

Payment Collection

COLLECTION GOALS

Management consultants for the medical profession say that if good financial practices are followed, the accounts receivable on a physician's books should equal no more than 2 to 3 months' gross charges, but if the receivables start falling below the average of 1 month's total charges, perhaps the collection procedures are too stringent. Guidelines can be determined by establishing two ratios. Evaluation of collection is based on the **collection ratio** and the **accounts receivable ratio.**

Collection Ratio

The collection ratio measures the effectiveness of the billing system. A minimum of 6 to 12 months' data should be used in computing the collection ratio. The basic formula for figuring the collection ratio is to divide the total collections by the net charges

> If you are unable to pay your account this month, please telephone this office (776-4900) before
> _____ and let us know how you plan to take care of it.
>
> Your balance due is $350.

FIGURE 19-4 Suggested note to patient for 60-day billing.

(gross charges minus any discounts) to reach a percentage figure. This calculation is illustrated in the following example:

EXAMPLE OF CALCULATING A COLLECTION RATIO

Gross Charges		$125,000
Less:		
Courtesy discounts	$5,000	
Third-party insurance allowance	6,000	
Other adjustments	1,000	
Total Adjustments		12,000
Net charges (gross charges minus adjustments)		
Total Collections		$113,000
$110,000 ÷ $113,000 = 97% collection ratio		110,000

Accounts Receivable Ratio

The accounts receivable ratio measures how fast outstanding accounts are being paid. The formula for figuring the accounts receivable ratio is to divide the current accounts receivable balance by the average gross monthly charges. A desirable accounts receivable ratio is less than 2 months. It is the medical assistant's responsibility to keep both the accounts receivable and collections within normal limits. The method of calculating the accounts receivable ratio is shown in the following example:

EXAMPLE OF CALCULATING ACCOUNTS RECEIVABLE RATIO

Annual Gross Charges	$125,000
Average Monthly Gross Charges (125,000 ÷ 12 months)	10,417
Current Acc/Rec Balance	16,000
Acc/Rec Ratio: 16,000 ÷ 10,417 = 1.54 months	

IMPORTANCE OF COLLECTING DELINQUENT ACCOUNTS

The reasons for pursuing collections go beyond the obvious one that a physician must be paid for services to pay expenses and continue to treat patients. Failure to collect can result in the loss of a patient. A person who owes money to the physician and is not prodded gently into payment may stay away in embarrassment or may even change physicians.

Noncollection of medical bills may also imply guilt. A patient may infer that the physician thought that the patient received inadequate or improper care, and a malpractice suit may result. It is also not fair to paying patients to make no attempt to collect from nonpaying patients. Abandoning accounts without collection follow-up encourages nonpayers, and, as a result, the paying patients indirectly **subsidize** the cost of medical care for those who can pay but do not.

Why Patients Do Not Pay

Most patients are honest. It is estimated that probably fewer than 4% never intend to pay. There may be a larger percentage who are financially "shipwrecked" and temporarily unable to pay. Also, a certain percentage of patients irresponsibly live beyond their incomes. According to the American Medical Association, the three most common reasons for patients' failure to pay are negligence, inability to pay, and unwillingness to pay.

Figures 19-4 and 19-5 illustrate notes that might be sent to patients to remind them of their financial obligations.

Know When to Say No

There must be some limit put on the time, effort, and expense invested in trying to collect an uncollectible account. Under some circumstances, it may be better simply to write off an unpaid account. An example of a letter that might be used to cancel the obligation and at the same time improve the image of the physician is shown in Figure 19-6.

> Every courtesy has been extended to you in arranging for payment of your long overdue account. Our auditor suggests that it no longer be carried on our books.
>
> Unless we hear from you by _____ , the account will be turned over to
> _____ for collection.

FIGURE 19-5 Suggested final letter to patient.

PROCEDURE 19-2
Collecting Delinquent Accounts

GOAL
To initiate proceedings to collect delinquent accounts.

EQUIPMENT AND SUPPLIES
Typewriter or computer
Telephone
Delinquent accounts

Stationery
Collection letter series
Agency's credit policy

PROCEDURAL STEPS
1 Assemble the delinquent accounts

2 Separate accounts according to the action required.
PURPOSE: It is more efficient to process as a group all accounts requiring the same activity.

3 Make telephone calls to those so designated.

4 Record responses on the ledger cards.
PURPOSE: For further action as necessary.

5 Review the accounts requiring collection letters.

6 Choose an appropriate letter from the collection series and individualize it for the account in question.
PURPOSE: Form letters may be used as a guide but should be individualized to suit the situation.

7 Prepare the collection letter(s).

8 Make a notation of the action taken on the ledger card.
PURPOSE: To avoid repetition of the same letter if further action is necessary.

Date

Patient Name
Street Address
City, State ZIP Code

Dear Patient:

Your balance of $200 has been on our books for 23 months.

In view of the financial circumstances that make payment for these past services difficult for you, Dr. Johnson has instructed me to consider the debt cancelled. We will no longer bill you for it.

Dr. Johnson wants you to feel free to call on him for any future service you may require.

Sincerely yours,

Office Manager for
E. F. Johnson, M.D.

FIGURE 19-6 Example of a letter that cancels a fee.

ACCOUNTS RECEIVABLE AGE ANALYSIS

Dr._____

Address_____   Date _____

Patient's name	Total account receivable	Distribution of accounts receivable by age				Remarks
		1-2-3 months	4-5-6 months	7-8-9-10-11-12 months	over 1 year	
A	450.00	100.00	350.00			
B	50.00	50.00				
C	100.00		75.00	25.00		
D	200.00		10.00	150.00	40.00	
E	550.00		550.00			
F	42.50	42.50				
G	65.00	20.00	45.00			
H	325.00	325.00				

FIGURE 19–7   Form for accounts receivable age analysis.

AGING ACCOUNTS RECEIVABLE

Aging is a term used for the procedure of classifying accounts receivable by age from the first date of billing. It should be done on a regular basis. Aging of accounts helps collection follow-up, because it enables the medical assistant to tell at a glance what accounts need attention in addition to a regular statement. Computer billing programs usually include this feature. With sufficient time, an **age analysis** may be accomplished manually (Fig. 19–7).

If the patient is billed on the day of service, the aging begins on that day; if the first billing is 30 days after service, the aging begins at 30 days. Some systems use a breakdown of Current, 30 days, 60 days, 90 days, and 90-plus days.

Looking at Figure 19–7, you see that

* Patient A has a balance of $450. Unless regular payments are being made, this account may be heading toward a collection problem because $350 of the balance is more than 3 months old.
* Patient B presents no problem because the entire balance is current.
* Patient C definitely is a potential problem even though the account is small. The entire balance is more than 3 months old, and one fourth of it is more than 6 months old.
* Patient D's account should never have been allowed to reach this stage of delinquency. If there had been a good collection policy established, it would not have happened.

The age analysis is simply a tool to show at a glance the status of each account. There is no need to do this every month if time is at a premium. If the accounts are aged quarterly you will stay on top of the problem. Usually, a coding system with metal clip-on tabs or adhesive peel-off labels on the ledger cards is used in conjunction with the age-analysis system.

To illustrate, after two statements have been sent, a green tab may be placed on the record, indicating that a courteous reminder was sent with the last statement. The following month the green tab may be replaced with a yellow tab to show that a second payment request was sent in the form of a polite letter or printed request. An orange tab may be substituted the next month, indicating that the patient received a letter requesting prompt attention to the account. Red tabs may be reserved for the accounts of patients who, as a last resort, have been notified of a specific time limit in which payment must be made, after which sterner measures will be taken. If you reach this stage in pursuing a particular account, make certain that you record the date of the time limit on the patient's ledger.

The law requires that once you have made a statement indicating that a specific action will be taken, you must follow through or be liable for the consequences under the law (Fair Debt Collection Practices Act 1977).

If you say, for example, "I am going to turn your account over for collection unless it is paid within 10 days," then you must do so. If you state in a collection letter that you will be taking the debtor to small claims court if the account is not paid by a certain date, then you must do as you say. The intent of the law is to prevent the collector from making idle threats or harassing a debtor. A patient may sue for harassment if such idle threats are made.

Memory Jogger

5 *Briefly describe the process and reason for "account aging."*

COLLECTION TECHNIQUES

Persuasive collection procedures include telephone calls, collection reminders and letters, and personal interviews. (See General Rules to Follow in Telephone Collections.)

GENERAL RULES TO FOLLOW IN TELEPHONE COLLECTIONS

What To Do

1 Call the patient when you can do so in privacy.
2 Call between 8 AM and 9 PM.
3 Determine the identity of the persons with whom you are speaking. If you ask, "Is this Mrs. Noble?" and she answers "Yes" it could be the patient's mother-in-law or daughter-in-law, who is also "Mrs. Noble." Use the person's full name.
4 Be dignified and respectful in your attitude. You can be friendly and formal at the same time.
5 Ask the patient if it is a convenient time to talk with you. Unless you have the attention of the called party, there is little to be gained by continuing. If you are told that you have called at an inopportune time, ask for a specific time when you may call back, or get a promise for the patient to call you at a specified time.
6 After a brief greeting, state the purpose of your call. Make no apology for calling but state your reason in a friendly, business-like way. You expect payment and are interested in helping the patient meet the financial obligation. "This is Alice, Dr. Brown's financial secretary. I'm calling about your account." A well-placed pause at this point in the call sometimes gets an immediate response from the debtor in regard to the nonpayment.
7 Assume a positive attitude. For example, convey the impression that you know the patient intended to pay and it is only a matter of working out some suitable arrangements.
8 Keep the conversation brief and to the point, and avoid threats of any kind.
9 Try to get a definite commitment—payment of a certain amount by a certain date.
10 Follow up on promises. This is best accomplished by a tickler file or a note on your calendar. If the payment does not arrive by the promised date, remind the patient with another call. If you fail to do this, your whole effort has been wasted.

WHAT NOT TO DO

1 Do not call between 9 PM and 8 AM. To do so may be considered harassment.
2 Do not make repeated telephone calls.
3 Do not call the debtor's place of work if you know that the employer prohibits personal calls.
4 If you do place a call to the debtor at work and the person cannot take the call, you can leave a message asking the debtor to "call Mrs. Black at 727-9238" without revealing the nature of the call—that is, do not state that the call is from "Dr. Jones's office" or "Dr. Jones's medical assistant."
5 Do not lose your temper or show hostility. An angry patient is a poor-paying patient. Insulted patients often do not pay at all.

Telephone Collection Calls

A telephone call at the right time, in the right manner, is more effective than a collection letter. The personal contact of a telephone call will bring in more money than if a call is not made. In the absence of time to make calls, the collection letter is the next best avenue. If collections are a serious problem, it may pay to hire an extra person to do the telephoning. Written notification is a must before making a final demand for payment indicating that legal or collection proceedings will be started. There are no hard and fast rules for pursuing collections by telephone. You must handle each case individually on the basis of your own acquaintance or experience with the person involved.

Collection Letters

Some consultants believe that a printed collection letter or reminder enclosed with a statement is more effective than a personal letter. Their attitude is that a patient may be embarrassed by a personal letter and feel that he or she has been singled out for attention. An impersonal printed message will probably encourage the debtor to send a payment. The printed form is a time saver and is recommended if a lack of time is contributing to poor collection follow-up. Standard printed forms are readily available; you can also design your own forms.

Letters that are friendly requests for an explanation of why payment has not been made are still effective in many cases. These letters should indicate that the physician is sincerely interested in the patient and wishes to help straighten out the financial obligations. The patient should be invited to visit the office to explain the reasons for nonpayment so that, if possible, special arrangements can be worked out. To give the patient an opportunity to save face, these letters can suggest that the patient may have overlooked previous statements.

On receipt of such a letter, most patients make some effort to explain their failure to make payment. If a patient really is having financial difficulties, the physician may be able to get public assistance for him or her. Or, if it is a temporary financial embarrassment, the physician and the patient may together be able to work out a satisfactory installment plan for payment.

The medical assistant often is given a free hand in designing collection patterns and composing collection letters. Many medical assistants compose a series of collection letters, using model letters that they have found to be effective. Such a series usually includes at least five letters in varying degrees of forcefulness (Fig. 19–8).

Sometimes even the person with poor paying habits will pay the bill if treated with respect and consideration. See Figure 19–9 for a suggested collection program.

OBSERVE ESTABLISHED COLLECTION POLICY The medical assistant should never go beyond the authority granted by the physician in pursuing col-

lections. If you have questions about special collection problems, always check with the physician before proceeding. This is particularly important with patients whom you do not know personally—for example, patients whom the physician has seen in the hospital or at home and others for whom you have no credit history. It is difficult to say whether pressing collections too hard loses more good will of patients than not pursuing collections diligently enough. The physician and the medical assistant together should agree on general collection policies as outlined earlier in this chapter, and then the policies should be followed. In all cases in which an account is to be assigned to a collection agency, be certain that the physician is aware of it.

WHO SIGNS COLLECTION LETTERS? In most medical offices, the medical assistant signs collection letters with the identification "Assistant to Dr.

1. Your account has always been paid promptly in the past, so this must be an oversight. Please accept this note as a friendly reminder of your account due in the amount of $_____ .

2. Since your care in this office in March, we have had no word from you in regard to how you are feeling or your account due. If it is impossible for you to pay the full amount of $_____ at this time, please call this office before June 15 so that satisfactory arrangements can be worked out.

3. Medical bills are payable at the time of service unless special credit arrangements are made. Please send your check in full or call this office before June 30.

4. If you have some question about your statement, we will be happy to answer it for you. If not, may we have a payment before the end of this month?

5. Unless some definite arrangement is made to reduce your balance of $_____ , we can no longer carry your account on our books. Delinquent accounts are turned over to our collection agency on the 25th of the month.

6. **When a payment plan has been established, it can be reinforced by recognizing the first remittance with a letter of acknowledgment:**

   Thank you for the recent payment of $_____ on your account. We are glad to cooperate with you in this arrangement for clearing your account. We will look for your next check at about the same time next month, and your final payment the following month.

7. **When a payment schedule has been arranged by a telephone call, it can be confirmed by letter.**

   As agreed upon in our telephone conversation today, we will expect you to mail a payment of $50 on February 10; $50 on March 10; and the balance on April 10. If some emergency should prevent your making one of these payments on time, please notify us immediately by telephone.

DO'S AND DON'TS

DO:

1. Individualize letters to suit the situation.

2. Design your early letters as mere reminders of debt.

3. Always imply that the patient has good intentions to pay, until lack of response over a period of time proves otherwise.

4. Send letters with a firmer tone only after you have sent one or two friendly reminders.

DON'T

1. Use the same collection letter for a patient with good paying habits as for one who is known to neglect financial obligations.

2. Place an overdue notice of any kind on a postcard or on the outside of an envelope. This is an **invasion of privacy.**

FIGURE 19–8 Suggestions for composing collection letters.

GOAL	TIME	PROCEDURE
Inform patient of expected charges	Prior to or at time of service	Personal contact
Confirmation of charges	At time of service or next billing cycle	Billing statement
Reminder of charges or new balance	30 days after first billing	Billing statement with notation "Second Statement"
Determine whether there is a problem with payment or service	Prior to third billing	Telephone patient to arrange payment commitment
If previous step was unsuccessful or not completed	At 60 days	Third billing with note (see Fig. 19-4)
Ask for definite date and dollar amount of payment	Prior to fourth billing	Telephone patient; must have definite plan
Final notice 15 days before sending to collection	At 90 days	Fourth billing; send final notice (see Fig. 19-5) by certified mail with return receipt requested
	At 105 days	Send to collector

FIGURE 19–9 Suggested collection program.

Brown" or "Financial Secretary" below the typewritten signature. Some physicians may wish to personally sign these communications, but generally the medical assistant who handles the accounts also signs the collection letters.

Personal Interviews

Personal interviews with patients can sometimes be more effective than a whole series of collection letters. By talking to a patient face to face, you can come to an understanding of the problem more quickly and reach an agreement about future payment plans.

Occasionally, a patient may undergo a long course of treatment and yet make no attempt to pay anything on account. Perhaps such a patient is only waiting for the physician or the medical assistant to suggest that a payment be made. When there is advance knowledge that the patient will require extensive treatment, the matter of payment should be discussed early in the course of treatment, the credit policy explained, and some agreement reached as to a payment plan.

Because the fee for medical services is far more intangible than that of any commercial account, collection efforts must not be delayed too long. Any responsible, sincere patient will call or write the physician's office after receiving a second statement and explain the delay in payment or ask for a payment plan.

If it becomes necessary to refer the account to a collector, a good agency should have a 35% to 40% recovery rate with an account that is assigned within 4 or 5 months. This may drop to 25% if the account is held only a few more months. If recovery by the agency is greater than 40%, it may indicate that the collection effort by the medical assistant needs to be intensified.

The value of medical accounts diminishes in direct proportion to the length of time that has elapsed since service was rendered. Do not fight the law of diminishing returns. All collection activity is costly. Know when to stop and call on the services of a professional agency.

Memory Jogger

6 *What are the procedural options for the medical assistant in pursuing collections?*

SPECIAL COLLECTION SITUATIONS

Tracing "Skips"

When a statement is returned marked "Moved—no forwarding address," you may consider this account as a "skip." This generally is accepted as an indication that the patient is attempting to avoid liability for debts. Some so-called skips are innocent errors. The person may have been careless in not leaving a forwarding address. Or the mistake may have occurred in the physician's office; the wrong name or address may have been placed on the statement.

However, immediate action should be taken in regard to returned statements. Do not wait until the next billing time to attempt to trace the debtor (see Suggestions for Tracing Skips).

SUGGESTIONS FOR TRACING SKIPS

1 Examine the patient's original office registration card.
2 Call the telephone number listed on the card. Occasionally a patient may move without leaving a forwarding address but will transfer the old telephone number. Or the new telephone number will be given when you call the old number.
3 If you are unable to contact the individual by telephone, make a few discreet calls to the references listed on the registration card to get leads.
4 Check the *City Directory* to secure the names and telephone numbers of neighbors or the landlord, and contact these persons to secure information about the debtor's whereabouts.
5 Do not inform a third party that the person owes you money. Simply state that you are trying to locate or verify the location of the individual.
6 Check the debtor's place of employment for information. If the person is a specialist in his or her field of work, the local union or similar organizations may be contacted. Although they may not give you the person's current address, they will relay the message that you are seeking to contact him or her. Often, people will be stirred into paying a bill if they think that their employer may learn of their payment failure.
7 Do not communicate with a third party more than once. This is specifically forbidden by law (Public Law 95-109, Sec. 804) unless the third party requests the collector to do so.

The tracing of skips is a challenge to any medical assistant. A certified letter can be sent; by paying additional fees, you can request the Postal Service to obtain a receipt including the address where the letter was delivered. The certified letter may be sent in a plain envelope so that the patient will not refuse to accept the letter because of the return address.

If all your attempts fail, turn the account over to your collection agency without delay. Do not keep a skip account too long, because the trail may become so cold as time elapses that even collection experts will be unable to follow it.

Claims Against Estates

A bill owed by a deceased patient may be handled a little differently than regular bills. Courtesy dictates that a bill not be sent during the initial period of bereavement, but do not delay more than 30 days. The person responsible for settling the affairs of the estate will be assembling outstanding accounts and will expect to receive the medical bills along with all others. Address the statement to

Estate of (name of patient)
c/o (spouse or next of kin, if known)
Patient's last known address

Do not address the statement to a relative unless you have a signed agreement that that person will be responsible. If for some reason the statement cannot be addressed as just suggested (e.g., if the patient was in a convalescent home and you do not know the name of a relative), you may seek information from the county seat in the county in which the estate is being settled.

A will is generally filed within 30 days of a death. A request to the Probate Department of the Superior Court, County Recorder's Office, will usually provide you with the name of the executor or administrator. The time limits for filing an estate claim are determined by the state in which the decedent resided.

After the name of the administrator or executor of the estate has been obtained, a duplicate itemized statement of the account should be sent to that person by certified mail, return receipt requested, so that you will know who received it. If no response is received in 10 days, you should contact the executor or the county clerk where the estate is being settled and obtain forms for filing claim against the estate. (Some states do not have special claim forms but will accept simple itemized statements.) This claim against the estate must be made within a certain length of time, varying from 2 to 36 months, depending on the state in which it is filed.

The executor of the estate will either accept or reject the claim and, if it is accepted, will send an acknowledgment of the debt. Payment is often delayed, owing to the legal complications in settling an estate, but if the claim has been accepted, you will receive your money in due time. If the claim is rejected and you have full justification for claiming the bill, you must file claim against the executor within a limited time, according to state laws. The time limit in such cases starts with the date on the letter of rejection that was sent you in response to your original claim.

Because states have different time limits and statutes in regard to such matters, it is advisable for the medical assistant to contact the physician's attorney or the local court for the exact procedure to follow.

Bankruptcy

Bankruptcy laws were passed to secure equal distribution of the assets of an individual among the individual's creditors. Bankruptcy laws are federal and are applicable in all states. When you are notified that a patient has declared bankruptcy, you should no longer send statements or make any attempt to collect on the account from the patient.

Chapter VII bankruptcy is usually a "no asset" situation. Because the physician's fee is an unsecured debt, there is little purpose in pursuing collection.

Chapter XIII is known as "Adjustment of Debts of an Individual with Regular Income," according to the Revised Bankruptcy Act of October 1, 1979. Under Chapter XIII, the patient/debtor pays a fixed amount (agreed on by the court) to the trustee in bankruptcy. This is then passed on to the creditors. During this period, none of the creditors can attach the debtor's wages or otherwise attempt to collect the debt. It is sometimes beneficial to file a claim under Chapter XIII because small payments will be made by the debtor under the supervision of the court over a period of 3 years.

STATUTES OF LIMITATIONS

A **statute of limitations** assigns a certain time after which rights cannot be enforced by action.

Malpractice Statutes

In many states, there are statutes of limitations applicable to malpractice lawsuits, which set a limit to the time during which malpractice actions can be filed. It is usually best to wait until this time has passed before pressing the account of a patient who may feel he or she is entitled to sue the physician. However, this should not be made a blanket policy; each case should be judged on its own merit.

Collection Statutes

Statutes of limitations affecting collections prescribe the time within which a legal collection suit may be rendered against a debtor; the term *outlaw* is sometimes used to refer to debts on which the time limit has passed. This legal time limit varies according to the state in which the debt is incurred. Table 19–1 lists the time limits for collections in the various states. It should be noted that if the debtor moves out of state, either temporarily or permanently, the time spent out of state is not included in the time limit. Only the time during which the debtor resides within the state is included in the statute.

The time limit may vary according to the class of account. Generally, accounts may be placed in one of three classes:

* Open book accounts
* Written contracts
* Single-entry accounts

OPEN BOOK ACCOUNTS Open book accounts are accounts on the books that are open to charges

TABLE 19–1 **Statute of Limitations**

Location	Open Accounts (Years)	Contracts in Writing (Years)
Alabama	3	6
Alaska	6	6
Arizona	3	6
Arkansas	3	5
California	4	4
Colorado	6	6
Connecticut	6	6
Delaware	3	6
District of Columbia	3	3
Florida	4	5
Georgia	4	6
Hawaii	6	6
Idaho	4	5
Illinois	5	10
Indiana	6	10
Iowa	5	10
Kansas	3	5
Kentucky	5	15
Louisiana	3	10
Maine	6	6
Maryland	3	3
Massachusetts	6	6
Michigan	6	6
Minnesota	6	6
Mississippi	3	6
Missouri	5	10
Montana	5	8
Nebraska	4	5
Nevada	4	6
New Hampshire	6	6
New Jersey	6	6
New Mexico	4	6
New York	6	6
North Carolina	3	3
North Dakota	6	6
Ohio	6	15
Oklahoma	3	5
Oregon	6	6
Pennsylvania	6	6
Rhode Island	6	6
South Carolina	6	6
South Dakota	6	6
Tennessee	6	6
Texas	4	4
Utah	4	6
Vermont	6	6
Virginia	3	5
Washington	3	6
West Virginia	5	10
Wisconsin	6	6
Wyoming	8	10
Puerto Rico	15	—

From Summary of Collection Laws published in the American Collectors Association, Inc., 1986 Membership Roster. (Reprinted with permission of American Collectors Association, Inc., Minneapolis, MN.)

made from time to time. The bill for each illness or treatment is computed separately, and the last date of entry—debit or credit—for that specific illness is the time designated by the statute of limitations for starting that specific debt. It is almost impossible to have a time limit on an account of a patient with a chronic condition, because there is no actual termination of the illness or treatment unless the patient changes physicians or dies. When legal time limits are set, they usually refer to these "open book accounts."

WRITTEN CONTRACTS Written contracts often have the same time limit as open book accounts, but in some states they have a longer time limit. The time limit on written contracts starts from the date due.

SINGLE-ENTRY ACCOUNTS Single-entry accounts are accounts with only one entry or charge. These accounts are usually short-lived and are for small amounts. Some states, such as California, place a shorter statute of limitations span on such accounts.

In many states, even though the legal time limit set by the statutes has passed, the account may be reopened and the date extended if you are able to obtain a written acknowledgment of the debt due. For instance, a letter from the patient stating "Yes, I know I owe you $150, but I do not intend paying Dr. Brown" is an acknowledgment of the debt. If this letter is signed and dated, keep it and contact your collector. On the basis of this letter, the collector can then proceed with collection. Also, a small payment on the account will extend the statute expiration date. Photocopy these small checks for proof of payment, should proof become necessary.

Memory Jogger

7 *Define statute of limitations.*

Using Outside Collection Assistance

When you have done everything possible internally to follow up on an outstanding account and have not received payment, the question arises as to what step to take next.

- Should your facility sue for the payment?
- Should the account be sent to a collection agency?
- Should the account be written off as a bad debt?

Before forcing an account, you must first consider the time element: Has the patient been given a fair chance to pay this bill? Have you sent statements regularly and used a systematic method of following the account? Ask yourself if there might be a misunderstanding about the fee charged. Did you fully itemize the first statement? A large unexplained bill may frighten a patient into making no payments at all because the whole balance looks too large.

If you have used correct registration forms to secure advance credit information, you should know the financial abilities of the patient to pay. However, illness may have caused a loss of salary and re-

sulted in temporary inability to pay. Try to thoroughly analyze the situation.

Could the patient have been dissatisfied with the care received? For some unknown reason, a patient may feel that he or she was not treated correctly. Perhaps the patient expected a complete cure too soon. Only an explanation of the condition, prognosis, and care can enlighten such patients, and this is best handled by the physician. If payment of a bill is pressed too hard and the patient is dissatisfied for some reason, a malpractice suit may be filed by the patient to "get even."

COLLECTING THROUGH THE COURT SYSTEM

Making the Decision to Sue

Will a physician lose more good will by suing for a bill than by writing it off as a loss? One management official has related that, strangely enough, when a physician-client sued two patients for large amounts, the patients lost the cases, paid up, and were back in the office for treatment very shortly! However, most physicians believe it is unwise to resort to the court to collect medical bills unless there are extraordinary circumstances.

An account must be considered a 100% loss to the physician before legal proceedings are started. Remember that you should never threaten to instigate legal proceedings unless you are prepared to carry out the threat and have the physician's consent to issue such a warning.

If the physician decides in favor of a lawsuit, investigate thoroughly before taking action. Litigation to collect a bill is generally in order when the

1. Patient can afford to pay without hardship.
2. Physician can produce office records that support the bill.
3. Physician can justify the size of the bill by comparison with fee practices in the community.
4. Patient's general condition after treatment is satisfactory.
5. Persuasive powers of an ethical collection agency have been exhausted, and the agency advises suing.
6. Patient can be given ample warning of the physician's intention to sue.
7. Defendant (whether a patient or a parent or legal guardian) is legally liable for the services rendered to the patient.
8. Defendant is not judgment proof.*
9. Statute of limitations has ruled out any possible malpractice action.
10. Physician is not bubbling over with indignation and is not in a "he-can't-do-this-to-me" frame of mind.

---

*The Soldiers and Sailors Civil Relief Act (1940) protects the rights of servicemen and women on active duty.

The experienced practitioner establishes these 10 "whens" before plunging into costly litigation.

Small Claims Court

Many medical practices find the small claims court a satisfactory and inexpensive way to collect delinquent accounts. The law places a limit on the amount of debt for which relief may be sought in the small claims court. Because this varies from state to state (from $300 to $5000) and in some instances even within a state, this limit should be checked locally before seeking recovery in this manner.

Parties to small claims actions cannot be represented by an attorney at the trial but may send another person to court in their behalf to produce records supporting the claim. Physicians often send their bookkeeper or medical assistant with records of unpaid accounts to show the judge.

If the court awards a judgment for the amount owed, the plaintiff in small claims court may also recover the costs of the suit. For a very small investment in time and money, the physician who uses this method has

- Saved the time of a regular court action
- Had no attorney's fee to pay
- Not sacrificed the commission charged by a collection agency

After being awarded a judgment, you must still collect the money. The only person in a small claims action who has the right of appeal is the defendant. An appeal by the defendant may have the judgment set aside. The plaintiff cannot file an appeal in a small claims action; the decision of the court is final.

The necessary papers for filing action and full instructions on the course to follow may be obtained from the clerk of the small claims court. The medical assistant who has never appeared in the court would probably be wise to attend once as only a spectator, to preview the procedure and feel more at ease when appearing for the physician.

A collection agency to which an account may have been assigned may not file or handle a small claims action. It must either sue in the regular municipal or justice court or attempt to collect the debt in some other manner.

USING A COLLECTION AGENCY

The medical assistant should try every means possible to collect accounts before they become delinquent. But as soon as the account is determined uncollectible through your office—that is, the patient has failed to respond to your final letter or has failed to fulfill a second promise on payment—send the account to the collector without delay. Skips should be assigned immediately.

Even though collection by an agency will mean sacrificing from 40% to 60% of the amount owed, further delay will only reduce the chances of recovery by the professional collector. If the agency finds that the case deserves special consideration, it will seek the physician's advice before proceeding further.

Selecting a Collection Agency

There are a number of agencies either owned and operated as an integral part of the county medical society or operated separately from the medical society but supervised by the medical profession. These bureaus provide specialized medical collection services.

Another type of collection agency is a division of the local credit association, recognized by the National Retail Credit Association. If the local credit association does not maintain a collection department, it will be able to recommend a reputable one. A nationally recognized credit association has considerable responsibility and a high standard to maintain. These factors serve as monitors to its reliability.

The most common type of collection agency throughout the United States is the privately owned and operated agency. Many of these work with the local professional societies and strive to keep their work on a high ethical standard. Because a few bureaus are unethical and unscrupulous in their tactics, care should be taken to be sure that the one you choose is reliable and ethical. For the sake of comparison, many health care facilities use two or three agencies.

Responsibilities to the Collection Agency

When you select a reputable agency and decide to make use of its services, you must be prepared to provide the agency with all the necessary data to enable it to begin prompt collection procedures on overdue accounts. The agency should receive

- Full name of the debtor
- Name of the spouse
- Last known address
- Full amount of the debt
- Date of the last entry on account (debit or credit)
- Occupation of the debtor
- Business address
- Any other pertinent data

After an account has been released to a collection agency, your office makes no further collection attempts. Once the agency has begun its work, follow these guidelines and procedures:

1. Send no more statements.
2. Mark the patient's ledger or stamp it so that you know it is now in the hands of the collector.
3. Refer the patient to the agency if he or she contacts you in regard to the account.
4. Promptly report any payments made directly to

your office (a percentage of this payment is due the agency).

5. Call the agency if you obtain any information that will be of value in tracing or collecting the account.

6. Do not push the agency with frequent calls. The representatives of the agency will report to you regularly and keep you posted on collection progress.

LEGAL AND ETHICAL ISSUES

Regularity in billing accounts is controlled by the Fair Credit Billing Act of October 28, 1975, which states that when a billing date for an account has been established, future mailings must not vary more than 5 days without notification to the debtor (patient). If there is a balance due or a credit balance of one dollar or more, the account must be billed every 30 days .

A bill for a minor must be addressed to a parent or legal guardian unless the minor is emancipated.

A threat to take any action against a debtor that cannot legally be taken or that is not intended to be taken is a violation of the federal Fair Debt Collection Practices Act 1977 Section 807 (5).

A person who has declared bankruptcy is protected from any further attempts to collect a debt, and the physician should discontinue sending bills.

Representation by an attorney is prohibited in actions of the small claims court.

We have checked and verified all statements made in this chapter about collection law and legal procedures. However, laws do change, and it is recommended that you check with your local state regulations and laws to verify points pertinent to your special area. State law takes precedence over federal law if the state law is stronger. For a general textbook of this nature, it is impossible to check each of these state requirements to determine which are stronger and which would prevail over federal Public Law 95–109.

CRITICAL THINKING

1 Some medical assistants are uncomfortable about asking a patient for payment. Examine your own feelings, leading to ease of making collections. Understand why the physician is justified in the need for payment, and how to explain this to the patient if questioned.

2 Study the age analysis chart in Figure 19–7. Evaluate the accounts of patients E, F, G, H.

HOW DID I DO? Answers to Memory Joggers

1 No further billing and bookkeeping expenses, and no risk of loss.

2 Provides basis for judging accounts objectively and equitably.

3 The Fair Credit Billing Act requires that the date of mailing a statement must not vary more than 5 days without notification to the debtor.

4 When the minor is emancipated.

5 Aging is a procedure of classifying accounts receivable by the length of time they have been owed and the probability of their being collectible.

6 Printed collection letter or reminder, personal letter, personal interview, telephone.

7 A certain time after which rights cannot be enforced by action.

REFERENCES

American Medical Association: The Business Side of Medical Practice, Chicago, AMA, 1989.
Fair Credit Billing Act, October 28, 1975.
Bankruptcy Act (Title II, U.S. Code), October 1, 1979.

Health Insurance and Managed Care

Sue Hunt, MA, RN, CMA

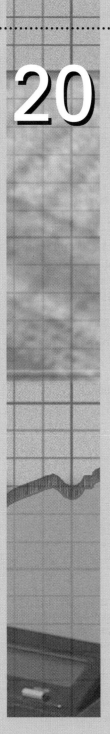

20

LEARNING OBJECTIVES

Cognitive: On successful completion of this chapter you should be able to:

1 Define the terms listed in the Vocabulary.
2 Cite three advantages of group insurance policies over individual policies.
3 Name seven major types of health insurance benefits.
4 State the meaning of the birthday law.
5 State the basic differences between indemnity and service benefit plans.
6 Describe the major government insurance plans.
7 Discuss the implications of managed care for the medical assistant.
8 Explain the differences between health maintenance organizations (HMOs), independent practice associations (IPAs), and preferred provider organizations (PPOs).
9 Describe the role of the medical assistant in obtaining referrals and authorizations for care.
10 Identify the legal implications of the medical records audit.

VOCABULARY

assignment of insurance benefits Statement authorizing the insurance company to pay benefits directly to the physician

beneficiary Person receiving the benefits of an insurance policy

birthday rule Rule governing the hierarchy of coordination of benefits

capitation Reimbursement to a health care provider as a fixed amount per member in a given time period

claim A demand to the insurer by the insured person for the payment of benefits under a policy

co-insurance Policy provision by which both the insured person and the insurer share in a specified ratio of the expenses resulting from an illness or injury

coordination of benefits The provision in an insurance contract that limits benefits to 100% of the cost

copayment A fixed dollar amount that the insured person must pay each time service is received

deductible A statement in an insurance policy that the insuring company will pay the expenses incurred after the insured person has paid a specified amount

disability The condition resulting from illness or injury that makes an individual unable to be employed

fee schedule A list of services or procedures indemnified by the insurance company and of the specific dollar amounts that will be paid for each service

fringe benefit A benefit granted by an employer that involves a money cost but does not affect the basic wage rates of employees

group policy Policy that covers a group (e.g., all employees of one company) under a master contract

indemnity Benefit paid by an insurer for a loss insured under a policy

individual policy Policy usually held by a person who does not qualify for a group policy

medically indigent Able to take care of ordinary living expenses but unable to afford medical care

member physician A physician who has agreed to accept the contracts of an insurer, usually including accepting the insurance benefits as payment in full

premium The periodic payment required to keep a policy in force

prepaid plan A plan that provides all covered services to a policyholder for payment of a monthly fee

rider Legal document that modifies the protection of a policy

service benefit plan Plan that agrees to pay for certain surgical and medical services and that is not restricted to a fee schedule

subscriber Person named as principal in an insurance contract

utilization review Approval for services by an outside group

Health insurance is an important factor in the practice of medicine. As a medical assistant, you must understand insurance terminology, types of insurance coverage, the importance of obtaining consent for release of information, the effect of **assignment of insurance benefits,** and how to handle a **claim.** You must also be able to communicate with patients about processing their insurance.

SKILLS AND RESPONSIBILITIES

INSURANCE CLAIM RESPONSIBILITIES

- Obtaining authorizations and referrals
- Preparing insurance claim forms
- Maintaining an insurance claims register
- Tracing unpaid claims
- Evaluating claims rejection
- Reporting procedures to prepaid care plans
- Translating medical terminology into procedural and diagnostic codes

Fifty years ago, health insurance as we know it now was uncommon. Today, most patients who come into a health care facility have some kind of health insurance coverage, either privately or through government-sponsored programs. Although the rapid growth of health insurance coverage is a recent phenomenon brought about by economic necessity, the concept of health insurance is not new. The first company organized specifically to write health insurance was founded in 1847. The nation's earliest accident insurance company came into being in 1850 in response to public demand for coverage against frequent rail and steamboat accidents of the mid-19th century. By the turn of the 20th century, 47 American companies were issuing accident insurance.

In its early stages, the emphasis of health insurance was directed toward replacement of income rather than toward hospital or surgical benefits. The early insurance company policy protected the policyholder against loss of earned income due to a limited number of diseases, including typhus, typhoid, scarlet fever, smallpox, diphtheria, diabetes, and a few others. Emphasis on insurance as a means of replacing income lost due to illness continued until 1929, the start of the Great Depression.

At this time, a group of schoolteachers formed an arrangement with Baylor Hospital in Dallas, Texas, to provide themselves with hospital care on a prepayment basis. This was the origin of the Blue Cross service concept for provision of hospital care.

A further major change occurred during World War II when the freezing of industrial wages made the **fringe benefit** a significant element of collective bargaining. Group health insurance became a large part of the fringe benefit package.

Memory Jogger

1 *Name seven tasks you may be expected to perform to process insurance.*

The Purpose of Health Insurance

Voluntary health insurance is designed to cover the cost of accidents or illness. In addition, there is an increasing trend for insurance policies to cover services that prevent illness (e.g., immunizations) or lead to early diagnosis (e.g., mammograms). Procedures that are not medically necessary (e.g., cosmetic surgery) or whose effectiveness is not proven (e.g., experimental procedures) are usually not covered.

COST OF COVERAGE

Few insurance policies pay all expenses resulting from accident or illness. The basic cost of health care coverage is a **premium,** monthly or annual, for which the insurer agrees to provide certain benefits. The real cost to the individual at the time of treatment includes

- Deductibles
- Copayment or co-insurance
- Services not covered

The **deductible** is that portion of the bill that a subscriber must pay before insurance coverage is effective. The amount of the deductible is stated in the contract.

A **copayment** is a contribution the subscriber must make to cover some portion of each bill. This could be $2 to $15 for each office visit. **Co-insurance** is a percentage of the total cost. The **subscriber** must also pay for services not covered by the insurance policy, such as eye examinations or dental care.

COORDINATION OF BENEFITS

Coordination of benefits (COB) or provisions to prevent duplicate payments for the same service are included in most group contracts. The purpose of COB provisions is to limit the benefits to 100% of the cost. If a plan does not have COB provisions, it becomes the primary payer and pays benefits first. Laws establishing which payer is primary, including the birthday law, were enacted in January 1987 in many states. In the case of an employed person who is eligible for Medicare benefits, the employer's plan is the primary carrier and Medicare is the supplemental carrier. In many families, both husband and wife are wage earners and, frequently, both are eligible for health insurance benefits through their own employment and that of their spouses.

COB follows the rules of the plan that is the primary payer. If both plans have COB provisions:

- The policyholder's own plan is primary for that individual. An exception occurs if the policyholder is laid off or retired and not a Medicare recipient. In this case, the policyholder's plan pays second.
- The primary coverage for dependents of policyholders is determined by the **birthday rule.** The insurance plan of the policyholder whose birthday comes first in the calendar year (month and day, not year) provides primary coverage for each dependent.
- If neither of the above situations applies, the plan that has been in existence longer is the primary payer.

The primary plan for dependents of legally separated or divorced parents is more complicated.

- The birthday rule is in effect if the parent who has custody of the dependent has not remarried. If the custodial parent has remarried, that parent's plan is primary for that dependent.
- If one parent has been decreed by the court as the responsible party, that parent's policy is primary. This is not always the parent with custody of the child.
- If one of the plans originated in a state that does not have the COB law, the plan that did originate in a state with a COB law will determine the order of benefits.

All of this emphasizes the need to determine whether there is a birthday rule in your state.

Memory Jogger

 2 *What are the real costs of coverage to an individual at the time of treatment?*

Availability of Health Insurance

Health insurance is available through a **group policy, individual policy,** and subscription to a **prepaid plan.** Many people are covered by government plans.

GROUP POLICIES

Insurance written under a group policy covers a group of people under a master contract, which is generally issued to an employer for the benefit of the employees. The individual employee may be given a certificate of insurance containing information regarding the master policy and indicating that the individual is covered under the policy. Professional associations also frequently offer group insurance as a benefit of membership.

Group coverage usually provides greater benefits at lower premiums, and a physical examination is seldom required for the enrollees. Every person in a group contract has identical coverage.

Memory Jogger

3 *Explain what the birthday rule means.*

INDIVIDUAL POLICIES

Individuals who do not qualify for inclusion in a group policy may apply to companies that offer individual policies. The applicant may be required to have a physical examination before acceptance and, if there is an unusual risk, may be denied insurance or may have to accept a **rider** or limitation on the policy. In any event, the individual premium will probably be greater and the benefits less than in a group policy.

GOVERNMENT PLANS

The federal government first became responsible for insuring a large group of people in 1956 with pas-

sage of Public Law 569. This law authorized dependents of military personnel to receive treatment by civilian physicians at the expense of the government. We know this today as the Civilian Health and Medical Program of the Uniformed Services (CHAMPUS).

In 1965 the federal government provided for another group, namely, the **medically indigent,** through a program that is still known as Medicaid. Title XIX of Public Law 89–97, under the Social Security Amendments of 1965, provided for agreements with states for assistance from the federal government to provide medical care for people who could not afford it.

Coverage for the patient older than age 65 years, called Medicare, went into effect on July 1, 1966. This plan was established under Social Security. The group of people eligible to receive Medicare was expanded in 1973 to cover disabled persons younger than 65 who had been receiving Social Security benefits, railroad retirement, or civil service retirement. This included disabled workers of any age, disabled widows, disabled dependent widowers and adults disabled before age 18 whose parents are eligible for or are retired on Social Security benefits, children and adults with end-stage renal disease, and kidney donors (including all expenses related to the kidney transplant).

The passage of the Health Maintenance Organization (HMO) Act in 1973 provided for federal aid to health insurance prepayment plans that met certain criteria. This brought about an accelerated growth of HMOs, which are organizations that provide for comprehensive health care to an enrolled group for a fixed periodic payment.

Title VI of the Social Security Amendments Act of 1983 contained the prospective payment system (PPS) for hospitals, which would begin the radical restructuring of the payment system to hospitals for Medicare inpatient services.

The most fundamental change in the determination of physicians' fees under Medicare since its inception was the resource-based relative value scale (RBRVS) reimbursement system put into effect in 1992.

Many large groups of people are covered by governmental insurance plans. The patient who is older than age 65 probably is covered by Part B of Medicare. The medically indigent patient may be eligible for Medicaid with or without Medicare. Dependents of military personnel are covered by CHAMPUS; surviving spouses and dependent children of veterans who died as a result of service-connected disabilities are covered by the Civilian Health and Medical Program of the Veterans Administration (CHAMPVA). Many wage earners are protected against the loss of wages and the cost of medical care resulting from occupational accident or disease through workers' compensation insurance. All of these plans are dealt with in more detail later in this chapter.

Memory Jogger

④ *What does medically indigent mean?*

Types of Insurance Benefits

An insurance package is tailored to the needs of each individual or group policy, and the combinations of benefits are limitless. A policy may contain any one or any combination of the following kinds of benefits.

HOSPITALIZATION

Hospital coverage pays the cost of all or part of the insured person's hospital room and board and special hospital services. Hospital insurance policies frequently set a maximum amount payable per day and a maximum number of days of hospital care. Some insurance companies require that the hospital be an accredited or a licensed hospital. Most hospital plans exclude admission for diagnostic studies.

SURGICAL

Surgical coverage pays all or part of the surgeon's fee; some plans also pay for an assistant surgeon. Surgery includes any incision or excision, removal of foreign bodies, aspiration, suturing, and reduction of fractures. The surgery may be accomplished in the hospital, in a doctor's office, or elsewhere. The insurer frequently provides the subscriber with a surgical fee schedule that sets forth the amount the insurer will pay for commonly performed procedures.

BASIC MEDICAL

Medical coverage pays all or part of the physician's fee for nonsurgical services, including hospital, home, and office visits. Usually there is a deductible amount payable by the patient as well as a copayment or co-insurance each time service is received. The insurance plan may include provision for diagnostic laboratory, x-ray, and pathology fees. Some medical plans do not cover routine physical examinations when the patient does not have a specific complaint or illness.

MAJOR MEDICAL

Major medical insurance (formerly called catastrophic coverage) provides protection against especially heavy medical bills resulting from catastrophic or prolonged illnesses. It may be a supplement to basic medical coverage or a comprehensive integrated program providing both basic and major medical protection.

DISABILITY (LOSS OF INCOME) PROTECTION

Weekly or monthly cash benefits are provided to employed policyholders who become unable to work owing to an accident or illness. Many policies do not start payment until after a specified number of days or until a certain number of sick leave days have been used. Payment is made directly to the patient and is intended to replace loss of income resulting from illness. It is not intended for payment of specific medical bills.

Memory Jogger

⑤ *What does basic medical mean?*

DENTAL CARE

Dental coverage is included in many fringe benefit packages. Some policies are based on a copayment and incentive program, with the company's copayment increasing each year until 100% coverage is reached.

VISION CARE

Vision care insurance may include reimbursement for all or for a percentage of the cost for refraction, lenses, and frames.

MEDICARE SUPPLEMENT

These are contracts insuring persons 65 years of age or older that supplement the coverage provided by Medicare. Federal regulation now requires these contracts to be uniform in benefits to decrease confusion for the purchaser.

SPECIAL CLASS INSURANCE

Applicants for health insurance who cannot qualify for a standard policy by reason of health may be issued special class insurance with limited coverage.

SPECIAL RISK INSURANCE

This insurance protects a person in the event of a certain type of accident, such as automobile or airplane crashes, or for certain diseases, such as tuberculosis or cancer. There is usually a maximum benefit.

LIABILITY INSURANCE

There are many types of liability insurance, including automobile, business, and homeowners' policies. Liability policies often include benefits for medical expenses payable to individuals who are injured in the insured person's home or car, without regard to the insured person's actual legal liability for the accident.

LIFE INSURANCE

Life insurance policies sometimes provide monthly cash benefits if the policyholder becomes permanently and totally disabled. Sometimes, the proceeds from life insurance are used to meet the expenses of the insured person's last illness.

How Benefits Are Determined

Insurance benefits may be determined and paid in one of several ways:

- By indemnity schedules
- By service benefit plans
- By determination of the usual, customary, and reasonable fee
- By relative value studies

INDEMNITY SCHEDULES

In **indemnity** plans, the insurer agrees to pay the subscriber a set amount of money for a given procedure or service. The insured person is given a schedule of indemnities (**fee schedule**) when the policy is purchased.

Indemnity plans do not agree to pay for the complete services rendered. Often there is a difference in the amount paid by the insurance company and the amount of the physician's fee. For example, the insurer may agree to pay up to $1000 for a specific operation, with no consideration for the time or complications of the surgery. If the physician charges $1200, the difference of $200 is the responsibility of the patient.

This type of plan takes the major expense out of medical bills and helps to keep the premiums down. The amount of the premium often determines the schedule of benefits. Indemnity benefits are usually paid to the person insured unless that person has authorized payment directly to the provider.

SERVICE BENEFIT PLANS

In **service benefit plans,** the insuring company agrees to pay for certain surgical or medical services without additional cost to the person insured. There is no set fee schedule.

In a service benefit plan, surgery with complications would warrant a higher fee than an uncomplicated procedure. Premiums are sometimes higher for this type of coverage, but often payments are larger. Frequently, the payment for benefits is sent directly to the physician and is considered full payment for the services rendered.

USUAL, CUSTOMARY, AND REASONABLE FEE

Some insurance companies agree to pay on the basis of all or a percentage of the physician's usual, customary, and reasonable fee. Charges for a specific service are compared to a database of charges for the same service to other patients by the same physician and to patients by other physicians in the same geographic area. The insurance company determines whether the charge is usual, customary, and reasonable. Any amount over the limit determined by the insurance company will not be paid.

RESOURCE-BASED RELATIVE VALUE SCALE

This is the fee schedule that is the basis for payment to physicians for services provided under Medicare Part B since 1992. This system was implemented to standardize payments with an adjustment for overhead costs in different geographic areas. More specific information regarding RBRVS is provided in Chapter 21.

Memory Jogger

6 *Name four ways benefits are determined.*

Kinds of Plans

BLUE CROSS AND BLUE SHIELD

In the early 1930s, hospitals introduced Blue Cross plans to provide coverage for hospital costs. Today, there are local Blue Cross plans operating in all states of the United States, the District of Columbia, Canada, Puerto Rico, and Jamaica.

In 1939, state medical societies in California and Michigan began sponsoring health plans to provide medical and surgical services; these became known as Blue Shield plans. Other states soon followed, and today Blue Shield is the largest medical prepayment system in the country.

Early in its development, Blue Shield was often known as the doctor's plan. A **member physician** agreed to bill Blue Shield for services to subscribers and abide by other prearranged procedures. Under many Blue Shield contracts, physicians accept Blue Shield's payment as payment in full for covered services. Blue Shield and its member physicians agree on methods of reimbursement in advance of the service performed.

In many plans, Blue Shield provides the medical and surgical coverage and Blue Cross provides hospital coverage. However, in some areas, Blue Cross plans write medical and surgical insurance in addition to providing hospital coverage. Conversely, some Blue Shield plans offer hospital insurance as well as medical and surgical coverage.

Blue Cross benefits are normally paid to the provider of service. In some cases, a check issued jointly to the provider and the person insured is sent to the latter, who must then endorse and forward it to the provider. Blue Shield makes direct payment to member physicians. For services of a nonmember physician, the payment is sent to the subscriber.

BC/BS identification cards usually carry the subscriber's name and identification number with a three-character alphabetical prefix. The letters are an important part of the number and must be included on the claim form (Fig. 20–1).

BLUE CARD

The Blue Shield Reciprocity has been replaced by an improved service known as the Blue Card Program. It is designed to serve subscribers while they are traveling or covered by a Blue Plan in another area. The Blue Card may cover Blue Shield only, Blue Cross only, or a combination of the two programs.

FOUNDATIONS FOR MEDICAL CARE

A foundation for medical care is a management system for community health services. It takes the form of an organization created by local physicians through their medical society, and it concerns itself with the quality and cost of medical care. Under the foundation concept, the following procedure occurs:

1. An insurance company sells and negotiates the policy. It collects the premiums, assumes all the risks, and reimburses the foundation for the cost of the claims office.
2. The foundation sets policy standards; receives, processes, reviews, and pays claims to doctors;

sets maximum fees based on current fees in the area; elects doctor-members yearly; and continually studies local medical-economic problems.
3. Member doctors agree to accept foundation fees as full payment under foundation-approved policies. The local medical society legally controls the foundation and selects foundation trustees.
4. The patient selects the doctor of his or her own choice; the patient or the patient's union or employer pays the premium directly to the insurance company.

COMMERCIAL INSURERS

Many people are covered by health insurance issued by private (commercial) insurance companies. Physicians and medical societies control neither the premiums paid nor the benefits received from such policies. For traditional types of policies payment is normally made to the subscriber unless the subscriber has authorized that payment be made directly to the physician. For HMOs, payment is made directly to the physician.

GOVERNMENT PLANS

Medicare

There are two distinct parts (A and B) to the Medicare program.

PART A: HOSPITAL INSURANCE Retired people 65 years of age and older and other people who receive monthly Social Security or railroad retirement checks are automatically enrolled for hospital insurance benefits and pay no premiums for this insurance. Part A is financed by special contributions paid by employed individuals as deductions from their salary, with matching contributions from their employers. These sums are collected along with regular Social Security contributions from wages and self-employment income earned during a person's working years. There is a significant deductible that the hospitalized patient must pay toward the hospital expenses.

Medicare health insurance cards identify if a person has Part A alone or has both Part A and Part B insurance. A patient whose Medicare claim number ends in the letter "A" will have the same Social Security number and Medicare number. If the person has different Social Security numbers and Medicare numbers, the Medicare number ends in a "B" or a "D" (Fig. 20–2).

PART B: MEDICAL INSURANCE Those persons who are eligible for Part A are eligible for Part B but must apply for this coverage and pay a monthly premium. Some federal employees and former fed-

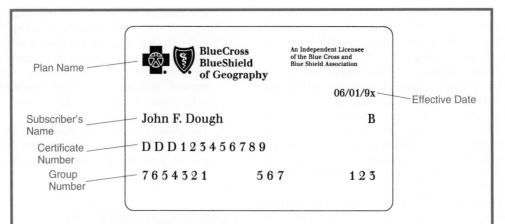

Blue Cross and Blue Shield Plan

Blue Cross Plan

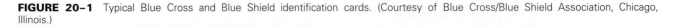

FIGURE 20–1 Typical Blue Cross and Blue Shield identification cards. (Courtesy of Blue Cross/Blue Shield Association, Chicago, Illinois.)

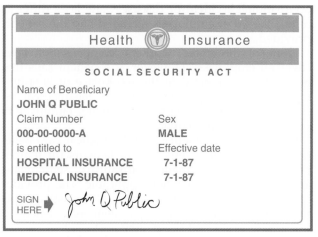

FIGURE 20–2 Medicare identification card.

eral employees who are not eligible for Social Security benefits and Part A may still enroll in Part B. Certain disabled persons younger than age 65 years are also eligible for Medicare.

The patient with Medicare Part B has to meet an annual deductible before benefits become available, after which Medicare pays 80% of the covered benefits. Usually the physician accepts assignment of benefits for Medicare patients and is paid directly. In these cases the physician must accept the payment that Medicare allows and bills the patient for 20% of the charge allowed by Medicare. If the physician does not accept assignment, the patient must pay the entire bill (which cannot be greater than the limit set by Medicare for nonparticipating physicians), and the patient will receive a check from Medicare.

Many Medicare enrollees also carry private supplemental insurance that pays the deductible and the 20% copayment.

Medicaid

Title XIX of Public Law 89–97 under the Social Security Amendments of 1965 provides for agreements with states for assistance from the federal government in providing health care for the medically indigent. All states and the District of Columbia have Medicaid programs, but wide variations may exist among these programs.

The federal government provides basic funding to the state, after which the states individually elect whether to provide funds for extension of benefits. The state determines the type and extent of medical care that will be covered within the minimum requirements established by the federal government. Some local areas and states are developing HMOs that serve only the patients who qualify for Medicaid.

The physician may accept or decline to treat Medicaid patients. The physician who does accept Medicaid patients automatically agrees to accept Medi-

caid payment as payment in full for covered services. The patient cannot be billed for the difference between the Medicaid fee and the physician's normal fee. The patient can be billed for any services that are not covered by Medicaid. Eligibility for benefits is determined by the respective states.

> **EXAMPLES OF INDIVIDUALS WHO QUALIFY FOR ELIGIBILITY BENEFITS**
>
> - Persons receiving certain types of federal and state aid
> - Persons who are medically needy (i.e., they can provide for the expenses of daily living but are unable to afford medical care)
> - Recipients of Aid to Families with Dependent Children
> - Persons who receive Supplemental Security Income (SSI)
> - Qualified Medicare Beneficiaries (QMB) (pays Medicare Part B premiums, deductibles, and co-insurance for qualified low-income elderly)
> - Persons in institutions or other long-term care in nursing facilities and intermediate care facilities
> - Medicaid purchase of COBRA coverage (low income persons who lose employer health insurance coverage)

A benefits identification card (BIC), which looks like a white credit card, or sticker/label showing proof of eligibility is usually issued to the beneficiary. The BIC is verified by a point of service (POS) device similar to a credit card verification. The medical assistant must verify coverage each time the patient comes into the office before being seen if the state uses a BIC.

Medi/Medi

Some patients who qualify for Medicare are still unable to pay the portion for which they are responsible and may qualify for both Medicare and Medicaid. Medicare is the primary coverage, and any residual is paid by the Medicaid assistance program. Claims submitted for coverage under Medicare and Medicaid are sometimes referred to as crossover claims.

Memory Jogger

7 *What does BIC stand for?*

Military Medical Benefits

CHAMPUS In 1956, the passage of Law 569 authorized dependents of military personnel to receive in-hospital treatment by civilian physicians at the expense of the government. This program was first

...ied Medicare but was later changed to CHAMPUS.

On September 30, 1966, the Military Medical Benefits Amendment Act of 1966 became law. This act added outpatient care benefits, including prescription drugs, to the in-hospital benefits previously allowed. Military retirees and their dependents as well as dependents of deceased members became eligible for outpatient benefits in January 1967.

To receive CHAMPUS benefits, eligible persons must be enrolled in the Defense Enrollment Eligibility Reporting System (DEERS), a computerized database that is used for verifying eligibility.

Benefits under CHAMPUS are limited to (1) dependents of active-duty personnel, (2) retirees and their dependents, and (3) dependents of service personnel who have died in active duty.

CHAMPVA In 1973, a program similar to CHAMPUS was established for the spouses and dependent children of veterans suffering total, permanent, service-connected disabilities and for the surviving spouses and dependent children of veterans who have died as a result of service-connected disabilities. This is called the Civilian Health and Medical Program of the Veterans Administration (CHAMPVA).

Eligibility is determined, and identification cards are issued, by the nearest Veterans Affairs medical center. The insured persons then are free to choose their own private physicians. Benefits and cost-sharing features are the same as those for CHAMPUS beneficiaries who are military retirees or their dependents and dependents of deceased members of the military.*

CHAMPUS/TRICARE MANAGED CARE In 1993 the Department of Defense contracted to provide an alternative managed care system for CHAMPUS beneficiaries in the states of California and Hawaii. It has continued to expand to other states and is expected to be available in all 50 states before 2000. Only CHAMPUS-eligible persons have the option of TRICARE Managed Care. It is not available to CHAMPVA or Medicare recipients. CHAMPUS/TRICARE offers three options: TRICARE/PRIME (HMO), TRICARE/EXTRA (PPO), and TRICARE STANDARD, which is the same as standard CHAMPUS.

WORKERS' COMPENSATION

All state legislatures have passed workers' compensation laws to protect wage earners against the loss of wages and the cost of medical care resulting from occupational accident or disease. State laws differ as to the classes of employees included and the benefits provided.

None of the states' workers' compensation laws cover all employees. However, if a patient says that he or she was injured in the workplace or is suffering from a work-associated illness, the medical assistant should check with the patient's employer to verify the insurance coverage.

Compensation benefits include medical care benefits, weekly income replacement benefits for temporary disability, permanent **disability** settlements, and survivor benefits when applicable. The provider of service (e.g., doctor, hospital, therapist) accepts the workers' compensation payment as payment in full and does not bill the patient.

Time limitations are set forth for the prompt reporting of workers' compensation cases. The employee is obligated to promptly notify the employer; the employer, in turn, must notify the insurance company and must refer the employee to a source of medical care. In some states, the employer and the insurance company have the right to select the physician who will treat the patient. In essence, the purpose of workers' compensation laws is to provide prompt medical care to the injured or ill worker so that the person may be restored to health and return to full earning capacity in as short a time as possible.

LIFE INSURANCE

When an individual whom the physician is treating or has treated in the past makes application for life insurance, the insuring company naturally wants to know the current state of the applicant's health and any significant past medical history.

To get an account of the applicant's current state of health, the insurance company authorizes a health care professional (physician or nurse, depending on the state) to perform physical examinations of prospective clients.

The insurance company's agent arranges the applicant's appointment for the physical examination and supplies the necessary forms for completion. After the examination, a report is sent to the insurance company. The company may require that the forms be completed in the examiner's own handwriting. The insurance company pays a stipulated amount on receipt of the report.

For a summary of the applicant's past medical history, the agent asks the applicant to supply the names and addresses of any physicians consulted in the past. The company, in turn, requests reports from these physicians. Your physician may receive a request for such information concerning a current or previous patient. Before completing the form, make certain that the applicant has signed an authorization for release of information to that insurance carrier.

---

*Further information regarding these military medical benefit programs may be obtained by writing to OCHAMPUS, Aurora, CO 80045-6900.

The request form usually has a voucher check for a minimal fee attached. The physician may accept the proffered fee or, if it is inadequate, may bill the insurance company for balance of fee. If the bill is reasonable, it is paid without question.

DISABILITY INSURANCE

MANDATED Several states require that employees be covered by nonindustrial disability (time loss) insurance. A small percentage (ranging from 0.3% to 1.2%) of the employee's salary may be deducted to cover the cost of this insurance. All regular employees, part or full time, are covered until they retire.

The weekly benefits are based on the employee's salary and calculated using a predetermined formula. There is a waiting period before benefits begin (usually 7 days) and a time limit ranging from 26 to 52 weeks for benefits to continue.

VOLUNTARY In states that do not have mandated disability insurance, employees or groups may seek coverage from a commercial carrier.

Managed Care

What is managed care? *Managed care* is a term used for a variety of prepaid health plans developed to provide health services at low cost. Under managed care, a medical group such as a health maintenance organization (HMO) or an independent practice association (IPA) is contracted to assume some of the responsibilities of the insurance company, that is, claims processing, provider relations, member services, utilization review, and eligibility. The primary care physician (PCP), selected by the patient, manages all patient services.

There has been mass confusion at times of what an HMO is. Some will refer to their insurance company as their HMO, some will refer to their PCP as their HMO, and some will refer to their medical group as their HMO. At first, an HMO and IPA were both simply two entities of medical groups; but with the daily changes of managed care, the entire organization is now considered as an HMO with different functions (Fig. 20–3).

In the traditional type of HMO, the HMO builds a medical group of physicians (PCPs and specialists) who agree to be paid on a per-patient basis instead of a fee-for-service basis. The HMO contracts with employers to provide health service for their employees. The member of an HMO selects a PCP from the medical group. Under an HMO without a foundation, the HMO is responsible for all but limited administrative needs of a PCP, including processing of **capitation** and/or fee-for-service checks.

In an IPA, an organization of physicians (a foundation for medical care) will contract with several employers to provide health services in the same way as an HMO. The IPA contracts with physicians, specialists, hospitals, and laboratories in the community and the member/patient will select a PCP under the IPA. Under an IPA, physicians or group practices will contract to tap into the IPA's health plans (insurance contracts). In return, the IPA will provide member physicians with administrative services either partially or in full. The IPA will receive all capitation monies, keep a contracted percentage for its services, process all the capitation checks, and will forward all the printed checks to the administrator for approval.

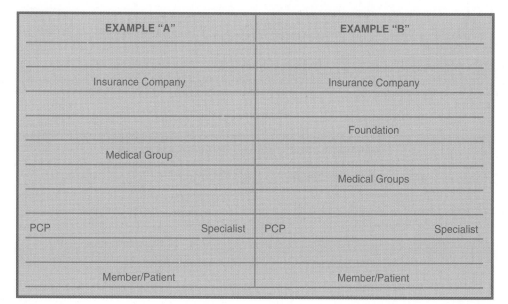

EXAMPLE "A"	EXAMPLE "B"
Insurance Company	Insurance Company
	Foundation
Medical Group	Medical Groups
PCP Specialist	PCP Specialist
Member/Patient	Member/Patient

FIGURE 20–3 Examples of organizational levels of medical groups. *A,* Without foundation. *B,* With foundation.

INSURANCES ACCEPTED BY PHYSICIAN(S); CREDENTIALED			
NAME	ADDRESS	PR CONTACT NAME AND TELEPHONE #	MS CONTACT NAME AND TELEPHONE #

FIGURE 20–4   Telephone list for provider relations (PR) and member services (MS).

CONTRACTED HOSPITAL(S)				
	NAME	ADDRESS	TELEPHONE	CONTACT
1				
2				
3				
4				

A

CONTRACTED URGENT CARE CENTER(S) - ANCILLARY				
	NAME	ADDRESS	TELEPHONE	CONTACT
1				
2				
3				
4				

B

FIGURE 20–5   *A,* Telephone directory for contracted hospitals. *B,* Telephone directory for contracted urgent care centers.

ANCILLARY PROVIDERS

RADIOLOGY - usually capitated

	NAME	ADDRESS	TELEPHONE	CONTACT
1				
2				
3				

LAB(S) - usually capitated

	NAME	ADDRESS	TELEPHONE	CONTACT
1				
2				
3				

HOME CARE SERVICES - available through medical group

	NAME	ADDRESS	TELEPHONE	CONTACT
1				
2				
3				

FIGURE 20–6   Lists for ancillary providers.

When you work in a physician's office, you will most likely be working with one or more managed care plans. You will need to maintain a list of telephone and fax numbers for the following: provider relations, member services, claims department, utilization review/utilization management, eligibility, and medical director (Figs. 20–4 through 20–6).

HEALTH MAINTENANCE ORGANIZATION

The HMO is what first comes to mind when we speak of prepaid plans. An HMO plan agrees to provide specific services to every enrolled member for a prepaid fee. When a health insurance carrier is involved, it contracts to pay in advance for the full range of health services to which the insured is entitled under the terms of the health insurance contract.

Public Law 93-222, the HMO Assistance Act, was enacted in 1973 to encourage and promote the growth of HMOs as a means of health care cost containment. Many Medicare recipients endorse their benefits over to an HMO for fully prepaid medical care. Employers who provide health care benefits to employees are required to offer federally qualified HMOs as an option.

Several types of HMOs are

- Prepaid group practice model, in which physicians form a group and contract with a health plan. The physicians are not paid by the health plan and, therefore, can concentrate on practicing medicine.
- Staff model, in which a health plan hires physicians directly and pays them a salary.
- Independent practice association, in which the physicians are not employees and are not paid salaries. Instead, they are paid fees for their services out of a fund drawn from the premiums collected by an organization that markets the health plan minus a discount of up to 30% to cover operating deficits. At the end of the year, the physicians share in any surplus or deficit.
- Network HMO, which contracts with two or more group practices to provide health services.

Examples of HMO plans are

Kaiser Permanente

Blue Cross/Blue Shield HMO USA

CHAMPUS/TRICARE Prime, TRICARE/Extra and TRICARE/Standard

Medicare HMO risk plans or HMO cost plans

Medicaid (Medi-Cal in California)

INDEPENDENT PRACTICE ASSOCIATION

An IPA is a closed-panel HMO. Instead of maintaining its own staff and clinic buildings, the IPA contracts with independently practicing physicians who continue to practice in their own offices. The IPA may pay each doctor a set amount per patient in advance (capitation), or the fees charged for services to group members may be billed directly to the IPA rather than to the patient. Fees for services to nonmember patients are handled the same as any other fee for service. The physician may be contracted with several IPAs.

Memory Jogger

8 *Name three HMO plans.*

PREFERRED PROVIDER ORGANIZATION

The PPO preserves the fee-for-service concept that is desirable in the eyes of many physicians. An insurer, representing its clients, contracts with a group of providers (physicians) who agree on a predetermined list of charges for all services, including those for complex and unusual procedures.

The care is not prepaid. Usually, there are deductibles of 20% to 25% of the predetermined charge that the patient pays; the insurer pays the balance. A provider who joins a PPO does not need to alter the manner of providing care and continues to treat and bill the regular patients on a fee-for-service basis. When a patient covered under a PPO plan comes for treatment, the physician treats the patient and bills the PPO.

Working with Managed Care Plans

PRECERTIFICATION OR PREAUTHORIZATION

Most managed care systems require preauthorization for a patient to be referred to a specialist or even for certain laboratory tests or other procedures. It is necessary when a new patient makes an appointment to ask what type of insurance the patient has. If the patient belongs to an HMO you should check that plan contract for precertification or preauthorization requirements. If you are not sure of the requirements, call the plan and keep a record of the requirements on a reference guide that you prepare with the following information:

- Plan name
- Address
- Telephone number(s)
- Name and phone number of contact person
- Copay amount or deductible
- Hospital benefits for inpatient and outpatient surgery
- Second opinion, preauthorization requirements, telephone number, and assistant surgeon with percentage
- Participating hospitals, x-ray providers, laboratories, and physicians

SKILLS AND RESPONSIBILITIES

NEW PATIENT INSURANCE VERIFICATION PROCEDURE

1 When a patient calls for an appointment, identify what type of insurance the patient has or what HMO the patient belongs to.
2 When the patient arrives for the appointment, photocopy both sides of the patient ID card, because amounts to be paid may appear on the back side for hospital, office, or the emergency department.
3 Give the patient a letter to read and sign outlining the plan requirements and possible restrictions or noncovered items.
4 When referrals are required, explain the procedure to the patient so that it is understood that without the referral, it is the patient's responsibility to pay for the physician's services.
5 Collect any copays or deductibles.

PROVIDER RELATIONS

The provider relations department is designed to assist the physician's office with any inquiries he or she may have about capitation, contract, credentialing, physician appeals, formularies, and so forth. Whenever questions arise concerning a member/patient, the physician's office should contact the appropriate department (member services eligibility or the insurance company). *Do not* refer a patient to this department.

MEMBER SERVICES

This department was designed to assist the member/patient with any inquiries and/or concerns that may arise. Some HMOs will have one department that is a combination of provider relations and member services where a physician's office is able to check the status of their claims.

CLAIMS DEPARTMENT

Although this department was designed primarily to process all medical claims, the setup will vary from medical group to medical group. *If you provided services that required an authorization, always submit a copy of the authorization.* You need to determine where to forward claims and what kind of documentation is required for each managed care plan with which your office has a contract. Payments for managed care plans may be made either on a capitation basis (that is, a monthly check based on the number of patients in the plan) or based on the services that have been rendered to the patient (that is, a monthly check with an explanation of benefits [EOB] to indicate how much was paid for each service rendered to each patient). The EOB will have all the information from the claim and a code that specifies that the claim was processed and forwarded to the insurance company for processing and payment.

UTILIZATION MANAGEMENT

Review of care by health care professionals who do not provide the care is a necessary component of managed care to control costs. A **utilization review** committee reviews individual cases to make sure that the medical care services are medically necessary and to study how providers use medical care resources. This department reviews all the physician's referrals, emergency department visits, and urgent care. After review, this department will either approve or deny the referral, so it is important to submit exact documentation and precise statements. You will be able to contact this department directly. Never refer a member/patient to this department.

ELIGIBILITY SERVICES

Eligibility services was designed to assist the physician's office in checking eligibility of a patient/member. If the member is not in the database, this department is responsible to contact the insurance company and enter the information into the database.

MEDICAL DIRECTOR

The medical director is a highly qualified physician who works with every department in the medical group, including utilization review management. When certain referrals, questions, and/or concerns arise, the medical director will contact the PCP and will make a final decision based on the information obtained from the PCP.

FORMULARY

A formulary is a list of oral and parenteral medications that are covered by a member's (patient's) health plan. Every physician should have a copy of a formulary (one for every health plan with which he or she is connected). If you do not have one, contact your medical group's provider relations manager.

If a medication is in question, contact the plan's provider relations department and it will either give you an answer or will contact the insurance company.

Referrals and Authorizations

Managed care changes on a day-to-day basis. To compete within this market, some insurance companies have added a benefit that will allow a member/patient to self-refer (an authorization is not required to see a specialist). Many plans for senior citizens now have a self-referral and a copay as well as some other insurance coverage.

The following information will apply if you are working for a primary care physician, internist, family practitioner, general practitioner, pediatrician, and sometimes obstetrician or gynecologist.

Referral is a term used in managed care to refer a patient from the PCP to a specialist (Fig. 20–7). When completing a referral form, it is imperative that all necessary information be included. For example

> Referring physician ⇒ Specialist being referred to ⇒ Diagnosis ⇒ Treatment (medication ⇒ past and present) ⇒ Chart notes (if necessary) ⇒ Minor surgical procedures

If a referral is denied because of insufficient information or no medical necessity, the PCP's office will be notified. Some medical groups will notify both the PCP and the patient. When the PCP's office provides the medical group with the necessary information, the referral will be reviewed again.

A referral can take a few minutes to a few days to be reviewed and approved or denied. There are three types of referrals:

1. *Regular* referral usually takes 3 to 10 working days. This type of referral is used when a patient has not responded to any of a PCP's treat-

LIST OF SPECIALTIES AVAILABLE THROUGH OUR MEDICAL GROUP			
Acupuncture	Y	N	Otorhinolaryngology
Allergy/Immunology			Pathology
Anesthesiology			Pediatrics
Cardiovascular Diseases			Pediatric Allergy
Critical Care Medicine			Pediatric Cardiology
Dermatology			Pediatric - Dental Trauma
Dermatopathology			Pediatric Dermatology
Emergency Medicine			Pediatric Endocrinology
Endocrinology			Pediatric Gastroenterology
Family/General Practice			Pediatric Genetics
Gastroenterology			Pediatric Hematology/Oncology
Gynecology			Pediatrics, Infectious Disease
Hematology			Pediatrics, Nephrology
Hepatology			Pediatric Neurology
Hyperbaric Medicine			Pediatric Neurosurgery
Internal Medicine			Pediatric Ophthalmology
Maternal and Fetal Medicine			Pediatric Orthopedic Surgery
Neonatal-Perinatal Medicine			Pediatric Otorhinolaryngology
Nephrology			Pediatric Plastic Surgery
Neurology			Pediatric Podiatry
Obstetrics and Gynecology			Pediatric Psychiatry
Oncology			Pediatric Psychology
Ophthalmology			Pediatric Pulmonology
Ophthalmic Plastic Reconstructive and Orbital Surgery			Pediatric Rheumatology
Orthopedic Surgery			Pediatric Surgery
Pediatric Urology			Surgery, Colon and Rectal
Podiatry			Surgery, Head and Neck
Psychiatry			Surgery, Neurological
Psychiatry, Child and Adolescent			Surgery, Oncology
Pulmonary Diseases			Surgery, Maxillofacial
Radiology, Diagnostic			Surgery, Orthopedic
Radiology, Oncology			Surgery, Orthopedic/Oncology
Rheumatology			Surgery, Facial Plastic, and Otorhinolaryngology
Sleep Disorders			Surgery, General Vascular
Sports Medicine			Urology
Surgery, Cardiovascular and Thoracic			
OTHER			

FIGURE 20–7 Keeping a record of authorized specialty referrals.

ment and/or medication, and the physician believes that the patient needs to see a specialist to continue treatment.

2. An *urgent* referral will usually take 24+ hours. This type of referral is used when an urgent matter occurs and is not life threatening.

3. A *STAT* referral can be approved by telephone immediately after faxing it to the utilization review department. A STAT referral is used in an emergency situation as indicated by the physician, such as a matter of life or death, miscarriage, loss of limb, or other conditions of similar magnitude. Usually the physician will refer the patient by telephone and will fax the information with the referral afterward.

A regular referral is the most common and can be troublesome. Most managed care plans require you to contact the member services department to check the status of a referral. A cardinal rule is to never tell the patient that the referral has been approved unless you have a hard copy of the **authorization.** *Authorization* is a term used by managed care for an approved referral. A referral becomes an authorization after it is reviewed by utilization management/review and/or the medical director and approved.

When a referral is approved the PCP's office will receive by mail or fax a copy of the authorization. Always review the authorization in full. The patient will receive a letter with an authorization number and the approved services. The patient must present the authorization to the specialist's office receptionist on the day the services will be provided. An authorization provides the following information to both the PCP and the specialist:

1. An authorization number, which could be alpha, numeric, or alphanumeric.
2. The date on which it was received by utilization management, the date on which it was approved, and the expiration date.
   a. An authorization is good for 60 days.
   b. If the services are provided after the expiration date, the services will be denied. If this happens, you need to contact utilization management or member services and ask for an extension and answer a few questions. Sometimes you may have to involve the patient and/or specialist's office.
   c. If the authorization expires and services have not been provided, you can request an extension. Utilization management will change the expiration date and will fax a copy to the PCP and specialist or will generate a new authorization with a new number.
3. A diagnosis code.
4. The name, address, and telephone number of the contracted specialist where the services will be provided. Sometimes the PCP will refer the patient to a specialist but will not receive approval for that specialist and must get approval

for another. Always be sure that any specialist to whom your physician refers patients is contracted with the same managed care plan as the PCP.

5. The comment(s) section is the most critical area of a referral because this area will designate what services are approved.
   a. The specified number of authorized visits to the specialist.
   b. An authorization may be issued for (1) evaluation only, (2) evaluation and treatment plan, (3) evaluation and biopsy, (4) evaluation and one injection, etc.
   c. Authorization for an evaluation only and/or treatment plan. When this authorization appears, the medical assistant must inform the patient that there will not be any treatment—only an evaluation and/or a treatment plan.

Memory Jogger

10 *Name the three types of referrals.*

Guidelines for the Assistant in Specialty Practice

If you work for a specialist you do not have to worry about the referral process—only the authorizations.

SKILLS AND RESPONSIBILITIES

GUIDELINES FOR THE MEDICAL ASSISTANT FOR PROCESSING AUTHORIZATIONS

1 Always review the authorization thoroughly before providing services.

2 Deny services if a patient comes in for an appointment without an authorization. Contact the managed care plan and request a copy of the authorization.

3 If you do provide services to the patient, and then discover that the services were not authorized, you cannot bill the patient for any services provided. You can try to get the service authorized by working with the PCP, the member/patient, and the managed care plan, but most of the time you will eventually have to write off the charges. This will not please your employer.

4 Have the patient sign a form agreeing to pay for any services not covered by insurance.

ALLERGIES: _____

_____

_____

PATIENT NAME: _____
PHONE NO. _____

PRESCRIPTIONS

DATE	MEDICATION	AMOUNT	DOSE	START	STOP	REFILLS	INITIALS

FIGURE 20–8 Form for keeping a record of a patient's prescriptions.

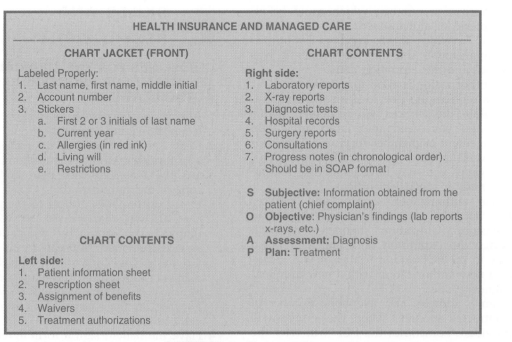

HEALTH INSURANCE AND MANAGED CARE

CHART JACKET (FRONT)

Labeled Properly:
1. Last name, first name, middle initial
2. Account number
3. Stickers
   a. First 2 or 3 initials of last name
   b. Current year
   c. Allergies (in red ink)
   d. Living will
   e. Restrictions

CHART CONTENTS

Left side:
1. Patient information sheet
2. Prescription sheet
3. Assignment of benefits
4. Waivers
5. Treatment authorizations

CHART CONTENTS

Right side:
1. Laboratory reports
2. X-ray reports
3. Diagnostic tests
4. Hospital records
5. Surgery reports
6. Consultations
7. Progress notes (in chronological order). Should be in SOAP format

S **Subjective:** Information obtained from the patient (chief complaint)
O **Objective:** Physician's findings (lab reports x-rays, etc.)
A **Assessment:** Diagnosis
P **Plan:** Treatment

FIGURE 20–9 Chart assembly.

Medical Records Audit

Medical records can be audited at any time by the managed care carrier. The medical record (chart) is a legal document that supports the patient/physician relationship. The managed care carrier has the right to access any chart for audit purposes on demand. Therefore, the medical assistant must be certain that the record is properly assembled and maintained.

Auditors look for the following items:

A. Security of Records
 1. Can records be easily accessed by patients or others?
 2. What procedures are being taken to maintain confidentiality?
 3. Are records kept from harm's way?
 4. Are records in a jacket and the contents secured?
 5. Are active records separate from inactive records?
 6. Can records be easily obtained?
B. Documentation Requirements
 1. Is the chart organized and in chronologic order?
 2. Is the chart complete and does it contain the following information:
    a. Family history
    b. Personal history
    c. Past history
    d. Social history
    e. Menstrual and pregnancy history
 3. Is the patient's name on each page?
 4. Are all entries dated?
 5. Is the chart legible?
 6. Are all entries signed by the person making the entry?
 7. Is there proper documentation of weight, height, blood pressure, vital signs, etc., as mandated by the insurance carrier?
 8. Does the chart reflect the SOAP notes as well as patient education?
 9. Are the sections of the chart separated from one another?
 10. Is there an immunization log?
 11. Is there a chart of current medications?
 12. Are samples given to the patient properly documented?
 13. Are there copies of orders from consulting physicians, for blood work, for x-rays, prescriptions, etc.?
 14. Does the documentation for prescriptions contain the following information (Fig. 20–8):
    a. Name of patient
    b. Date
    c. Drug
    d. Strength of drug
    e. Amount dispensed
    f. Number of refills
    g. Instructions to the patient
    h. Who ordered the prescription
    i. The name of the person calling in the prescription
 15. Are missed appointments documented in the chart?
 16. Are there growth charts for pediatric patients?
 17. Has the physician initialed all reports, tests, procedures, etc., after reviewing them?

See Figure 20–9 for an example of setting up the patient record.

LEGAL AND ETHICAL ISSUES

It is the medical assistant's responsibility to become well acquainted with the various insurance plans utilized by the patients. The medical assistant must be knowledgeable or be able to find the requirements for referral or authorization of patient care. The medical assistant must explain insurance submission policies and patient financial responsibilities before care. Signatures to authorize insurance billing, supplying information to insurance companies, and accepting assignment of benefits (if appropriate) should be obtained from all new patients. Managed care can create a physician/patient barrier that did not exist during the fee-for-service era. An extra effort in human relations on the part of the medical assistant can overcome this barrier and put the patient at ease.

CRITICAL THINKING

1 A patient enters your office stating she has an HMO of which your physician is not a member. How would you deal with this situation?

HOW DID I DO? Answers to Memory Joggers

1 Seven tasks a medical assistant may have to perform are to
 a. Obtain authorizations and referrals
 b. Prepare insurance claim forms
 c. Maintain an insurance claims register
 d. Trace unpaid claims
 e. Evaluate claims rejection
 f. Report procedures to prepaid care plans
 g. Translate medical terminology into procedural and diagnostic codes

2 Deductibles, copayment, and services not covered.

3 The insurance plan of the policyholder whose birthday comes first in the calendar year (month and day, not year) provides primary coverage for each dependent.

4 Medically indigent is someone who is able to take care of ordinary living expenses but is unable to afford medical care.

5 Basic medical means that insurance pays all or part of the physician's fee for nonsurgical services, including hospital, home and office visits, depending on the coverage. It may also include diagnostic laboratory, x-ray, and pathology fees.

6 Benefits are determined by indemnity schedules, by service benefits plans, by determination of the usual, customary and reasonable fee, and by relative value studies.

7 BIC stands for benefits identification card used in California.

8 HMO plans are Kaiser Permanente, Blue Cross/Blue Shield HMO USA, TRICARE Prime, TRICARE Extra, TRICARE Standard, Medicare HMO risk plans, or HMO cost plans; and Medicaid has various plans.

9 *a.* Verify name of HMO when patient makes appointment.
b. Photocopy ID card.
c. Have patient read and sign a letter outlining plan and or restrictions.
d. Explain the necessity for referral authorization.
e. Collect copay or deductible.

10 *a.* Regular
b. Urgent
c. Stat

REFERENCES

American Medical Association: American Medical News. Chicago, AMA, published weekly.
Fordney M: Insurance Handbook for the Medical Office, 5th ed. Philadelphia, WB Saunders, 1997.

Coding and Claims Processing

Sue Hunt, MA, RN, CMA

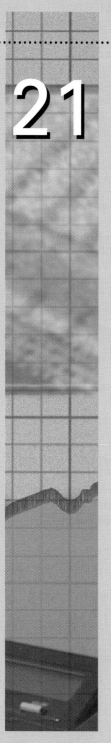

21

LEARNING OBJECTIVES

Cognitive: On successful completion of this chapter you should be able to:

1 Define and spell the terms listed in the Vocabulary.

2 Identify four purposes of numerical diagnostic and procedural coding.

3 Name the principal coding systems that link the medical profession and the insurance system.

4 List 10 reasons for possible rejection of insurance claims.

5 State the maximum billing period for Medicare claims.

6 Explain why a patient's care under workers' compensation should be recorded separately from his or her care as a private patient.

7 List and briefly describe three types of managed care organizations.

Performance: On successful completion of this chapter you should be able to:

1 Identify and complete the appropriate insurance forms for patients covered by
a Medicare
b CHAMPUS
c Workers' compensation
d Blue Cross and Blue Shield

2 Calculate the billing for patients whose insurance includes deductibles and copayments or co-insurance.

VOCABULARY

ancillary diagnostic services Services that support patient diagnoses (e.g., laboratory or x-ray)

ancillary therapeutic services Services that support patient treatment (e.g., specialists, surgery)

coding Converting verbal descriptions of diseases, injuries, and procedures into numerical and alphanumerical designations

comorbidities Preexisting conditions that will, because of their presence with a specific principal diagnosis, cause an increase in length of stay by at least 1 day in approximately 75% of the cases

complications Conditions that arise during the hospital stay that prolong the length of stay by at least 1 day in approximately 75% of the cases

crossover claim Claim for benefits under both Medicare and Medicaid

discharge face sheet Summary of the hospital stay prepared at the time of the patient's discharge from the hospital

electronic billing Submission of a claim via computer to computer

established patient A patient who has received care from the physician within the past 3 years or other specified period

etiology Classifying a claim according to the cause of the disorder

fiscal intermediary An organization that handles claims from hospitals, nursing facilities, intermediate and long-term care facilities, and home health care agencies

grouper Computer software program that is used by the fiscal intermediary in all cases to assign discharges to the appropriate DRGs using the following information abstracted from the inpatient bill: patient's age, sex, principal diagnosis, principal procedures performed, and discharge status

International Classification of Diseases, Ninth Revision, Clinical Modification (ICD-9-CM) System for classifying diseases to facilitate collection of uniform and comparable health information

major diagnostic categories (MDCs) Broad clinical categories differentiated from all others based on body system involvement and disease etiology

mandated Required by an authority or law

new patient A patient who has not received any professional services from the physician in the past 3 years or other specified period

nonparticipating provider (non-par) A physician who does not accept assignment under Medicare or the Blue Plans

participating provider (par) A physician who accepts assignment under Medicare or the Blue Plans

peer review organization (PRO) Entity composed of a substantial number of licensed doctors of medicine and osteopathy engaged in the practice of medicine or surgery in the area, or an entity that has available to it the services of a sufficient number of physicians engaged in the practice of medicine or surgery, to assure the adequate peer review of the services provided by the various medical specialties and subspecialties

preauthorization Permission by the insurance carrier obtained before giving certain treatment to a patient

preexisting condition Physical condition of an insured person that existed before the issuance of the insurance policy

principal diagnosis That condition that after study is determined to be chiefly responsible for occasioning the admission of the patient to the hospital

professional standards review organization (PSRO) A group of physicians working with the government to review cases for hospital admission and discharge under government guidelines; sometimes referred to as peer review

Tax Equity and Fiscal Responsibility Act (TEFRA) Signed into federal law in 1982 and contains provisions for major changes in Medicare reimbursement

uniform hospital discharge data set (UHDDS) A minimum data set required to be collected for each Medicare patient on discharge

In recent years the process of submitting insurance claims for payment has become more complicated. After a patient receives service, the office computes charges and adds them to the patient's ledger. If the patient has insurance, a claim is prepared to submit to the insurance company. To facilitate the processing of large numbers of claims insurance companies increasingly require numerical codes for diagnoses and procedures. The insurance company wants to have a means of reviewing quickly that the patient received appropriate services and identifying exactly what services were provided to a given patient. Converting verbal descriptions of diseases, injuries, and procedures into numerical designations is the essence of **coding.**

Numerical diagnostic procedural coding was developed for a number of reasons:

- Tracking disease processes
- Classification of medical procedures
- Medical research
- Evaluation of hospital utilization

This transference of words to numbers also facilitated the use of computers in claims processing. Without the use of computers, it would be impossible to take care of the 60,000 to 65,000 claims processed each day in an average mid-sized claims processing center.

Fee Schedules

RELATIVE VALUE SCALE (RVS)

The RVS was pioneered by the California Medical Association in 1956 to help physicians establish rational, relative fees. Other states soon followed suit. Hundreds of the most commonly performed procedures were compiled, given procedure numbers similar to those in the American Medical Association's *Current Procedural Terminology,* and assigned a unit value. The assigned unit value represented the value of that procedure in relation to other procedures commonly performed. Although no monetary value was placed on the units, many insurance companies used the RVS to determine benefits by applying a conversion factor to assign a monetary value to the unit value. In 1978, the Federal Trade Commission (FTC) interpreted the California RVS as a fee-setting instrument and prohibited its publication and distribution. The FTC was attempting to make medical practice more competitive by ruling against the setting of fees and by encouraging physicians to advertise.

Memory Jogger

1 *Name four reasons that coding was developed.*

RESOURCE-BASED RELATIVE VALUE SCALE (RBRVS)

We have now come full circle and are again practicing under relative value scales nationally. The RBRVS is one of the outcomes of the Medicare Physician Payment Reform that was enacted in the Omnibus Budget Reconciliation Act of 1989 (OBRA '89). Since the beginning of Medicare, Part B of the program has paid physicians using a fee-for-service system based on customary, prevailing, and reasonable charges. The RBRVS, effective in 1992, has changed this. The RBRVS consists of three parts:

1. Physician work
2. Charge-based professional liability expenses
3. Charge-based overhead

The physician work component includes the degree of effort invested by the physician in a particular service or procedure and the time it consumed. The professional liability and overhead components are computed by the Health Care Financing Administration (HCFA).

The fee schedule is designed to provide national uniform payments after being adjusted to reflect the differences in practice costs across geographic areas. The fee schedule includes a conversion factor, which is a single national number applied to all services paid under the fee schedule.

Procedural Coding

PHYSICIANS' CURRENT PROCEDURAL TERMINOLOGY (CPT-4)

The *CPT-4 Manual* is a listing of descriptive terms and identifying codes that is used for reporting medical services and procedures performed by physicians. The purpose of the terminology is to provide a uniform language that accurately identifies medical, surgical, and diagnostic services and that can be used as an effective means for reliable, nationwide communication among physicians, patients, and third parties. The *CPT Manual* was developed initially in 1966 by the American Medical Association. There have been several revisions, and it is updated yearly. It is organized into six sections:

1. Evaluation and Management	99201–99499
2. Anesthesiology	00100–01999
3. Surgery	10040–69979
4. Radiology	70010–79999
5. Pathology and Laboratory	80000–89399
6. Medicine	90701–99199

Evaluation and Management has various categories divided into three to five levels based on key components, contributory factors, and the face-to-face time of the services. The three key components the physician uses to select the appropriate level of services are (1) the level of history, (2) the level of examination, and (3) the complexity of medical decision-making. When seeing a **new patient,** all three key components must be met. When seeing an **established patient,** only two of the three components need to be met. Time is considered only if over 50% of the encounter was spent in counseling.

New codes for services and procedures are identified in the *CPT Manual* by the following symbols:

A bullet (●) in front of a code number indicates a new code.

A triangle (▲) in front of a code number indicates that the description for the code has been changed or modified.

A star (★) placed after a code number indicates that a procedure is not subject to the surgical package concept.

The *CPT Manual* is divided into sections, subsections, subheadings, and categories.

Section: Surgery
    Subsection: Respiratory System
        Subheading: Lung
            Category: Excision

An alphabetical index of procedures is located at the back of the *CPT-4 Manual.* At the beginning of each section are guidelines that explain items unique to that section that should be reviewed by the coder. A number of specific code numbers have been designated for reporting unlisted procedures. Use of an unlisted code requires a special report. Two-digit modifiers may be attached to the five-digit code to indicate that the service or procedure has been altered. For example, -50 indicates multiple or bilateral procedures, -52 indicates reduced service, -62 indicates two surgeons, and -80 indicates surgical assistant services.

Books with revised CPT codes are published yearly in the last quarter after Congress has approved the changes and use of new numbers recommended by the American Medical Association.

Memory Jogger

2 *Name the six sections of the* CPT-4 Manual.

HCPCS CODING SYSTEM

Medicare carriers have converted to the HCFA's Common Procedure Coding System (HCPCS) (pronounced Hic-Pics). HCPCS, which is based on the current edition of the *CPT,* is a five-digit alphanumerical coding system that can accommodate the

addition of modifiers. There are three levels of codes assigned and maintained by Medicare carriers:

- Level I codes include 95% to 98% of all Medicare Part B procedural codes and comprise only CPT codes (excluding those for anesthesiology, which is currently designated by surgery codes).
- Level II codes are assigned by the HCFA and are consistent nationwide. These codes are for physician and nonphysician services not contained in the CPT system; they are alphanumerical, ranging from A0000 to V9999.
- Level III codes are assigned and maintained by each local fiscal intermediary. These codes represent services that are not included in the CPT system and are not common to all carriers. These codes range from W0000 to Z9999.

Diagnostic Coding

INTERNATIONAL CLASSIFICATION OF DISEASES, NINTH REVISION, CLINICAL MODIFICATION (ICD-9-CM)

The *International Classification of Diseases, Ninth Revision, Clinical Modification (ICD-9-CM)* is published in three volumes:

Volume 1 (Diseases: Tabular (Numerical) Index)
Volume 2 (Disease: Alphabetical List)
Volume 3 (Tabular List and Alphabetical Index of Procedures)
Volumes 1 and 2 are used in the physician's office to complete insurance claims. Volume 3 is used primarily in hospitals.

The *ICD-9-CM* is used by health care providers in coding and reporting clinical information required for participation in Medicare and Medicaid programs and for statistical tabulation. Each single disease entity has been assigned a three-digit category. A fourth digit is added to provide specificity to the diagnosis regarding **etiology,** site, or manifestations. In certain cases, a fifth digit is required. It is important to use the correct code because the insurance carrier bases its payment for services on their medical justification or necessity. If the claim contains an incomplete or incorrect code, the insurance company may consider the service unnecessary.

The *ICD-9-CM* lists what is wrong with the patient and what initially brought the patient to see the doctor. The list of diagnoses includes

- Diseases
- Conditions
- Accidents
- Injuries
- Poisonings
- All diagnoses

Although diagnostic coding dates back to 17th century England, and the first *International Classifica-*

tion of Diseases (ICD) was published by the World Health Organization (WHO) in 1948, the *ICD-9* took on new significance in 1988 when Congress passed the Medicare Catastrophic Coverage Act. Since 1989, the HCFA has **mandated** the use of *ICD-9-CM* codes on every Medicare Part B claim. New numbers are published yearly.

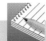

SKILLS AND RESPONSIBILITIES

CODING GUIDELINES

1 Billers must use the appropriate code or codes from 001.0 through V82.9 to identify diagnoses, symptoms, conditions, or other reasons for the encounter/visit.

2 List first the *ICD-9-CM* code for diagnosis, condition, problem, or other reason for encounter/visit shown in the medical record to be chiefly responsible for the services provided. List additional codes that describe any coexisting conditions.

3 Codes must be used at their highest level of specificity, e.g.:
  • Assign three-digit codes only if there are no fourth-digit codes within that code category.
  • Assign fourth-digit codes only if there is no fifth-digit subclassification for that category.
  • Assign the fifth-digit subclassification code for those categories where it exists.

4 Do not code diagnoses documented as Probable, Suspected, Questionable, or Rule Out, as if they are established. Rather, code the condition(s) to the highest degree of certainty for that encounter/visit, such as Symptoms, Signs, Abnormal Test Results, or other reason for the visit (e.g., chest pain, fever).

5 Chronic disease treated on an ongoing basis may be coded and reported as many times as the patient receives treatment and care for the condition(s).

6 For patients receiving **ancillary diagnostic services** only during an encounter/visit, the appropriate V code for the examination is sequenced first and the diagnosis or problem for which the services are being performed is sequenced second.

7 For patients receiving **ancillary therapeutic services** only during an encounter/visit, the appropriate V code for the service is listed first and the diagnosis or problem for which the services are being performed is listed second.

8 For surgery, code the diagnosis for which the surgery was performed. If the postopera-

tive diagnosis is known to be different from the preoperative at the time the claim is filed, select the postoperative diagnosis for coding.

9 Code all documented conditions that coexist at the time of the encounter/visit and that require or affect patient care, treatment, or management. Do not code conditions previously treated and no longer existing.

10 E codes are supplementary and used to describe a variety of external causes of injuries and poisonings.

11 E codes should not be listed as primary diagnoses; they are supplementary. Although not usually required, these codes are sometimes useful to clarify the cause of a disease or injury.

Memory Jogger

3 *Which volume number of the* ICD-9-CM *has the alphabetical listing?*

Guidelines for Claims Processing

GATHERING DATA AND MATERIALS

When the first appointment is made, the medical assistant should ask the patient for all insurance information. The information obtained for the patient record (see Chapter 15) is used for processing the insurance claim. Verify that it is current.

SKILLS AND RESPONSIBILITIES

GUIDELINES FOR THE MEDICAL ASSISTANT FOR CLAIMS PROCESSING

• If the patient has an identification card, it should first be examined to determine that the coverage is current and then photocopied for the office record.

• If more than one insurance policy is involved, obtain the name, address, group, and policy number for each company.

• Obtain the name of the subscriber if it is someone other than the patient.

• Obtain a signed authorization form for releasing information if you are submitting the insurance claim for the patient.

FIGURE 21–1 Health insurance claim form.

CLAIM FORMS

Universal Health Insurance Claim Form

The HCFA designed the basic claim form HCFA-1500 (Fig. 21–1) for the Medicare and Medicaid claims of physicians and other suppliers (see Procedure 21–1). It has also been adopted by the Civilian Health and Medical Program of the Uniformed Services (CHAMPUS) and has received the approval of the American Medical Association Council on Medical Services. Form HCFA-1500 answers the needs of most health care insurers and is referred to as the universal health insurance claim form. One exception is that it is not used to claim reimbursement for ambulance services.

Some commercial insurance companies provide their own forms. When filing a claim with such a company, you can complete the HCFA-1500 form and attach it to the commercial form for submission to the insurance carrier. Because many insurance carriers are using optical character recognition (OCR) scanners to transfer the information on claim forms to their computers' memories, the original form printed in red must be used.

THE SUPERBILL

A private insurance carrier may send its own form to the patient. Rather than completing this form, the office that uses the superbill discussed in Chapter 19 can usually simply attach a copy to the insurance form or give an extra copy of the superbill to the patient if he or she is to submit the claim form. Make certain that the code descriptions on the superbill match those listed in the latest CPT code book.

ASSIGNMENT OF BENEFITS

Some insurance companies honor requests for assignment of benefits to the physician. The medical assistant should request that the patient complete an assignment of benefits form (Fig. 21–2). This is an authorization to the insurance company to make payment directly to the physician. In the case of private insurance it is the patient's responsibility to pay any balance that is not covered by the insurance.

In the case of government-sponsored insurance agreeing to accept assignment of benefits, the physician will accept the fee determination of the plan and the insurance carrier will pay its portion of the fee directly to the physician. The patient can only be billed based on the amount allowed by the insurance plan. See a more complete description below under Medicare billing.

Keeping current with insurance information and changes is no small part of the medical assistant's responsibility. The procedure manual should be updated as changes occur (Fig. 21–3). Government programs are frequently modified, and these changes are reported in bulletins sent to all physicians. *Read these bulletins carefully and save those that contain pertinent information.*

Attend workshops offered to medical assistants and physicians in your area whenever possible and keep the information in a notebook or folder.

TRACKING INSURANCE CLAIMS

Keep a log of insurance claims as they are received and processed (Fig. 21–4). Date-stamp the forms as they are received and enter the information on the log. This log will enable you to determine immediately whether a claim form has been completed and mailed.

- If possible, set aside a definite time for completing insurance claims.
- Have a central location for all insurance forms.
- Have readily available the necessary manuals, code books, and other references needed.
- Create a master list of codes most often used by the practice, including fourth and fifth digits, if appropriate.

ASSIGNMENT OF INSURANCE BENEFITS

I, the undersigned, represent that I have insurance coverage with and do hereby authorize
_____ to pay and assign directly to _____
(NAME OF COMPANY)   (NAME OF DOCTOR)
all surgical and/or medical benefits, if any, otherwise payable to me for services as described on the attached forms hereof, but not to exceed the charges for those services. I understand that I am financially responsible for all charges whether or not paid by said insurance. I hereby authorize said assignee to release all information necessary to secure the payment of said benefits.

Date _____ Signed _____

FIGURE 21–2 Assignment of benefits form.

INSURANCE CARRIER Name and Address	Department and Individual to Contact	POLICYHOLDER Individual to Contact	Group or Policy Number	SPECIAL NOTES
BLUE SHIELD PO Box 12345 Anytown, USA	Tom Jones Professional Relations 123-456-7890	Aerospace Industries Joan Crawford 123-888-3030	AI-89037	Tom Jones will speak to groups or give personal assistance in office
		Bell Burgers Nancy Donovan 123-465-2210	BB-3415Z	Scheduled benefits
OCCIDENTAL PO Box 42873 Anytown, USA	Cathy Redding Claims Dept. 213-440-3131	Town School Dist. Mary Embers 312-055-3210	Group No. 4414	Does not pay for assistant surgeon

FIGURE 21–3   Page from procedure manual. Insurance problems can be diminished by knowing whom to contact at the insurance carrier and the policyholder.

- Make it a practice to complete the forms as soon as possible after service is rendered, usually at the end of the day.
- Use the superbill or HCFA-1500 form as often as possible.
- Complete the forms by category (e.g., all Blue Cross, all Medicare).
- Set the tabulator stops on the typewriter or word processor for the form being completed. Make a note of these stops so they can easily be set up when completing the same kind of form again.
- If using a computer billing program to print insurance forms, the computer will store insurance information on outstanding claims that can be printed in batches using the HCFA-1500 forms. Adjust the printer so that the information prints correctly on the form.
- Transmit claims electronically whenever possible.

INSURANCE CLAIM REGISTER					
PATIENT	INSURANCE COMPANY	DATE FILED	AMOUNT BILLED	AMOUNT PAID	DIFFERENCE

FIGURE 21–4   Insurance log showing the date each claim was filed, the amount billed, the amount paid, and the difference that must be either discounted or billed to the patient.

RECORDS RELEASE　　　　　　　　　　　　　Date _____

To _____
　　　　　　　　　　　　　　　　DOCTOR

_____
　　　　　　　　　　　　　　　　ADDRESS

I hereby authorize and request you to release

to _____
　　　　　　　　　　　　　　　　DOCTOR

_____
　　　　　　　　　　　　　　　　ADDRESS

the complete medical records in your possession, concerning my illness and/or treatment during

the period from _____ to _____

　　　　　　　　　　　　　Signed _____
　　　　　　　　　　　　　　　　　　　(PATIENT OR NEAREST RELATIVE)

_____ Relationship _____
　　　WITNESS

FORM 122 - Eastman, Inc.

FIGURE 21–5 Authorization form for release of medical information.

COMPLETING THE HCFA-1500 FORM

1 If you plan to mail the form directly to the insurance company, be sure that the patient has signed the Authorization to Release Information form (Fig. 21–5)
2 Make sure that Medicare patients sign an Extended Signature Authorization form (Fig. 21–6)
3 Typewrite all claim forms and keep a photocopy or computer printout of each.
4 Use accepted diagnostic and procedure codes, and be certain that the procedures are consistent with the diagnoses.

5 List all procedures performed, one procedure per line. Be specific. If a laceration was treated, give the location, length, and depth; the number of sutures required; and the duration of treatment involved. If a sterile surgical tray was used for office surgery, itemize and bill as a separate fee. If a treatment injection was given, state the injected material and the amount given.
6 Attach a copy of the x-ray report, hospital report, and/or consultant's report in complicated cases.
7 State the physician's usual and customary fee on all claim forms, regardless of what payment is expected.

MEDICARE LIFETIME ASSIGNMENT

Name of beneficiary: _____

Medicare number: _____

I request that payment of authorized Medicare benefits be made to me or on my behalf to (physician/supplier name) for any services furnished me by that provider. I authorize any holder of medical information about me to release to the Health Care Financing Administration and its agents any information needed to determine benefits or the benefits payable for related services.

This authorization is in effect until I choose to revoke it.*

Signed: _____ Date: _____

*If you are a patient in a hospital or skilled nursing facility, this authorization is in effect for the period of your confinement.

FIGURE 21–6 Patient's extended signature authorization for Medicare claims.

8 Never alter a claim as to services performed, date of service, or fees established.

9 If more than one visit per day was required, state the times of day so that the claims processor will know they were separate procedures and attach a letter of medical necessity on the physician's letterhead.

10 Fill in all blanks. Type DNA (does not apply) or NA (not applicable) or simple dash lines (–) rather than leave an item blank. This is confirmation that the item was not overlooked.

ELECTRONIC CLAIMS SUBMISSION

The medical practice that is computerized probably uses the computer for processing electronic claims (E-claims). This may be handled in several ways (e.g., transmitting data via modem or by recording data on computer disk or tape and sending it to the payer or intermediary).

An obvious advantage of **electronic billing** is the amount of time saved with its use. The system interrupts the transmission of incomplete or incorrect data, giving the biller the opportunity for on-the-spot correction. The sender knows immediately whether the insurance company is accepting the claim. Another advantage of electronic billing is that it speeds up the date of payment, which results in an increase in cash flow to the practice.

Electronic transfer of information is also advantageous to the payer. The HCFA is a strong advocate and has long given preference to the processors of E-claims. By 2000, all providers of Medicare and Medicaid must file their claims electronically.

Not all claims are suitable for electronic submission. For example, those claims that are complicated and require a cover letter or those that require some kind of attachment must be sent on hard copy (paper) by mail or messenger.

CLAIM REJECTION

If a claim form is not sufficiently detailed, complete, and accurate, it may be rejected by the insurance company.

EXAMPLES OF THE REASONS FOR CLAIM REJECTION

- Diagnosis is missing or incomplete
- Diagnosis is not coded accurately
- Diagnosis does not correspond with treatment
- Charges are not itemized
- Patient's group, member, or policy number is missing or incorrect
- Patient's portion of the form is incomplete, or the patient's signature is missing
- Patient's date of birth is missing
- Fee is not listed
- Dates are incorrect or missing
- Physician's signature or address is missing

Memory Jogger

4 *If a diagnosis is missing from an insurance claim, what will be the result?*

Billing Requirements

MEDICARE

Under Medicare, the physician may be a **participating provider** or a **nonparticipating provider** (sometimes referred to as **par** and **non-par providers**). Both are required by law to file the HCFA-1500 insurance claim for all eligible patients. The office may also file for a secondary carrier.

A participating provider accepts assignment on Medicare claims. The allowance payment comes directly to the physician and is accepted as payment in full. The patient is still responsible for paying the deductible and the 20% co-insurance to the physician.

A nonparticipating provider is not required to accept assignment. If such is the case, the patient is responsible for the balance after Medicare makes its payment. The allowable payment to the non-par provider is less than the payment to the par provider.

The non-par provider who plans to perform elective surgery on a Medicare patient that costs $500 or more is subject to Medicare's $500 surgery rule (Fig. 21–7). The provider must prepare a financial statement showing the type of surgery to be performed, the estimated charge, the estimated payment from Medicare, and the patient's probable out-of-pocket expense. This statement must be signed by the patient. Give one photocopy to the patient and file another with the patient's chart.

Claims for Medicare must be filed by December 31 of the year following that in which the services were rendered. For example, care rendered in 1999 must be billed no later than December 31, 2000.

MEDICAID

A physician is free to accept or to refuse to treat a patient under Medicaid. However, if the patient is accepted, requirements for rendering service and billing for services are strict and must be closely followed:

The patient's identification card must be current. Some include labels that must be attached to the

Dear Patient:

I do not plan to accept assignment for your surgery. The law requires that where assignment is not taken and the charge is $500 or more, the following information must be provided prior to your surgery. These estimates assume you have met the annual Part B Medicare deductible.

Type of surgery _____

Estimated charge $ _____

Estimated Medicare payment $ _____

Your estimated payment $ _____

(This includes your Medicare co-insurance)

Physician's Signature _____

I have read and understand the above information.

X _____   _____

(Patient's Signature)   (Date)

FIGURE 21-7 Non-par provider's financial statement that is used to comply with Medicare's $500 surgery rule.

billing form. Others have a benefits identification card (BIC) that must be verified before seeing the patient.

Preauthorization may be required for the service, for which a form is completed. For an emergency situation, authorization may be secured by telephone but must be followed up with the appropriate form.

Claims are submitted on the HCFA-1500 form or a similar form required by the individual state for optical scanning. There will be a time limit for billing after the termination of which the claim may be rejected, depending on the state regulations. It is important that the medical assistant check the local regulations and keep current on requirements. Some Medicaid patients have been shifted to HMOs, and their bills should be sent to the HMO not the Medicaid fiscal agent.

Physicians who accept Medicaid are required to accept assignment of benefits and are not allowed to bill the patient beyond what Medicaid allows.

Memory Jogger

5 *Describe Medicare's $500 surgery rule.*

MEDI/MEDI

The HCFA-1500 form is used, and the physician must always accept assignment. Failure to indicate acceptance of assignment will result in a Medicare payment going to the patient and in rejection of the claim by Medicaid. A label from the patient's ID card or a photocopy of the current card may be required.

The claim form is first processed through Medicare and is then automatically forwarded to Medicaid. It is not necessary to prepare two claims forms. This is sometimes referred to as a **crossover claim.**

Memory Jogger

6 *What does HCPCS stand for?*

BLUE PLANS

When a patient is covered under a Blue Plan, claims should be submitted as soon as possible after the service is provided. Many of the Blue Plans have adopted use of the HCFA-1500 form. Check with the local office or representative in your area.

Like Medicare, the Blue Plans have arrangements with participating and nonparticipating providers. Usually the participating provider is paid directly for covered services and agrees not to bill the patient for any difference between the provider's fee and the allowed fee.

The Blue Plans have provider manuals that describe coverage and coding features of the Plan. These manuals are periodically revised. Contact your local representative if your manual might be outdated.

CIVILIAN HEALTH AND MEDICAL PROGRAM OF THE UNIFORMED SERVICES (CHAMPUS) AND CIVILIAN HEALTH AND MEDICAL PROGRAM OF THE VETERANS ADMINISTRATION (CHAMPVA)

Use form HCFA-1500 for the covered portion of the fee. Like Medicare, if the physician accepts assignment, the patient should be billed for the entire deductible but can only be billed for the co-insurance portion of the charge allowed by CHAMPUS or CHAMPVA. If the physician does not accept assignment, the patient submits claim forms with the physician's itemized statement to the insurance company and is responsible for the total deductible and co-insurance. The claim must be filed no later than December 31 of the year following that in which services were provided.

WORKERS' COMPENSATION

Records for the workers' compensation case (sometimes referred to as an industrial case) should be kept separate from the physician's regular patient histories. If the patient who is seen for an industrial injury has previously been treated as a private patient, a new chart and ledger should be started that will be used only for the treatment rendered under conditions of the workers' compensation law.

The insurance carrier may request and is entitled to receive copies of all records pertaining to the industrial injury but not the records of a private patient. *Information in the records of a private patient is privileged information and may be released only with the patient's consent.* There could be a lawsuit or a hearing before a referee or appeals board for which records are subpoenaed. If separate records are kept, there is no question of privilege involved.

The employer and the physician who sees the injured or ill worker first are required, in most states, to file a report with the insurance carrier within a specified length of time. The medical assistant should make a minimum of five copies of this report. The insurance company usually requires at least two copies. One copy goes to the state regulatory body. The employer may get a copy, and one file copy should remain with the physician's record. This report must be personally signed by the physician and should contain the following information:

- The history of the case as obtained from the patient, with notation of any **preexisting condition** (injuries or diseases)
- The patient's symptoms and physical complaints
- Complete physical findings, including laboratory and x-ray results
- A tentative diagnosis
- An estimate of the type and extent of the disability. In cases in which permanent disability has resulted, there should be a careful survey and the extent of disability should be given.
- Treatment indicated, including type, frequency, and duration. It may be necessary to attach a letter giving more detailed information to assist in making an evaluation of the case.
- If the patient is unable to return to work, the probable date that he or she will be able to return to work

The insurance carrier may supply its own billing forms. Payment is usually made on the basis of a fee schedule. Any charges in excess of the fee schedule must be fully explained and documented. In billing for the service, use the coding system specified in your state. Itemize the statement, including any drugs and dressings used.

In severe or prolonged cases, supplementary reports and billing should be sent to the insurance carrier at least once per month. At the termination of treatment, a final report and bill are sent to the insurance carrier. Do not bill the patient.

PROCEDURE 21–1
Completing Insurance Forms

GOAL
To complete an insurance claim form for services.

EQUIPMENT AND SUPPLIES
Patient chart
HCFA-1500 claim form

Patient ledger
Typewriter or computer

PROCEDURAL STEPS

A Ask for patient's identification card
PURPOSE: To determine whether the patient is insured.

B Photocopy card and place the copy in the patient's file.
PURPOSE: If questions arise, the office has an exact copy of the insurance information.

C Have the patient sign an Extended Signature Authorization form.
PURPOSE: This form grants lifetime authorization for the physician to submit assigned or unassigned claims on the beneficiary's behalf. (It must be canceled on the patient's request.)

D Complete the following entries (blocks 1–33) on the HCFA-1500 form:

Continued

1 Check the appropriate boxes for all types of health insurance coverage applicable to the claim.

1A Enter the insured person's identification number (and all letters) as it appears on the person's insurance card.

2 Enter the patient's full name (last name, then first name and middle initial) exactly as it appears on the insurance card.

3 Enter six-digit birth date and sex.

4 Enter word "SAME" if patient and insured are the same person, or enter the full name of the insured person (last name, then first name and middle initial).

5 Enter the patient's permanent mailing address and telephone number. (Do not use P.O. box for address.)

6 Enter patient's relationship to the policyholder by checking the correct box.

7 Enter the word "SAME" if the patient and insured live at the same address. Otherwise enter the mailing address of the policy holder. If CHAMPUS, put the sponsor's military address.

8 Check the appropriate boxes to identify the patient's marital and employment status.

9 Complete this block only if the patient has other insurance coverage. Otherwise enter NA on the first line of this block. On the first line of the block enter the name of the insured person (last name, then first name and middle initial).
   A Enter the policy or group number including letters.
   B Enter date of birth and sex.
   C Enter employer's name or school name.
   D Enter insurance plan or program name.

10 Check the appropriate boxes (YES or NO).
   A If the patient's condition is related to employment, check YES and submit the claim to workers' compensation.
   B If the patient's condition is related to a vehicular accident, check YES and include the two-letter code for the state where the accident occurred.
   C If the patient's condition is related to an accident other than a vehicular accident, check YES.
   D Generally this box is used exclusively for Medicaid. Enter the patient's Medicaid number preceded by "MCD."

11 This block must be completed for Medicare. If the patient has insurance that is primary to Medicare, complete blocks 11A through 11C. If other insurance is not primary to Medicare, enter "NONE." Indicate "CHAMPUS" in this block if the patient has Medicare. The block should be filled out with the information of the insured person.

12 If the patient has signed an "Authorization for Release of Medical Information," fill in this box with "SIGNATURE ON FILE" or "SOF." If the claim will be filed electronically, it is necessary to have the signature on file. If the claim will be sent through the mail, the patient can sign the form.

13 Reserve for the patient's signature if a Medicare supplement policy is indicated in block 9; or if the patient has signed a separate Medicare or Medigap authorization, enter "SIGNATURE ON FILE." If the claim is to Medicaid, the POE sticker goes here.

14 For Medicare, CHAMPUS, or commercial insurance, enter the date of the patient's current illness; or for pregnancy, enter the date of the last menstrual period.

15 For Medicare, Medicaid, or Blue Cross/Blue Shield, leave blank. For CHAMPUS, workers' compensation, or commercial insurance, fill in if appropriate.

16 For Medicare or commercial insurance, enter the dates the patient cannot work, if employed. This box may also be filled in for workers' compensation.

17 Enter the HCFA-assigned unique provider identification number of the physician. This is written as a 10-digit number: the first seven characters are the provider's number, the next is a check digit, and the last two characters identify the provider's location.

18 Complete this block when the medical service is related to hospitalization (enter admission and discharge dates).

Continued

19 Consult the billing manual of the particular insurance to determine what may be needed in this box.

20 Complete when billing for diagnostic tests. Check "NO" if all laboratory tests included on the claim form were completed in the physician's office. Check "YES" if laboratory tests were done outside the office and billed to the physician's office. Fill in the amount of the bill. If "YES" is checked, the charge for each test should be entered in box 24D and the name of the outside laboratory should be entered in block 32.

21 Enter ICD-9-CM diagnosis codes beginning with the primary diagnosis and up to three other diagnoses that justify the procedures entered in block 24. If more than four diagnoses are needed, fill out a second claim form. Do not use decimal points.

22 Complete only for Medicaid.

23 For Medicare, Medicaid and CHAMPUS enter the prior authorization number (PRO), a 10-digit number if required for the procedure.

24 One procedure may be listed per line for blocks 24A through 24K.
    24A Enter the month, day, and year for each procedure or service. If the from and to dates are the same, enter only the from date. If the same service or procedure with identical charges is provided on consecutive days, both the from and to dates should be entered.
    24B Enter the code for the place of service.
    24C Enter CHAMPUS, Medicaid, and workers' compensation service codes.
    24D Enter procedure codes, either CPT codes or HCPCS codes, depending on the requirements of the insurance. Enter the five-digit code and modifiers if needed, without decimal points.
    24E Enter the number 1, 2, 3, or 4 that points to the diagnosis code for the procedure in box 21 that justifies the medical necessity for performing the procedure. Do not use the actual codes in this box.
    24F Enter the fee for each service. Do not enter dollar signs or decimal points.
    24G Enter the number of days or units being billed.
    24H This box is used only for Medicaid. EPSDT refers to a Medicaid early, periodic, screening, diagnosis, and treatment. Enter "E" for these services or "F" for family planning.
    24I Check this box for commercial insurance or Medicaid if care was given in an emergency department.
    24J For Medicaid, check if coordination of benefits.
    24K For Medicare, CHAMPUS, and commercial insurance, enter the employer identification number (EIN) or the HCFA-assigned unique provider identification number (UPIN) of the provider when the physician is in a group practice. Enter the first two digits in box 24J and the remaining eight digits in box 24K.

25 Enter the physician's federal tax ID number. This may be the EIN or the Social Security number (SSN).

26 Enter the number assigned to the patient if the practice uses numerical identification numbers or if the claim is filed electronically.

27 For Medicare or CHAMPUS, check "YES" or "NO" to indicate whether the physician accepts assignment of benefits. For Medicaid and Medicare/Medicaid, the physician must check "YES."

28 Enter the total charge for services. This block must be completed.

29 For Medicare, enter the amount paid by the patient with the exception of the 20% co-insurance and deductible. For CHAMPUS, enter the amount paid by the patient or other insurance. For Medicaid, enter payment by insurance other than Medicare.

30 Enter the balance due.

Continued

31 Show the signature of the physician or that of his or her representative. Most insurance companies will accept a stamp if it fits in the box. Type the provider's name underneath (not the practice name.)

32 Enter the name and address of the facility if other than home or office. If you checked "YES" in box 20, you must enter the name and address of the laboratory that performed diagnostic tests billed on this form.

33 Enter the billing name, address and telephone number for the physician. Enter the UPIN number for a physician in solo practice or the group PIN number if the physician practices as part of a group.

Health Care and Cost Containment

HEALTH CARE REFORM

Since World War II, group insurance has been a significant fringe benefit in collective bargaining. In the fee-for-service concept of the 1960s to 1980s, the patient saw the doctor, received care, and then received a bill for the service. Insurance programs were first designed simply to pay those bills. The patient who had insurance paid an annual premium, and in return the insurance company paid at least a portion of the bill. Much of the fee-for-service care has been provided by Medicare, Medicaid, and the Blue Plans, but all of these plans are now utilizing cost-containment alternatives to fee for service.

During the 1990s, a major restructuring of the U.S. health care system was brought about because

- A growing percentage of Americans were not covered by private or government insurance.
- Employers were having to pay escalating health care premiums and did not want to cut wages. They wanted methods to lower the cost of employee health care.
- The government needed to reduce the deficit by keeping down increases in Medicaid and Medicare programs.
- Physicians and hospital costs were soaring out of sight due to inflation, expensive equipment, medications, and so on.
- Patients were reluctant to pay for physical examinations and immunizations, which were not usually covered by traditional insurance policies, and sometimes conditions were not diagnosed as early as desirable.

Over 70% of insurance has become HMO and is no longer fee for service.

MANAGEMENT OF HMO PLANS

If claims are not being paid promptly or correctly, the medical assistant should take steps to resolve the problem.

SKILLS AND RESPONSIBILITIES

GUIDE TO RESOLVING UNPAID OR INCORRECTLY PAID CLAIMS

1 Take examples to the next renegotiating session when the physician's contract expires.
2 Send a statement to the director notifying him or her that if the bill is not paid you will contact the employer's benefits manager or patient notifying him or her of the slow payments. Tell that person that the physician may not renew the contract and the director may need to find another physician.
3 Write to the plan representative.

PEER REVIEW ORGANIZATIONS

A **peer review organization (PRO)** is an outgrowth of a 1972 amendment to the Social Security Act that brought about the formation of federal **professional standards review organizations (PSROs),** whose purposes were to monitor the validity of diagnoses and the quality of care and to evaluate the appropriateness of hospital admissions and discharges of patients covered by government-sponsored health insurance. The effectiveness of PSROs was continually debated, and they were gradually phased out.

In 1982 PROs were legislated as part of the **Tax Equity and Fiscal Responsibility Act (TEFRA).** The purpose of a PRO is identical to that of the PSRO. The primary difference is that the PROs are mostly limited to a single group within a state. PRO contracts are awarded by the HCFA to physician-based organizations within each state, and the mechanics of PROs vary slightly from state to state. In an attempt to control costs, an insurance carrier may require prior authorization from the PRO before a patient is hospitalized for elective medical or surgical care. If the patient's condition can be adequately and safely treated on an outpatient basis, payment for hospitalization will not be approved. It is important that the medical assistant be aware of the types of admission cases that require previous authorization and that the authorization be obtained before the admission date.

PROSPECTIVE PAYMENT SYSTEM

In April 1983, the Social Security Amendments Act of 1983 (Public Law 98-21) was signed into law. Title VI of this law contained the prospective payment system (PPS) for hospitals, which would begin the radical restructuring of the payment system to hospitals for Medicare inpatient services.

As identified by HCFA, a major objective of the PPS was to establish the government as a prudent buyer of health care while maintaining beneficiaries' access to quality care. The prudent buyer objective was to be accomplished by paying Medicare providers a predetermined specific rate per discharge for diagnoses rather than on the basis of reasonable costs.

If a hospital does not contract with a PRO, it is not eligible for payment from the Medicare program. The law provides authority to grant waivers from the PPS if a state has an approved hospital reimbursement control system. Additional criteria must be met by a state to receive approval and a waiver from the federal PPS.

Diagnosis-Related Groups (DRGs)

The DRG classification forms the basis for payment under the PPS. It is based on an average cost for the patient's problem, as opposed to the traditional method of payment based on actual costs incurred in the provision of care. Payment to the hospital of a DRG amount generally constitutes payment in full for services rendered to Medicare patients.

The DRG system classifies patients on the basis of diagnosis and was developed by Yale University researchers in the 1970s as a mechanism for utilization review. DRGs are derived from taking all possible diagnoses identified in the ICD-9-CM system, classifying them into 25 **major diagnostic categories** (MDCs) based on organ system, and further breaking them into 495 **distinct groupings,** each of which is said to be medically meaningful. The principal diagnosis is the most critical factor in the assignment of DRGs. All diagnoses must reflect information contained in the patient's medical record.

To assign a case to a DRG, five pieces of information are necessary:

1. Patient's **principal diagnosis** and up to four **complications** or **comorbidities**
2. Treatment procedures performed
3. Patient's age

4. Patient's sex
5. Patient's discharge status

Physician's Responsibility

The major factor determining the assignment of a DRG is the physician's assessment of the principal diagnosis. It is the physician's responsibility to record the principal diagnosis as well as the other determining factors on a **discharge face sheet.** It is extremely important that the principal diagnosis, as stated by the physician, correspond to the various tests, procedures, and notes contained within the complete medical record.

Once the discharge face sheet has been completed by the physician, the chart is forwarded to the hospital's medical records department for review and coding. The codes contained in the *ICD-9-CM* are used for determining the DRG and, therefore, must be entered in the appropriate section of the discharge face sheet.

From the medical records department the information is forwarded to the financial office for completion of the bill to be submitted to the **fiscal intermediary.** The fiscal intermediary, through the use of a **grouper** computer program, determines the appropriate DRG and then calculates the payment to the hospital.

Memory Jogger

7 *What is the major factor in determining the assignment of a DRG?*

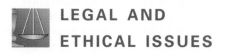

LEGAL AND
ETHICAL ISSUES

The practice of medicine and the responsibilities of the medical assistant, are greatly affected by the legislative process. It is extremely important to stay current on the laws that affect medicine, and in particular the coding process.

The person who is responsible for coding procedures must be very careful. It is the physician's responsibility to identify the patient's diagnosis and identify the procedures that have been performed. Often these codes are preprinted on the encounter form or superbill and/or in the computer, but if they are not, the medical assistant must identify the correct code. An incorrect code used for billing a service can be considered a fraud, especially if it is a recurrent offense.

In addition, the medical assistant must be sure to obtain patient signatures permitting insurance billing and to obtain proper authorizations from insurance carriers whenever required.

CRITICAL THINKING

1 Using your *CPT Manual,* code the following:
The physician is called to the ICU at the local hospital to see a patient in coronary crisis. The physician spends 1 hour at the patient's bedside stabilizing him.
Code: _____

2 An established patient is one who has received professional services from the physician or another physician of the same specialty in the same group within _____.

3 Using your *ICD-9-CM Manual,* code the following:
a. Bacterial endocarditis due to AIDS
Code: _____
b. Herniated disk, L4S1
Code: _____
c. Congestive heart failure with hypertension
Code: _____

HOW DID I DO? Answer to Memory Joggers

1 Tracking disease processes, classification of medical procedures, medical research, and evaluation of hospital utilization

2 Evaluation and Management, Anesthesiology, Surgery, Radiology, Pathology and Laboratory, and Medicine

3 Volume 2

4 The claim could be returned or rejected, or the physician could be fined if the claim were for Medicare.

5 If elective surgery is necessary on a Medicare patient, the provider must prepare a financial statement showing the type of surgery to be performed, the estimated charge, the estimated payment from Medicare, and the patient's probable out-of-pocket expenses. This statement must be signed by the patient. Put a copy in the patient's chart and give the patient a copy.

6 Health Care Financing Administration Common Procedure Coding system

7 The principal diagnosis

REFERENCES

American Medical Association: DRGs and the Prospective Payment System: A Guide for Physicians. Chicago, AMA, 1984.

American Medical Association: Physician's Current Procedural Terminology, 4th ed. Chicago, AMA, 1997.

American Medical Association: American Medical News, a weekly newspaper.

Fordney M: Insurance Handbook for the Medical Office, 5th ed. Philadelphia, WB Saunders, 1997.

Gosfield AG: RBRVS Special Report. Salt Lake City, Med-Index Publications, 1991.

HCPCS 1991–1992, 3rd ed. Salt Lake City, Med-Index Publications, 1997.

Reimbursement Strategies. Salt Lake City, Med-Index Publications, 1991.

SECTION 6

Advanced Administrative Skills

CURRICULUM CONTENT/COMPETENCIES

Chapter 22 Editorial Duties and Travel Arrangements
- Perform basic clerical functions
- Schedule, coordinate, and monitor appointments
- Develop educational materials
- Conduct continuing education activities

Chapter 23 Facility Environment
- Maintain supply inventory
- Comply with established risk management and safety procedures
- Maintain and dispose of regulated substances in compliance with government guidelines
- Negotiate leases and prices for equipment and supply contracts

Chapter 24 Management Responsibilities
- Orient and train personnel
- Interview and recommend job applicants
- Supervise personnel
- Process payroll
- Develop and maintain personnel, policy, and procedure manuals

Assisting with Library, Research, Travel, and Meetings

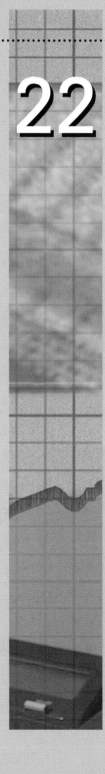

22

LEARNING OBJECTIVES

Cognitive: On successful completion of this chapter you should be able to:

1 Define and spell the terms listed in the Vocabulary.
2 Originate and maintain a card catalog for a personal library.
3 Discuss the nature and importance of an abstract.
4 List the four items to include on a cross-reference card for a general reference file.
5 Name five items of information to include on a diagnostic file card.
6 Name two of the largest medical databases for electronic retrieval of information.
7 List the seven items of information needed for each bibliography reference.
8 Briefly outline the general procedure for preparing a manuscript for publication.
9 List the five items that should be included in the first paragraph of meeting minutes.

Performance: On successful completion of this chapter you should be able to:

1 Prepare cards for an abstract file.
2 Set up a diagnostic file, including subject cards and the necessary subheadings to accommodate the patient charts.
3 Retype a manuscript that has been edited using proofreader's marks.
4 Type a speech in correct format and estimate the time necessary for delivery.
5 Make travel arrangements for a proposed trip.
6 Prepare a typewritten itinerary.
7 Make arrangements for a group meeting.
8 From a rough draft, type the minutes of a meeting in correct form, including the secretary's signature.

VOCABULARY

abstract A written summary of the key points of a book, paper, or case history

agenda A list of the specific items under each division of the order of business that is to be presented at a business meeting

bibliography A list of the works that are referred to in a text or that were consulted by the author in producing a text

colloquialisms Expressions that are acceptable and correct in ordinary conversation or informal speeches but unsuitable for formal speech or writing

draft A preliminary outline or writing that the author expects to amend or revise

footnotes Comments placed at the bottom of a page that would be distracting if placed within the main text

galley proofs Printer's proofs taken from composed type before page composition

legend Heading or title of a figure

manuscript Written or typewritten document, as distinguished from printed copy

monograph Learned treatise on a small area of knowledge; a written account of a single thing or class of things

order of business List of the different divisions of business in the order in which each is to be addressed at a business meeting

periodicals Journals published with a fixed interval (greater than 1 day) between their issues or numbers

reprints Reproductions of printed matter

synopsis Summary of the main points of a longer text

treatise Systematic exposition or argument in writing

The medical profession is unique in that the physician traditionally shares with others, through writing and speaking, the discoveries, information, and observations gained in practice, research, and private study. The medical assistant who becomes proficient in maintaining the physician's personal library and in assisting with the preparation of articles and speeches can be of immeasurable help in these endeavors.

The Physician's Library

The books that a physician acquires while in medical school are the nucleus of a personal library that will grow over the years. New books reflecting the changes in medicine and the physician's special interests are continually added (Fig. 22–1). The physician may accumulate a file of professional journals such as the *Journal of the American Medical Association* (JAMA), the journal of the state medical society, specialty journals, trade journals, and even informative material provided by pharmaceutical companies.

Journals should be bound at regular intervals, generally by volume, to preserve the individual copies. The medical assistant may be responsible for having the journals bound regularly and consistently. Most journals in the medical field publish indexes, annually, semiannually, or quarterly. The index should be bound with the journal pages. In most cities, the binding of **periodicals** can be done locally. The hospital librarian is a good source of information for locating a bookbinder.

ORGANIZING THE LIBRARY

Although the physician's library may not be large, it must be systematically organized so that information is readily accessible.

In setting up or rearranging a small library, books should be classified by subject groupings that reflect

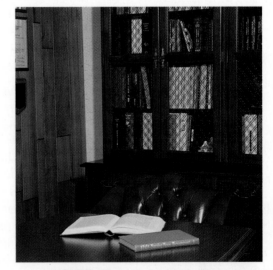

FIGURE 22–1 A physician's library.

medical specialties. Those dealing with related topics should be placed together. Journals and periodicals are usually arranged alphabetically.

CATALOGING OF BOOKS

The books should be indexed, either in a card catalog or in a computer database. A 3 × 5-inch card file is practical for this purpose. Generally, three or more cards should be prepared for each book (Fig. 22–2):

- Title card
- Subject card
- Author card(s)

Here is how to index a book in this manner, using the book you are reading as an example:

1. Prepare a title card with the heading "The Administrative Medical Assistant."
2. Prepare a subject card with the heading "Medical Assisting."
3. Prepare author card with the heading Kinn, Mary E.
4. The cards may then be filed alphabetically or, preferably, in a file divided into sections for title, subject, and author. With such a file and cross-reference system, any book can be located very quickly.

Administrative Medical Assistant, The, 4th Edition

Mary E. Kinn
Philadelphia, W. B. Saunders Company, 1999

Textbook and reference covering all administrative phases of medical assisting in the physician's office

TITLE CARD

Medical Assisting

The Administrative Medical Assistant, 4th Edition,
Philadelphia, W. B. Saunders Company, 1999

Mary E. Kinn

SUBJECT CARD

Kinn, Mary E.

The Administrative Medical Assistant, 4th Edition,
Philadelphia, W. B. Saunders Company, 1999

1. Medical Assisting

AUTHOR CARD

FIGURE 22–2 Title, subject, and author cards for referencing a book in a personal library.

Memory Jogger

1 *What is the purpose of indexing the contents of a personal library?*

PERIODICAL FILE

One of the physician's greatest challenges is keeping up with medical literature, particularly the articles that appear regularly in the periodicals. It is unlikely that the physician will want to maintain a complete index of all articles appearing in these periodicals, but most will want to keep track of those articles that are of particular interest. Abstracts are of great value in the continuing task of keeping abreast of scientific developments.

Preparation of an Abstract

An **abstract** is a **synopsis** of a book, paper, or case history. It is brief, indicates the nature of the article, and summarizes the most important points and conclusions. Abstracts prepared by professionals are found in many medical journals as a service to the individual physician.

Many physicians prepare abstracts of the articles that they find of particular value; and in some offices, the medical assistant is trained to do abstracting for the physician. A medical assistant who can prepare a good abstract of an article can save the physician from reading 10 to 20 pages of the original article and can help focus attention on information of particular interest in the article.

Abstracts must clearly indicate the nature of the information contained in the article. Each should note

- Any new procedures
- Results of studies and experiments
- Conclusions noted

The length and character of the article determine the type and length of the abstract. In most scientific articles, the conclusions of the writer are summarized at the end of the piece. This summary is of great help in preparing an abstract.

The abstracts are typed on cards, with the text of the abstract preceded by the following information:

- Title of the article
- Surname and initials of the author
- Name of the publication
- Volume number
- Inclusive page numbers
- Month and year

The cards are then filed. If abstract cards are kept, it is not necessary to clip and file the actual articles separately. The journals in which they appear can be kept in the usual alphabetical order.

Memory Jogger

 Name the three classes of information that should be included in an abstract.

OTHER REFERENCE FILES

Physicians frequently need a variety of miscellaneous medical information in addition to book collections and periodicals and their indexes. For this reason, they may develop a separate reference file of valuable information. Often, this consists of pages photocopied from journals or reference books.

The physician and the medical assistant together may set up a subject index for filing the material and a cross-reference card file for easily locating the information. Begin by tabbing file dividers with the main topics and folders with subheadings. When an article or item is photocopied, a card is prepared with the title of the article or chapter, author's name, periodical or book in which it appears, and the date of publication. The copy of the reference material is then filed in the appropriate folder and the card filed by subject for easy reference. As new developments occur, later articles may be filed and the outdated material discarded.

DIAGNOSTIC FILES

Physicians often draw material for their writing and speaking from the case histories of their own patients. For this reason, many physicians like to set up diagnostic files so that they can quickly pull out information on, for example, the incidence of certain side effects among patients treated with a specific medication. The medical assistant must be familiar with medical terminology to maintain this kind of file.

The system used can vary, but subject cards generally have a main heading with the name of the disease or surgical procedure and subheadings for various aspects of the disease or procedure. The patient cards list the patient's name, diagnosis, and type of treatment.

EXAMPLE OF MAIN HEADING WITH SUBHEADINGS

BLOOD DISEASES
Anemia
Granulocytosis
Hemophilia
Leukemia
Polycythemia
Thalassemia
Toxemia

EXAMPLE OF A PATIENT'S CARD FILED UNDER ANEMIA

Anemia
Patient name: Date:
Diagnosis:
Treatment:
Prognosis:
Other pertinent information:

By keeping a file such as this, a physician can readily obtain the charts of all patients with a specified condition from the history files. This is particularly valuable to physicians who do a great deal of teaching, writing, or research. In the physician's office equipped with a computer, it is very easy to keep a detailed diagnostic file using these same principles.

LIBRARY FOR PATIENTS

A small library of educational information for patients may be maintained by the medical assistant. This library generally contains some books written in language that the average patient can understand as well as a number of pamphlets and reprints that the patient can take home. This might include information on such subjects as diabetes, heart disease, skin conditions, the danger signals of cancer, lung disease, first aid, and other subjects of interest to many patients, depending on the type of practice. The specialist may have information dealing specifically with his or her specialty. A library service such as this saves the physician considerable time in repeating simple educational information and is generally welcomed by the patients. Maintaining the library for patients may be a joint effort of physician and staff. Any items added to the library should first be approved by the physician.

Research

The medical assistant who is employed by a physician who teaches, writes, or lectures frequently may be called on to assist with the preparation of papers. The duties might include

- Preparing a list of references for a presentation or a paper for publication
- Doing actual research
- Preparing abstracts

Any medical assistant who is called on to assume such responsibilities must know how to make the best use of the available library and Internet reference facilities.

USING LIBRARY FACILITIES

Almost all physicians, even those practicing in rural areas, have access to medical libraries. The physician who practices in a metropolitan area or near a medical center such as one affiliated with a university is particularly fortunate, because outstanding library facilities are readily at his or her disposal.

All general hospitals maintain medical libraries consisting of a basic collection of carefully selected, authoritative medical textbooks and reference works of the latest edition as well as files of current journals. The Medical Library Association sets standards for member libraries.

A physician usually has access to a county society library or can use the package library services of the state society. In addition, extension library facilities can be used to obtain information from special supplemental collections. The American Medical Association, for example, and some specialty societies, offer periodical lending services and package library services to their members.

The National Library of Medicine has established a system whereby physicians may get materials from a regional medical library program when information is not available locally. In those instances when the regional program cannot satisfy the need, the request is channeled to the National Library of Medicine.

All libraries systematically organize the books, periodicals, and other materials in a fairly uniform manner so that the information can be easily located and is accessible. The medical assistant who finds it necessary to go to a library to do special work should seek out the librarian or an assistant and get an idea of what the library has to offer with respect to materials and their arrangement, privileges, rules, and regulations for use of the library. After a brief discussion, the trained medical librarian usually can suggest shortcuts that are of great help in locating references or doing research.

Memory Jogger

3 *List the three research activities that a medical assistant might assume in medical research.*

Card Catalog (Computer)

Any book, monograph, treatise, handbook, dictionary, and encyclopedia contained in a library is indexed by author and subject and sometimes by title in the card catalog. Although we still refer to it as the "card" catalog, in reality, the index is now usually accessed via a computer terminal. This catalog is really an index of the book contents of the library. Cards are arranged alphabetically (with subject, author, and title cards alphabetized in one series) or

are alphabetized within separate sections for subject, author, or title.

CLASSIFICATION SYSTEMS There are a number of systems for classifying library books. In library procedure, classification means putting together materials on a given subject with related materials placed nearby. Medical libraries use various classification systems. The two most used systems are the Dewey decimal system and the Library of Congress classification system.

The Dewey decimal system is used not only in medical but also in all types of libraries. This system uses decimal numbers to indicate specific subjects and arranges the book collection in numerical sequence for easy location. For example, "616" indicates "Pathology, Diseases, Treatment."

EXAMPLE OF HOW THE DEWEY DECIMAL SYSTEM WORKS	
616.1	Diseases of the cardiovascular system
616.9	Communicable and other diseases
616.96	Parasitic diseases
616.99	Other general diseases
616.992	Neoplasms and neoplastic diseases

The Library of Congress classification system consists of a number of separate, mutually exclusive classifications based on combination of letters of the alphabet and numerals.

EXAMPLE OF LIBRARY OF CONGRESS SYSTEM	
QR	Bacteriology
RD	Surgery
RC 321–431	Diseases of the nervous system

HOW THE CARD CATALOG CAN HELP YOU LOCATE BOOKS No matter which system of classification is used, its main purpose is to help those who use the library to locate volumes quickly. The symbol for the particular book, whether it be a numeral, a letter, or a combination of numerals and letters, appears on the entry for the book in the card catalog. This symbol is called a classification mark. It also appears on the spine of the volume.

To locate a volume, check the classification mark on the card catalog entry and, if an open-shelf system is used, find that shelf in the library where corresponding symbols appear. If a closed-shelf system is used in the library, give the number of the book and its title to a librarian who will locate it for you.

Memory Jogger

4 *What is the purpose of a card catalog?*

Periodical Indexes

The bulk of current medical literature appears in medical journals, and some reference system for organizing and accessing the thousands of articles is necessary. The majority of journals publish their own indexes, one for each volume, sometimes with an annual index. If you know the name of the journal that published the article you are looking for, this is the fastest way to locate it. Otherwise, composite indexes may be consulted.

CLINICAL MEDICINE The monthly *Index Medicus* and the annual *Cumulated Index Medicus,* published by the National Library of Medicine, include author and subject indexes for over 3000 periodicals. They are international in scope, representing foreign publications and languages as well as publications in English.

The monthly *Abridged Index Medicus* and the annual *Cumulated Abridged Index Medicus* are smaller versions of *Index Medicus* and *Cumulated Index Medicus* and are limited to indexing 100 major periodicals in the medical field. These periodicals are readily available in the majority of medical libraries. The computer equivalent of both the *Index Medicus* and the *Abridged Index Medicus* is MEDLINE.

NURSING AND ALLIED HEALTH The *Cumulative Index to Nursing & Allied Health Literature* is published by Glendale Adventist Medical Center.* This index is very comprehensive and is the only thorough source for coverage of allied health. It is published bimonthly with an annual cumulation. The computer equivalent is Nursing & Allied Health Index on Bibliographic Retrieval System (BRS) and Dialog.

The *International Nursing Index* is published quarterly, with an annual cumulation, by the *American Journal of Nursing.* The computer equivalent is MEDLINE.

---

*1509 Wilson Terrace, Glendale, CA 91206.

Bibliography Search

Information for a **bibliography** may be obtained either by a manual search through indexes or by a computer search.

For a manual search, you must look under the subject closest to the one on which you need information, then copy down all the information (author, title of journal, and complete bibliographic information, including volume number, pages, and date).

Most of the world's literature is now accessible through various vendors that provide computer access to specialized files. There are thousands of these databases. The major vendors in health care facilities are

- National Library of Medicine
- Dialog Information Services, Inc.
- Bibliographic Retrieval System (BRS)
- Systems Development Corporation (SDC)

The National Library of Medicine is the least expensive of these four vendors.

PREPARING A BIBLIOGRAPHY Utilizing the various reference sources of the medical library, you can make up a bibliography or list of references on a specific topic with comparatively little difficulty. It does take time, and the list of references must be accurate. Many researchers recommend listing each reference separately on a card or in a small looseleaf notebook (Fig. 22–3). This simplifies the actual preparation of the formal bibliography that always accompanies any published medical paper. Note the following information for each reference:

1. Author
2. Subject
3. Title of book or article
4. Publisher or periodical
5. Volume number
6. Date of publication
7. Page numbers

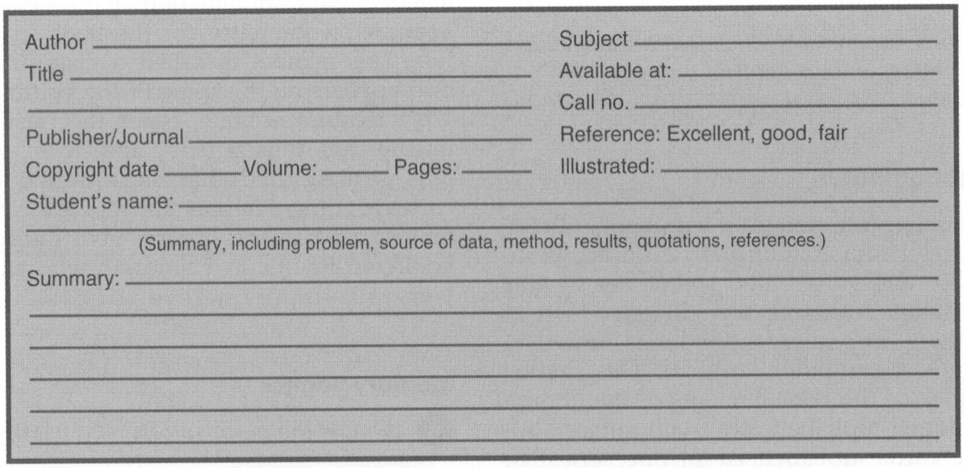

Author _____   Subject _____
Title _____   Available at: _____
_____   Call no. _____
Publisher/Journal _____   Reference: Excellent, good, fair
Copyright date ____ Volume: ____ Pages: ____   Illustrated: _____
Student's name: _____

(Summary, including problem, source of data, method, results, quotations, references.)
Summary: _____

FIGURE 22–3 Card for reporting bibliographic data.

Sometimes card catalogs and other periodical references list brief summaries of the specific reference cited; this information is also helpful in research and should be noted.

Some libraries prepare medical bibliographies free of charge or for a small fee. Some also abstract or review literature, translate articles, and collect case reports. The library of the American College of Surgeons, for example, offers this service at a modest fee to its members. The American Medical Association also offers this service to its members.

ELECTRONIC RETRIEVAL OF INFORMATION

The individual physician or health care facility with a computer, a modem, telecommunications software, and a telephone line may subscribe to one or more information utilities. Some of the medically oriented utilities are

- GTE   Medical Information Network (MINET)
- BRS   Colleague Medical
- DIALOG

Through GTE access may be made to EMPIRES (Excerpta Medica Physician Information Retrieval and Education Service), the American Medical Association's clinical literature database that contains current and historical citations and abstracts from over 300 key medical journals.

The development of databases and electronic retrieval systems has provided an invaluable service to the medical profession by making possible easy access to references on an unlimited number of medical subjects. It is also possible for subscribers to read the complete text of books, journals, and other publications.

Principal Medical Resources

Two of the largest medical databases are MEDLINE and EMBASE, each of which includes citations and abstracts from thousands of publications.

MEDLINE is one of a family of several databases known as MEDLARS (MEDical Literature Analysis and Retrieval System). It is produced by the National Library of Medicine (NLM), which is part of the National Institutes of Health, a federal agency in Bethesda, Maryland. *Index Medicus* is produced from this computer file.

EMBASE is produced by Excerpta Medica, and the *Excerpta Medica Index* is produced from this database.

Both MEDLINE and EMBASE are bibliographic indexes, not full-text databases. The computer search generates a bibliography of literature. The searcher must then locate a copy of the article. Some files provide abstracts that are available online. Articles not available from a health care library can usually be requested through the library as an interlibrary loan.

AMA/NET   The American Medical Association offers an online information service called AMA/Net free to its members. The subscriber to this service has instant access to millions of published documents. MEDLINE and EMPIRES are two of the sources available through this service. AMA/Net also offers continuing medical education programs, several sources of medical news, and an electronic mail system.

AAMA   Members of the American Association of Medical Assistants may contact the Association or network with other members nationwide through the Internet at www.aama-ntl.org.

Other Reference Sources

There are a number of other specialized reference volumes that a medical librarian may use to locate literature. The Monthly Catalog of U.S. Government Publications, for example, contains certain medical listings and is sometimes valuable in research work. In securing biographical information about physicians or other professionals, it is often necessary to turn to such books as the *Directory of Medical Specialists*, *American Men of Science*, the *American Medical Directory*, or *Who's Who Among Physicians and Surgeons*. Encyclopedias such as *Encyclopedia Britannica* and the *Practical Medicine* series also are sometimes helpful in obtaining basic information.

Memory Jogger

5   *Name the two largest medical databases.*

Manuscript Preparation

In most cases, the medical assistant's tasks in connection with the preparation of a lecture or a **manuscript** for publication are mainly the gathering of references and facts; the physician is responsible for the actual writing. However, because some physicians ask their medical assistants to serve in the capacity of editorial assistants and to smooth out and actually edit their copy before submitting it for publication, a basic understanding of the style, format, and characteristics of medical papers is helpful.

SPEECHES

Not all papers are intended for publication. Some are prepared for presentation before medical and scientific meetings. Speeches should be typed and double-spaced; in some offices a jumbo or magna type machine is used so that the speech is easy to read. Special large-type elements, such as the IBM Orator, are available for single-element or daisy wheel typewriters. All computer word processing programs have a vast selection of print type and size.

At the bottom of each page, in the lower right-hand corner, type the first two or three words that appear at the beginning of the next page. The final draft of the paper should be carefully checked for any typographical errors.

The speaker at a large meeting is usually allotted 10 to 20 minutes to present a paper. At county society and small meetings, the speaker may have from 30 minutes to an hour for the presentation. Check in advance to find out exactly how much time will be allowed. The physician or the medical assistant should time the speech. On average, it takes about 2 minutes to read a page of copy on which there are 200 to 250 words. If slides or other exhibits are planned, arrangements for showing this material must be made in advance and the necessary time allowed.

MANUSCRIPT STYLE

Each medical journal has its own style for published papers. The individual hoping to publish in a specific journal should request a copy of the journal's guidelines for manuscripts in advance and then prepare the manuscript accordingly to minimize editorial changes. However, there are certain fairly uniform procedures to be followed in the preparation of a manuscript to be submitted for publication.

A good medical paper must present established new facts, modes, or practices; principles of value; results of suitable original research; or a review of facts on a subject from which the reader can draw a legitimate conclusion. The subject should be limited to a definite area or problem before writing is begun, and the purpose should be determined in advance.

The typical medical article begins with an introductory section outlining the nature of the material or problem to be covered, follows with actual discussion of the subject, and concludes with a summary in which conclusions are usually noted in numerical form. The format for case reports is somewhat similar. Case reports based on clinical information should be written clearly in smooth narrative style and should not read like a collection of telegraphic notes. There should be a clear presentation of the sequence of events. A brief abstract summarizing the article may appear at the beginning or end of any article. This summary should be rigidly condensed and should contain the deductions as well as clearly reflect the author's viewpoint. Only the actual conclusions reached should be numbered.

The writing in a scientific paper should be simple and straightforward. Excess words should be ruthlessly pared from the article. Grammatical construction must facilitate direct, clear expression. The paper should be well organized and proceed smoothly from beginning to end. Slang, **colloquialisms,** personal allusions, and reminiscences should generally be avoided in papers for publication, although they are often acceptable and add a friendly tone to a paper to be delivered in person before a medical meeting.

DRAFTING, REVISING, AND FINAL COPY

A **draft** of a paper may be made before the final copy. Sometimes several drafts are made. Using an electronic word processor or computer can greatly reduce the laborious retyping of manuscripts, but the author may still want a printout of each revision. Sometimes different colors of paper are used to distinguish between each draft. Double- or triple-space drafts to allow plenty of room for the author's revisions.

An important step in the preparation of any manuscript is a careful revision of copy. This is a duty sometimes delegated to the medical assistant or secretary.

SKILLS AND RESPONSIBILITIES

MAKING REVISIONS TO A SCIENTIFIC PAPER

- Organization—Determine that information moves from topic to topic in an organized, logical sequence.
- Accuracy—Check for accuracy by referring to reference material or querying physician.
- Content—Verify that content is complete by comparing with outline or summary.
- Conciseness—Confirm that explanations are straightforward and free of unnecessary wording.
- Correct sentence construction and grammar— Review for any errors in grammar or awkwardly constructed sentences.
- Clarity and smoothness—Read through for a sense of clarity in the explanation of material and ease in moving from one idea to another.

Check for correct spelling, using the computer spell check, a medical dictionary, and a standard dictionary.

Prepare the final copy using a good-quality $8\frac{1}{2} \times$ 11-inch white paper. Print on one side of the paper only. Double-space the copy, allowing a margin of at least 1 inch at each side and at the bottom. Double-spacing provides space for the editor who receives the manuscript to make corrections or insert instructions for the publisher. Unless otherwise instructed, number each page in the upper right-hand corner.

The original manuscript is submitted to the publisher, and the author should retain one or more copies. If the manuscript is on disk or tape, one printout is sufficient to retain in the file.

FOOTNOTES

When a paper is based on a study of the writing of others, it is necessary to acknowledge the sources used. In medical and scientific papers, **footnotes** usually provide exact references to sources of material. Forms of footnotes differ slightly, depending on the style of the periodical; but, in general, a footnote contains the following information:

- Author's name
- Title of the work cited
- Facts of publication
- Exact page from which the citation was taken

The first time a book or article is mentioned in a footnote, all the information about the publication should appear in the footnote; after that, references to the same source can be shortened to the author's last name and the page number cited. When a periodical is concerned, a later reference need contain only the author's name, the journal name, and the page number.

Detailed information about footnote preparation can be obtained from *The Chicago Manual of Style* or one of several published reference manuals for office workers (Table 22–1).

FINAL BIBLIOGRAPHY

All scientific papers should carry a complete bibliography of source materials. List only those sources that directly pertain to the paper and that were used

in its preparation. The form of bibliographies is fairly uniform.

LISTING FOR PERIODICALS

- Author's name and initials
- Title of the article
- Name of the periodical
- Volume number
- Pages cited
- Date of publication

LISTING FOR BOOK REFERENCES

- Author's name and initials
- Title of the book
- Edition (only after the first edition)
- Place of publication
- Name of publisher
- Year of publication

Bibliographies may be arranged alphabetically according to author's name or numerically as the references appear in the text. Whatever form and punctuation are used should be consistent through the entire listing.

ILLUSTRATIONS

All drawings, photographs, and other illustrative material submitted with a manuscript should be placed on separate sheets and keyed to the manuscript. In other words, illustrations should be numbered and indications should be noted in the manuscript as to where each illustration will be placed. Do not include such materials in the body of the manuscript. The explanation of the drawing or illustration should appear in a caption, or **legend.**

Glossy black and white or color photographs reproduce best. Captions for photographs should be typed on separate sheets or may be attached with rubber cement below the photograph. On the back of the photograph, the author's name and the number of the illustration should be penciled lightly. Do not use paper clips on photographs. Credit lines should be given for copyrighted or commercial photographs or illustrations. If x-ray films are submitted, make sure the prints are shiny; indicate on the back where they may be cropped but leave localizing landmarks.

Charts and line drawings must be carefully prepared to achieve good reproduction. Such drawings preferably should be done with India or black ink on heavy white bond paper. Present-day techniques point to preparation of these items using a com-

TABLE 22–1 Abbreviations Used in Manuscript Preparation

Abbreviation	Meaning
cf.	compare
e.g.	for example
et al.	and other people
ibid.	in the same place
i.e.	that is
loc. cit.	in the place cited
op. cit.	in the work cited
sic	intentionally so written
q.v.	which see

puter. Charts should be condensed and simplified as much as possible. Letters and identifying numerals can be placed on the face of the chart with the explanation in the legend below.

Tables should be prepared in a uniform style on separate sheets, using a typewriter or computer. Each table should be numbered consecutively and have a descriptive heading.

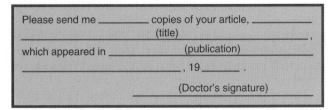

FIGURE 22–4 Typical card for ordering reprints.

Memory Jogger

6 *List the six items of information that should be included in a bibliographical book reference.*

MAILING THE MANUSCRIPT

Generally, manuscripts should not be folded but should be mailed flat in a large envelope. Sometimes a paper of fewer than four pages can be folded twice and mailed in a regular business envelope, or a manuscript of four to eight pages can be folded once and mailed in a 6 × 9-inch envelope. A letter stating that the manuscript is being submitted for publication should be included. Photographs and illustrations should be mailed flat, between sheets of protective cardboard.

GALLEY PROOFS

A paper accepted for publication will be set in type, and proofs of the article will usually be returned by the editor to the author for checking. Because changes in a manuscript once it is set in type are costly, revisions should be limited to correction of errors and minor changes.

If possible, work as a team when checking **galley proofs,** with one person holding the proofs and the other person reading from the original copy. Check for typographic errors, omitted lines and words, and so forth. When correcting proofs, use a different-colored pencil from the one used by the proofreader on the publication. Corrections should be entered in the margins of the proof, next to the line with the error to be corrected. A knowledge of proofreader's marks is helpful (see Chapter 12).

One corrected set of galley proofs should be returned to the editor, and one set of proofs should be retained by the author. If a second set of proofs is sent later, check the first corrected set against the second set to make sure that all corrections have been made.

INDEXING

Often it is necessary to provide an index for a long paper or a book. An author and subject index can be made from page proofs. One system for indexing is to use slips of paper or 3 × 5-inch cards. Each index entry is listed on a separate card or slip; this simplifies alphabetizing under major headings later. The whole index can then be typed from the alphabetized cards. Manuscripts prepared by computer can be indexed quickly and accurately with the necessary software.

REPRINTS

At the time an article is set in type, the author should order all needed **reprints,** because type is often destroyed after the original press run. The medical assistant generally handles the ordering of the reprints, which may be as many as 500 copies or more. The order should be adequate to cover any future needs. Most physicians send copies of their articles to colleagues, to physicians who have evidenced an interest in their work, and to hospitals and teaching institutions with which they have had contact (Fig. 22–4). They probably maintain a card file of names and addresses of those to whom they wish to send reprints.

Addresses in the card file should be checked from time to time in the *American Medical Directory* or by scanning membership and request lists. Some record of reprint mailing should be kept, and acknowledgments should be checked. A person who does not acknowledge two or three reprints should be taken off the mailing list.

An enclosure card, printed in advance, is sent by some authors with a copy of the reprint. Others prefer to enclose a short letter stating that the reprint is a complimentary copy.

Travel and Meeting Arrangements

TRANSPORTATION AND LODGING

The medical assistant may be expected to make transportation and lodging arrangements for the physician for out-of-town meetings (see Procedure 22–1). Although the physician who is located in a

PROCEDURE 22-1
Making Travel Arrangements

GOAL
To make travel arrangements for the physician from his or her city of residence to Toronto, Canada

EQUIPMENT AND SUPPLIES

Travel plan
Telephone
Telephone directory

Typewriter or computer
Typing paper

PROCEDURAL STEPS

1 Verify the details of planned trip:
- Desired date and time of departure
- Desired date and time of return
- Preferred mode of transportation
- Number in party
- Preferred lodging and price range

2 Telephone travel agency to arrange for transportation and lodging reservations.

3 Arrange for traveler's checks if desired.

4 Pick up tickets or arrange for their delivery

5 Check tickets to confirm conformance with the travel plan.
PURPOSE To avoid any error due to misunderstanding and to verify compliance with requests.

6 Check to see that hotel reservations are confirmed.

7 Prepare an itinerary, including all the necessary information:
- Date and time of departure
- Flight numbers or identifying information of other modes of travel.
- Mode of transportation to hotel(s).
- Name, address, and telephone number of hotel(s), with confirmation numbers if available.
- Date and time of return.

8 Place one copy of itinerary in the office file.
PURPOSE It may be necessary to contact the traveler or to forward mail.

9 Give several copies of the itinerary to the traveler.
PURPOSE The traveler may wish to have extra copies for family or friends.

---

metropolitan area probably uses a travel agent for most travel arrangements, the medical assistant may be responsible for working with the travel agent and preparing the detailed itinerary.

When not working with a travel agent, the medical assistant may be expected to personally make the hotel and transportation arrangements. A person who is sufficiently skilled in computer operations may be able to accomplish both without outside help. One should keep a file of the telephone numbers of airlines and hotels that have been found satisfactory or been recommended. When a reservation has been made, ask for the confirmation number. When traveling by automobile, the literature and maps provided by an auto club can be very useful.

ITINERARY

When all arrangements are final, prepare the itinerary. Keep one copy in the office file. Give the original to the physician plus any copies that may be requested for family members or other individuals. Since it is sometimes necessary to contact the physician while traveling, it is important that the itinerary be carefully prepared, including locations and telephone numbers.

MEETING CALENDAR

A calendar of all meetings that the physician plans to attend should be kept by the medical assistant, with both the physician and the medical assistant retaining a copy. The calendar can be merely a sheet of paper but should include the following information for each event:

- Name of the meeting
- Date
- Place
- Time

Any changes or additions to the calendar should be made on both copies as notices are received. A reminder to the physician a few days in advance of each meeting is usually appreciated.

MEETING RESPONSIBILITIES

A physician often accepts official responsibilities in his or her professional society or on the hospital board. The administrative medical assistant for this physician may be expected to assist in arranging meetings, preparing an agenda, and typing minutes of the meeting dictated by the physician (see Procedure 22–2).

The medical assistant who takes an active part in a professional society for medical assistants will have personal use for these skills as well.

Arranging a Meeting

When arranging a meeting you need to know

- The purpose of the meeting
- The number of persons expected to attend
- Whether a meal is to be included
- The expected duration of the meeting
- The date, time, and place
- The list of persons to be notified

Choosing the Location

Some groups meet regularly and use the same facility each time. In this case, it is necessary merely to confirm the date and time with the facility. If a meal is to be served, the menu, price, and approximate number expected to attend must be determined. If a new location is being used, you need to verify that

- The space is adequate
- Any necessary electronic equipment is available
- Parking facilities are available if needed
- Lighting and ventilation are adequate
- Menus are available if a meal is to be included

Preparing the Notice of Meeting

Meeting notices are usually mailed to all members of the group. For a small committee meeting, the members may be notified by telephone. If there is to be a speaker, the name of the speaker and the topic are included in the meeting notice. The notice must include the date, time, and place of the meeting.

Preparing the Agenda

Organizations whose bylaws specify *Robert's Rules of Order, Newly Revised,* as the parliamentary authority and that have not adopted a special order of business use the following prescribed **order of business:**

1. Reading and approval of the minutes
2. Reports of officers, boards, and standing committees
3. Reports of special (select or ad hoc) committees
4. Special orders
5. Unfinished business and general orders
6. New business

The order of business lists the different divisions of business in the order in which each will be called for at business meetings.

An **agenda** is a list of the specific items under each division of the order of business that the officers or board plan to present at a meeting. The medical assistant who is expected to prepare the agenda should determine what topics are to be discussed, type them in the prescribed order, and duplicate enough copies for the meeting. For a large group, the program is usually printed. For the smaller group, photocopies are satisfactory.

Memory Jogger

7 *How does an agenda differ from an order of business?*

Preparing the Minutes

The record of the proceedings of a meeting is called the minutes. The minutes contain mainly a record of what was done at the meeting, not what was said by the members.

The first paragraph of the minutes should contain the following information:

- Kind of meeting (e.g., regular, special)
- Name of the association
- Date, time, and place of the meeting
- The fact that the regular chairman and secretary were present or, in their absence, the names of the persons who substituted for them
- Whether the minutes of the previous meeting were read and approved

The body of the minutes should contain a separate paragraph for each subject matter. It should include all main motions, including (a) the wording in which each motion was adopted or otherwise dis-

PPROCEDURE 22-2
Arranging a Group Meeting

GOAL
To arrange a breakfast meeting for the physician's hospital committee

EQUIPMENT AND SUPPLIES
Directory of committee members
Meeting plan
Telephone

Typewriter or computer
Post cards

PROCEDURAL STEPS

1 Verify the proposed date and time for the meeting.

2 Gather details for meeting arrangements
- Purpose of the meeting
- Expected attendance
- Name of the speaker, if any, and the program topic
- Expected duration of the meeting

3 Arrange for a meeting room based on the requirements

4 Mail notice of the meeting to members and invited guests. Include:
- Date
- Time
- Place
- Name of the speaker and the topic
- Cost, if any
- Registration information

5 Arrange for any necessary equipment (e.g., microphone, projector, and screen).

6 Notify the meeting place of the number of reservations, if required.

7 Arrange for registration check-in.

8 Prepare the agenda.

9 Give the required number of copies of the agenda to physician.

---

posed of, (b) the disposition of the motion, and (c) the name of the mover. The name of the seconder of a motion should not be entered in the minutes unless ordered by the assembly. The body of the minutes should also include any points of order and appeals, whether they were sustained or lost, and the reasons given by the chair for the ruling. The minutes may include the name and subject of a guest speaker, but no attempt should be made to summarize the speech. The last paragraph should state the hour of adjournment.

The minutes should be signed by the secretary. In some organizations the president also signs the minutes. The practice of including the words "Respectfully submitted" is obsolete and should not be used.

The medical assistant who might be expected to type the minutes of meetings should consult an authoritative book on the subject and prepare a model

to follow in typing the minutes of each meeting so that every set of minutes will be in the same style.

Memory Jogger

8 *Under what circumstance is the name of the seconder of a motion included in the minutes?*

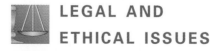

LEGAL AND
ETHICAL ISSUES

The medical assistant can provide a significant contribution by helping the physician fulfill his or her obligation to keep current with medical progress. In so doing, the medical assistant is also gaining insight into new developments.

CRITICAL THINKING

1 Select a short article from a professional journal and prepare an abstract using the suggested form in this chapter.

2 Suggest specific items that might be placed in a library for patients.

3 What items would *not* be displayed?

4 Describe how the typing of a speech that is to be presented at a professional meeting might differ from an ordinary typewritten page.

5 What advance information is needed before arranging a group meeting?

HOW DID I DO? Answers to Memory Joggers

1 The purpose of indexing is to provide ready access to information being sought.

2 *a.* New procedures
b. Results of studies and/or experiments
c. Any conclusions noted

3 *a.* Prepare a list of references

b. Perform actual research
c. Prepare abstracts

4 The purpose of a card catalog is to provide a means of locating information quickly.

5 The two largest medical databases are MEDLINE and EMBASE

6 *a.* Author's name and initials
b. Title of book
c. Edition number (after the first edition)
d. Place of publication
e. Name of publisher
f. Year of publication

7 The agenda is a list of the specific items under each division of the order of business.

8 The name of the seconder of a motion is included in the minutes only when ordered by the assembly.

REFERENCES

Baldwin F, McInerney S: Infomedicine. Boston, Little, Brown & Co., 1996.
Robert's Rules of Order, Newly Revised. Glenview, IL, Scott, Foresman & Co., 1990.
Sabin WA: The Gregg Reference Manual, 7th ed. New York, McGraw-Hill, 1994.

Facility Environment

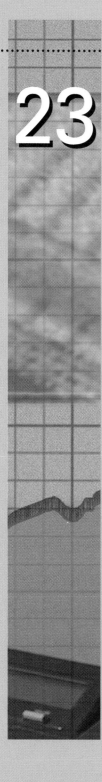

23

LEARNING OBJECTIVES

Cognitive: On successful completion of this chapter you should be able to:

1 Define and spell the terms listed in the Vocabulary.
2 List seven items of concern in controlling the general environment of a health care facility.
3 Discuss the utilization of various areas of the facility.
4 Describe how the medical assistant would arrange for and supervise a maintenance service.
5 Explain the inventory process.
6 Explain the importance of the instructions and warranties accompanying new equipment purchases.
7 Cite precautions to be observed in storing poisons, narcotics, acids and caustics, and flammable items.
8 Discuss the procedure for storing supplies and drug samples.
9 List six possible safety hazards in a health care facility.
10 Discuss the importance of and procedures to observe in routine office security.

Performance: On successful completion of this chapter you should be able to:

1 Write instructions for a maintenance service.
2 Set up an equipment inventory.
3 Organize, store, and dispose of drug samples.
4 Establish and maintain a supply inventory and ordering system.

VOCABULARY

capital purchase The purchase of a major item of furniture or equipment

categorically Pertaining to a division in any classification system

caustics Substances that corrode or eat away tissues

expendable Concerning supplies or equipment that is normally used up or consumed in service

inventory A list of articles in stock, with the description and quantity of each

reputable Honorable; having a good reputation

Planning and Organizing Facilities

The same principles of organization and planning that guide the business management of a medical office are essential in the organization and care of the facilities and supplies. A comfortable, attractive, clean environment lifts the spirits of patients and contributes to the efficiency and enthusiasm of the staff.

GENERAL ENVIRONMENT

TEMPERATURE The ideal temperature for a reception room is about 74° F. Working areas can be somewhat cooler. There should be a constant exchange of air by means of open windows or air conditioning. However, you should guard against drafts, because people who are ill are very susceptible to chills.

LIGHTING Working areas need to be well lighted. Fluorescent lights are usually preferable, because their light is uniform and they do not give off heat. Lamps in the reception area can be decorative, but they are useful only if carefully chosen and properly placed. They should be at reading height. If they are too high, they will shine into the eyes of others in the room. Lighting, furnishings, and comfort of the reception room are fully discussed in Chapter 8.

WALLS AND FLOOR COVERINGS Carpeting is usually chosen for floor covering in the reception area and often in the physician's consultation room. Unsecured rugs should never be used in a medical facility. In the clinical areas, a smooth washable floor covering, such as vinyl or tile, is generally more satisfactory. If wax is used on the floor covering, it should be the nonskid variety.

Wallpaper can add a pleasant atmosphere in the reception area. In the administrative and clinical areas, a good quality wall paint in soft colors is attractive, easily cleaned, and long lasting.

TRAFFIC CONTROL The furnishings in the entrance and reception areas should be arranged to allow easy traffic without crowding in any one area. The reception desk must be placed so that anyone coming into the office can easily spot the desk and so that the medical assistant at the desk can view the entire reception area (see Chapter 8). In the inner office, the physician and other members of the staff should be able to pass from one station to another without creating a roadblock.

SOUND CONTROL Walls should be soundproof, if possible, to prevent voices and conversations from being heard from one room to another.

PRIVACY Treatment rooms should be arranged so that the patient is out of view if it should become necessary to open the door to a hallway.

EFFICIENCY The physician and medical assistant must be able to move easily within each room and have access to equipment and supplies as needed.

Memory Jogger

1 *Briefly describe several general features of the medical facility that are essential to a comfortable and efficient working environment.*

AREA UTILIZATION AND CARE

The medical facility, whether large or small, is separated by utilization into the following areas:

- Reception
- Administration
- Clinical activities
- Lavatories
- Storage and utility

The overall cleaning and maintenance of these areas is probably being done by an outside service under the direction of the medical assistant or office manager. However, additional individual attention is required by members of the staff. In some instances, particularly in less populated areas, it may be the sole responsibility of the medical assistant.

Good housekeeping begins with having a place

for everything and with keeping everything clean and ready for use. Good housekeeping saves time and energy, conserves property, and eliminates incorrect use of materials. Poor housekeeping holds potential dangers for patients, physicians, and assistants alike.

Reception Area

The importance of a neat, attractive reception room was discussed in Chapter 8. Draperies, carpet, and upholstery should be cleaned at regular intervals in addition to the daily maintenance.

Administration Area

The administration area includes the receptionist desk; the records storage; telephone equipment; business machines such as typewriters, computers, calculators, photocopier, and fax machine; and so forth. This area should be separated from the reception room by a locked door. Records and business papers on the receptionist's desk should be placed in desk trays where they will be safe and out of sight of visitors during the day and in locked files at night. Personal items should be put away in a drawer or locker.

Clinical Area

The clinical area includes the physician's consultation room, which is used for patient interviews and for the physician's private study; patient examination and treatment rooms; and a recovery room where patients may rest after therapy or minor surgery.

CONSULTATION ROOM The physician's consultation room should always be kept neat and clean. Give this room a quick onceover after each patient visit and remove any evidence of the departing patient. Follow the preferences of the physician with respect to straightening the desk or other furnishings.

Memory Jogger

2 *Why is good housekeeping a high-priority item in a health care facility?*

EXAMINATION AND TREATMENT ROOMS Examination and treatment rooms are designed for utility; only necessary equipment and supplies should be placed here (Fig. 23–1). Instruments, medications, and other supplies are in cabinets or drawers. Supply cabinets should be checked daily before the first patient arrives (Fig. 23–2). The room must be straightened and all counter tops and the sink wiped clean after each patient. Disposable gowns,

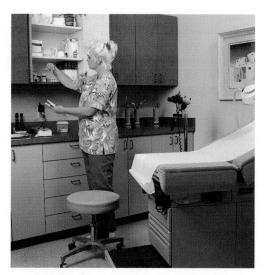

FIGURE 23-1 Patient examination room.

towels, and tissues must be discarded, fresh linens provided, and the room left spotless. The temperature in these rooms is crucial to the comfort of the patients, who are often asked to disrobe and put on a gown—and sometimes left waiting.

LABORATORY The laboratory may be anything from a small closet to a large room or suite of rooms. It must be kept clean, with everything in its place, for accurate work to be accomplished.

Adequate ventilation in the laboratory is especially important. There are many odors from the laboratory to which the staff becomes accustomed but which may be disagreeable to patients.

Contamination control must be exercised according to the current regulations of the Occupational Safety and Health Administration (OSHA), which are available from the U.S. Department of Labor. The department issues standards that employers and employees must follow, and site visits are made to

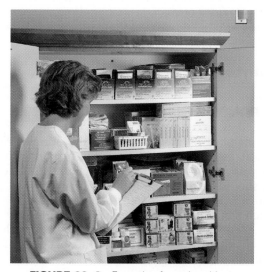

FIGURE 23-2 Example of supply cabinet.

ensure compliance. One of the most important is the exposure control plan. The facility's exposure control plan must be written and available to all employees and should be included in the policy and procedures manual (see Chapter 24). Some states have their own OSHA-approved occupational safety and health regulations, which may be even more stringent than the federal standards.

RECOVERY ROOM The recovery room should be comfortable, clean, and quiet. Facilities should be provided so that patient can relax and keep warm. Interesting reading material will help the time pass more pleasantly. If the patient wishes to sleep, provide a light blanket and see that no one enters the room.

Lavatories

In the small solo practice office, the lavatory may be shared by staff and patients. In this situation, every member of the staff should be instructed to leave the room meticulously clean. Larger medical facilities provide a separate lavatory for patients. This room must be checked by the medical assistant after each use to be certain it is left clean and that all supplies are replenished as needed.

Storage and Utility Rooms

There must be storage space for office and medical supplies, cleaning equipment and supplies, staff lockers or coat hooks, and so forth. The size of these spaces will vary, but whatever area is available must be kept organized and supplies and other items kept in order. Storage and utility rooms are generally kept closed to all except the staff.

Memory Jogger

3 *Name an important part of the OSHA regulations that should be included in the office policy and procedures manual.*

Maintenance

RESPONSIBILITIES OF STAFF

One member of the staff, often the administrative medical assistant, is delegated the responsibility of overseeing the maintenance of the premises. The details should be outlined in the office policy and procedures manual (see Chapter 24).

Each staff member will probably wish to tidy and dust his or her own desk or work station, with the administrative medical assistant taking care of the physician's desk.

The clinical medical assistant is usually the one who periodically cleans the interior of cabinets and drawers in the examination and treatment rooms. This should be done only when there is time to complete the job.

SKILLS AND RESPONSIBILITIES

PROPER METHOD OF CLEANING CABINET AND DRAWER INTERIORS

1 Do one shelf at a time.
2 Start at the top.
3 Remove all items from the shelf and place them on a table in the same order as on the shelf.
4 Wash the shelf with warm water and soap and rinse it well. Dry the shelf.
5 Clean and polish the instruments and check for faults. Examine hinges and blades.
6 Check all labels on containers for clarity. Reglue labels, if necessary. Examine supplies for expiration dates, quantity, and deterioration. Make a list of those items that should be reordered.
7 Replace the supplies in their original places on the shelf.

Clean the tops of cabinets and the undersides of towel and tape dispensers as necessary. These areas are frequently overlooked in the daily cleaning.

Maintenance services do not usually include as part of their service such tasks as cleaning mirrors, replacing light bulbs, cleaning the refrigerator, daily cleaning of sinks, straightening magazines, and watering plants. These and numerous other occasional as well as daily jobs are performed by the office staff.

Memory Jogger

4 *You are assigned to clean the cabinets in an examination room. Where would you start?*

INSTRUCTIONS TO MAINTENANCE SERVICE

Every member of the staff must be alert to any problem of cleanliness or safety that might be overlooked by the maintenance service and report the condition to the medical assistant in charge. The staff member who has the responsibility for instructing the maintenance service must be able to plan and be explicit in giving instructions:

SKILLS AND RESPONSIBILITIES

SYSTEM OF INSTRUCTING MAINTENANCE SERVICES

- Prepare a written list of the service that you expect.
- Go over it with the service people.
- Be specific about any areas that are not to be entered or disturbed.
- Set up a regular schedule.
- Evaluate the service regularly.
- Communicate your pleasure or displeasure promptly to the person in charge of performing the service.

Furniture and Equipment

The physician, individually or as a member of a group practice, has a large investment in the furnishings and equipment necessary to carry on a medical practice. The medical assistant has a responsibility to properly use and care for any piece of equipment to preserve its useful life.

ACQUISITION

When a new piece of equipment is acquired, read the instructions thoroughly and carefully. Do not attempt to assemble or use items before consulting the instructions. Keep the purchase invoice on file. The date of purchase and the cost are required for insurance and for depreciation credit on income tax.

WARRANTY REQUIREMENTS

If there is a warranty card with the item, copy the code number, fill in the blanks, and mail it as instructed.

SERVICE

Keep a service file for equipment that will need regular servicing.

SERVICE FILE CONTENTS

- Warranty dates
- Frequency of service
- When and by whom the unit was last serviced
- Cost of service

File all instructions in a special folder and save them for future reference or for your successors.

INVENTORY

It is good business to **inventory** all equipment and supplies once per year. If you have an office computer, keep the inventory on disk for easy access and updating.

First, list all **capital purchases,** such as furniture, medical and surgical instruments, sterilizers and autoclaves, laboratory equipment, business machines, and any major pieces of artwork or artifacts. These items are permanent and usually expensive. List the date of purchase of each item, along with its original price.

Next, list the smaller, less costly items that are considered **expendable,** such as small instruments, syringes, and thermometers.

Last, estimate the usable supplies and drugs on hand. Keep this inventory to check against the inventory for the coming year. An inventory is valuable in preparing income tax, and especially in case of office burglary or loss from other causes.

Memory Jogger

5 *Why is an annual inventory of equipment and supplies important? What is included?*

Supplies

SELECTING SUPPLIES AND SUPPLIERS

Supplies are those items that are expendable and must be ordered fairly frequently.

ADMINISTRATIVE FUNCTION SUPPLIES

- Stationery and filing supplies
- Appointment books and cards
- Accounting supplies
- Small desk items, such as paper clips, staples, typewriter ribbons, pens, and pencils

CLINICAL AREA SUPPLIES

- Examination and treatment items, such as disposable scopes, specula, lubricants, tongue blades, applicators, syringes and needles, dressings, and bandages
- Paper gowns, drapes, towels
- Autoclaving and sterilizing supplies

GENERAL USAGE SUPPLIES

- Soap and towels for lavatories
- Cleaning supplies
- Tissues
- Items for the staff lounge

In general, the person who will use the item is the best person to select what is to be ordered, but it is probably best for only one person to be in charge of ordering all supplies. The purchasing agent in the local hospital is a good source of information on supplies and suppliers.

Because such a variety of supplies is needed, you will probably use more than one supplier. Study the market and find the items that are best suited to the practice with respect to quality and packaging, and order from the suppliers who offer the best service and prices. You should make periodic price checks, but do not sacrifice convenience and service for the sake of saving a few pennies.

ORDERING SUPPLIES

There should be an established method for ordering supplies. Keep a list or running inventory from which you can note diminishing supplies and determine when to reorder (Figs. 23–3 and 23–4; see

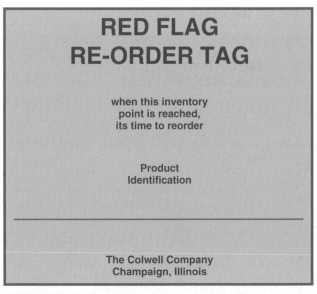

RED FLAG RE-ORDER TAG

when this inventory point is reached, its time to reorder

Product Identification

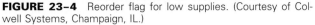

The Colwell Company Champaign, Illinois

FIGURE 23–4 Reorder flag for low supplies. (Courtesy of Colwell Systems, Champaign, IL.)

Procedure 23–1). Representatives of supply houses regularly call at physicians' offices and are often very helpful in suggesting new items and answering questions about what is available to meet your needs. Mail-order houses also send catalogs describing a great variety of equipment and supplies that can be ordered by mail.

ORDER	(ITEM NAME)	3-ply Disposable Drape Sheets (white) 7459								**ON ORDER**	
ORDER QUANTITY 300								REORDER POINT 100			
ORDER	QTY	REC'D	COST	PREPAID	ON ACCT	ORDER	QTY	REC'D	COST	PREPAID	ON ACCT
1/25	300	2/10	64.95	X							

INVENTORY COUNT	JAN	FEB	MAR	APR	MAY	JUNE	JULY	AUG	SEPT	OCT	NOV	DEC
20 00	200											
20 00												

ORDER SOURCE	UNIT PRICE
The Colwell Company	100 - $23.95
201 Kenyon Road	300 - $64.95
Champaign, IL 61820	

FORM 2450 COLWELL CO., CHAMPAIGN, ILLINOIS

FIGURE 23–3 Preprinted form for inventory control. (Courtesy of Colwell Systems, Champaign, IL.)

It is advisable to establish good credit with several reputable supply companies, both local and mail order, to provide a choice of vendors. However, do not shift your purchases from company to company without good reason. The loyal customer usually receives better service and may enjoy special privileges, such as being given the option of trying a piece of equipment before actually agreeing to purchase it.

Attention to detail in ordering will speed delivery and ensure greater accuracy. Use the actual title of the supply being ordered, including any special name, size, color, and so forth. The order should state whether payment is enclosed or whether the purchase is to be charged to the physician's account.

PREVENTION OF WASTE

In some cases, the unit cost of an item may be reduced by purchasing in larger quantities, but this is not always a saving. Make this decision only after considering the following guidelines.

GUIDELINES FOR PURCHASING LARGE QUANTITIES

- Will the supply be used in a reasonable length of time?
- Will it spoil or deteriorate?
- Is there sufficient space for storage?
- Will the practice continue to use the product?

RECEIVING AND STORING

RECEIVING All orders should be placed in the storage area when they arrive and opened only when you have time to check the contents. Compare the items in the package with your original purchase order and the invoice included with the shipment. Check for correct items, sizes, and styles as well as the number or amount received.

If you have any questions regarding the order or if you have a complaint to make, gather the following information before contacting the supplier.

INFORMATION NEEDED TO CORRESPOND WITH A SUPPLIER

- Invoice number
- Date ordered
- Name of person who placed the order

List on paper your questions and the information you desire. If a catalog was used in placing the order, open your copy to the correct page and secure any additional pertinent information. With all this information at hand, you can make a professional inquiry by letter or telephone.

When you are satisfied that the order is correct and complete, make the necessary notations on the inventory and order cards and place the items in their designated storage areas.

Memory Jogger

6 *When a shipment of supplies arrives, what three procedures will you do before placing the items in their designated storage areas?*

STORING Follow good housekeeping standards in storing supplies. Place supplies where they are most accessible yet protected from damage and exposure to moisture, heat, light, and air. Most drugs and solutions should be stored in a cool, dark cupboard, because direct light and sunlight cause drug deterioration. If drugs are to be stored for some time, the stoppers should be dipped in paraffin to seal them from the air. Do not fill these bottles to the very top; leave a little room for expansion.

Poisons should be stored in a locked compartment and kept separate from products used routinely. Have a distinct label or cap for poisons. A bright red color for their labels or caps may be useful. Narcotics must be stored in a secure place out of sight. Acids and **caustics** should have special resistant lids; never use metal lids for these substances. Do not store strong acids next to alkalis. Flammable items must be stored away from heat (Fig. 23–5).

PRODUCT	STORAGE	SPECIAL INSTRUCTIONS
Poisons	In locked case	Separate from products used routinely
Narcotics	Secure cabinet	Out of sight
Acids and caustics	Separate from alkalis	Special resistant lid; no metal lids
Inflammables	Away from heat	
Long-term storage solutions	Cool, dark cupboard	1. Dip stoppers in paraffin to air-seal 2. Leave some open space at top for expansion

FIGURE 23–5 Storage of drugs and solutions.

PROCEDURE 23-1

Establishing and Maintaining a Supply Inventory and Ordering System

GOAL

To establish an inventory of all expendable supplies in the physician's office and follow an efficient plan of order control using a card system.

EQUIPMENT AND SUPPLIES

File box
Inventory and order control cards
List of supplies on hand

Metal tabs
Reorder tags
Pen or pencil

PROCEDURAL STEPS

1 Write the name of each item on a separate card.
   PURPOSE: To establish a record of all items in inventory.

2 Write the amount of each item on hand in the space provided.
   PURPOSE: To establish beginning inventory.

3 Place a reorder tag at the point where the supply should be replenished.
   PURPOSE: The tag will serve as an alert that supply is low.

4 Place a metal tab over the *order* section of the card.
   PURPOSE: The metal tab will be a reminder to include this item in the next order.

5 When the order has been placed, note the date and quantity ordered and move the tab to the *on order* section of the card.

6 When the order is received, note the date and quantity in the appropriate column, remove the tab, and refile the card.
   NOTE: If the order is only partially filled, let the tab remain until the order is complete.

CARING FOR LABELS

If a bottle is to be used for a long time, the label should be indestructible. The original label should be treated for preservation when it is first received. When using the contents of the bottle, pour away from the label side to prevent any dripping on the label. Plastic screw caps protect the lip of the bottle and keep it clean.

 Safety Alert: When a label shows signs of wear or mutilation, or is difficult to read, replace the entire bottle and solution for safety purposes.

DRUG SAMPLES

Samples of drugs and medications that are suitable to the physician's practice should be organized **categorically** in a sample cupboard or drawer.

Place all similar drugs together, preferably in boxes of similar size and shape, with the tops open and plainly labeled on the outside. Clear plastic boxes are excellent for this type of storage. Color-coded labels are an additional help in identification.

Keep all the sedative samples in one box, all stimulant samples in another, and so forth. It is good practice to band together drug samples that have the same code number or expiration date. Rotate the drugs by placing the most recently received items in back of those that were previously on hand. At regular intervals, check all samples for expiration dates, and properly dispose of those that have expired.

Memory Jogger

7 *What action should you take when a drug container label shows signs of wear or mutilation?*

The Doctor's Bag

Although the physician who makes house calls has become a rarity, the practice is not entirely extinct and is even making a comeback in some areas. Any

Blood pressure set	Sterile syringes and needles (disposable)	Probe
Stethoscope		Tourniquet
Thermometers (oral and rectal)	Sterile swabs	Percussion hammer
Flashlight or penlight	Sterile dressings	Illuminated diagnostic set
Sterile gloves and lubricant	Tongue depressors	(otoscope and ophthal-
Wooden applicators	Scissors	moscope)
Assorted bandages	Sterile dressing forceps	Sterile tissue forceps
Adhesive tape (assorted widths)	Aspiration equipment	Medications:
Safety pins	Microscopic slides and fixative	Epinephrine
Towel	Containers for specimens	Digitalis
Ballpoint pens	Culture tubes for throat cultures	Antibiotics
Prescription pads	Sterile stuture set	Antihistamines
Sterile hemostatic forceps	Sterile scalpel	Alcohol and/or skin dis-
		infectant
		Sterilizing solution
		Spirits of ammonia

FIGURE 23–6 Basic inventory of items commonly found in a doctor's bag.

medical assistant who is given the responsibility of keeping the doctor's bag ready for use must regard it seriously and give it close and continual attention.

The items that are included in the bag depend on professional requirements, the kinds of emergencies that are responded to, and the personal preferences of the person using it. That person could be the physician, a physician assistant, a nurse practitioner, or an emergency medical technician. A basic inventory of items commonly found in a doctor's bag are listed in Figure 23–6.

As a guide, keep an inventory of the bag's contents posted inside a cupboard above the place where you check and clean the bag. When checking the bag after a patient has been tended to, remove any specimens and see that they are properly labeled with the patient's full name, the date, and the type of test if the specimen is to be sent out for examination.

If any instruments or gloves have been used, remove them and replace with sterile ones. Even if this equipment has not been used, it should be sterilized weekly. Keep the containers of alcohol, germicides, and other substances filled, and check containers often for any leakage. Allow a small space for heat expansion in containers of fluid.

Safety and Security Considerations

DETECTION OF HAZARDS

The physician and every member of the staff should continually monitor possible hazards to themselves and the patients.

The reception room and public areas of the facility are particularly vulnerable. Are the chairs in the reception room safe for children, for an exceptionally heavy patient, or for a physically disadvantaged patient? Are there any exposed telephone or light cords that could cause someone to trip? Are there lamps that could tip?

In the examining rooms, be especially careful to put away any sharp instruments, hazardous liquids, or medications. Any spills on the floor should be wiped immediately to prevent slipping or a fall. Keep prescription pads out of sight.

Are the stairways and entrances to the facility well lighted and safe? Are there any known hazards in the parking area?

DRUG ENFORCEMENT ADMINISTRATION REGULATIONS

A physician who has controlled substances (narcotics) stored on the premises must keep these drugs in a locked cabinet or safe. Any loss of controlled drugs by theft must be reported to the regional office of the Drug Enforcement Administration at the time the theft is discovered. The local police department and the state bureau of narcotics enforcement should also be notified (see Chapter 6).

SMOKE ALARMS AND FIRE EXTINGUISHERS

Smoke alarms are required in all new buildings and should be installed in every existing medical facility. Their functioning must be checked regularly to ensure effectiveness if they should be needed. There should be a fire extinguisher readily accessible to any part of the facility.

FIRE EXITS

Fire exits should be clearly marked and the staff instructed on evacuation procedures in case of fire.

CONTACT WITH SECURITY SYSTEM MANAGEMENT

If the physician's office is located in a multiple-unit building or medical complex, know whom to contact if a security emergency should occur. Have the telephone number handy for local fire and police departments (i.e., 911 in many areas).

ROUTINE OFFICE SECURITY

Within the office, all valuables should be kept out of sight. A frequent target of thieves is the medical assistant's handbag, which is often left under a desk or table, where it can be easily spotted by an intruder.

It is important to secure all entrances, windows as well as doors. Have good double locks installed by a reliable locksmith. It may be well worth the cost to consult a professional security service and follow its advice. Making an office burglar proof is impossible, but entry can be made difficult; and this, in itself, usually discourages the amateur.

Outside sensor lights with unbreakable shields are extremely helpful. Leaving a light burning and a radio playing inside the office are additional deterrents. Tell the local police or the building security force which lights will always be left on.

Alarms can be helpful if they are reliable and are not easily disconnected by an expert. Loud local alarms are usually sufficient to frighten off a prowler. It is possible, if greater security is needed, to install an alarm system that will ring in the local police station or at a special security office.

Police departments urge that all valuables be protected by etching them with personal identification, such as the owner's name or Social Security number. This is easily done with an electric engraving tool that cuts into the equipment, and the marking is practically impossible to eradicate. Even if an attempt is made to scratch it off, a sufficient impression will be left so that police, with the aid of a special chemical, can bring the engraved characters up again (Fig. 23–7).

The most effective step in protecting your premises against break-ins is to remember to check carefully at the end of every day to make certain that all doors and windows are double locked.

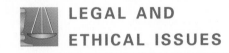

LEGAL AND ETHICAL ISSUES

The physician can be the victim of a lawsuit if a patient is injured on the premises. The medical assistant should report or eliminate any hazard observed.

Patients are entitled to confidentiality. Be aware of sound control and visual privacy.

Keep current and abide by OSHA regulations.

CRITICAL THINKING

1 When you are visiting a professional office, observe the physical arrangements and try to think of ways the office could be made more efficient or more user-friendly.

2 Become informed on security procedures by examining your own living quarters. How might security be improved?

HOW DID I DO? Answers to Memory Joggers

1 Answers will vary but should include room temperature, lighting, and sound control.

2 Good housekeeping: saves time, conserves property, and eliminates incorrect use of materials. Poor housekeeping: could create physical danger for all occupants.

3 Exposure control plan.

4 Start at the top so that any drippings or dust will not fall on clean areas.

5 The inventory is valuable in preparing income tax reports and for reimbursement in case of loss and should include capital purchases, expendable equipment, and usable supplies.

6 *a.* Place in storage area until time to open packages.
b. Compare items in packages with original purchase order.
c. Check for correct items, sizes, and styles.

7 Replace entire bottle and solution for safety purposes.

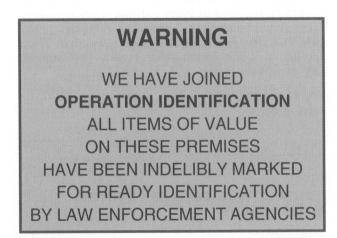

FIGURE 23–7 Warning sign indicating that valuables have been marked for the purpose of identification.

REFERENCES

American Medical Association: Managing the Medical Practice. Norcross, GA, Coker Publishing Company, 1996.
Andress A: Manual of Medical Office Management. Philadelphia, WB Saunders, 1996.

Management Responsibilities

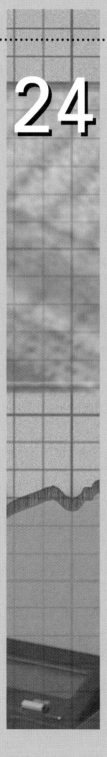

24

LEARNING OBJECTIVES

Cognitive: On successful completion of this chapter you should be able to:

1 Define and spell the terms listed in the Vocabulary.
2 State the purpose and goals of medical office management.
3 Discuss the desirable qualities of an office manager and their importance in the selection of a supervisor.
4 Identify the goals of an office policy manual and how they may be achieved.
5 Explain how a procedure manual differs from a policy manual.
6 Discuss the steps in the hiring and dismissal of employees.
7 List five kinds of staff meetings.
8 Discuss the concept of practice development and its importance.
9 List at least 10 features of a patient information folder.
10 State two advantages of patient instruction sheets.
11 Discuss the supervisor's role in financial management.
12 Identify the source of reference for information on employer taxes and deposit requirements.

Performance: On successful completion of this chapter you should be able to:

1 Interview an applicant for a position, utilizing the guidelines in this chapter.
2 Prepare an outline of contents for a basic office policy manual.
3 Write a procedure sheet for a specific task.
4 Outline a patient information folder.
5 Outline a financial policies folder.
6 Write a patient instruction sheet.

VOCABULARY

ancillary Subordinate; auxiliary

appraisal Setting a value on or judging as to quality

candid Frank; straightforward

circumvention Going around or avoidance

discrimination A distinction based on race, religion, sex, or some other factor, especially one resulting in unfair or injurious treatment of an individual belonging to a specific group

disseminate To broadcast or spread over a considerable area

insubordination Refusing to submit to authority

meticulous Extremely careful of small details

motivation The process of inciting a person to some action or behavior

orientation The determination or adjustment of one's intellectual or emotional position with reference to circumstances

philosophy The general laws that furnish the rational explanation of anything

probationary Pertaining to a trial period to ascertain fitness for a job

recruitment The supplying of new members or employees.

Purpose of Management

The purpose of management in a medical practice is to provide a quiet, functional environment in which the physician or physicians can see and treat patients, provide competent medical care, safely store health information, and bill and collect for services to continue practicing medicine. We have learned that the daily functioning of a medical facility involves a multitude of details and that good management does not just happen.

Memory Jogger

1 *What are the three basic purposes of medical office management?*

WHO'S IN CHARGE?

If there is only one medical assistant, that person must be able to assume many of the management responsibilities with cooperation from the physician. When there are two medical assistants, one administrative and one clinical, it is often the administrative medical assistant who is expected to assume the management duties. In the office with a larger staff, a line of authority must be established.

A facility with three or more employees should have one person designated as supervisor or office manager. This individual should have management skills and the ability to deal with personnel matters. Other employees answer to the supervisor, the supervisor answers to the physician or physicians. This sets up an orderly way for

- The office staff to consult with the physician regarding administrative or clinical problems, complaints, or grievances

- The physician to check on the operation of the office, **disseminate** information on policy changes, and correct errors or grievances

The career of medical assisting becomes more challenging with the passing years. On the plus side, it also offers more opportunities for advancement than ever before. The recently graduated medical assistant whose first position possibly was as a receptionist may systematically be given more responsibilities and eventually become the office manager of a large staff. The single most critical short supply in health manpower is executive level personnel, specifically, individuals competent to develop and operate a health maintenance organization or prepaid group practice.

AVOIDING MANAGEMENT PROBLEMS

Management problems can often be avoided by carefully defining the areas of authority and responsibility of each employee. Many physicians say that friction between workers is their most common personnel problem. A definite chain of command must be established, and the physician must not undermine the supervisor's authority by **circumvention.** When employees know what is expected of them, they can plan both their daily and long-term work more effectively.

Qualities of a Supervisor

The selection of the right person to supervise the employees is critical. The supervisor may come from within the ranks or may be selected as a new member of the staff. Some employees do not wish to assume management responsibilities; others may not have the necessary qualifications.

PERSONAL QUALITIES

SUPERVISORY QUALITIES
- Leadership ability
- Good judgment
- Good health
- Ability to organize
- Ability to learn and improve
- Original ideas
- A sense of fairness
- Strength to stand firm on policy, but enough flexibility to recognize when an exception should be made

The management aspect of a medical practice is becoming more complex every year. Practice management consultants frequently conduct seminars for medical office personnel. These are often arranged through a chapter of the American Association of Medical Assistants or the local medical society.

Management Duties

Medical office administrative procedures fall into three broad categories: patient scheduling, health information management, and practice management. We have dealt in detail with the first two categories in previous chapters. It is the third category—practice management process—that concerns us here.

The practice manager's duties vary with the practice but may include any or all of the responsibilities listed under Personnel Management.

SKILLS AND RESPONSIBILITIES

PERSONNEL MANAGEMENT
- Prepare and update policy and procedure manuals and job descriptions
- Recruitment
- Orientation and training
- Performance and salary review
- Dismissal
- Plan staff meetings
- Maintain staff harmony
- Establish work flow guidelines
- Improve office efficiency
- Supervise purchase and care of equipment
- Patient education
- Eliminate time-wasting tasks for the physician
- Practice marketing

FINANCIAL MANAGEMENT
- Supervise cash transactions
- Maintain payroll records
- Manage employee benefits

OFFICE POLICY AND PROCEDURES MANUALS

Personnel management can best be accomplished with the backup of a well-designed policy manual and a detailed procedure manual.

A policy manual is informational, tells "what to do," and often has an opening statement of the philosophy of the practice, for example:

> The patient is the most important person in this office.
> The patient is the purpose of our being here.
> The patient shall receive our most courteous and attentive treatment at all times.

A procedure manual supplements the policy manual by telling "how to do it." Sometimes the two manuals are combined. The procedure manual will contain a job description for each position in the practice and detailed steps for carrying out each task.

Memory Jogger

2 Briefly state the difference between a policy manual and a procedure manual.

Office Policy Manual

The policy manual must be designed for a specific facility with its important goals and considerations outlined. It must be
- Comprehensive but flexible
- Easy to read
- Conform with professional ethics
- Reviewed frequently and kept up-to-date as changes occur

A well-designed policy manual will accomplish several results reflecting the expectations of the office:
- Solidifying what may have been vague thoughts into definite statements of policy
- Communicating these statements in exactly the same way to every employee
- Providing a permanent record of these policies

The manual may well be the office manager's best friend by serving as a clear and concise guide for policy information. It can serve as
- An informational guide for the new employee
- A ready reference for a temporary employee
- A reminder of policies for the regular employee
- A back-up for expectations when or if a controversy occurs

Development of the Policy Manual

Begin with the opening statement of the philosophy of the practice. Follow the opening statement with a staff chart that shows the line of authority and states who has authority to enforce the policies. Continue with professional information for each physician on the staff, including education and specialty board achievements, hospital staff memberships, memberships in professional societies, state license number, and narcotic registry number.

What are the expectations regarding the personal appearance of employees? Guidelines regarding appropriate dress, use of makeup, nail polish, perfume, cleanliness, grooming, and hygiene are difficult to discuss on a personal basis but can be matter-of-fact in an office manual.

Describe the work week, listing the daily office hours and any days off, the daily appointment schedule, and where the physician can be reached with messages or emergencies. Specify the time allowed each day for lunch and breaks and whether they must be taken at specific times.

Discuss the provisions for sick leave, emergency leave, and any other absences. Are medical services provided by the professional staff free to employees? Are they discounted? When is the employee eligible for benefits?

Describe the vacation policy, including how much vacation time the employee is allowed in terms of number of working days, who authorizes it, and whether there are any restrictions as to when vacation time may be taken. List the holidays observed.

Are there other benefits for employees, such as payment of professional dues, health insurance, uniform allowances, pension plan, profit sharing, and free parking?

Is time off given for education courses or for attending professional organization conventions or seminars? If so, is this time counted as paid time or as vacation time?

Does the office pay for courses, professional memberships, and expenses incurred at professional conventions?

When is payday? What is the policy on overtime? Are there annual bonuses? If so, how are they determined? What is the policy for performance reviews, salary reviews, and merit increases (Fig. 24–1)?

How much notice is expected if an employee wishes to quit? Can the employee who resigns receive severance pay? What are the grounds for immediate dismissal? How are complaints and grievances handled?

Office Procedure Manual

The office procedure manual supplements the office policy manual. It will contain a job description for each position in the practice and procedure sheets for carrying out each task.

Job Description

A job description is a detailed account of the duties and the qualifications for a specific position. In some cases it should state both primary and secondary responsibilities, emphasizing that the employee must be flexible. Job descriptions may change with personnel changes. No two people have the same capabilities and interests, and there is no need to try to mold a person to a job description when a simple shift in duties may accomplish a happier result. For instance, an administrative assistant might normally be expected to complete the computer sheets at the end of the day; but if a clinical assistant has special aptitude for this and really enjoys the task, there is no reason that this change in responsibility should not be made. Note it on the job description so that there is no confusion about who is responsible (Fig. 24–2). Following the list of duties, there should be a procedure sheet for each task.

Name _____ Soc. Sec. No. _____

Job classification _____

Employment date _____ Starting salary _____

    Salary checks are issued every (week) (two weeks) (semi-monthly) (month) on _____ (day or date).
    Increase-in-pay review will be conducted six months after the completion of three-month probationary period and each six months thereafter.
    Date of first pay review _____
    Current maximum salary for this job classification $ _____
        Revised _____ $ _____
        Revised _____ $ _____

SALARY SCHEDULE

Date	Amount of increase	Total salary
_____	_____	_____
_____	_____	_____
_____	_____	_____
_____	_____	_____

FIGURE 24–1 Example of page from an office policy manual.

JOB DESCRIPTION   OFFICE MANAGER

The office manager is responsible for the coordination of all office activities, including recruitment and training of personnel, practice management, and financial procedures.

QUALIFICATIONS: CMA or degree in business administration
                  Previous medical office experience
                  Supervisory experience helpful

REPORTS TO: Physician

SPECIFIC TASKS: 1. Prepare annual budget
                   2. Prepare monthly profit and loss statement
                   3. Approve all expenditures
                   4. Review and dispose of delinquent accounts
                   5. Approve all write-offs
                   6. Maintain liaison with accountant
                   7. Recruit, hire, and fire
                   8. Conduct performance appraisals and report to physician
                   9. Arrange personnel vacations and keep records of leave days
                  10. Assist in improving work flow and office efficiencies
                  11. Supervise purchase and repair of equipment
                  12. Purchase and supervise storage of supplies
                  13. Arrange for practice insurance
                  14. Conduct regular staff meetings
                  15. Maintain current office policy and procedure manuals
                  16. Prepare patient education materials as needed

SUPERVISES: Administrative and Clinical Assistants
                  Service Personnel

Date of Revision: _____

FIGURE 24–2 Example of job description.

Procedure Sheets

A procedure sheet is a verbal flow chart that lists step-by-step the logical sequence of activities involved in a given task. An employee should be able to perform the task by following the written instructions (Fig. 24–3). Procedure writing is sometimes difficult because, once we become proficient, we tend to take for granted many of the simpler steps involved in performing a task. After a task has been learned, it is unnecessary to refer to the procedure sheet for instructions, but the detailed procedure sheet is invaluable in training the new recruit and in assisting the temporary employee.

Memory Jogger

3 *What are the two categories of information that are included in an office procedure manual?*

PROCEDURE SHEET   PROCESS INCOMING MAIL

1. Assemble all necessary tools and supplies: letter opener, paper clips, stapler, mending tape, date stamp.
2. Open all mail except letters marked personal.
3. Check to be sure writer's address is on letter before destroying envelope. Staple envelope to letter if address is missing.
4. Paper clip enclosures to letter (or note their absence if they are not enclosed).
5. Date stamp the letter or piece of mail.
6. Set aside cash receipts for processing.
7. Route insurance claim forms and inquiries to insurance clerk.
8. Arrange mail with second and third class on bottom, then first class, with any personal mail on top.
9. Place entire stack in mail tray on right side of physician's desk.

FIGURE 24–3 Example of procedure sheet.

Benefits and Subject Matter

Job descriptions and procedure sheets help the employee achieve expectations. Practice management specialists say that the most common remark from a discharged employee is "I didn't know I was supposed to. . . ." A written job description may also help avoid legal problems with an employee who is dismissed for not meeting performance standards.

A great deal of instruction can be incorporated into a procedure manual. Preferred performance procedures, both administrative and clinical, should be spelled out in detail, including the following information:

- A checklist of daily, weekly, monthly, quarterly, and yearly duties
- How much time is allotted for new patients? Established patients? Postoperative patients?
- How are records prepared and filed? A description of the filing system may save the day if a temporary employee needs to find something in the file during the regular medical assistant's absence.
- How is the telephone to be answered? Which calls are put through to the physician immediately, and which may the medical assistant handle? Include a list of the names and telephone numbers of persons who are called frequently — for example, consulting physicians, hospitals, laboratories, and the physician's spouse.
- Billing and collection procedures. Is billing done weekly, twice monthly, monthly? Are the statements prepared in the office? By what method? Is a collection agency used? Which one? What procedure is used for copays? What is the procedure for referrals?
- Completed samples of forms that need to be filled out and samples of correspondence (these provide excellent visual instruction)
- What kind of setup does the physician prefer for office surgeries or treatments? Is there a card index showing these setups? If so, where is it kept?
- Where and how are supplies ordered and stored? Include the name, address, and telephone number of every supplier. Also include an inventory of major equipment with serial numbers, where and when the equipment was purchased, and a telephone number for servicing.
- Any special duties the physician expects of the medical assistant, such as organizational activities or making travel arrangements

Management studies indicate that, in the multiple-employee facility, it is good practice to have an understudy for each position who can substitute in an emergency. A well-documented procedure manual that is kept current ensures continuity when one employee must, on occasion, fill in for or assist another.

Development of a procedure manual is a good discussion item for staff meetings; the cooperation of the staff is essential if the project is to be successful. Keep it simple to update by using a three-ring binder. Include date of revision. Be sure to destroy old pages when revisions are made. One complete master copy should remain in the custody of the office manager and one with the physician. Each employee should have a copy of the portion that pertains to his or her specific job.

RECRUITMENT

The office manager can be expected to initiate the recruitment and screening of prospective employees. Careful judgment and objectivity must be used in the search for an employee who is suitable for the practice. When possible, have the prospective employee complete an application form (Fig. 24–4) and screen it well before the initial interview.

Preliminary Steps

Before interviewing any applicant, the interviewer needs to know

- What personal qualities and abilities the applicant must have
- The responsibilities of the position
- Salary range
- How soon the position will be open

Add any other specifications for the position. Then, after reviewing the policy manual, prepare an outline for guidance in selecting prospective applicants.

EXAMPLE OF GUIDELINES IN SELECTING PROSPECTIVE APPLICANTS

- Do the applicant's appearance and personal grooming meet the standards set forth in the policy manual?
- Has the applicant been previously employed? What duties were performed?
- If previously employed, how long was the applicant in the last position? Why did the applicant leave?
- What are the applicant's skills? Do these meet the requirements for the position as set forth in the office procedure manual? Does the applicant seem to accept and enjoy responsibility?
- What is the applicant's formal education? Certified Medical Assistant? If not certified, is the applicant interested in taking the certifying examination? Is the applicant a member of a professional organization? Does he or she attend meetings?

APPLICATION FOR POSITION / Medical or Dental Office
AN EQUAL OPPORTUNITY EMPLOYER

(In answering questions, use extra blank sheet if necessary)

No employee, applicant, or candidate for promotion, training or other advantage shall be discriminated against (or given preference) because of race, color, religion, sex, age, physical handicap, veteran status, or national origin.

PLEASE READ CAREFULLY AND WRITE OR PRINT ANSWERS TO ALL QUESTIONS. DO NOT TYPE.

Date of Application

A. PERSONAL INFORMATION

Name - Last   First   Middle   Social Security No.   Area Code/Phone No. ( )

Present Address: - Street   (Apt #)   City   State   Zip   How Long At This Address?

Previous Address: - Street   City   State   Zip   Person to notify in case of Emergency or Accident - Name:
From: To: Address: Telephone:

B. EMPLOYMENT INFORMATION

For What Position Are You Applying?:   ☐ Full-Time ☐ Part-Time ☐ Either   Date Available For Employment?:   Wage/Salary Expectations:

List Hrs./Days You Prefer To Work   List Any Hrs./Days You Are Not Available: (Except for times required for religious practices or observances)   Can You Work Overtime, If Necessary? ☐ Yes ☐ No

Are You Employed Now?: ☐ Yes ☐ No   If So, May We Inquire Of Your Present Employer?: ☐ No ☐ Yes, If Yes: Name Of Employer: Phone Number: ( )

Have You Ever Been Bonded? ☐ Yes ☐ No   If Required For Position, Are You Bondable? ☐ Yes ☐ No ☐ Uncertain   Have You Applied For A Position With This Office Before? ☐ No ☐ Yes If Yes, When?:

Referred By / Or Where Did You Learn Of This Job?:

Can You, Upon Employment, Submit Verification Of Your Legal Right To Work In The United States?: ☐ Yes ☐ No
Submit Proof That You Meet Legal Age Requirement For Employment? ☐ Yes ☐ No

Language(s) Applicant Speaks or Writes (If Use Of A Language Other Than English is Relevant To The Job For Which The Applicant Is Applying:

C. EDUCATIONAL HISTORY

Name & Address Of Schools Attended (Include Current)	Dates From	Thru	Highest Grade/Level Completed	Diploma/Degree(s) Obtained/Areas of Study
High School				
College				Degree/Major
Post Graduate				Degree/Major
Other				Course/Diploma/License/ Certificate

Specific Training, Education, Or Experiences Which Will Assist You In The Job For Which You Have Applied.

Future Educational Plans

D. SPECIAL SKILLS

CHECK BELOW THE KINDS OF WORK YOU HAVE DONE: ☐ MEDICAL INSURANCE FORMS   ☐ RECEPTIONIST

☐ BLOOD COUNTS	☐ DENTAL ASSISTANT	☐ MEDICAL TERMINOLOGY	☐ TELEPHONES
☐ BOOKKEEPING	☐ DENTAL HYGIENIST	☐ MEDICAL TRANSCRIPTION	☐ TYPING
☐ COLLECTIONS	☐ FILING	☐ NURSING	☐ STENOGRAPHY
☐ COMPOSING LETTERS	☐ INJECTIONS	☐ PHLEBOTOMY (Draw Blood)	☐ URINALYSIS
☐ COMPUTER INPUT	☐ INSTRUMENT STERILIZATION	☐ POSTING	☐ X-RAY

OFFICE EQUIPMENT USED: ☐ COMPUTER   ☐ DICTATING EQUIPMENT   ☐ WORD PROCESSOR   ☐ OTHER:

Other Kinds Of Tasks Performed Or Skills That May Be Applicable To Position: Typing Speed   Shorthand Speed

ORDER # 72-110 • © 1976 BIBBERO SYSTEMS, INC. • PETALUMA, CA. • (REV. 1/95)
TO REORDER CALL TOLL FREE: (800) BIBBERO (800-242-2376) OR FAX (800) 242-9330   MFG IN U.S.A.

(PLEASE COMPLETE OTHER SIDE)

FIGURE 24–4 Application for position in medical office. (Courtesy of Bibbero Systems, Inc., Petaluma, California (800) 242-2376, Fax (800) 242-9330.)

Illustration continued on following page

E. EMPLOYMENT RECORD

LIST MOST RECENT EMPLOYMENT FIRST

May We Contact Your Previous Employer(s) For A Reference? ☐ Yes ☐ No

1) Employer

Work Performed. Be Specific:

Address   Street   City   State   Zip Code

Phone Number

( )

Type of Business	Dates	Mo.	Yr.		Mo.	Yr.
	From			To		

Your Position

Hourly Rate/Salary

Starting   Final

Supervisor's Name

Reason For Leaving

2) Employer

Worked Performed. Be Specific:

Address   Street   City   State   Zip Code

Phone Number

( )

Type of Business	Dates	Mo.	Yr.		Mo.	Yr.
	From			To		

Your Position

Hourly Rate/Salary

Starting   Final

Supervisor's Name

Reason For Leaving

3) Employer

Worked Performed. Be Specific:

Address   Street   City   State   Zip Code

Phone Number

( )

Type of Business	Dates	Mo.	Yr.		Mo.	Yr.
	From			To		

Your Position

Hourly Rate/Salary

Starting   Final

Supervisor's Name

Reason For Leaving

F. REFERENCES — FRIENDS / ACQUAINTANCES NON-RELATED

(1) _____

Name   Address   Telephone Number   (☐ Work ☐ Home)   Occupation   Years Acquainted

(1) _____

Name   Address   Telephone Number   (☐ Work ☐ Home)   Occupation   Years Acquainted

Please Feel Free To Add Any Information Which You Feel Will Help Us Consider You For Employment

READ THE FOLLOWING CAREFULLY, THEN SIGN AND DATE THE APPLICATION

"I certify that all answers given by me on this application are true, correct and complete to the best of my knowledge. I acknowledge notice that the information contained in this application is subject to check. I agree that, if hired, my continued employment may be contingent upon the accuracy of that information. If employed, I further agree to comply with Company/Office rules and regulations."

Signature: _____   Date: _____

FIGURE 24–4 *continued*

ARRANGING THE PERSONAL INTERVIEW

If the applicant sent a letter asking for an interview, note whether the letter was correctly typed, included the essential information, and provided a personal data sheet (see Chapter 2). Forget the applicant who sends a letter handwritten in pencil. By telephoning the applicant, you will have an opportunity to judge the telephone voice. If it is poor, you may not wish to consider the applicant further.

Set a time for the personal interview when you most likely will be able to give the applicant your undivided attention. However, an applicant who is being considered for employment should have an opportunity to see your office when there is a fairly normal amount of activity. The prospective employee who is interviewed in a peaceful, quiet office on the physician's day out may not be prepared for the activity on a normal working day.

Before interviewing any applicant, make certain that you are thoroughly familiar with the federal, state, and local fair-employment practice laws affecting hiring practices. Both men and women are receiving protection from on-the-job discrimination, sexual harassment, mandatory lie detector tests, and unfair discharge.

Illegal questions are sometimes asked on preprinted employment applications or during interviews. Title VII of the Civil Rights Act of 1964, as amended by the Equal Employment Opportunity Act of 1972, prohibits inquiries into an applicant's race, color, sex, religion, and national origin. Inquiries regarding medical history, arrest records, or former drug use are also illegal. Most states have laws designed to protect the rights of job applicants, and these laws may impose additional restrictions.

Either send the applicant an application form to be completed and brought in at the time of the interview or allow ample time for its completion on the day of the interview. The application form can serve as a check of the applicant's penmanship and thoroughness as well as a permanent record for your files. If you wish it to be completed in the applicant's own handwriting, be sure to state this on the instructions. The applicant should be meticulous about following instructions and filling in all the blanks.

Memory Jogger

4 *List five items of personal information that are prohibited from being requested under the Equal Employment Opportunity Act.*

The Interview

First, make certain that the applicant feels at ease. You might shake his or her hand and ask a few social questions before starting the interview. In general, follow good manners and see that the person to be interviewed is comfortable.

Begin with a few open-ended questions that cannot be answered with a simple "yes" or "no," such as "What did you do in your last employment?" When interviewing a recent graduate who does not have experience, you might ask, "What was your favorite class?"

As you speak with the applicant, make a mental note of whether the applicant displays essential personal qualities.

PERSONAL QUALITIES

APPEALING PERSONAL QUALITIES IN AN APPLICANT
- Converses easily
- Is a good listener
- Is free of annoying mannerisms
- Has a ready smile
- Is interested enough to ask as well as to answer questions
- Appears interested in the office and in the physician's specialty

Avoid questions that involve the applicant's privacy. Your questions should be related to the available position and the applicant's ability to do the job. An interview should be a two-way exchange of information between the applicant and the interviewer.

If the applicant appears to be one who will receive serious consideration, you have the responsibility of explaining what will be expected in the way of duties; office policies regarding appearance, working hours, overtime, time off, and vacations; what initial salary is offered and any fringe benefits; and the office policy on increases. If you fail to mention these items, the applicant may be hesitant to inquire.

If your employer is a member of a credit bureau, it may be advisable to request the applicant's permission to check his or her credit rating, especially if handling office finances will be one of the responsibilities. It can safely be assumed that one who is unable to handle personal financial affairs will be a poor risk in handling office finances.

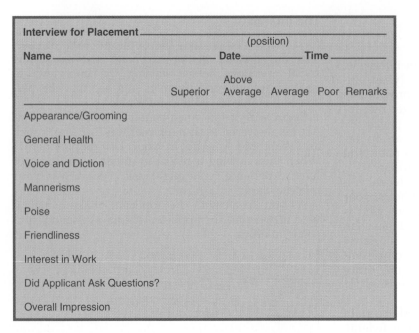

Interview for Placement _____					
(position)					
Name _____ Date _____ Time _____					
	Superior	Above Average	Average	Poor	Remarks
Appearance/Grooming					
General Health					
Voice and Diction					
Mannerisms					
Poise					
Friendliness					
Interest in Work					
Did Applicant Ask Questions?					
Overall Impression					

FIGURE 24–5 Form for applicant rating after interview.

Review the job description for the position being filled. This is essential if you are to be certain that the person being interviewed understands the required duties and responsibilities. Ask if the applicant has any questions, and close the interview on a positive note.

During the hiring proceedings, you may wish to invite the prospective employee to lunch with the staff or for coffee in the more relaxed atmosphere of the employee lounge. This presents an opportunity to discover whether the applicant's personality will mesh with the atmosphere of the office.

Follow-Up Activities

When the interview is over, take a few moments immediately to rate the applicant on your checklist. Jot down some notes to refresh your memory when you refer this applicant to the physician for the final interview. Do not trust your impressions to memory, especially if several applicants will be interviewed. Figure 24–5 is a suggested checklist that may be modified to suit your own circumstances.

Checking References

It is always advisable to carefully check all references and to follow through on any leads for information. It is best to use the telephone in checking references because people are sometimes less than candid in a letter; furthermore, letter writing is time consuming and you may not get a reply.

Prepare a checklist before you place the call. When you talk with the person called, be sure to "listen between the lines." Note the tone of the re-

plies to your questions. Do not ask questions that might incriminate the person answering them. You might ask the following questions as an introduction:

1. When did (the applicant) work for you?
2. How long?
3. What were the duties and responsibilities?
4. Did the employee assume responsibility well?

Hiring

When a decision has been reached to hire someone, notify the applicant of the decision and state when the applicant will be expected to report for work. Remember to notify all others who have applied. They may have hesitated to accept other interviews in the hope of hearing from you. It is unfair to keep individuals who are seeking employment "on the string." Good etiquette requires that you drop them a note or call by telephone and say that the position is filled. Thank the individual for applying, and say that you will keep his or her application on file.

ORIENTATION AND TRAINING

Recruitment does not end with the hiring. Some preliminary orientation and training will help new employees to understand what is expected and to develop their full potential. Acquaint the new employee with such aspects of the office as:

- Staff
- Physical environment
- Nature of the practice and specialty. Explain

what types of patients are dealt with and how the staff is expected to interact with them.

- Office policies. Have the employee read the policy manual and then discuss it.
- Long-range expectations

PERFORMANCE AND SALARY REVIEW

A new employee should be granted a probationary period. Sixty to 90 days has been traditional, but many employers believe that 2 weeks is sufficient to determine whether the employee will be able to learn and adapt to the position.

A definite date for a performance review at the end of the probationary period should be set at the time of employment. This review should not be squeezed in between patient visits or be given a token few minutes at the end of a day. There should be ample time to relax and talk. At this time, the new employee is told how well expectations have been met and whether there are any deficiencies. Then give the employee an opportunity to ask questions. Sometimes an employee fails to perform because of never having been told what was expected.

The performance **appraisal** includes a judgment of both the quality and quantity of work, personal appearance, attitudes and team spirit, dependability, self-discipline, **motivation,** attendance, and any other qualities essential to satisfactory performance of the job in question.

Although the probationary period does not always allow time to fully train an individual for a specific position, it is fair to assume that the potential for being a satisfactory employee can be judged at this time. Now is the time to talk out any problems and make suggestions for improvement.

The supervisor is responsible for ongoing performance appraisals of all employees, complimenting whenever possible and appropriate and offering helpful criticism when necessary. A formal performance appraisal at the end of the probationary period and at regular 6-month intervals thereafter, with a report to the physician employer, is helpful in the employee's salary review (Fig. 24–6).

DISMISSAL

The necessity for dismissing an employee is unpleasant at best, but if the ground rules are decided on in advance, written into the policy manual, and explained to all employees, the problem is partially solved. The policies must be applied equally and impartially to all. The final decision for dismissal will probably be made by the physician but may be based on the recommendation of the office manager/supervisor. The person who does the hiring should do the firing.

The probationary employee who does not prove satisfactory should be dismissed at the end of the probationary period, with tact and a full explanation of the reasons for dismissal. In all fairness, an individual should be told why the employment is ended and not be given weak excuses or untruths that do not help to correct deficiencies. If you are not straightforward in telling an employee the reason for dismissal, you are not helping that person to grow (Fig. 24–7).

An employee who has been in service for some time and is offering unsatisfactory performance should be warned and given an explanation of the specific improvements expected. If a second chance does not produce improvement in performance or attitude, then dismissal must follow. It should be done privately, with tact and consideration.

Most practice consultants believe that firing should come close to the end of the day, after all other employees have left, and that the break should be clean and immediate. If the office policy provides for 2 weeks' notice, give 2 weeks' pay. A dismissed employee should not be allowed to train or influence a replacement.

The exit meeting should be planned just as carefully as the employment interview. Be honest with the employee. Discuss the employee's assets as well as liabilities and give the reasons for the termination before you announce the dismissal. There is no need to dwell on the employee's deficiencies. These should have been thoroughly discussed at the warning interview, and the employee need only be told that the necessary improvements have not been made. Do listen to the employee's feedback. This may reveal some important administrative problems that need correction (Fig. 24–8).

After you dismiss an employee, do not leave that person in the office unattended. Request and get the office keys before giving a dismissed employee the final paycheck. And do not offer to give the employee a good reference unless you can do it sincerely.

Certain breaches of conduct, such as embezzlement and blatant insubordination or violation of patient confidentiality, are grounds for immediate dismissal without warning.

Occasionally, an employee voluntarily terminates a job without giving a valid reason. The physician or office manager may wish to follow up with a letter to the former employee to seek out any problem that may have prompted the resignation (Fig. 24–9).

Memory Jogger

5 *What courtesy should be extended to a long-term employee whose performance is unsatisfactory?*

Text continued on page 379

PERFORMANCE EVALUATION AND DEVELOPMENT PLAN
(OFFICE AND CLERICAL)

NAME: _____   DATE OF EVALUATION: _____

DATE OF HIRE: _____   DEPARTMENT: _____

JOB TITLE: _____   SUPERVISOR: _____

DATE APPOINTED THIS JOB: _____   MANAGER: _____

LAST REVIEW DATE: _____   LAST REVIEW RATING: _____

NEXT REVIEW DATE: _____   CURRENT REVIEW RATING: _____

PURPOSE

The purpose of this evaluation is to:

1. SET GOALS WITHIN SCOPE OF PRESENT JOB.
2. COMMUNICATE OPENLY ABOUT PERFORMANCE.
3. EVALUATE PAST PERFORMANCE.
4. DISCUSS FUTURE DEVELOPMENT PLANS FOR GROWTH.

INSTRUCTIONS

1. Supervisor to review form prior to completion. If specific items are not applicable they should be left blank.

2. Supervisor and employee to review job description prior to review.

3. In "COMMENTS" section supervisor may indicate which factors should be more heavily weighted in this particular evaluation.

4. Comments should be specific and job-related. All appropriate evaluation factors should be commented on to some degree.

I. POSITION OBJECTIVES AND MAJOR RESPONSIBILITIES. Summarize specific responsibilities of the job.

_____

_____

_____

II. ACCOMPLISHMENTS AND/OR IMPROVEMENTS. What specific accomplishments and/or improvements has employee made since last review with respect to set goals?

_____

_____

PLEASE CONSIDER THE EMPLOYEE'S DEMONSTRATED PERFORMANCE AND MARK THE CIRCLE WHICH MOST CLOSELY DESCRIBES THAT PERFORMANCE.

4 - Performance consistently far exceeds expectations and requirements.
3 - Performance consistently exceeds normal expectations and job requirements.
2 - Performance consistently meets expectations and job requirements
1 - Performance usually meets expectations and minimum job requirements.
0 - Performance does not meet job requirements.

– CONTINUED, NEXT PAGE –

FORM # 72-119 © 1987 BIBBERO SYSTEMS, INC. PETALUMA, CA

TO REORDER CALL TOLL FREE:
800-BIBBERO /(800 242-2376) OR
FAX: (800) 242-9330 MFG IN U.S.A.

FIGURE 24–6 Performance evaluation and development plan. (Courtesy of Bibbero Systems, Inc., Petaluma, California (800) 242-2376, Fax (800) 242-9330.)

7. DEPENDABILITY: CONSIDER ATTENDANCE, PUNCTUALITY, IDLE TIME AND RELIANCE WHICH CAN BE PLACED ON EMPLOYEE TO PERSEVERE AND CARRY THROUGH TO COMPLETION ALL ASSIGNED TASKS

○ 0   ○ 1   ○ 2   ○ 3   ○ 4

_____

_____

_____

8. COMPLIANCE WITH COMPANY POLICIES: DOES THE EMPLOYEE COMPLY WITH RULES AND REGULATIONS WHICH APPLY TO SAFETY, FAIR EMPLOYMENT PRACTICES AND GENERAL ADMINISTRATIVE PROCEDURE.

○ 0   ○ 1   ○ 2   ○ 3   ○ 4

_____

_____

_____

9. SPECIFIC PERFORMANCE	1	2	3	4	**COMMENTS**
A. Ability to handle scheduling:					
B. Willingness to work OT when necessary:					
C. Handling of calls and follow-up:					
D. Maintenance of equipment:					
E. Ability to handle patient complaints:					
F. Tact in dealing with patients:					
G. Speed (in specific technical procedures):					
H. Secretarial accuracy:					
I. Professional terminology:					
J. Assisting procedures:					
K. Laboratory techniques:					
L. X-ray techniques:					
M. Physical therapy:					
N. Collections:					
O. Medical Insurance:					
P. Bookkeeping:					

10. PERSONAL	1	2	3	4	**COMMENTS**
A. Grooming:					
B. Professional conduct:					
C. Energy, enthusiasm:					
D. Ability to handle stress:					

ADDITIONAL COMMENTS: _____

_____

_____

_____

_____

FORM # 72-119 © 1987 BIBBERO SYSTEMS, INC. PETALUMA, CA

FIGURE 24–6 *continued*

TERMINATION / REHIRE EVALUATION FORM

Employee Name_____ Social Security No._____

Department _____ Title _____

Termination Date _____

Reason for Termination: _____Resigned _____Laid Off_____Retired

Evaluation of Job Performance	Excellent	Very Good	Average	Poor	Unacceptable
Quality (accuracy, etc.)	☐	☐	☐	☐	☐
Quantity (productivity, consistency, etc.)	☐	☐	☐	☐	☐
Knowledge of Duties	☐	☐	☐	☐	☐
Reliability (absenteeism)	☐	☐	☐	☐	☐
Punctuality	☐	☐	☐	☐	☐
Ability to Cooperate with Co-workers	☐	☐	☐	☐	☐
Relationship with Patients	☐	☐	☐	☐	☐
Overall Attitude (willingness and commitment)	☐	☐	☐	☐	☐
Initiative	☐	☐	☐	☐	☐
Judgment	☐	☐	☐	☐	☐

Recommendation for Rehiring: _____

_____

_____

Comments:_____

_____

_____

_____

_____

_____

_____

_____

_____ Date _____

Supervisor's Signature

FORM # 72-123   PERSONNEL RECORDS ORGANIZING SYSTEMS • © 1987 BIBBERO SYSTEMS, INC. • PETALUMA, CA.
TO REORDER CALL TOLL FREE: (800) BIBBERO (800-242-2376) OR FAX (800) 242-9330.   Mfg In U.S.A.

FIGURE 24–7 Termination/rehire evaluation form at end of probationary period. (Courtesy of Bibbero Systems, Inc., Petaluma, California (800) 242-2376, Fax (800) 242-9330.)

EXIT INTERVIEW QUESTIONNAIRE

Employee Name (Optional) _____ Date _____

Job Title _____ Department _____

Immediate Supervisor _____ Dates of Employment _____

SSN# _____ EMP. ID# _____

I. Please rate the following conditions.

	Excellent	Very Good	Average	Poor	Unacceptable
Employer in General	☐	☐	☐	☐	☐
Administration	☐	☐	☐	☐	☐
Policies and Procedures	☐	☐	☐	☐	☐
New Employee Orientation	☐	☐	☐	☐	☐
Wages	☐	☐	☐	☐	☐
Vacation	☐	☐	☐	☐	☐
Holidays	☐	☐	☐	☐	☐
Sick Leave	☐	☐	☐	☐	☐
Other Benefits	☐	☐	☐	☐	☐
Immediate Supervisor	☐	☐	☐	☐	☐
Management	☐	☐	☐	☐	☐
Challenge of Position	☐	☐	☐	☐	☐
Satisfaction of Position	☐	☐	☐	☐	☐
Advancement	☐	☐	☐	☐	☐
Training Programs	☐	☐	☐	☐	☐
Co-workers	☐	☐	☐	☐	☐
Professional Staff	☐	☐	☐	☐	☐
Working Conditions (Physical)	☐	☐	☐	☐	☐
Hours	☐	☐	☐	☐	☐
Days	☐	☐	☐	☐	☐
Work Load	☐	☐	☐	☐	☐
Pressures / Stress	☐	☐	☐	☐	☐
Morale of Staff	☐	☐	☐	☐	☐

Specific comments on any of the above factors: _____

_____

_____

_____

II. Please rate the following conditions in your department.

	Excellent	Very Good	Average	Poor	Unacceptable
Orientation Program	☐	☐	☐	☐	☐
Intra-departmental Communication	☐	☐	☐	☐	☐
Inter-departmental Cooperation	☐	☐	☐	☐	☐
Opportunities for Training and Development	☐	☐	☐	☐	☐
Morale of Co-workers	☐	☐	☐	☐	☐

Specific comments on any of the above factors: _____

_____

_____

_____

ORDER # 72-122 PERSONNEL RECORD SYSTEM • © 1984 BIBBERO SYSTEMS, INC. • PETALUMA, CA.
TO REORDER CALL TOLL FREE: (800) BIBBERO (800-242-2376) OR FAX (800) 242-9330 (Rev. 5/96) MFG IN U.S.A.

FIGURE 24–8 Exit interview questionnaire after voluntary termination of employment. (Courtesy of Bibbero Systems, Inc., Petaluma, California (800) 242-2376, Fax (800) 242-9330.)

Illustration continued on following page

III. Please rate your immediate supervisor.

	Excellent	Very Good	Average	Poor	Unacceptable
Follows Policies & Procedures	☐	☐	☐	☐	☐
Follows Regulations of Department	☐	☐	☐	☐	☐
Fair & Equal to Employees	☐	☐	☐	☐	☐
Assigns Work Fairly	☐	☐	☐	☐	☐
Provides Adequate Training	☐	☐	☐	☐	☐
Open to Suggestions	☐	☐	☐	☐	☐
Encourages and Praises Staff	☐	☐	☐	☐	☐
Encourages Team Effort and Cooperation	☐	☐	☐	☐	☐
Resolves Complaints & Problems	☐	☐	☐	☐	☐
Encourages Advancement	☐	☐	☐	☐	☐
Assigns Responsibility Equally	☐	☐	☐	☐	☐
Demands Realistic Standards	☐	☐	☐	☐	☐

Specific comments on any of the above factors: _____
_____
_____

IV. Please answer following general questions.

a. Why were you interested in working here?_____
_____

b. Were you satisfied with your job here? _____
_____

c. Positive conditions of work here?_____
_____

d. Would you recommend employment here?   _____Yes   _____ No

Why? _____
_____

e. Please specify your reasons for leaving?
Moving to another location _____
Work schedule_____
Personal (family) _____
Supervision _____
Opportunity for Advancement _____
Transportation _____
Marriage _____
Pregnancy _____
Attend School _____
Retirement (voluntary) _____
Dissatisfied _____
Another Position _____
Other (Specify) _____
Conditions or benefits of new employment that you have found more appealing: _____
_____
_____

f. Suggestions for general improvements here or specifically within your department: _____

ORDER # **72-122** PERSONNEL RECORD SYSTEM • © 1984 BIBBERO SYSTEMS, INC. • PETALUMA, CA.
TO REORDER CALL TOLL FREE: (800) BIBBERO (800-242-2376) OR FAX (800) 242-9330 (Rev. 5/96)   MFG IN U.S.A.

FIGURE 24–8 *continued*

Dear _____

Since your decision to leave our employ a few weeks ago, I have been concerned about your reasons for doing so. There may have been more than one reason—and one of them may have been dissatisfaction with the working conditions.

If there was in fact some reason for dissatisfaction that influenced your decision to leave our employ, I would appreciate your passing it along to me, so that I may avoid losing other valuable employees in the future.

Please drop me a note, telephone, or come in if you wish. I assure you that any comments you care to make will be treated with respect and appreciation.

Cordially yours,

FIGURE 24–9 Example of letter from physician to employee who resigned suddenly.

Business Management

STAFF MEETINGS

There must be some formal mechanism for keeping the office manager and other key employees current on the daily business affairs of the practice. One of the most common complaints from office personnel is that of being unable to discuss problems with the physician. The solution to this problem may be to hold regular staff meetings, which may be scheduled as frequently as weekly but should be no less often than quarterly. Some of the best ideas on improvement come from the office staff, and expressing ideas should be encouraged.

The simplest technique is to set aside a specific time for regular meetings at an hour when the most people can attend with the least disruption. The meetings need not be long or overly formal, but to be effective they must be planned and organized.

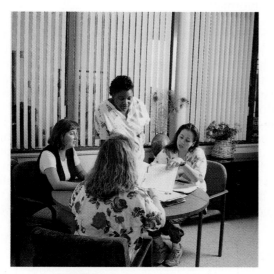

FIGURE 24–10 Staff meeting.

There must be a leader, and a secretary should be appointed to take notes. The effectiveness of the leader, a person who can balance firmness with fairness, is an important aspect of the meeting. This is usually either the physician or the office manager/supervisor. All members of the staff should be encouraged to submit ideas for discussion.

Draw up a simple outline of the issues you want to discuss and prepare any supporting data needed for the meeting. There are many kinds of staff meetings. They may be purely informational, or problem solving, or brainstorming; they may be work sessions for updating manuals, training seminars, or whatever is necessary to that individual practice. The staff should meet to discuss new ideas and any changes in office procedures and to resolve any problems. The staff meeting must not be allowed to deteriorate into a gripe session. Individual complaints should be handled privately.

The meeting must have a set agenda, with time for topics that need discussion on a regular basis, as well as time to handle any current problems. The agenda might be similar to that of any business meeting:

1. Reading of the last meeting's minutes
2. Discussion of any unfinished business
3. Discussion of any problems in the clinical area
4. Discussion of any problems in the administrative area
5. Discussion of any problems in common areas
6. Adjournment

Some physicians like to combine the staff meeting with a breakfast or lunch. The time or place is not important as long as it is "neutral" and suits the practice and the meetings are conducted regularly, democratically, and without interruption (Fig. 24–10). There must be follow-up to the items discussed; otherwise, the only result will be frustration and a reluctance to discuss problems at future meetings.

Memory Jogger

6 *Why is it important to have an agenda for a staff meeting?*

PRACTICE DEVELOPMENT

The business manager will play a large role in practice development, or "practice marketing" as it is often referred to. Practice development techniques are the outcome of a conscious need to improve the professional image, to increase exposure to the public, and to attract and keep patients. With the expansion of managed care in the health care industry, the average physician receives less income, has increased costs, and works a more competitive practice environment. In many instances it has become necessary to make slight changes in office hours to accommodate the patient population, including, in some cases, providing for evening and weekend hours or even house calls.

The medical assistant with management responsibilities can encourage the physician to participate in community affairs. For example, the practice might offer to give mass inoculations when needed, serve as a consultant in area health fairs, or speak on health topics to civic and professional groups. Some physicians gain public exposure by writing articles or a question-and-answer column for an area newspaper. Local events may suggest other ways of promoting the practice.

Communication with the patient is essential. The medical practice with a computer and word processing software can easily generate a newsletter several times a year containing information pertaining to the practice specialty or advances in health care in general. A letter to the patient and one to the patient's referring physician after a consultation are greatly appreciated by both and are easily and quickly accomplished with electronic equipment. Holiday and birthday remembrances are another easy way of keeping the patient aware of the practice and conveying your concern.

The first, last, and most important rule of marketing a medical practice, of course, is to treat the patients well, because the best source of patients consists of referrals from existing satisfied patients.

Memory Jogger

7 *Memorize the most important rule of marketing a medical practice.*

PATIENT EDUCATION

Patients have many common concerns about the physician's policies, such as office hours, what is included in his or her specialty, directions for reaching the office, parking facilities, emergency services, answering service, cancellations, house calls, prescription renewals, and payment of fees. You can satisfy the patients' concerns and save your own time by putting these policies in writing and giving a copy to every patient.

Many management experts recommend that two separate folders or pamphlets be prepared—one devoted to general office information and another to financial policies.

Patient Information Folder

Only a very small percentage of practices have a booklet that explains the information basic to the operational and service aspects of the practice. Yet, a patient information folder can easily be compiled by the physician and staff cooperatively in a staff meeting. Experience has shown that if such a folder is given to every new patient, the number of incoming phone calls can be reduced by an average of 20% to 30%. It can also reduce misunderstanding and forgotten instructions. The folder must of necessity be tailored to the specific practice.

The patient information folder should be an introduction to the practice and, if possible, mailed to a new patient before the first visit. A supply may also be left with referring physicians' offices to be given to patients coming to your office. It should be designed to easily fit into a No. 10 business envelope.

The cover should show the name of the practice, its location, and the practice logo, if there is one. Consider using a photo of the medical building for easy identification by the new patient.

A statement of philosophy is frequently included in the introduction, followed by a description of the practice.

> The doctors and staff would like to welcome you to our office. We work as a team with the goal of providing prompt and thorough care of your problems. We are always working to improve our care and service in any way possible.
>
> Our practice is limited exclusively to the musculoskeletal system and its disorders. Therefore, it is important for each patient to have a primary care physician such as a pediatrician, family physician, or internist to oversee the primary medical care for the entire patient. Our role is most effective as a consultant to your primary care physician.

Describe the office policy regarding appointments and cancellations, telephone calls, and the function of the answering service. If a separate "business only" telephone line is available, be sure to include this information.

> This office has two receptionists available to answer phone calls during regular office hours. The office is very busy, and you will occasionally be asked to hold for a brief period. Please be patient with this. If you wish to speak to a doctor, your call will usually be returned during the next available break period or at the end of the office day. We receive many calls during the day, and it is unfair to the patients who have scheduled appointments to continually interrupt the doctor for telephone calls. Therefore, the receptionist will usually take a message and your call will be returned as soon as possible. Please inform the receptionist if your problem is urgent and she will let the doctor know this.

Describe any **ancillary** or laboratory services provided, how test results are reported, and your policy on prescription renewals.

Patients need to know the provisions for emergency procedures: What hospitals does the practice use regularly? What is the night and weekend coverage? Hospitalization procedures and postoperative care and follow-up may also be included.

> One of the doctors in the group is always on call for emergency situations. You may reach him by calling our office phone number (714) 333–2323, and the answering service will put you in touch with the doctor on call at that time. Our doctors are on staff at St. Joseph Hospital (714-222-3333) and, for children, Children's Hospital of Orange County, 714-222-4444. In case of emergency, call 911.

List all physicians in the practice; state their educational backgrounds, training, and board certifications; and define their specialties. List the names of key clinical and administrative staff members, such as registered nurses and nurse practitioners, medical assistants, the office manager, and the business manager. Provide the practice address, a map of how to get there, and information about the parking facilities.

Don't just stack these folders in the reception room for patients to pick up. Have the receptionist write the patient's name on the folder and hand it to the patient when he or she registers for the first appointment and suggest that the patient keep it for future reference.

Memory Jogger

8 *In what ways does a patient information folder improve medical care?*

Financial Policy Folder

A separate small folder of information covering the financial policies of the office can eliminate many questions and possible misunderstandings. Tailor the financial policy folder to your specific practice. Keep it small enough to fit into the billing envelope, and send it out with the first monthly statement. If the practice sends out a "welcome" package before the patient's first visit, include the financial policy folder. Otherwise, present one at the first visit.

Spell out policies regarding billing and collection procedures, and make it clear that patients are responsible for the uninsured portion of the fees. If you expect payment at the time of service, put this in the folder. Keep the language simple and straightforward so that the message is clear.

> **FINANCIAL POLICY**
>
> We ask that our services be paid for at the time they are rendered. You will be provided with a superbill so that you may bill your insurance company and be reimbursed for services paid at the time of your visit. Simply attach the superbill to your insurance form and mail it to the insurance company. The appropriate diagnoses and charges will be on the superbill. There is usually a greater charge for the initial visit because this involves more time than follow-up visits. If you are sent to an outside office for laboratory testing or special x-rays, you will be billed separately from that office. We will be available to help if special circumstances arise involving difficulty with forms or receiving reimbursement. We will bill your insurance if you have a special situation such as surgery, prepaid health plans, Medicaid, CCS, or Senior Savers. We will complete disability papers as promptly as possible. However, you must obtain the necessary forms from your employer or the disability office.

The financial policy folder should also clearly state that the ultimate responsibility for payment lies with the patient.

Patient Instruction Sheets

In most medical offices there are patient procedures that occur over and over again. Instead of attempting to orally instruct a patient each time, why not develop clearly stated instruction sheets that you can review with the patient and then give the patient the written instructions to take home?

> **EXAMPLES OF PROCEDURES TO BE LISTED IN INSTRUCTION SHEETS**
>
> - Preparation for x-ray or laboratory tests
> - Preoperative and postoperative instructions
> - Diet sheets
> - Performing an enema
> - Dressing a wound
> - Taking medications
> - Using a cane, crutches, walker, or wheelchair
> - Care of casts
> - Exercise therapy

Financial Management

A physician in a solo practice or small partnership may prefer to handle most financial aspects of the practice personally or may place that responsibility in the hands of a certified public accountant or management consultant. In this situation, the medical assistant's involvement may be limited to the billing and bookkeeping activities discussed in previous chapters.

The medical assistant who is able to handle more responsibility will probably have the opportunity to do so. This could be the most challenging part of the position and may include any or all of the following activities:

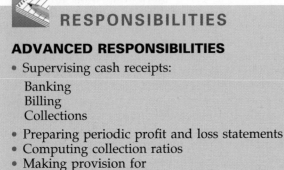

SKILLS AND RESPONSIBILITIES

ADVANCED RESPONSIBILITIES

- Supervising cash receipts:
  Banking
  Billing
  Collections
- Preparing periodic profit and loss statements
- Computing collection ratios
- Making provision for
  Practice insurance
  Professional liability
  Workers' compensation
  Employee's health benefits
  Disability insurance
  Unemployment insurance
- Writing payroll checks
- Paying bills
- Preparing reports for governmental agencies
- Serving as liaison with the accountant

PAYROLL RECORDS

Handling payroll records, whether for one employee or dozens of employees, involves frequent reporting activities. If it were necessary only to write a check to each employee for the agreed-upon salary for a given pay period, no discussion of payroll records would be necessary. But government regulations require the withholding of taxes from employees and payment of certain taxes due from both employees and employers.

To comply with government regulations, complete records must be kept for every employee. You must keep all records of employment taxes for at least 4 years. These should be available for review by the Internal Revenue Service (IRS). Such records include the following:

- Social Security number of the employee
- Number of withholding allowances claimed
- Amount of gross salary
- All deductions for Social Security and Medicare taxes; federal, state, and city or other subdivision withholding taxes; state disability insur-

ance; and state unemployment tax, where applicable

Memory Jogger

9 *How long must employee financial records be kept?*

PAYROLL REPORTING FORMS

Each employee and each employer must have a tax identification number. The Social Security number is the employee's tax identification number. Any person who does not have a Social Security number should apply for one, using Form SS-5 available from any Social Security Administration office.

The employer applies for a number for federal tax accounting purposes using Form SS-4, available at Social Security Administration offices or by calling 1-800-TAX-FORM. In states that require employer reports, a state employer number must also be obtained.

Before the end of the first pay period, the employee should complete an Employee's Withholding Allowance Certificate (Form W-4) showing the number of withholding allowances claimed (Fig. 24–11). Otherwise, the employer must indicate withholding on the basis of a single person with no exemptions.

The employee should complete a new form when changes occur in marital status or in the number of allowances claimed. Each employee is entitled to one personal allowance and one for each qualified dependent. The employee may elect to take fewer or no allowances, in which case the tax withheld will be greater and a refund may be due when the employee's annual tax report is filed. If an employee claims more than 10 withholding allowances or an exemption from withholding and his or her wages would normally be more than $200 per week, the employer is required to send to the IRS copies of these W-4 forms.

A supply of all the necessary forms for filing federal returns, preprinted with the employer's name, will be furnished to an employer who has applied for an employer identification number. Extra forms may be obtained from the IRS office.

INCOME TAX WITHHOLDING

Employers are required by law to withhold certain amounts from employees' earnings and to report and forward these amounts to be applied toward payment of income tax. The amount to be withheld is based on the following:

- Total earnings of the employee
- Number of withholding allowances claimed

- Marital status of the employee
- Length of the pay period involved

The *Federal Employer's Tax Guide* includes tables to be used in determining the amount to be withheld. Sample pages are shown in Figure 24–12. There is one table for single persons and unmarried heads of households and one for married persons. The tables cover monthly, semimonthly, biweekly, weekly, and daily or miscellaneous periods.

Memory Jogger

10 *What four items determine the amount of income tax withholding for each employee?*

EMPLOYER'S INCOME TAX

The physician who is practicing as an individual is not subject to withholding tax but is expected to make an estimated tax payment four times a year. The accountant prepares four copies of Form 1040-S, Declaration of Estimated Tax for Individuals, for the ensuing year when the annual income tax return is prepared. The first form and the quarterly estimated tax for the next year is filed at the same time as the tax return. The remaining three forms, with the estimated tax due, must be filed on June 15, September 15, and January 15. It may be the business manager's responsibility to see that these returns are filed when due. The employer also contributes to Social Security and Medicare in the form of a self-employment tax.

SOCIAL SECURITY, MEDICARE, AND INCOME TAX WITHHOLDING

The Federal Insurance Contributions Act (FICA) provides for a federal system of old-age, survivors, disability, and hospital insurance. The tax rate is reviewed frequently and is subject to change by Congress. In 1998, the wage base for Social Security tax is $68,400 and the tax rate is 6.2% each for employers and employees. All wages (no ceiling) are subject to the Medicare tax at a rate of 1.45% each for both employees and employers.

QUARTERLY RETURNS

Each quarter of the year, all employers who are subject to income tax withholding (including withholding on sick pay and supplemental unemployment benefits) of Social Security and Medicare taxes must file an Employer's Quarterly Federal Tax Return on or before the last day of the first month after the end of the quarter (Fig. 24–13). Due dates

for this return and full payment of the tax are April 30, July 31, October 31, and January 31. If deposits equaling full payment of taxes due have been made, the due date for the return is extended 10 days.

ANNUAL RETURNS

The employer is required to furnish two copies of Form W-2 Wage and Tax Statement to each employee from whom income tax or Social Security tax has been withheld or from whom income tax would have been withheld if the employee had claimed no more than one withholding allowance. The forms should be given to employees by January 31.

If employment ends before December 31, the employer may give the W-2 form to the terminated employee any time after employment ends. If the employee asks for Form W-2, the employer should give the employee the completed copies within 30 days of the request or the final wage payment, whichever is later.

Employers must file Form W-3, Transmittal of Income and Tax Statement, annually, to transmit wage and income tax withheld statements (Forms W-2) to the Social Security Administration. These forms are processed by the Social Security Administration, which then furnishes the IRS with the income tax data that it needs from those forms. Form W-3 and its attachments must be filed separately from Form 941 on or before the last day of February after the calendar year for which the W-2 forms are prepared.

HOW TO DEPOSIT

In general, the employer must deposit income tax withheld and both the employer and employee Social Security and Medicare taxes by mailing or delivering a check, money order, or cash to an authorized financial institution or Federal Reserve bank, using Form 8109, Federal Tax Deposit (FTD) Coupon. However, some taxpayers are required to deposit by electronic funds transfer. If the total deposits of Social Security, Medicare, railroad retirement, and withheld income taxes were more than $50,000 in 1996, then all depository tax liabilities that occur after 1997 must be made by electronic deposits. The Electronic Federal Tax Payment System (EFTPS) must be used to make electronic deposits. Failure to do so may result in being subject to a 10% penalty.

FEDERAL UNEMPLOYMENT TAX

Employers also contribute under the Federal Unemployment Tax Act (FUTA). Generally, credit can be taken against the FUTA tax for amounts paid into a state unemployment fund up to a certain percentage. Employers are responsible for paying the FUTA

Text continued on page 391

Personal Allowances Worksheet

A   Enter "1" for **yourself** if no one else can claim you as a dependent . . . . **A** _____

B   Enter "1" if: { • You are single and have only one job; or
      • You are married, have only one job, and your spouse does not work; or   } . . **B** _____
      • Your wages from a second job or your spouse's wages (or the total of both) are $1,000 or less. }

C   Enter "1" for your **spouse**. But, you may choose to enter -0- if you are married and have either a working spouse or
      more than one job. (This may help you avoid having too little tax withheld.). . . . . **C** _____

D   Enter number of **dependents** (other than your spouse or yourself) you will claim on your tax return . . . . . . **D** _____

E   Enter "1" if you will file as **head of household** on your tax return (see conditions under **Head of household** above) . **E** _____

F   Enter "1" if you have at least $1,500 of **child or dependent care expenses** for which you plan to claim a credit . . **F** _____

G   **New—Child Tax Credit:**   • If your total income will be between $16,500 and $47,000 ($21,000 and $60,000 if married),
      enter "1" for each eligible child.   • If your total income will be between $47,000 and $80,000 ($60,000 and $115,000 if
      married), enter "1" if you have two or three eligible children, or enter "2" if you have four or more . . . . **G** _____

H   Add lines A through G and enter total here. **Note:** This amount may be different from the number of exemptions you claim on your return. ▶ **H** _____

For accuracy,   { • If you plan to **itemize or claim adjustments to income** and want to reduce your withholding, see the Deductions
complete all   and Adjustments Worksheet on page 2.
worksheets   • If you are **single,** have **more than one job,** and your combined earnings from all jobs exceed $32,000 OR if you
that apply.   are **married** and have a **working spouse or more than one job,** and the combined earnings from all jobs exceed
                  $55,000, see the Two-Earner/Two-Job Worksheet on page 2 to avoid having too little tax withheld.
              • If **neither** of the above situations applies, **stop here** and enter the number from line H on line 5 of Form W-4 below.

- - - - - - - - - - - - - - - - - -   **Cut here and give the certificate to your employer. Keep the top part for your records.**   - - - - - - - - - - - - - - - -

Form **W-4**

Department of the Treasury
Internal Revenue Service

Employee's Withholding Allowance Certificate

▶ **For Privacy Act and Paperwork Reduction Act Notice, see page 2.**

OMB No. 1545-0010

19**98**

1 Type or print your first name and middle initial Last name	**2** Your social security number

Home address (number and street or rural route)	**3** ☐ Single ☐ Married ☐ Married, but withhold at higher Single rate. **Note:** *If married, but legally separated, or spouse is a nonresident alien, check the Single box.*
City or town, state, and ZIP code	**4** If your last name differs from that on your social security card, check here and call 1-800-772-1213 for a new card . . . . ▶ ☐

5   Total number of allowances you are claiming (from line H above or from the worksheets on page 2 if they apply) .   **5** |

6   Additional amount, if any, you want withheld from each paycheck . . . .   **6** $ |

7   I claim exemption from withholding for 1998, and I certify that I meet **BOTH** of the following conditions for exemption:
      • Last year I had a right to a refund of **ALL** Federal income tax withheld because I had **NO** tax liability **AND**
      • This year I expect a refund of **ALL** Federal income tax withheld because I expect to have **NO** tax liability.
      If you meet both conditions, enter "EXEMPT" here . . . . ▶ **7** |

Under penalties of perjury, I certify that I am entitled to the number of withholding allowances claimed on this certificate or entitled to claim exempt status.

Employee's signature ▶   Date ▶ _____ , 19___

8   Employer's name and address (Employer: Complete 8 and 10 only if sending to the IRS) | **9**   Office code (optional) | **10**   Employer identification number |

Cat. No. 10220Q

FIGURE 24–11   Form W-4: Employee's Withholding Allowance Certificate.

Form W-4 (1998)   Page **2**

Deductions and Adjustments Worksheet

Note: *Use this worksheet only if you plan to itemize deductions or claim adjustments to income on your 1998 tax return.*

1   Enter an estimate of your 1998 itemized deductions. These include qualifying home mortgage interest, charitable contributions, state and local taxes (but not sales taxes), medical expenses in excess of 7.5% of your income, and miscellaneous deductions. (For 1998, you may have to reduce your itemized deductions if your income is over $124,500 ($62,250 if married filing separately). Get Pub. 919 for details.) ... **1** $ _____

2   Enter: $7,100 if married filing jointly or qualifying widow(er)
            $6,250 if head of household
            $4,250 if single
            $3,550 if married filing separately   .... **2** $ _____

3   **Subtract** line 2 from line 1. If line 2 is greater than line 1, enter -0- ... **3** $ _____

4   Enter an estimate of your 1998 adjustments to income, including alimony, deductible IRA contributions, and education loan interest ... **4** $ _____

5   **Add** lines 3 and 4 and enter the total ... **5** $ _____

6   Enter an estimate of your 1998 nonwage income (such as dividends or interest) ... **6** $ _____

7   **Subtract** line 6 from line 5. Enter the result, but not less than -0- ... **7** $ _____

8   **Divide** the amount on line 7 by $2,500 and enter the result here. Drop any fraction ... **8** _____

9   Enter the number from Personal Allowances Worksheet, line H, on page 1 ... **9** _____

10 **Add** lines 8 and 9 and enter the total here. If you plan to use the Two-Earner/Two-Job Worksheet, also enter this total on line 1 below. Otherwise, **stop here** and enter this total on Form W-4, line 5, on page 1 ... **10** _____

Two-Earner/Two-Job Worksheet

Note: *Use this worksheet only if the instructions for line H on page 1 direct you here.*

1   Enter the number from line H on page 1 (or from line 10 above if you used the Deductions and Adjustments Worksheet) **1** _____

2   Find the number in **Table 1** below that applies to the **LOWEST** paying job and enter it here ... **2** _____

3   If line 1 is **GREATER THAN OR EQUAL TO** line 2, subtract line 2 from line 1. Enter the result here (if zero, enter -0-) and on Form W-4, line 5, on page 1. **DO NOT** use the rest of this worksheet ... **3** _____

Note: *If line 1 is **LESS THAN** line 2, enter -0- on Form W-4, line 5, on page 1. Complete lines 4–9 to calculate the additional withholding amount necessary to avoid a year end tax bill.*

4   Enter the number from line 2 of this worksheet ... **4** _____

5   Enter the number from line 1 of this worksheet ... **5** _____

6   **Subtract** line 5 from line 4 ... **6** _____

7   Find the amount in **Table 2** below that applies to the **HIGHEST** paying job and enter it here ... **7** $ _____

8   **Multiply** line 7 by line 6 and enter the result here. This is the additional annual withholding amount needed ... **8** $ _____

9   Divide line 8 by the number of pay periods remaining in 1998. (For example, divide by 26 if you are paid every other week and you complete this form in December 1997.) Enter the result here and on Form W-4, line 6, page 1. This is the additional amount to be withheld from each paycheck ... **9** $ _____

Table 1: Two-Earner/Two-Job Worksheet

Married Filing Jointly				All Others			
If wages from **LOWEST** paying job are—	Enter on line 2 above	If wages from **LOWEST** paying job are—	Enter on line 2 above	If wages from **LOWEST** paying job are—	Enter on line 2 above	If wages from **LOWEST** paying job are—	Enter on line 2 above
0 - $4,000	0	38,001 - 43,000	8	0 - $5,000	0	70,001 - 85,000	8
4,001 - 7,000	1	43,001 - 54,000	9	5,001 - 11,000	1	85,001 - 100,000	9
7,001 - 12,000	2	54,001 - 62,000	10	11,001 - 16,000	2	100,001 and over	10
12,001 - 18,000	3	62,001 - 70,000	11	16,001 - 21,000	3		
18,001 - 24,000	4	70,001 - 85,000	12	21,001 - 25,000	4		
24,001 - 28,000	5	85,001 - 100,000	13	25,001 - 42,000	5		
28,001 - 33,000	6	100,001 - 110,000	14	42,001 - 55,000	6		
33,001 - 38,000	7	110,001 and over	15	55,001 - 70,000	7		

Table 2: Two-Earner/Two-Job Worksheet

Married Filing Jointly		All Others	
If wages from **HIGHEST** paying job are—	Enter on line 7 above	If wages from **HIGHEST** paying job are—	Enter on line 7 above
0 - $50,000	$400	0 - $30,000	$400
50,001 - 100,000	760	30,001 - 60,000	760
100,001 - 130,000	840	60,001 - 120,000	840
130,001 - 240,000	970	120,001 - 250,000	970
240,001 and over	1,070	250,001 and over	1,070

Privacy Act and Paperwork Reduction Act Notice. We ask for the information on this form to carry out the Internal Revenue laws of the United States. The Internal Revenue Code requires this information under sections 3402(f)(2)(A) and 6109 and their regulations. Failure to provide a completed form will result in your being treated as a single person who claims no withholding allowances. Routine uses of this information include giving it to the Department of Justice for civil and criminal litigation and to cities, states, and the District of Columbia for use in administering their tax laws.

You are not required to provide the information requested on a form that is subject to the Paperwork Reduction Act unless the form displays a valid OMB control number. Books or records relating to a form or its instructions must be retained as long as their contents may become material in the administration of any Internal Revenue law. Generally, tax returns and return information are confidential, as required by Code section 6103.

The time needed to complete this form will vary depending on individual circumstances. The estimated average time is: **Recordkeeping** 46 min., **Learning about the law or the form** 10 min., **Preparing the form** 1 hr., 10 min. If you have comments concerning the accuracy of these time estimates or suggestions for making this form simpler, we would be happy to hear from you. You can write to the Tax Forms Committee, Western Area Distribution Center, Rancho Cordova, CA 95743-0001. **DO NOT** send the tax form to this address. Instead, give it to your employer.

Printed on recycled paper   GPO: 1997-419-121

FIGURE 24–11 *continued*

SINGLE Persons—MONTHLY Payroll Period
(For Wages Paid in 1998)

If the wages are—		And the number of withholding allowances claimed is—										
At least	But less than	0	1	2	3	4	5	6	7	8	9	10
		The amount of income tax to be withheld is—										
$2,440	$2,480	364	302	268	235	201	167	133	100	66	32	0
2,480	2,520	375	312	274	241	207	173	139	106	72	38	4
2,520	2,560	387	324	280	247	213	179	145	112	78	44	10
2,560	2,600	398	335	286	253	219	185	151	118	84	50	16
2,600	2,640	409	346	292	259	225	191	157	124	90	56	22
2,640	2,680	420	357	298	265	231	197	163	130	96	62	28
2,680	2,720	431	368	305	271	237	203	169	136	102	68	34
2,720	2,760	443	380	317	277	243	209	175	142	108	74	40
2,760	2,800	454	391	328	283	249	215	181	148	114	80	46
2,800	2,840	465	402	339	289	255	221	187	154	120	86	52
2,840	2,880	476	413	350	295	261	227	193	160	126	92	58
2,880	2,920	487	424	361	301	267	233	199	166	132	98	64
2,920	2,960	499	436	373	310	273	239	205	172	138	104	70
2,960	3,000	510	447	384	321	279	245	211	178	144	110	76
3,000	3,040	521	458	395	332	285	251	217	184	150	116	82
3,040	3,080	532	469	406	343	291	257	223	190	156	122	88
3,080	3,120	543	480	417	354	297	263	229	196	162	128	94
3,120	3,160	555	492	429	366	303	269	235	202	168	134	100
3,160	3,200	566	503	440	377	314	275	241	208	174	140	106
3,200	3,240	577	514	451	388	325	281	247	214	180	146	112
3,240	3,280	588	525	462	399	336	287	253	220	186	152	118
3,280	3,320	599	536	473	410	347	293	259	226	192	158	124
3,320	3,360	611	548	485	422	359	299	265	232	198	164	130
3,360	3,400	622	559	496	433	370	307	271	238	204	170	136
3,400	3,440	633	570	507	444	381	318	277	244	210	176	142
3,440	3,480	644	581	518	455	392	329	283	250	216	182	148
3,480	3,520	655	592	529	466	403	340	289	256	222	188	154
3,520	3,560	667	604	541	478	415	352	295	262	228	194	160
3,560	3,600	678	615	552	489	426	363	301	268	234	200	166
3,600	3,640	689	626	563	500	437	374	311	274	240	206	172
3,640	3,680	700	637	574	511	448	385	322	280	246	212	178
3,680	3,720	711	648	585	522	459	396	333	286	252	218	184
3,720	3,760	723	660	597	534	471	408	345	292	258	224	190
3,760	3,800	734	671	608	545	482	419	356	298	264	230	196
3,800	3,840	745	682	619	556	493	430	367	304	270	236	202
3,840	3,880	756	693	630	567	504	441	378	315	276	242	208
3,880	3,920	767	704	641	578	515	452	389	326	282	248	214
3,920	3,960	779	716	653	590	527	464	401	338	288	254	220
3,960	4,000	790	727	664	601	538	475	412	349	294	260	226
4,000	4,040	801	738	675	612	549	486	423	360	300	266	232
4,040	4,080	812	749	686	623	560	497	434	371	308	272	238
4,080	4,120	823	760	697	634	571	508	445	382	319	278	244
4,120	4,160	835	772	709	646	583	520	457	394	331	284	250
4,160	4,200	846	783	720	657	594	531	468	405	342	290	256
4,200	4,240	857	794	731	668	605	542	479	416	353	296	262
4,240	4,280	868	805	742	679	616	553	490	427	364	302	268
4,280	4,320	879	816	753	690	627	564	501	438	375	312	274
4,320	4,360	891	828	765	702	639	576	513	450	387	324	280
4,360	4,400	902	839	776	713	650	587	524	461	398	335	286
4,400	4,440	913	850	787	724	661	598	535	472	409	346	292
4,440	4,480	924	861	798	735	672	609	546	483	420	357	298
4,480	4,520	935	872	809	746	683	620	557	494	431	368	305
4,520	4,560	947	884	821	758	695	632	569	506	443	380	317
4,560	4,600	958	895	832	769	706	643	580	517	454	391	328
4,600	4,640	969	906	843	780	717	654	591	528	465	402	339
4,640	4,680	980	917	854	791	728	665	602	539	476	413	350
4,680	4,720	991	928	865	802	739	676	613	550	487	424	361
4,720	4,760	1,003	940	877	814	751	688	625	562	499	436	373
4,760	4,800	1,014	951	888	825	762	699	636	573	510	447	384
4,800	4,840	1,026	962	899	836	773	710	647	584	521	458	395
4,840	4,880	1,038	973	910	847	784	721	658	595	532	469	406
4,880	4,920	1,051	984	921	858	795	732	669	606	543	480	417
4,920	4,960	1,063	996	933	870	807	744	681	618	555	492	429
4,960	5,000	1,076	1,007	944	881	818	755	692	629	566	503	440
5,000	5,040	1,088	1,018	955	892	829	766	703	640	577	514	451

$5,040 and over — Use Table 4(a) for a **SINGLE person** on page 34. Also see the instructions on page 32.

FIGURE 24–12 Pages from 1998 Withholding Tax Table.

MARRIED Persons—MONTHLY Payroll Period

(For Wages Paid in 1998)

If the wages are—		And the number of withholding allowances claimed is—										
At least	But less than	0	1	2	3	4	5	6	7	8	9	10
		The amount of income tax to be withheld is—										
$0	$540	0	0	0	0	0	0	0	0	0	0	0
540	560	2	0	0	0	0	0	0	0	0	0	0
560	580	5	0	0	0	0	0	0	0	0	0	0
580	600	8	0	0	0	0	0	0	0	0	0	0
600	640	12	0	0	0	0	0	0	0	0	0	0
640	680	18	0	0	0	0	0	0	0	0	0	0
680	720	24	0	0	0	0	0	0	0	0	0	0
720	760	30	0	0	0	0	0	0	0	0	0	0
760	800	36	3	0	0	0	0	0	0	0	0	0
800	840	42	9	0	0	0	0	0	0	0	0	0
840	880	48	15	0	0	0	0	0	0	0	0	0
880	920	54	21	0	0	0	0	0	0	0	0	0
920	960	60	27	0	0	0	0	0	0	0	0	0
960	1,000	66	33	0	0	0	0	0	0	0	0	0
1,000	1,040	72	39	5	0	0	0	0	0	0	0	0
1,040	1,080	78	45	11	0	0	0	0	0	0	0	0
1,080	1,120	84	51	17	0	0	0	0	0	0	0	0
1,120	1,160	90	57	23	0	0	0	0	0	0	0	0
1,160	1,200	96	63	29	0	0	0	0	0	0	0	0
1,200	1,240	102	69	35	1	0	0	0	0	0	0	0
1,240	1,280	108	75	41	7	0	0	0	0	0	0	0
1,280	1,320	114	81	47	13	0	0	0	0	0	0	0
1,320	1,360	120	87	53	19	0	0	0	0	0	0	0
1,360	1,400	126	93	59	25	0	0	0	0	0	0	0
1,400	1,440	132	99	65	31	0	0	0	0	0	0	0
1,440	1,480	138	105	71	37	3	0	0	0	0	0	0
1,480	1,520	144	111	77	43	9	0	0	0	0	0	0
1,520	1,560	150	117	83	49	15	0	0	0	0	0	0
1,560	1,600	156	123	89	55	21	0	0	0	0	0	0
1,600	1,640	162	129	95	61	27	0	0	0	0	0	0
1,640	1,680	168	135	101	67	33	0	0	0	0	0	0
1,680	1,720	174	141	107	73	39	6	0	0	0	0	0
1,720	1,760	180	147	113	79	45	12	0	0	0	0	0
1,760	1,800	186	153	119	85	51	18	0	0	0	0	0
1,800	1,840	192	159	125	91	57	24	0	0	0	0	0
1,840	1,880	198	165	131	97	63	30	0	0	0	0	0
1,880	1,920	204	171	137	103	69	36	2	0	0	0	0
1,920	1,960	210	177	143	109	75	42	8	0	0	0	0
1,960	2,000	216	183	149	115	81	48	14	0	0	0	0
2,000	2,040	222	189	155	121	87	54	20	0	0	0	0
2,040	2,080	228	195	161	127	93	60	26	0	0	0	0
2,080	2,120	234	201	167	133	99	66	32	0	0	0	0
2,120	2,160	240	207	173	139	105	72	38	4	0	0	0
2,160	2,200	246	213	179	145	111	78	44	10	0	0	0
2,200	2,240	252	219	185	151	117	84	50	16	0	0	0
2,240	2,280	258	225	191	157	123	90	56	22	0	0	0
2,280	2,320	264	231	197	163	129	96	62	28	0	0	0
2,320	2,360	270	237	203	169	135	102	68	34	0	0	0
2,360	2,400	276	243	209	175	141	108	74	40	6	0	0
2,400	2,440	282	249	215	181	147	114	80	46	12	0	0
2,440	2,480	288	255	221	187	153	120	86	52	18	0	0
2,480	2,520	294	261	227	193	159	126	92	58	24	0	0
2,520	2,560	300	267	233	199	165	132	98	64	30	0	0
2,560	2,600	306	273	239	205	171	138	104	70	36	3	0
2,600	2,640	312	279	245	211	177	144	110	76	42	9	0
2,640	2,680	318	285	251	217	183	150	116	82	48	15	0
2,680	2,720	324	291	257	223	189	156	122	88	54	21	0
2,720	2,760	330	297	263	229	195	162	128	94	60	27	0
2,760	2,800	336	303	269	235	201	168	134	100	66	33	0
2,800	2,840	342	309	275	241	207	174	140	106	72	39	5
2,840	2,880	348	315	281	247	213	180	146	112	78	45	11
2,880	2,920	354	321	287	253	219	186	152	118	84	51	17
2,920	2,960	360	327	293	259	225	192	158	124	90	57	23
2,960	3,000	366	333	299	265	231	198	164	130	96	63	29
3,000	3,040	372	339	305	271	237	204	170	136	102	69	35
3,040	3,080	378	345	311	277	243	210	176	142	108	75	41
3,080	3,120	384	351	317	283	249	216	182	148	114	81	47
3,120	3,160	390	357	323	289	255	222	188	154	120	87	53
3,160	3,200	396	363	329	295	261	228	194	160	126	93	59
3,200	3,240	402	369	335	301	267	234	200	166	132	99	65

FIGURE 24–12 *continued*

Form **941** (Rev. January 1998) Department of the Treasury Internal Revenue Service (O)	**Employer's Quarterly Federal Tax Return** ▶ **See separate instructions for information on completing this return.** **Please type or print.**	

Enter state code for state in which deposits were made ONLY if different from state in address to the right ▶ ⬚ (see page 3 of instructions).

Name (as distinguished from trade name)	Date quarter ended	OMB No. 1545-0029
Trade name, if any	Employer identification number	T FF FD FP
Address (number and street)	City, state, and ZIP code	I T

If address is different from prior return, check here ▶ ⬚

IRS Use

1 1 1 1 1 1 1 1 1 1	2	3 3 3 3 3 3 3 3	4 4 4	5 5 5
6 7 8 8 8 8 8 8 8 8		9 9 9 9 9	10 10 10 10 10 10 10 10 10	

If you do not have to file returns in the future, check here ▶ ⬚   and enter date final wages paid ▶

If you are a seasonal employer, see **Seasonal employers** on page 1 of the instructions and check here ▶

1	Number of employees in the pay period that includes March 12th . ▶	1		
2	Total wages and tips, plus other compensation		**2**	
3	Total income tax withheld from wages, tips, and sick pay		**3**	
4	Adjustment of withheld income tax for preceding quarters of calendar year		**4**	
5	Adjusted total of income tax withheld (line 3 as adjusted by line 4—see instructions) . . .		**5**	
6	Taxable social security wages	**6a**	× 12.4% (.124) =	**6b**	
	Taxable social security tips	**6c**	× 12.4% (.124) =	**6d**	
7	Taxable Medicare wages and tips . . .	**7a**	× 2.9% (.029) =	**7b**	
8	Total social security and Medicare taxes (add lines 6b, 6d, and 7b). Check here if wages are not subject to social security and/or Medicare tax . . . . ▶ ⬚		**8**	
9	Adjustment of social security and Medicare taxes (see instructions for required explanation) Sick Pay $ _____ ± Fractions of Cents $ _____ ± Other $ _____ =		**9**	
10	Adjusted total of social security and Medicare taxes (line 8 as adjusted by line 9—see instructions)		**10**	
11	**Total taxes** (add lines 5 and 10)		**11**	
12	Advance earned income credit (EIC) payments made to employees		**12**	
13	Net taxes (subtract line 12 from line 11). **This should equal line 17, column (d) below (or line D of Schedule B (Form 941))**		**13**	
14	Total deposits for quarter, including overpayment applied from a prior quarter		**14**	
15	**Balance due** (subtract line 14 from line 13). See instructions		**15**	
16	**Overpayment,** if line 14 is more than line 13, enter excess here ▶ $ _____ and check if to be: ⬚ Applied to next return **OR** ⬚ Refunded.			

- **All filers:** If line 13 is less than $500, you need not complete line 17 or Schedule B (Form 941).
- **Semiweekly schedule depositors:** Complete Schedule B (Form 941) and check here . . . . ▶ ⬚
- **Monthly schedule depositors:** Complete line 17, columns (a) through (d), and check here . . . . ▶ ⬚

17	**Monthly Summary of Federal Tax Liability.** Do not complete if you were a semiweekly schedule depositor.			
	(a) First month liability	**(b)** Second month liability	**(c)** Third month liability	**(d)** Total liability for quarter

Sign Here | Under penalties of perjury, I declare that I have examined this return, including accompanying schedules and statements, and to the best of my knowledge and belief, it is true, correct, and complete.

Signature ▶ _____   Print Your Name and Title ▶ _____   Date ▶ _____

For Privacy Act and Paperwork Reduction Act Notice, see page 4 of separate instructions.   Cat. No. 17001Z   Form **941** (Rev. 1-98)

FIGURE 24–13   Employer's Quarterly Federal Tax Return.

Form 941
Payment Voucher

Purpose of Form

Complete Form 941-V if you are making a payment with **Form 941,** Employer's Quarterly Federal Tax Return. We will use the completed voucher to credit your payment more promptly and accurately, and to improve our service to you.

If you have your return prepared by a third party and make a payment with that return, please provide this payment voucher to the return preparer.

Making Payments With Form 941

Make payments with Form 941 only if:

1. Your net taxes for the quarter (line 13 on Form 941) are less than $500 or

2. You are a monthly schedule depositor making a payment in accordance with the **accuracy of deposits** rule. (See section 11 of **Circular E,** Employer's Tax Guide, for details.) This amount may be $500 or more.

Otherwise, you must deposit the amount at an authorized financial institution or by electronic funds transfer. (See section 11 of Circular E for deposit instructions.) Do not use the Form 941-V payment voucher to make Federal tax deposits.

Caution: *If you pay amounts with Form 941 that should have been deposited, you may be subject to a penalty. See Circular E.*

*U.S. Government Printing Office: 1998 - 432-190/60347

Specific Instructions

Box 1—Amount paid. Enter the amount paid with Form 941.

Box 2. Enter the first four characters of your name as follows:

● **Individuals (sole proprietors, estates).** Use the first four letters of your last name (as shown in box 5).

● **Corporations.** Use the first four characters (letters or numbers) of your business name (as shown in box 5). Omit "The" if followed by more than one word.

● **Partnerships.** Use the first four characters of your trade name. If no trade name, enter the first four letters of the last name of the first listed partner.

Box 3—Employer identification number (EIN). If you do not have an EIN, apply for one on **Form SS-4,** Application for Employer Identification Number, and write "Applied for" and the date you applied in this entry space.

Box 4—Tax period. Darken the capsule identifying the quarter for which the payment is made. Darken only one capsule.

Box 5—Name and address. Enter your name and address as shown on Form 941.

● Make your check or money order payable to the Internal Revenue Service. Be sure to enter your EIN, "Form 941," and the tax period on your check or money order. Do not send cash. Please do not staple your payment to the voucher or the return.

● Detach the completed voucher and send it with your payment and Form 941 to the address provided in the separate **Instructions for Form 941.**

Printed on recycled paper

(Detach here)

Form 941-V	**Form 941 Payment Voucher**	OMB No. 1545-0029

Department of the Treasury
Internal Revenue Service

▶ Use this voucher when making a payment with your return.

1998

1 Enter the amount of the payment you are making	2 Enter the first four letters of your last name (business name if corporation or partnership)	3 Enter your employer identification number

▶ $

4 Tax period		5 Enter your business name (individual name if sole proprietor)
⊘ 1st Quarter	⊘ 3rd Quarter	Enter your address
⊘ 2nd Quarter	⊘ 4th Quarter	Enter your city, state, and ZIP code

For Privacy Act and Paperwork Reduction Act Notice, see Instructions for Form 941.

FIGURE 24–13 *continued*

Form **940**

Department of the Treasury
Internal Revenue Service (O)

**Employer's Annual Federal
Unemployment (FUTA) Tax Return**

▶ **For Paperwork Reduction Act Notice, see separate instructions.**

OMB No. 1545-0028

19**97**

T	
FF	
FD	
FP	
I	
T	

Name (as distinguished from trade name)   Calendar year

Trade name, if any

Address and ZIP code   Employer identification number

A Are you required to pay unemployment contributions to only one state? (If "No," skip questions B and C) . ☐ **Yes** ☐ **No**

B Did you pay all state unemployment contributions by February 2, 1998? ((1) If you deposited your total FUTA tax when due, check "Yes" if you paid all state unemployment contributions by February 10. (2) If a 0% experience rate is granted, check "Yes." (3) If "No," skip question C.) . . . . ☐ **Yes** ☐ **No**

C Were all wages that were taxable for FUTA tax also taxable for your state's unemployment tax? . . . . . ☐ **Yes** ☐ **No**

If you answered "No" to any of these questions, you must file Form 940. If you answered "Yes" to all the questions, you may file Form 940-EZ, which is a simplified version of Form 940. (Successor employers see **Special credit for successor employers** in the **Instructions for Form 940.**) You can get Form 940-EZ by calling 1-800-TAX-FORM (1-800-829-3676).

If you will not have to file returns in the future, check here, and complete and sign the return . . . . ▶ ☐
If this is an Amended Return, check here . . . . ▶ ☐

Part I   **Computation of Taxable Wages**

1 Total payments (including payments shown on lines 2 and 3) during the calendar year for services of employees . . . . | **1** |

2 Exempt payments. (Explain all exempt payments, attaching additional sheets if necessary.) ▶ --

----

Amount paid

| **2** | |

3 Payments for services of more than $7,000. Enter only amounts over the first $7,000 paid to each employee. Do not include any exempt payments from line 2. The $7,000 amount is the Federal wage base. Your state wage base may be different. **Do not use your state wage limitation** . | **3** | |

4 Total exempt payments (add lines 2 and 3) . . . . | **4** |

5 **Total taxable wages** (subtract line 4 from line 1) . . . . ▶ | **5** |

Be sure to complete both sides of this return, and sign in the space provided on the back.   Cat. No. 11234O   Form **940** (1997)

DETACH HERE

Form **940-V**

Department of the Treasury
Internal Revenue Service

Form 940 Payment Voucher

Use this voucher only when making a payment with your return.

OMB No. 1545-0028

19**97**

Complete boxes 1, 2, 3, and 4. Do not send cash, and do not staple your payment to this voucher. Make your check or money order payable to the **Internal Revenue Service.** Be sure to enter your employer identification number, "Form 940," and "1997" on your payment.

1 Enter the amount of the payment you are making

▶ $

2 Enter the first four letters of your last name
(business name if partnership or corporation)

3 Enter your employer identification number

Instructions for Box 2

—Individuals (sole proprietors, trusts, and estates)—
Enter the first four letters of your last name.

—Corporations and partnerships—Enter the first four characters of your business name (omit "The" if followed by more than one word).

4 Enter your business name (individual name for sole proprietors)

Enter your address

Enter your city, state, and ZIP code

FIGURE 24–14   Employer's Annual Federal Unemployment Tax (FUTA) Return.

Form 940 (1997)   Page **2**

Part II   Tax Due or Refund

| 1 | Gross FUTA tax. Multiply the wages in Part I, line 5, by .062 . . . . | 1 | |
| 2 | Maximum credit. Multiply the wages in Part I, line 5, by .054 . . . . | 2 | | |

3   Computation of tentative credit (Note: *All taxpayers must complete the applicable columns.***)**

(a) Name of state	(b) State reporting number(s) as shown on employer's state contribution returns	(c) Taxable payroll (as defined in state act)	(d) State experience rate period		(e) State experience rate	(f) Contributions if rate had been 5.4% (col. (c) x .054)	(g) Contributions payable at experience rate (col. (c) x col. (e))	(h) Additional credit (col. (f) minus col.(g)). If 0 or less, enter -0-.	(i) Contributions actually paid to state
			From	To					

3a	Totals . . . ▶								
3b	**Total tentative credit** (add line 3a, columns (h) and (i) only—see instructions for limitations on late payments) ▶								

4		
5		
6	**Credit:** Enter the smaller of the amount in Part II, line 2 or line 3b	6	
7	**Total FUTA tax** (subtract line 6 from line 1)	7	
8	Total FUTA tax deposited for the year, including any overpayment applied from a prior year . .	8	
9	**Balance due** (subtract line 8 from line 7). This should be $100 or less. Pay to the Internal Revenue Service. See page 4 of the **Instructions for Form 940** for details . . . . ▶	9	
10	**Overpayment** (subtract line 7 from line 8). Check if it is to be: ☐ **Applied to next return** or ☐ **Refunded** . . . . ▶	10	

Part III   Record of Quarterly Federal Unemployment Tax Liability *(Do not include state liability.)* Complete only if line 7 is over $100.

Quarter	First (Jan. 1–Mar. 31)	Second (Apr. 1–June 30)	Third (July 1–Sept. 30)	Fourth (Oct. 1–Dec. 31)	Total for year
Liability for quarter					

Under penalties of perjury, I declare that I have examined this return, including accompanying schedules and statements, and to the best of my knowledge and belief, it is true, correct, and complete, and that no part of any payment made to a state unemployment fund claimed as a credit was, or is to be, deducted from the payments to employees.

Signature ▶	Title (Owner, etc.) ▶	Date ▶

FIGURE 24–14 *continued*

tax; it must not be deducted from employees' wages. For 1998 the FUTA tax was 6.2% of the first $7,000 in wages paid to each employee during the calendar year.

For deposit purposes, the FUTA tax is figured quarterly, and any amount due must be paid by the last day of the first month after the quarter ends. The formula for determining the amount due is set forth in the Federal Employer's Tax Guide.

An annual FUTA return must be filed on Form 940 on or before January 31 following the close of the calendar year for which the tax is due. Any tax still due is payable with the return. Form 940 may be filed on or before February 10 following the close of the year, if all required deposits were made on time and if full payment of the tax due is deposited on or before January 31 (Fig. 24–14).

Memory Jogger

11 *Who is responsible for the payment of FUTA tax?*

STATE UNEMPLOYMENT TAXES

All of the states and the District of Columbia have unemployment compensation laws. In most states, the tax is imposed only on the employer, but a few states require employers to withhold a percentage of wages for unemployment compensation benefits.

An employer may be subject to federal unemployment tax and not subject to state unemployment tax. In some states, for instance, the employer with fewer than four employees is not subject to the state unemployment tax. The regulations for a specific state should be checked.

STATE DISABILITY INSURANCE

Some states require that employees be covered by disability or sick-pay insurance. The employer may be required to withhold a certain amount from the employee's salary to pay for this insurance.

Special Duties

Before closing the chapter, we should mention certain events that do not occur with regularity but that may confront the office manager at some time.

MOVING A PRACTICE

The thought of moving into a shiny new spacious office can be exciting. However, unless the move is planned in advance, moving day and the weeks that follow can be a nightmare.

Planning the New Quarters

Do some careful measuring to see how the furniture and equipment you plan to move will fit into the new quarters. If possible, draw the rooms to scale and show where each item is to be placed by the mover. Include the location of available electrical outlets in your floor plan. If new furniture, carpets, or equipment is needed, try to have them in place before moving day. Don't expect to have the new carpet installed the day of your move.

Establishing a Moving Date

Decide what day you will move and whether you will close the office for 1 day or several. Select a mover and confirm the date. Patients must be notified of the move. As soon as the moving date is established, post a notice in the office and draw the patients' attention to it. You may want to send announcement cards to the active patients. Many physicians place a notice in the local newspapers.

Notifying Utilities and Mailers

At least 60 days in advance of the move, start a change-of-address notification campaign. Notify publishers of journals and suppliers of catalogs. (Cards for changes of address are available from the post office.) Six weeks' notice is generally required on all subscriptions, and postage due on forwarded journals can be very expensive. Notify the telephone company and utility companies well in advance so that there will no break in service. File a change of address card with the local post office. Order stationery and business cards with the new address.

Packing

The moving company will supply packing cartons for you to use. Have each employee be responsible for packing and labeling the items from his or her own work area. Tag each carton with a number and keep a master list of what is in each numbered carton. This will help you find items that you need. Also, if a carton should be lost or mislaid, you will have a record of what was in it. If time allows, just before moving is a good time to cull material from the files and discard old journals, supply catalogs, and any obsolete supplies or equipment.

Moving Day Strategy

Prepare a written outline of the moving day strategy, indicating each person's responsibility, and give each member of the office staff a copy. It may be wise to work in shifts to avoid confusion, but have one person stationed at the new address to direct the movers when they arrive.

Follow-Up

After the move, be sure to mention the new address when patients call for appointments. This is often neglected, especially after a few months have passed, and is very upsetting to the patient who tries to check in at the former address.

CLOSING A PRACTICE

A medical practice may be closed because of retirement, death, a change in geographic location, or a change in profession. If the closing is unexpected, as in the case of sudden death of the physician, much of the burden falls on the staff. If the closing is voluntary and planned for, the physician may wish to consult an attorney or the local medical society for guidelines. The following information is useful in either event.

Advance Notice to Patients

The physician who anticipates retirement can begin cutting back the practice months in advance. Patients can be notified as they come in that the practice will be closing on a specified date and asked to begin arrangements for care from another physician. The physician can also ask that patients pay at the time of service, to minimize accounts receivable at the time of retirement.

Avoiding Abandonment Charge

To avoid a charge of abandonment, the physician should notify active patients by letter that the practice is being discontinued. The letter should be sent out at least 3 months in advance, if possible. If a patient has been discharged or has not been given care by the physician for at least 6 years, there is no obligation to send the notice.

Public Announcement

About 1 month after the physician begins telling patients of the closing, an announcement should be placed in a local newspaper, giving the closing date of the office, explaining any arrangements made for continuing care and thanking patients for their support in prior years.

Other Notices

Hospital affiliations should be informed early, particularly if the physician will be leaving the community. If the office space is being rented, be sure to notify the landlord in observance of the rental contract if there is one. Insurance carriers must be advised of the change. The state medical licensure board should be contacted. If the practice is incorporated, an attorney should be consulted about disincorporation.

Patient Transfer and Patient Records

If another physician is taking over the practice, tell the patient about the new physician. However, be sure to explain that the patient's records will be transferred to any physician the patient chooses and that the request for transfer of records must be in writing. For convenience, the physician can have a form available that needs only the patient's signature.

Although the records belong to the physician, they can legally be transferred to another physician only with the consent of the patient. Any records not transferred should be stored, either in bulk or on microfilm or disk, until the statutes of limitations for malpractice and abandonment have run out.

Memory Jogger

12 *What action is required before transferring a patient's records to another physician?*

Financial Concerns

Income tax returns and supporting documents should be kept for at least 3 years after the tax return was filed. Appoint someone to take care of any remaining outstanding accounts receivable.

Disposition of Controlled Substances

Check with the Drug Enforcement Administration (DEA) for current regulations on disposal of controlled substances and the physician's certificate of registration. Do not simply toss them out. The certificate will have to be sent to the DEA for cancellation, and then it will be returned. It may be necessary to produce an inventory of all controlled substances on hand when the practice is terminated, along with duplicate copies of the official order forms that were used to obtain them. Return any unused forms to the DEA. Do not use leftover prescription blanks for note pads. Burn or shred them to avoid misuse.

Professional Liability Insurance

The physician who is discontinuing active medical practice can safely drop the professional liability insurance. However, do not destroy any of the previous policies. Most professional liability claims are covered by the policy that was in effect at the time the alleged act of negligence took place. The suit may be filed many years later, and it is important that the old policy be available.

Furnishings and Equipment

Unfortunately, used office furniture and equipment do not bring much in the marketplace. If another physician is taking over the practice, the value of the furnishings and equipment can be negotiated. Many physicians donate their libraries to the local hospital and declare the gift as a deduction from their income tax. This is an item to check with the accountant.

A physician may reward loyal employees with severance pay. On average, this equals at least 1 month's salary plus prorated compensation for any unused vacation time. A letter of reference is usually offered.

There are many details to take care of in closing a medical practice. Contact the local medical society for further guidance.

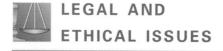 **LEGAL AND ETHICAL ISSUES**

The areas of authority and responsibility must be clearly defined to avoid management problems. Authority and responsibility are defined in the policy and procedures manual. This information must be available to every employee and updated on a regular basis.

The person in charge of hiring must be familiar with the Civil Rights Act of 1964, as amended by the Equal Opportunity Act of 1972 (available from EEOC, 2401 E Street, N.W., Washington, DC 20507).

A long-term employee whose performance declines should be counseled and given a chance to improve to attain specific practice goals.

CRITICAL THINKING

1 Practice your interviewing skills with another student, exchanging roles of interviewer and applicant.

2 Prepare a procedure sheet for a position that you would expect to seek.

3 Discuss with a colleague the ways in which a medical assistant could affect the success of the practice.

HOW DID I DO? Answers to Memory Joggers

1 The purpose of medical office management is to provide appropriate environment, safely store health information, and bill and collect for services.

2 The policy manual tells "what to do"; the procedures manual describes "how to do it."

3 Job descriptions and procedure sheets

4 Race, sex, religion, national origin

5 A warning and a full explanation of specific improvement expected

6 There should be an agenda for the staff meeting to prevent it from becoming a forum for individual complaints, which should be handled privately

7 The most important rule of marketing a medical practice is to "treat the patients well."

8 The patient information folder explains the philosophy and policies of practice and reduces misunderstanding and forgotten instructions.

9 At least 4 years

10 Total earnings, number of withholding allowances claimed, marital status, and length of pay period

11 Only the employer is responsible—not deducted from wages

12 Consent of the patient

REFERENCES

American Medical Association: Personnel Management in the Medical Practice. Norcross, GA, Coker Publishing, 1996.

U.S. Department of the Treasury, Internal Revenue Service: Circular E, 1998.

Notes

Assisting with Office Emergency Procedures

MaryAnn Woods, PhD, RN, CMA

25

LEARNING OBJECTIVES

Cognitive: On successful completion of this chapter you should be able to:

1 Describe the medical assistant's responsibilities in an emergency.
2 Recall two resources that can help to make your medical office accident proof.
3 List the basic items that must be included on an emergency cart.
4 Explain the purpose of a defibrillator in an emergency.
5 Recognize a choking victim.
6 Recall the conditions that necessitate the implementation of CPR.
7 List the major symptoms associated with heart attack.
8 Describe the emergency medical care that is usually given to victims of asthma, anaphylactic shock, convulsions, and hemorrhagic shock.
9 State the functions of a poison control center.
10 Define and spell vocabulary terms.

Performance: On successful completion of this chapter you should be able to:

1 Demonstrate triage techniques in a simulated emergency situation.
2 Accurately perform CPR using a simulated mannequin.

VOCABULARY

anaphylaxis Allergic condition caused by an antigen-antibody reaction; may cause shock, bronchoconstriction, airway obstruction, and loss of consciousness

apical pulse Pulse heard over the base (apex) of the heart

convulsion A series of involuntary contractions of the voluntary muscles

cyanosis Blue color of the mucous membranes and body extremities caused by lack of oxygen

diaphragmatic Pertaining to the primary muscle of respiration; separates the thoracic and the abdominal cavities

ecchymosis A hemorrhagic skin discoloration commonly called bruising

epistaxis Nosebleed

insulin shock Shock brought about by too much insulin, too little food, or excessive exercise; when untreated, it can result in death

mediastinum Space in the center of the chest under the sternum

paroxysm The sudden onset of symptoms, such as a spasm or seizure

sublingually Pertaining to under the tongue

syncope Loss of consciousness; fainting

syrup of ipecac A syrup given to induce vomiting

traumatic Pertaining to, resulting from, or causing physical injury or shock

triage To sort or to choose; to determine the priority of need for treatment

venom Poison transmitted through the bite or sting of spiders, snakes, and some insects

---

First aid is defined as the immediate care given to a person who has been injured or has suddenly taken ill. It includes well-chosen words of encouragement, a willingness to help, a promotion of confidence by the demonstration of competence, and the performance of temporary physical care to alleviate pain or a life-threatening situation. Knowledge of first aid and skill can often mean the difference between life and death, temporary and permanent disability, and rapid recovery and long-term hospitalization.

Frequently, the medical assistant may be responsible for initiating first aid in the office and continuing to administer first aid until the physician or trained medical teams arrive. Every medical assistant should successfully complete a course in cardiopulmonary resuscitation (CPR) and continue to hold a current CPR card as long as employed. Basic knowledge of CPR and life-support skills need to be updated on a regular basis because of recommended changes for procedures as new techniques are developed. Medical assistants should encourage their local medical assisting chapters to offer workshops conducted by physicians and emergency personnel from the community.

There are many acceptable approaches to emergency care. All offices need to establish written policies concerning the handling of medical emergencies. The medical assistant should consult with the physician-employer for his or her preferences in handling emergencies in that particular practice.

SKILLS AND RESPONSIBILITIES

MEDICAL ASSISTANT'S ROLE IN PERFORMING EMERGENCY PROCEDURES

1 Perform only the emergency procedures in which you are trained.
2 If an emergency occurs in the office, notify the physician.
3 If a physician cannot be located, then contact the local emergency medical services team.

Medical assistants do not assume the responsibility of diagnosing but are expected to make decisions based on their medical knowledge. A major goal in emergency care of the injured is to cause no further harm.

In a true emergency, the Good Samaritan law permits anyone to do whatever is reasonably necessary, provided that the care given is within the scope of competence of the person administering first aid. The law holds persons giving emergency care to be responsible for any injury that they cause as a result of their negligence or failure to exercise reasonable care. You, the medical assistant, are limited to the standards of your state laws, and your physician-employer is legally responsible for your mistakes.

Memory Jogger

1 *What is the primary responsibility of the medical assistant in an emergency?*

Making the Office Accident Proof

Usually, it is the medical assistant's responsibility to make the office as accident proof as possible. Do not use scatter rugs or delicate chairs, and be sure that floors are not slippery (Fig. 25–1). Keep cupboard doors and drawers closed. Wipe up spills immediately, and pick up dropped objects. All medications should be kept out of sight; dangerous drugs should be kept in locked cupboards. If there are children in the office, keep all sharp objects out of reach. Never leave a seriously ill patient or a restless, depressed, or unconscious patient unattended.

Planning Ahead

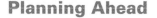

The office staff should discuss possible emergencies that may occur and have an emergency action plan to be used for rapid, systematic intervention. For instance, local industries may present unique problems that call for very specialized care. Plan for these, and ask the physician's advice on what procedures to follow. If there are several employees, each should be assigned specific duties. Organization and planning make the difference between systematic care for the patient and complete chaos.

Some offices have set up a team management system. This system designates one person to take immediate charge of the patient while another obtains needed materials and calls for assistance.

Memory Jogger

2 *What is the advantage of the team management system?*

USING COMMUNITY EMERGENCY SERVICES

Many communities have established an emergency medical services (EMS) system. This system includes an efficient communications network, such as the emergency telephone number 911, well-trained rescue personnel, properly equipped vehicles (Fig. 25–2), an emergency facility that is open 24 hours a day to provide advanced life support, and hospital intensive care for the victims.

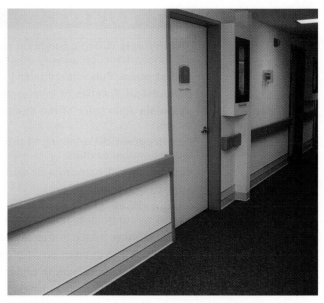

FIGURE 25–1 Keeping office accident proof with doors closed and hallway free of all equipment and unnecessary containers.

There are more than 300 poison control centers in the United States ready to provide emergency information for treating victims of poisonings. Many of the centers have toll-free lines. Some have systems for communicating with deaf persons.

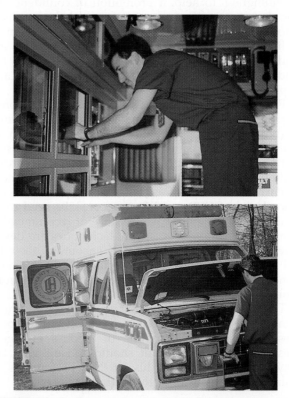

FIGURE 25–2 Emergency medical technicians inspecting ambulance before first run. (From Henry MC, Stapleton ER: EMT Prehospital Care, 2nd ed. Philadelphia, WB Saunders, 1997.)

Every office is required to post a list of local emergency numbers. This list should be in plain sight and should be known to all office personnel. Include on the list the local EMS system, poison control center, ambulance and rescue squad, fire department, and police department numbers.

Memory Jogger

3 *Name the local emergency agencies whose numbers should be posted in the medical office.*

Supplies and Equipment for Emergencies

EMERGENCY SUPPLIES

The emergency supplies consist of a properly equipped cart of first-aid items needed for a variety of emergencies (Fig. 25–3). The contents of the cart will vary to some degree, according to the type of emergencies each office encounters. This cart should be kept in an easily accessible place known to all personnel in the office. A firm rule must be made that no one borrows items from the cart. Medication expiration dates must be checked on a routine basis and the cart replenished with fresh supplies after every use.

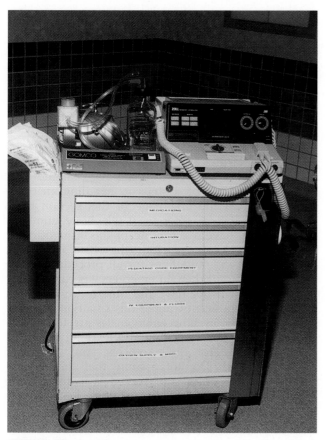

FIGURE 25–3 Office emergency cart with defibrillator. Drawers are marked for easy retrieval of emergency supplies.

BASIC EMERGENCY CART ITEMS

SUPPLIES

Adhesive tape in 1-inch and 2-inch widths
Alcohol (70%) and alcohol wipes
Antimicrobial skin ointment
Cotton balls and cotton swabs
Elastic bandages in 2-inch and 3-inch widths
Gauze pads, 2 × 2- and 4 × 4-inch widths
Gloves, sterile and nonsterile
Hot and cold packs (instant type)
Muslin sling or cravat bandage to be used as a tourniquet
Orange juice
Suction catheters
Sterile dressings (miscellaneous sizes, including two abdominal pads)
Syringes, hypodermic needles, and intravenous equipment in assorted sizes and gauges

MEDICATIONS

Activated charcoal, bottle of 30 to 50 g
Amobarbital (Amytal)
Antihistamine, injectable and oral
Apomorphine
Atropine
Dextrose
Diazepam (Valium)
Digoxin (Lanoxin)
Disposable syringe and needle units
Epinephrine (Adrenalin), injectable (dilution 1 : 000)
Furosemide (Lasix)
Glucagon
Isoproterenol (Isuprel) aerosol spray
Lidocaine (Xylocaine)
Metaraminol (Aramine)
Spirits of ammonia
Syrup of ipecac

EQUIPMENT

Airways in various sizes
Ambu-bag with assorted sizes of facial masks
Bandage scissors
Blood pressure cuff (pediatric, regular, and large adult sizes)
Bulb syringe
Stethoscope
Flashlight
Portable oxygen tank with regulator and mask
Nasogastric suction unit equipped with tubing
Defibrillator

Epinephrine is a vasoconstrictor used to check hemorrhage. It relaxes the bronchioles, is used to relieve asthmatic **paroxysm,** and is an emergency heart stimulant used to treat shock. Epinephrine should be in a ready-to-use cartridge syringe and needle unit. These are supplied in 1.0-mL cartridges.

Other drugs used are atropine, digoxin (Lanoxin), and lidocaine (Xylocaine). Atropine decreases secretions, increases respiration and heart rates, and is a smooth muscle relaxant. It dilates the pupil of the eye and is a general cerebral stimulant. Atropine relieves gastrointestinal cramps and hypermotility and may also be used to relieve pain locally. Digoxin is a cardiotonic. It is used to treat congestive heart failure and is good for emergency use because it has a relatively rapid action. Lidocaine is used intravenously to decrease heart arrhythmia and as both a local and a topical anesthetic.

Apomorphine is a prompt and effective emetic and is used in cases of poisoning when a stomach pump cannot be employed. **Syrup of ipecac** is also an emetic and one that many physicians recommend be kept on hand in the home for use in emergencies.

Antihistamines are used to counteract the effect of histamine and are used in the treatment of allergic reactions and **anaphylaxis.** Isoproterenol, an antispasmodic, is used in bronchial spasm and is also a cardiac stimulant. Some trade names for this product are Isuprel, Medihaler-Iso, and Norisodrine.

Other medications that may be found on a crash tray are metaraminol (Aramine) (50%, in a prefilled syringe), for severe shock; amobarbital sodium (Amytal) and diazepam (Valium), for convulsions and as sedatives; dextrose and insulin, to treat diabetic patients; and furosemide (Lasix), for congestive heart failure. Glucagon is primarily used to counteract severe hypoglycemic reactions in diabetic patients taking insulin.

Small cans of orange juice, with pull-tab openers, are handy for quick sugar administration in cases of diabetic patients experiencing **insulin shock.**

Most physicians and others involved in emergency care do not recommend a tourniquet because of the danger that may result from incorrect usage. A tourniquet that completely stops blood flow to the point of no measurable pulse is potentially hazardous and should be used very cautiously. It is much better to apply pressure directly over the bleeding area. Today, rather than a tourniquet, a constricting band is employed for the purpose of decreasing lymphatic and superficial venous blood flow for bites by insects and snakes. In these cases, the constricting band is applied just above the bite area.

As more patients come to clinics and physicians' offices to seek emergency care, the medical assistant will need to become even more familiar with specialized equipment on the emergency cart to help save lives. Figure 25–3 shows the outside and the inside of a typical emergency cart. The cart contains numerous locking drawers in which supplies and medicines are kept.

Memory Jogger

4 *When would you use the cans of orange juice on the emergency cart?*

DEFIBRILLATORS

The medical assistant who works in a large clinic, in a cardiology office, or in an urgent-care center may be required to assist the team with defibrillation of emergency patients. Defibrillators are instruments that send a massive jolt of electricity into the heart muscle by means of plates or paddles applied to the chest to reestablish the proper rhythm of the heartbeat. One paddle is placed to the right of the upper sternum, and the other is placed just to the left of the nipple, at the apex of the heart.

The office defibrillator is portable and is powered by standard 110-V current or batteries (see Fig. 25–3). The monitor has a nonfading display, and it is possible to freeze the monitor for prolonged viewing. If a permanent record of the victim's heart rate is desired, the machine can make a printed copy.

Memory Jogger

5 *What is the purpose of the defibrillator?*

General Rules for Emergencies

When first starting a new job, you should be shown a book of office protocols. In this book should be a section on the accepted steps in handling an office emergency. On the first page of this section there should be a list of emergency telephone numbers. Many offices have a duplicate of this list posted at the telephone locations within the office. This book is considered the guidelines for all procedures done within the office. When an emergency occurs, it may be that you will not have the time to go and look up how the physician wanted this situation handled. You need to know how emergencies are to be handled and this means reading and learning what this book contains and the protocols your employer wants followed. Do not assume that the method used in the last office you worked in is going to be exactly the same in this office. Assuming can cause situations that may be embarrassing or may even cause you to lose your job. *Be certain, read the book!*

When faced with an emergency there are some general rules that are universal.

SKILLS AND RESPONSIBILITIES

MEASURES TO TAKE IN EMERGENCY SITUATIONS

- Most importantly, stay calm. Reassure the patient and make him or her as comfortable as possible.
- Survey the situation to determine the nature of the emergency. Decide whether the need is immediate. This decision requires calm judgment and may call for some medical knowledge.
- Examine the scene. Quickly evaluate potential hazards, possible injuries, and any clues that you can determine from the overall appearance of the situation.
- Take immediate steps to remedy the situation. Calmly but firmly give specific instructions to the patient and to other office personnel. Never say, "Will someone call the doctor?" Say, "YOU call the doctor, YOU get a blanket, and YOU get the emergency cart."
- After the emergency is under control, make certain that all the events and the medications used are recorded accurately. Be precise when recording. Have statements of what happened and what events preceded the emergency.
- *Always follow Standard Precautions.* When an emergency occurs, it is impossible to determine the level of infection that you are encountering. A good rule to follow is if it is wet and it isn't yours, don't touch it without protecting yourself. All body fluids must be considered infectious, and the appropriate precautions must be employed.

Memory Jogger

6 *The first and most important rule in emergency situations is _____.*

Emergency Management

An emergency can occur at any time to anyone. The office emergency could involve a patient, a coworker, or the physician. In addition to emergencies that can occur within the office, others might occur outside the office. A person may fall, get hit by a car, or have a heart attack or stroke. Whatever the emergency, documentation becomes an important function in emergency care management.

BASIC INFORMATION THAT NEEDS TO BE COLLECTED

1 Patient's name, address, age, and health insurance information
2 Name and whereabouts of any person with the patient
3 Patient's vital signs and chief complaint
4 Sequence of events, beginning with how trauma occurred, any changes in the patient's overall condition, and any observations you have made regarding the patient's condition
5 Any procedures or techniques performed on the patient
6 If possible, any allergies, medications, or known health conditions

Stay with the patient until you have been relieved of your responsibility by the EMS provider or the physician. Never leave an injured patient alone.

The two primary functions of first aid remain constant. Never do anything that will worsen the situation, and provide the best care you can to correct any life-threatening situation.

Memory Jogger

7 *Name the two primary functions of first aid.*

Common Emergencies

FAINTING (SYNCOPE)

One of the most common emergency problems to confront the medical assistant is fainting. **Syncope** is usually caused by lack of oxygen in the blood, with a consequent lack of oxygen to the brain. Before fainting, a person may appear pale; may feel cold, weak, dizzy, or nauseated; and may have numbness of the extremities. Immediately lay the patient flat, with the head lower than the heart. Loosen all tight clothing, and maintain an open airway. Apply a cold washcloth to the forehead. If allowed, pass aromatic spirits of ammonia back and forth under the patient's nostrils, but be careful not to hold the ammonia too close to the nose. Obtain the patient's pulse, respiration rate, and blood pressure, and then report the findings to the physician. Keep the patient in a supine position for at least 10 minutes after consciousness has been regained.

If recovery is not prompt, summon the physician or emergency medical rescue team for transportation to the hospital. Syncope might be a brief episode in the development of a serious underlying illness.

EMERGENCY RESUSCITATION

Breathing may suddenly cease for a variety of reasons, including shock, disease, and trauma. The most obvious sign that breathing has stopped is when the chest is no longer moving. Artificial ventilation must be started immediately, because death may follow within 4 to 6 minutes.

Before beginning assessment of the patient, *put on gloves.* Check the patient responsiveness to determine the level of consciousness. Then check for breath sounds and heartbeat. Now check the airway. When it has been established that CPR must be started as a lifesaving measure, tell someone to call for emergency assistance and then begin the resuscitation procedure.

Establishing the Airway

The airway must be opened by positioning the patient on the back and relieving possible obstruction of the air passage by the tongue. Extreme caution must be used if there is any chance that the patient has suffered a cervical neck injury, as should be assumed in any accident. If neck injury is not suspected, the head is tilted by downward pressure on the forehead and upward pressure under the chin. If neck injury may be present, grasp the angle of the victim's lower jaw without extending the neck.

Resuscitation

Mouth-to-mouth resuscitation is begun if breathing does not follow opening of the airway. Position yourself on the side of the patient's head. One hand should continue pressing on the forehead and should also be turned so that the fingers can hold the nose shut. The other hand should continue lifting the chin upward. Place a CPR mouth barrier (Fig. 25–4) over the patient's face. Place your mouth over the tube in the barrier and give the victim two full breaths. Check for the carotid pulse. If the pulse is present, continue ventilating the lungs every 5 seconds. If the pulse is absent, you must provide artificial circulation in addition to artificial ventilation (see next section).

There are mouth-to-nose and mouth-to-stoma methods for resuscitation of victims with tracheotomies. The reader is referred to the American Red Cross *Standard First Aid Manual* or *American Heart CPR Manual* for specific procedures and precautions. Artificial airways may be inserted by trained personnel to establish or maintain breathing. Airways

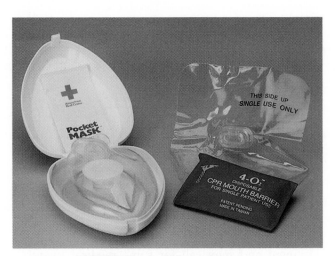

FIGURE 25–4 CPR mouth barriers.

of various types and sizes should be kept ready on the emergency cart (Fig. 25–5).

Memory Jogger

8 *How often must you ventilate the lungs?*

Cardiopulmonary Resuscitation

Cessation of breathing may be accompanied by a cessation of the heartbeat (cardiac arrest), which is identified by the lack of a pulse. Artificial ventilation must then be accompanied by external (closed) cardiac massage. This is called cardiopulmonary resuscitation, which is the combination of artificial circulation and artificial breathing (see Procedure 25–1).

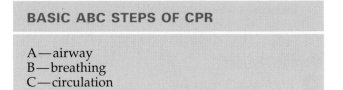

BASIC ABC STEPS OF CPR

A—airway
B—breathing
C—circulation

When both breathing and pulse stop, the victim has suffered sudden death. There are many causes of sudden death, including choking, drowning, poisoning, suffocation, electrocution, and smoke inhalation. CPR must be started immediately in an attempt to prevent death or permanent damage to body organs, especially the brain.

Because CPR may cause injuries to the ribs, heart, liver, lungs, and blood vessels, it should be performed only by individuals properly trained in the techniques and only if cardiac arrest has occurred. In CPR, the heart is compressed by downward pressure on the sternum, which should cause the blood to circulate. The proper position is for the heel of the one hand to be placed on the sternum, two fingerwidths above the lower notch where the ribs join.

The other hand is placed on top, and the rescuer presses straight down. The sternum will be depressed 1½ to 2 inches with sufficient pressure.

Compressions should be given at a rate of 80 to 100 compressions per minute (15 compressions should take 9 to 11 seconds). Compress down and up smoothly, keeping hand contact with the victim's chest at all times. After every 15 compressions, move back to the mouth, open the airway with the head-tilt/chin-lift, and breathe two full breaths into the victim. After four cycles have been completed, locate and check the carotid pulse, feeling for 5 seconds. Continue CPR until a qualified person can relieve you or until advanced life support is available.

CPR for infants and small children is similar to that for adults, but a few important differences must be remembered. When handling an infant be careful that you do not overextend the head when tilting it back (Fig. 25–5A). The infant's neck is so pliable that forceful backward tilting might block breathing passages instead of opening them. With an infant who is not breathing, be certain to cover both the mouth and the nose with your mouth and deliver two slow puffs that are just strong enough to make the chest rise. With a small child, pinch the nose, cover the mouth, and breathe as for an infant. In an infant, check the brachial pulse (see Fig. 25–5B) between the elbow and the shoulder. Use only the fingertips at the center of the sternum for compressions on the infant (see Fig. 25–5C). Compress the sternum between ½ and 1 inch, at a rate of at least 100 times per minute. Only the heel of one hand is used for compressions on a small child. Depress the sternum 1 to 1½ inches, at a rate of 80 to 100 times per minute. CPR for children older than 8 years of age is the same as that for adults.

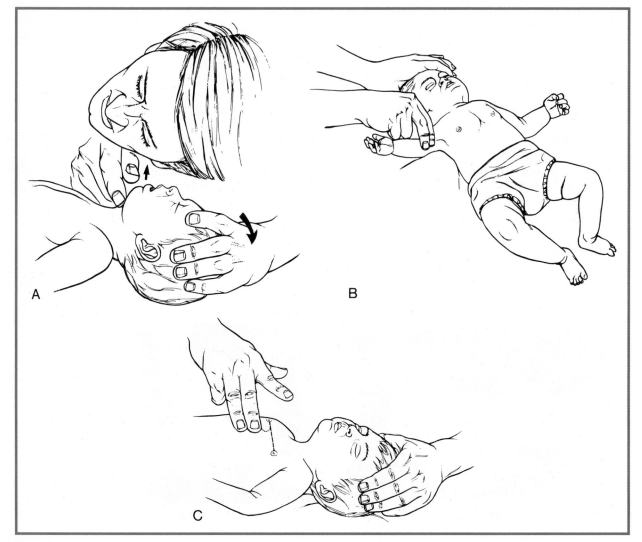

FIGURE 25–5 Modifications necessary for CPR on child. *A,* Chin lift in an infant. *B,* Placement of two fingers over medial aspect of upper arm halfway between elbow and axilla to locate pulse. *C,* To locate correct position for compression in an infant, place your index, middle, and ring fingers of the hand closest to infant's feet adjacent to nipple line and then lift index finger. (From Henry MC, Stapleton ER: EMT Prehospital Care, 2nd ed. Philadelphia, WB Saunders, 1997.)

PROCEDURE 25-1

Performing Cardiopulmonary Resuscitation

GOAL
To restore a victim's breathing and blood circulation when respiration and pulse stop.

EQUIPMENT AND SUPPLIES

Nonsterile gloves (sterile gloves may be preferred)
CPR mouth barrier

American Heart Association–approved mannequin equipped with a printout for demonstration of the proper technique for your instructor.

PROCEDURAL STEPS
(To be performed on an approved mannequin only.)

1 Begin a primary survey. Tap the victim and ask, Are you OK? Wait for victim to respond.
   PURPOSE: To determine whether the victim is conscious.

2 Shout for help. Put on gloves. Activate the EMS system.
   PURPOSE: To alert other rescue personnel to the problem.

3 Tilt the victim's head and lift the chin. Look, listen, and feel for signs of breathing. Place your ear over the mouth and listen for breathing. Watch the rising and falling of the chest for evidence of breathing (Figure 1).
   PURPOSE: To determine whether the victim is breathing and to open the airway.

4 Place the CPR mouth barrier over the victim's mouth and begin rescue breathing by pinching the nose tightly with your thumb and forefinger if none of the signs of breathing are present (Figure 2).
   PURPOSE: An airtight seal must be present so that air cannot escape through the nose when you perform mouth-to-mouth resuscitation.

5 Maintain an airtight seal with your mouth on the tube in the barrier that leads to the victim's mouth.

6 Give two full breaths.
   PURPOSE: May be sufficient stimulus to initiate breathing by the victim.

7 Check the carotid pulse. If a pulse is felt, continue resuscitation (Figure 3).
   PURPOSE: The pulse is easier to feel in this area.

Continued

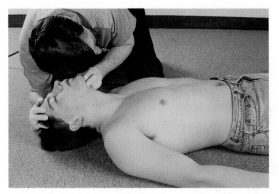

FIGURE 1

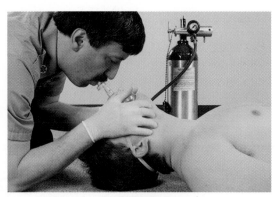

FIGURE 2

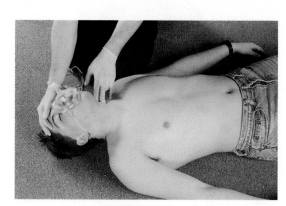

FIGURE 3

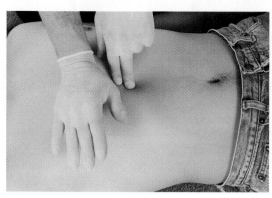

FIGURE 4

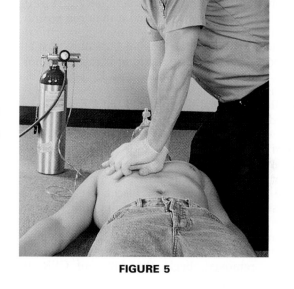

FIGURE 5

8 Continue mouth-to-mouth resuscitation at the rate of approximately one full breath every 5 seconds *if the pulse is present.*

9 Initiate CPR *if there is no pulse.*

10 Kneel at the victim's side opposite the chest. Move your fingers up the ribs to the point where the sternum and the ribs join. Your middle fingers should fit into the area and your index finger should be next to it across the sternum.

11 Place the heel of your hand on the chest midline over the sternum, just above your index finger (Figure 4).

12 Place your other hand on top of your first hand and lift your fingers upward off of the chest (Figure 5).
   PURPOSE: This position gives you the most control, allowing you to avoid injuring the victim's ribs as you compress the chest.

13 Bring your shoulders directly over the victim's sternum as you compress downward, and keep you arms straight.

14 Depress the sternum 1½ to 2 inches for an adult victim. Relax the pressure on the sternum after each compression but *do not remove your hands* from the victim's sternum.
   PURPOSE: The depth of compression is needed to circulate blood through the heart. Movement of the hands may cause injury to the victim.

15 After performing 15 compressions, open the airway and give two full, slow, breaths.

16 Complete three more cycles of compressions and breaths, ending with 2 breaths. Check for pulse and breathing for 5 seconds. If there is no pulse or breath, resume CPR at the rate of 15 compressions to two breaths. Always start and end each cycle with two full breaths. Continue giving CPR until the EMS relieves you.

CHOKING

Choking is caused by a foreign object, usually food, lodged in the upper airway. Often, exhalation can take place, but inhalation is blocked. Thus, the lungs quickly empty. The choking victim who has food or a foreign object lodged in the throat cannot speak, breathe, or cough. The victim may clutch the neck between the thumb and index finger (Fig. 25–6). This universal distress signal should be viewed as a sign that the victim needs help.

The face pales and turns blue. Eventually, there is loss of consciousness and cardiopulmonary arrest. If the object is not removed, the victim may die within 4 to 6 minutes.

If the victim has good air exchange or only partial obstruction and can speak, cough, or breathe, do not interfere. If the victim cannot speak, cough, or breathe, use the Heimlich maneuver. Give sub**diaphragmatic** abdominal thrusts until the foreign body is expelled or the victim becomes unconscious (Fig. 25–7). If the victim becomes unconscious, position the victim on his or her back and call out for help. Lift the jaw and sweep your finger in the victim's mouth in an attempt to remove the foreign body. Open the airway, and attempt rescue breathing. If you are still unsuccessful in removing the foreign body, use the Heimlich maneuver and give five subdiaphragmatic abdominal thrusts (Fig. 25–8). Repeat the sequence until you are successful. After the obstruction is removed, begin the ABCs of CPR, if necessary.

It is possible to perform the abdominal thrust maneuver on yourself if you are choking and there is no one nearby to help you. Press your fist into your upper abdomen with quick upward thrusts or lean forward and press the abdomen quickly against a firm object such as the back of a chair (Fig. 25–9).

To dislodge a foreign object from an infant, place the victim face down, over your forearm and across your thigh. The head should be lower than the trunk. Next, support the head and neck of the victim with one hand. Using the heel of the other hand, deliver four blows to the back, between the infant's shoulder blades (Fig. 25–10). Place the infant on his or her back, with the head lower than the trunk. Using two or three fingers, deliver four thrusts in the sternum area (Fig. 25–11). Repeat the sequence until the foreign body is expelled or the infant becomes unconscious.

If the infant becomes unconscious, position the infant on his or her back and call out for help. Sweep your finger through the mouth in an attempt to remove the foreign body (Fig. 25–12). Open the airway, and attempt rescue breathing. If you are still unsuccessful in removing the foreign body, perform the sequence of back blows and chest thrusts until you are successful. After the obstruction is removed, begin the ABCs of CPR, if necessary.

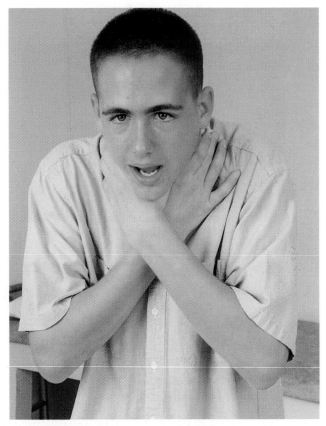

FIGURE 25–6 Universal choking distress signal.

Memory Jogger

9 *Demonstrate the universal distress signal for choking.*

CHEST PAIN

Chest pain can be associated with both heart and lung disease, as well as a few other conditions. It can be quite serious; all patients with chest pain are treated as cardiac emergencies until a physician has ruled out this diagnosis. The patient is often sweating and may have a gray, ashen appearance. The lips and fingernails may be blue (a sign of **cyanosis**) (Fig. 25–13). Frequently, the patient is clutching the chest in pain. This pain may radiate from the **mediastinum** down the left arm and up the left side of the neck. The pulse may be rapid and weak. Frequently, there is nausea.

Do not have the patient walk any distance. A wheelchair or a chair with rollers is an excellent method of moving this patient to a quiet room. The patient will probably prefer to have his or her head slightly elevated or even to be in a semi-sitting position. Keep the patient quiet and warm. Loosen all

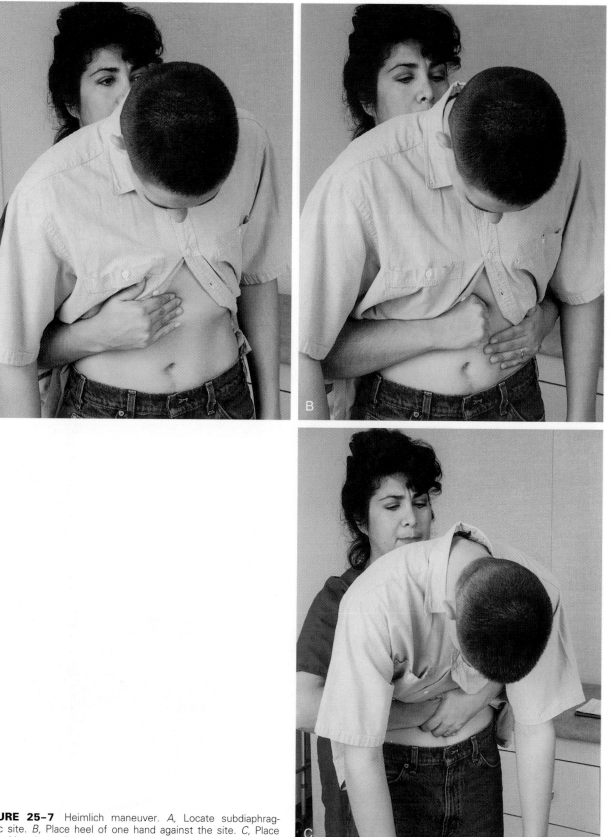

FIGURE 25–7 Heimlich maneuver. *A,* Locate subdiaphragmatic site. *B,* Place heel of one hand against the site. *C,* Place second hand over first hand and give abdominal thrusts.

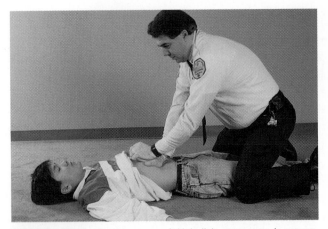

FIGURE 25–8 Performance of Heimlich maneuver in unconscious victim. (From Henry MC, Stapleton ER: EMT Prehospital Care, 2nd ed. Philadelphia, WB Saunders, 1997.)

tight clothing. Record **apical pulse** and radial pulse. Remember, you must use a stethoscope when obtaining an apical pulse. Administer oxygen if the physician has previously given these instructions. *Absolutely no smoking should be allowed by the patient*

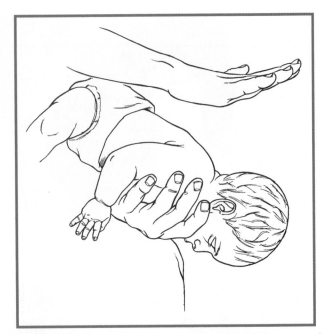

FIGURE 25–10 Back blows administered to infant supported on your arm and thigh. (From Henry MC, Stapleton ER: EMT Prehospital Care, 2nd ed. Philadelphia, WB Saunders, 1997.)

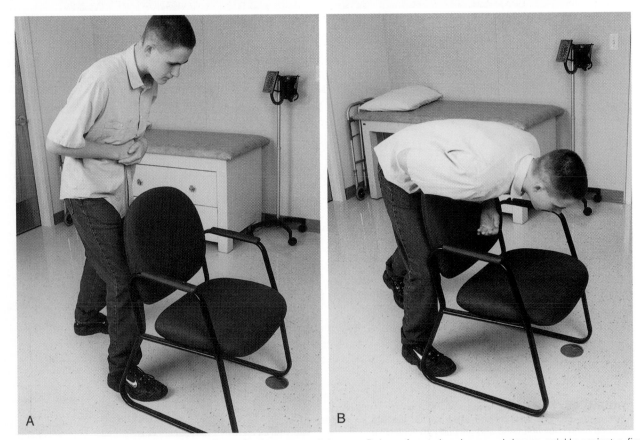

FIGURE 25–9 Self-induced Heimlich. *A,* Press fist into upper abdomen. *B,* Lean forward and press abdomen quickly against a firm object.

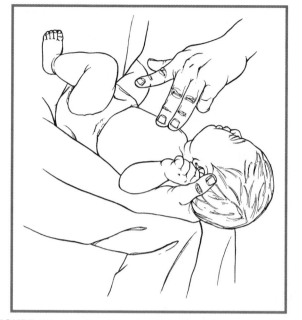

FIGURE 25-11 Chest thrusts administered in same position as cardiac compressions. (From Henry MC, Stapleton ER: EMT Prehospital Care, 2nd ed. Philadelphia, WB Saunders, 1997.)

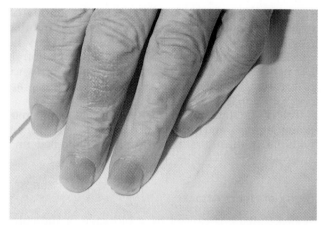

FIGURE 25-13 Cyanosis of nail beds. (From Henry MC, Stapleton ER: EMT Prehospital Care, 2nd ed. Philadelphia, WB Saunders, 1997.)

or by anyone within the vicinity. Bring the emergency cart into the room and open the medication drawer so that the physician is able to quickly prepare the medication(s) needed. This may be epinephrine (Adrenalin), atropine, digitalis, calcium chloride 10%, or morphine. If the patient is conscious, ask him or her about any medication that he or she may be carrying. If this is patient with an established heart disorder, the patient may be carrying nitroglycerin tablets. Nitroglycerin tablets are administered **sublingually,** and you may give them to the patient with the patient's consent (Fig. 25-14). Do not give the patient alcohol, food, or water by mouth without the physician's permission. Do not give spirits of ammonia.

If the physician is in the office or is on the way, connect the patient to the electrocardiograph and

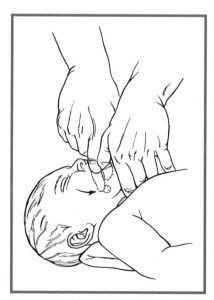

FIGURE 25-12 Finger sweep in infant should be done while maintaining jaw lift. (From Henry MC, Stapleton ER: EMT Prehospital Care, 2nd ed. Philadelphia, WB Saunders, 1997.)

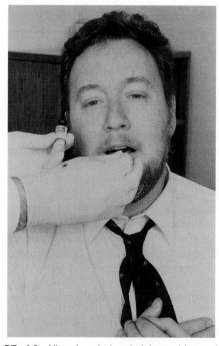

FIGURE 25-14 Nitroglycerin is administered beneath patient's tongue. (From Henry MC, Stapleton ER: EMT Prehospital Care, 2nd ed. Philadelphia, WB Saunders, 1997.)

record a few tracings. Lead II is usually considered to be the monitoring lead. If the physician cannot be reached, call the emergency rescue team. It may be necessary to start mouth-to-mouth resuscitation if the patient is unconscious and there is no evidence of breathing. If chest pain progresses to cardiac arrest, CPR must be performed.

The office staff must remain calm and offer emotional support and reassurance, because all patients with heart disorders are extremely frightened and anxious.

Signs of Heart Attack

A heart attack is caused by a blockage of the coronary arteries so that the blood supply to the heart muscles is stopped. The most common signal of heart attack is an uncomfortable pressure, squeezing, fullness, or pain in the center of the chest, in the mediastinal area. This may spread to the shoulder, neck, jaw, or arms. The pain may not be severe. Other symptoms include

- Sweating
- Nausea
- Indigestion
- Shortness of breath
- Cold and clammy skin
- A feeling of weakness
- Extreme apprehension

Memory Jogger

(10) *How are nitroglycerin tablets administered?*

CEREBROVASCULAR ACCIDENT (STROKE)

Cerebrovascular accident (CVA) is a disorder of the blood vessels serving the brain that results in an impairment of the blood supply to a part of the brain. The term *stroke* is often applied to this problem. This interruption in the normal circulation of blood through the brain leads to a sudden loss of consciousness and some degree of paralysis, which may be temporary or permanent depending on the severity of the oxygen deprivation of the brain cells.

Usually, minor strokes do not produce unconsciousness and the symptoms depend on the location of the hemorrhage and the amount of brain damage. Symptoms of a minor stroke include

- Headache
- Confusion
- Slight dizziness
- Ringing in the ears

This may be followed by minor difficulties in speech, memory changes, weakness of the extremities, and some disturbance of personality. Symptoms of a major stroke include

- Unconsciousness
- Paralysis on one side of the body
- Difficulty in breathing and swallowing
- Loss of bladder and bowel control
- Unequal pupil size
- Slurring of speech

Treatment

The patient should be protected against any further injury or physical exertion. Keep the patient lying down and covered lightly. Maintain an open airway. Position the head so that any secretions will drain from the side of the mouth to prevent choking. Do not give the patient anything to eat or drink. Vital signs should be taken at regular intervals and recorded for the physician. Have an ambulance take the patient to the hospital as soon as possible.

POISONINGS

All poisonings are considered medical emergencies. Poisoning can occur by mouth, absorption, inhalation, and injection. Over-the-counter medications such as acetaminophen, iron tablets, aspirin, or ibuprofen cause the majority of poisoning cases seen in young children. Other typical household poisons include medicines, detergents, cleaners, disinfectants, bleaches, insecticides, ammonia, glues, cosmetics, and poisonous plants (Fig. 25–15). Signs and symptoms of poisoning vary greatly and include

- Open bottles of medicines or chemicals
- Stains on clothing
- Burns on hands and mouth
- Changes in skin color
- Nausea
- Shallow breathing
- Convulsions
- Stomach cramps
- Heavy perspiration
- Dizziness
- Drowsiness
- Unconsciousness

When a person calls the office to report a poisoning, certain information needs to be obtained (see What to Ask When a Poisoning Is Reported).

WHAT TO ASK WHEN A POISONING IS REPORTED

1 The location and the phone number
2 The name of the poison taken
3 How much was taken
4 How long ago the poison was taken

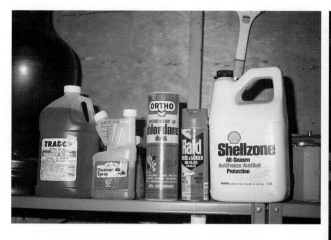
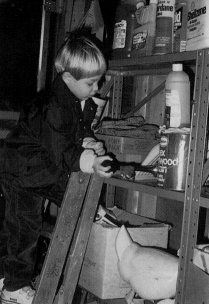

FIGURE 25–15 Hazardous household materials. (From Henry MC, Stapleton ER: EMT Prehospital Care, 2nd ed. Philadelphia, WB Saunders, 1997.)

5 Whether vomiting has occurred
6 The name, weight, and age of the victim
7 Any first aid being given

Instruct the caller *not* to hang up and *not* to leave the victim unattended. Call the local poison control center. Quickly forward all directions to the caller. Tell the caller to bring the container of poison or of vomitus to the office or hospital.

Treatment

Speed is essential in administering first aid in poisonings. In all cases, it is most important to dilute the poison, to induce vomiting (except when the person has swallowed a corrosive poison), and to seek medical attention. Generally, it is safe to try to dilute the poison with 1 or 2 cups of water or milk. It is important to dilute the poison before vomiting is induced. Do not induce vomiting if the victim is unconscious or having a **convulsion.** Do not attempt to induce vomiting when the victim has swallowed a strong corrosive or petroleum product. Give 1 tablespoon of syrup of ipecac with two cups of water to induce dilution of the poison and vomiting. If vomiting does not occur after 20 minutes, repeat the procedure. It may be necessary to make the victim gag to start vomiting. The gag reflex is started by touching the back of the tongue lightly. Encourage the victim to drink fluids until the emesis is reasonably clear. When vomiting has stopped, administer 30 to 50 g of activated charcoal, which absorbs any residual toxic substance and inhibits the absorption of poisons.

Memory Jogger

11 *How can poisoning occur?*

ANIMAL BITES

Any animal bite (including human) that breaks the skin should be seen by a physician and reported to the authorities. The animal must be identified and confined for quarantine. The animal should not be killed because a positive rabies identification is almost impossible to make if the animal has been dead for a period of time. Many pet owners will not admit that their pet has bitten a person because they fear that the animal will be killed. Assure them that the health department authorities only want to confine the animal for observation.

Treatment

The bite should be washed thoroughly with soap and water and should be treated as an infected wound would be treated. The victim should be seen by a physician.

INSECT BITES AND STINGS

This type of injury occurs when the insect either bites or stings the victim. **Venom** is injected into the tissue of the victim, which results in a internal body response to a foreign protein. Some of the more common types of bites and stings are those of mosquitoes, bees, wasps, hornets, spiders, fire ants, ticks, and fleas. Bites also can be caused by black widow spiders, brown recluse spiders, and scorpions.

Treatment

Remove the stinger, if there is one, by gently brushing it off or by using forceps or tweezers. Be careful not to squeeze the stinger. This injects more venom into the skin. Place the forceps as close to the skin as possible, not over the stinger sac, and gently remove the stinger. Apply ice in a towel or a plastic bag around the area, to relieve the pain and slow the absorption of the venom. Calamine lotion or a paste of baking soda may be applied to relieve itching. Keep the patient's activities to a minimum to slow down circulation and, thus, the spread of the venom.

If the patient has a history of allergies, especially to insect venom, he or she should be transported to the nearest hospital for immediate care. This patient may experience dyspnea and a decrease in blood pressure. A wet, itchy, swollen rash may occur. The victim may complain of shortness of breath or difficulty in breathing. Sometimes, there is edema of the lips and the face. Difficulty in talking is a sign of edema in the throat. In this situation, there is the possibility of complete airway obstruction. These are signs of a true emergency. Epinephrine and oxygen should be ready for immediate administration on the physician's orders. Antihistamines may be used, as well as cortisone, but the action of these agents is considerably slower than that of epinephrine. If the patient experiences acute anaphylactic shock, death may occur within 1 hour without the intervention of a physician.

SHOCK

Shock is a condition that produces a depressed state of many vital body functions. It is a physiologic reaction resulting from a **traumatic** condition to the body. Shock is often caused by an injury, accident, hemorrhage, illness, surgical operation, or overdose of drugs or by burns, pain, fear, or emotional stress. Shock may be immediate or delayed, mild or severe, and even fatal.

SIGNS OF SHOCK

- Paleness
- Clamminess
- Dilated pupils
- Weak and rapid pulse
- Low blood pressure
- Thirst
- Lethargy
- Feeling of faintness
- Labored breathing

Treatment

Ensure an open airway, and check for breathing and circulation. Place the patient on his or her back, with the legs elevated. Loosen all tight clothing. Cover the patient with a blanket for warmth. Do not move the patient unnecessarily. Fluids may be given by mouth if not contraindicated or if medical care will be delayed for more than 60 minutes. Because there are so many different causes of shock, it is advisable to administer only basic first-aid care and to have the patient transported to the hospital.

Memory Jogger

12 *What are the nine signs of shock?*

ASTHMATIC ATTACK

Asthma is a condition characterized by wheezing, coughing, choking, and shortness of breath resulting from spasmodic constriction of the bronchi in the lungs. Attacks vary greatly. Severe attacks rarely last for more than a few hours, but milder symptoms may persist much longer.

Some asthmatic patients carry respiratory inhalators with them. You may assist them with using their inhalators. A bronchodilator such as epinephrine or aminophylline may be ordered by the physician. Other medications are used to thin the mucus in the air passages so that the patient can clear the lungs more easily.

An asthmatic patient should be warned of the hazards of overstimulation of the body, such as exercise and emotional upsets causing laughing or crying. Explain the importance of relaxation to the patient with asthma.

SEIZURES

Seizures may be idiopathic or as a result of trauma, injury, or metabolic alterations such as hypoglycemia or hypocalcemia. A febrile seizure is transient and occurs with a rapid rise in fever over 101.8° F (38.8° C). Febrile seizures occur in children between 6 months and 5 years of age.

Seizures are frightening to witness, but usually the patient is not suffering, nor is there great danger. Establishing a tranquil environment is an essential component of caring for patients experiencing seizures.

Treatment

Loosen clothing but do not attempt to restrain the patient's movements, except to prevent injury. Remove anything that might be in the way that could cause harm. Always protect the head. Give neither fluids nor medication by mouth. If the patient remains unconscious after the jerking has subsided, position the patient in a semi-prone position to maintain an open airway and to allow drainage of excess saliva. Do not attempt to place anything between the teeth during the convulsion because forcing an object through a tightly clenched mouth may damage the teeth. After the seizure is over, let the patient rest or sleep in a quiet room. Follow the physician's directives and assist in every way that you can. If the physician is not in the office, check the protocol section in the office procedure manual. A general rule is to call 911 for emergency assistance if

- The patient has not regained consciousness within 10 to 15 minutes
- The seizure does not stop within a few minutes
- The patient begins a second seizure immediately after the primary one
- The patient is pregnant
- There are signs of head trauma
- The patient is a known diabetic
- This seizure is expected to be a febrile seizure

ABDOMINAL PAIN

Abdominal pain is any pain or discomfort in the abdomen.

CAUSES OF ABDOMINAL PAIN

- Stress
- Hemorrhage
- Ulcers
- Excessive eating, drinking, or smoking
- Inflammation
- Obstruction
- Tumors

All abdominal pain should be investigated. Severe and persistent abdominal pain, especially when accompanied by fever, should receive medical attention as soon as possible.

Treatment

Treatment varies with the cause of the pain. Keep the patient warm and quiet. Have an emesis basin available. Administer nothing by mouth. Do not apply heat to the abdomen unless so instructed by the physician. Check and record the patient's vital signs.

OBSTETRIC EMERGENCIES

The types of problems found in an obstetrics office are unique to this specialty. Every medical assistant employed in an office where the physician delivers babies should be trained to handle emergencies. The

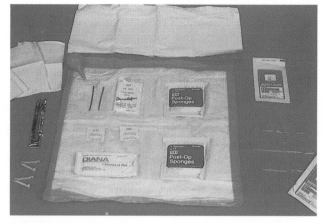

FIGURE 25–16 Emergency obstetrics kit. (From Henry MC, Stapleton ER: EMT Prehospital Care, 2nd ed. Philadelphia, WB Saunders, 1997.)

majority of these problems will be presented to you over the telephone. If a physician is in the office, those calls should be transferred to him or her immediately.

If a pregnant patient calls to report vaginal bleeding, you must ask some specific questions. Is the bleeding like a menstrual flow or is it a gushing type of hemorrhage? Is it painful or without any pain? If the bleeding is gushing, the patient must be told to lie down immediately while you send for an ambulance. In such a situation, the mother and baby could bleed to death in a matter of a few minutes as the result of pregnancy complications such as a ruptured uterus. If the bleeding is like a normal menstrual flow, have the patient go to bed, with the foot of the bed elevated. Tell her that you will report this to the physician immediately. If the tissue passed is liver-like, it may be a blood clot; white tissue may be fetus. No matter what the appearance of the tissue, have the patient take it with her to the hospital.

If the patient comes to the office and the physician informs you that she is delivering her baby right now, the physician will need an emergency obstetrics kit (Fig. 25–16). Get the kit and prepare to assist immediately. Unwrap the OB kit, being sure to keep sterile items sterile. This kit contains all of the supplies needed for the delivery. If there is time, place the apron and the goggles on the physician for protection against communicable diseases. Assist physician and offer encouragement and moral support to the mother. Watch the time and record the moment the child takes the first breath as the time of birth.

SPRAINS

A sprain is an acute partial tear of a muscle, a tendon, or a ligament. Sprains may also cause damage to blood vessels and surrounding nerve tissue. The victim may develop edema, ecchymosis, and sharp, radiating pain. It may be difficult to move or bear weight on the injured joint. When sprains are caused by chronic overuse, they typically cause stiffness, tenderness, and soreness.

Treatment

Treatment of sprains entails elevation, mild compression, and immediate application of ice. There is considerable advantage if the ice is applied within 20 to 30 minutes after the injury has occurred. The ice should remain on the part for 24 hours, with the injured area elevated. After 24 to 36 hours, application of mild heat is usually indicated. The patient may be advised to immobilize the part.

FRACTURES

A fracture is a break or crack in a bone and can result from trauma or disease. Fractures are always very painful, and the patient will have great difficulty in moving the injured part of the body.

Treatment

When a patient with a fracture is brought into the office, the medical assistant should make the patient as comfortable as possible. Place the patient in a position that does not place strain on the area. First aid includes preventing movement of the injured part, elevation of the affected extremity, application of ice, and control of any bleeding. Notify the physician immediately and proceed according to the orders given to you.

BURNS

Burns are among the most frequent cause of injuries in the United States. Burn injuries can result from flame, heat, scalds, electricity, chemicals, or radiation. The extent of the surface area burned, plus the depth and nature of the burn, is directly proportional to the extent of the pain. The skin surface may be reddened, blistered, or charred.

The depth and extent of burns are the major determinants in classifying the severity of a burn. Only second- and third-degree burns are counted when assessing the extent of the burn because first-degree burns do not result in loss of skin function.

Treatment

First aid for burns includes relief of the pain, prevention of infection, and treatment of shock. Burns are extremely painful and dangerous. Bring the emergency cart into the area and open the medication drawer. Next lay out sterile dressings and bandages and a pair of sterile gloves for the physi-

cian. Remove loose clothing from the burned area but do not attempt to pick pieces of charred fabric out of the wound site. Stay with the patient and assist the physician in a quiet and efficient manner.

Memory Jogger

13 *Burn pain is directly proportional to _____.*

LACERATIONS

Lacerations are a common presentation in the primary care physician's office. A lacerated wound displays a jagged or irregular tearing of the tissues. The severity depends on the mechanism of injury, the site of the injury, the extent of the injury, and the introduction of foreign bodies or contamination into the wound. It is important to consider damage to blood vessels, nerves, bones, joints, and organs within the body cavities.

Treatment

Notify the physician immediately. Have the patient lie down. Keep the patient quiet. Cover the injured area with a sterile dressing; use a dressing that is thick enough to absorb the bleeding. If bleeding persists or is profuse, apply direct pressure to the dressing and also to the area just above the wound. The injured part of the body should be elevated above the level of the victim's heart. Be sure to make an effort to reassure the victim and explain your actions as much as possible. Ask the patient when he or she received the last tetanus shot and record the date in the patient's record. If it has been more than 10 years, the physician will probably want a booster shot given.

Wounds that are not bleeding severely and that do not involve deep tissues should be cleansed. Wash in and around the wound with soap and water to remove bacteria and other foreign matter. If the laceration is extremely dirty, wait for the physician to arrive and tell you how to proceed with the cleansing of the wound. The physician may want to irrigate with sterile normal saline solution and/or rinse the wound thoroughly with clean water and blot dry.

The basic dressing includes a sterile gauze or other absorbent material that is applied directly to the wound. The dressing selected may vary in size and thickness according to the wound. A butterfly closure strip may be used over small lacerations, to hold the edges together. If the wound is superficial and has straight edges, it may be closed with a microporous tape, which eliminates the discomfort of suturing and suture removal as well as some of the potential risks of infected sutures. Figure 25–17

LACERATIONS

What you need to know . . .

It is important to prevent infection and to allow your cut to heal. Call your doctor or return to him or her immediately if any of the "danger signs" occur.

Return for recheck in _____ days
Return for suture removal in _____ days

Danger signs to watch for . . .

1. Increasing pain, swelling, redness, and warmth in the injured area.
2. Pus in or around the cut.
3. Fever greater than 100°F (38°C).
4. Blood soaking through the dressing.

If any of these signs occur, contact your doctor or return to the Emergency Department.

What to do at home . . .

1. Take all medicines exactly as directed.
2. Raise the injured area above your heart level for 1 to 2 days.
3. Keep the wound and bandage clean and dry. For cuts on the face, a bandage is often not necessary. All finger dressings must be changed within 24 hours.
4. Remove the bandage/dressing in 24 hours.
5. After 24 hours, you may shower or bathe. Begin cleaning the wound with clear water twice each day to remove crusting and scabbing. Then apply ointment (Polysporin).
6. Prevent sunburn. Use a sunscreen for 6 months (e.g., Pre-Sun or Eclipse).
7. If you have a private doctor or are a member of an HMO (e.g., Kaiser), you should call for an appointment for your recheck and suture removal. If you can't get an appointment, you are welcome to return here to complete your care.

Please remember . . .

1. The exam and treatment you have just received are not intended to provide complete medical care. You need to call your doctor to schedule a follow-up visit.

2. The X-rays or E.C.G. taken today will be reviewed by a specialist. If there is any change in your diagnosis, we will contact you.

FIGURE 25–17 Laceration educational material for home care of wound.

shows an excellent method of informing patients as to the nature of their injury and of both the office and the home treatment required. If you work in a multicultural community, forms should be printed in different languages for non-English–speaking patients.

Memory Jogger

14 *Describe a lacerated wound.*

NOSEBLEEDS (EPISTAXIS)

Nosebleed, or **epistaxis,** is a hemorrhage usually resulting from the rupture of small vessels within the nose. Nosebleeds can result from injury, disease, strenuous activity, high altitudes, exposure to cold, and overuse of blood-thinning medications such as aspirin.

Treatment

Keep the patient quiet and in a sitting position. Apply direct pressure to the affected nostril by pinching the nose. Continue the pressure for 5 minutes to allow clotting to take place. Repeat if bleeding cannot be controlled, insert a clean pad of gauze into the nostril and notify the physician. If the physician is not available, proceed with standard EMS protocols.

HEMORRHAGES

Bleeding may be external or internal. Those administering first aid can do little about internal bleeding, except to keep the patient quiet and warm to minimize shock and get medical help immediately. External bleeding is not as complex as internal bleeding in that you can frequently see the source of the bleeding. Shock and loss of consciousness may occur from a rapid loss of blood in a short time.

Treatment

There are four practical ways of controlling severe bleeding. The first technique is to use direct pressure over the area by applying a sterile dressing. If blood soaks through the entire pad, do not remove the pad but add additional pads of thick cloth and continue direct pressure. The second method is elevation of the injured part. Elevation uses the forces of gravity to control blood flow. The third method is to apply pressure over the nearest pressure point between the bleeding area and the heart. This compresses the main artery supplying the affected limb. The last resort is the application of a tourniquet. The use of a tourniquet is dangerous and should be used only for a life-threatening hemorrhage. By deciding to use a tourniquet, you have made a decision that the patient will bleed to death without it. In the medical office this decision would be the physician's.

Memory Jogger

15 *What is the first technique used in controlling bleeding?*

HEAD INJURIES

The severity of a head injury can vary greatly. With a head injury, the patient may appear normal; may experience dizziness, severe headache, mental confusion, or memory loss; or may even be unconscious. The loss of consciousness may be brief or prolonged; it may appear immediately or may be delayed. The victim may experience vomiting, loss of bladder and bowel control, and bleeding from the nose, mouth, or ears. The pupils of the eyes may be of unequal diameters.

Treatment

All head injuries must be considered serious. Notify the physician or contact the EMS immediately. Have the victim lie flat. If there is difficulty in breathing, raise the head and shoulders slightly. If there is evidence of neck injury, do not attempt to move the victim, contact the physician and assist with the patient assessment.

Do not administer anything by mouth. Keep the patient warm and quiet. Watch the pupils of the eyes, and record any changes. Obtain the vital signs. Control any hemorrhage. Record the extent and duration of any unconsciousness.

FOREIGN BODIES IN THE EYE

The eye is a delicate organ whose unique structure demands special handling. This kind of emergency is most uncomfortable, and it is often extremely difficult to keep the patient from rubbing the eye. Tell the patient not to touch the eye in any way. If the doctor has given you prior permission, you may put a few drops of ophthalmic topical anesthetic in the eye. The patient will greatly appreciate this and will experience almost immediate relief. The eye may be rinsed with tepid tap water in an attempt to remove the object. Unless the foreign object is clearly visible, do not attempt to search for it or to remove it.

Treatment

The medical assistant should never attempt to remove a foreign body from the cornea. The patient should be placed in a darkened room to wait. Have plenty of tissues available. If there is a contusion and swelling, cold wet compresses will help. If you have been trained to turn an upper eyelid out, then do so gently and search for the foreign body. Be very careful not to place any pressure on the eye. If the foreign body cannot be found, then ask the patient to close the eyes. Cover both eyes with eye pads and hold them in place with a strip of tape until the physician arrives.

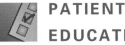

PATIENT EDUCATION

Emergencies can occur in the home, while on vacation, or in the physician's office. Patients need to be instructed in handling an emergency, both by example and through actual instruction. The medical assistant must remain calm, **triage** the situation, call for help, and be prepared to administer appropriate first-aid intervention. This attitude helps the patient learn how to report and handle an emergency. You can give patients brochures that instruct them in home safety.

Accidents are the leading cause of death among children younger than 15 years of age. Even more common are home accidents that cause injuries that do not kill but require hospitalization. More than one-half million of such accidents occur each year. The Children's Bureau of the Department of Health, Education, and Welfare has published pamphlets containing helpful tips on preventing accidents. Child-resistant bottle caps, safer toys, better-educated parents, more responsible toy manufacturers, and government regulations have helped to cut dramatically the number of childhood deaths and injuries. Most states require car safety seats for children younger than 4 years of age or who weigh less than 30 pounds. Parents should be encouraged to use car safety seats, make their homes accident proof, purchase safe toys, become familiar with basic first-aid procedures, and know the local emergency numbers. If you are employed in pediatrics or family practice specialties, you may be called on to educate families in these matters.

Remember to keep your American Red Cross and American Heart Association cards current. Take advantage of community workshops to maintain and extend your skills. Post a list of community safety workshops in an area where it can be seen by patients, and encourage them to attend. Your participation in emergency care workshops and your encouragement to have others participate may help to save lives.

LEGAL AND ETHICAL ISSUES

Most states have enacted Good Samaritan laws to encourage health care professionals to provide medical assistance at the scene of an accident without fear of being sued for negligence. These statutes vary greatly, but all seem to have the intent of protecting the caregiver. It is helpful for the medical assistant to understand the legal responsibilities and the rights of the caregiver. A physician or other health care professional is not legally obligated to give emergency care, regardless of the ethical and moral considerations. Legal liability is limited to gross neglect of the victim or willfully causing further injury to the victim. As a caregiver, you are required to act as a reasonable person and cannot be held liable for personal injury resulting from an act of omission. The Good Samaritan statutes provide for the evaluation of the caregiver's judgment.

If you have never been trained in CPR, you cannot be expected to perform the procedure. However, in many states, a health care provider with CPR training and skills who is present at the scene can be declared negligent if cardiac arrest occurs and he or she does not administer CPR to the victim.

Remember, if the victim is conscious or if a member of his or her immediate family is present, obtain a verbal consent for the emergency care procedure before you begin. Consent is implied if the patient is unconscious and no family member is present.

Many types of emergencies can be handled in the physician's office, and in an emergency situation the patient's life is often determined by the decisions that must be made quickly. You may be called on within the next few minutes to make a decision that could affect the outcome of someone's future. Do you believe that you could make this decision calmly and accurately? If you believe that you could not handle this type of decision making, now is the time to discuss this with your instructor and obtain the necessary help to ensure your ability in handling your first and subsequent emergencies.

CRITICAL THINKING

1 How would you triage an emergency situation?

2 Make an emergency phone list for your home telephone.

HOW DID I DO? Answers to Memory Joggers

1 The medical assistant is expected to make decisions based on his or her medical knowledge in an emergency situation.

2 The team management system allows one person to take immediate charge while another obtains needed materials and calls for assistance.

3 Local emergency numbers should include the EMS system, poison control center, ambulance and rescue squad, fire department, and police department.

4 Orange juice is given to diabetic patients experiencing insulin shock.

5 The defibrillator is used to reestablish the proper rhythm of the heartbeat.

6 The first and most important rule is to stay calm.

7 The two primary functions of first aid are never do anything that will worsen the situation and provide the best care you can.

8 Ventilate the lungs every 5 seconds.

9 The universal distress signal is clutching the neck between the thumb and index fingers.

10 Nitroglycerin tables are administered sublingually (under the tongue).

11 Poisoning can occur by mouth, absorption, inhalation, and injection.

12 Signs of shock include paleness, clamminess, dilated pupils, weak and rapid pulse, low blood pressure, thirst, lethargy, a feeling of faintness, and labored breathing.

13 The extent of the surface area burned, plus the depth and nature of the burn, is directly proportionate to the extent of the pain.

14 A lacerated wound displays a jagged or irregular tearing of the tissues.

15 The first technique used in controlling bleeding is direct pressure over the injured area by applying a sterile dressing.

Combining Forms in Medical Terminology*

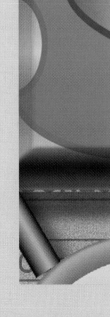

The following is a list of combining forms encountered frequently in the vocabulary of medicine. A dash or dashes are appended to indicate whether the form usually precedes (as *ante-*) or follows (as *-agra*) the other elements of the compound or usually appears between the other elements (as *-em-*). Following each combining form, the first item of information is the Greek or Latin word, or both a Greek and a Latin word, from which it is derived. Those words that are not printed in Greek characters are Latin. Information necessary to an understanding of the form appears next in parentheses. Then the meaning or meanings of the word are given, followed where appropriate by reference to a synonymous combining form. Finally, an example is given to illustrate the use of the combining form in a compound English derivative.

a-	α- (*n* is added before words beginning with a vowel) negative prefix. Cf. in-[3]. *a*metria
ab-	*ab* away from. Cf. apo-. *ab*ducent
abdomin-	*abdomen, abdominis. abdomin*oscopy
ac-	See ad-. *ac*cretion
acet-	*acetum* vinegar. *acet*ometer
acid-	*acidus* sour. *acid*uric
acou-	ἀκούω hear. *acou*esthesia. (Also spelled acu-)
acr-	ἄκρον extremity, peak. *acro-* megaly
act-	*ago, actus* do, drive, act. re*act*ion
actin-	ἀκτίς, ἀκτῖνος ray, radius, Cf. radi-. *actin*ogenesis
acu-	See acou-. osteo*acu*sis
ad-	*ad* (*d* changes to *c, f, g, p, s,* or *t* before words beginning with those consonants) to. *ad*renal
aden-	ἀδήν gland. Cf. gland-. *aden*oma
adip-	*adeps, adipis* fat. Cf. lip- and stear-. *adip*ocellular
aer-	ἀήρ air. an*aer*obiosis
aesthe-	See esthe-. *aesthe*sioneurosis
af-	See ad-. *af*ferent
ag-	See ad-. *ag*glutinant
-agogue	ἀγωγός leading, inducing. galact*agogue*
-agra	ἄγρα catching, seizure, pod*agra*
alb-	*albus* white. Cf. leuk-. *alb*ocinereous
alg-	ἄλγος pain. neur*alg*ia
all-	ἄλλος other, different, *all*ergy
alve-	*alveus* trough, channel, cavity. *al*veolar

*Compiled by Lloyd W. Daly, A.M., Ph.D., Litt.D., Allen Memorial Professor of Greek, University of Pennsylvania. *In* Dorland's Pocket Medical Dictionary, 21st ed. Philadelphia, W. B. Saunders Co., 1968.

amph-	See amphi-. *amph*eclexis
amphi-	ἀμφί (*i* is dropped before words beginning with a vowel) both, doubly. *amphi*celous
amyl-	ἄμυλον starch. *amylo*synthesis
an-¹	See ana-. *an*agogic
an.-²	See a-. *an*omalous
ana-	ἀνά (final *a* is dropped before words beginning with a vowel) up, positive, *ana*phoresis
ancyl-	See ankyl-. *ancylo*stomiasis
andr-	ἀνήρ, ἀνδρός man. gyn*andr*oid
angi-	ἀγγεῖον vessel. Cf. vas-. *angi*emphraxis
ankyl-	ἀγκύλος crooked, looped, *ankylo*dactylia. (Also spelled ancyl-)
ant-	See anti-. *ant*ophthalmic
ante-	*ante* before. *ante*flexion
anti-	ἀντί (*i* is dropped before words beginning with a vowel) against, counter. Cf. contra-. *antipyr*ogenic
antr-	ἄντρον cavern. *antr*odynia
ap-¹	See apo-. *ap*heter
ap-²	See ad-. *ap*pend
-aph	ἅπτω, ἀφ- touch. dys*aph*ia. (See also hapt-)
apo-	ἀπό (*o* is dropped before words beginning with a vowel) away from, detached. Cf. ab-. *apo*physis
arachn-	ἀράχνη spider. *arachn*odactyly
arch-	ἀρχή beginning, origin. *arch*enteron
arter(i)-	ἀρτηρία elevator (?), artery. *arterio*sclerosis, per*i*arteritis
arthr-	ἄρθρον joint. Cf. articul-. syn*arthr*osis
articul-	*articulus* joint. Cf. arthr-. dis*articul*ation
as-	See ad-. *as*similation
at-	See ad-. *at*trition
aur-	*auris* ear. Cf. ot-. *aur*inasal
aux-	αὔξω increase. enter*aux*e
ax-	ἄξων or *axis* axis. *ax*ofugal
axon-	ἄξων axis. *axon*ometer
ba-	βαίνω, βα- go, walk, stand. hypno*ba*tia
bacill-	*bacillus* small staff, rod. Cf. bacter-. antino*bacill*osis
bacter-	βακτήριον small staff, rod. Cf. bacill-. *bacterio*phage
ball-	βάλλω, βολ- throw. *ball*istics. (See also bol-)
bar-	βάρος weight. pedo*bar*ometer
bi-¹	βίος life. Cf. vit-. aero*bi*c
bi-²	*bi-* two (see also di-¹). *bi*lobate
bil-	*bilis* bile. Cf. chol-. *bil*iary
blast-	βλαστός bud, child, a growing thing in its early stages. Cf. germ-. *blast*oma, zygoto*blast*.
blep-	βλέπω look, see. hemia*blep*sia
blephar-	βλέφαρον (from βλέπω; see blep-)eyelid. Cf. cili-. *blephar*oncus
bol-	See ball-. em*bol*ism
brachi-	βραχίων arm. *brachi*ocephalic
brachy-	βραχύς short. *brachy*cephalic
brady-	βραδύς slow. *brady*cardia
brom-	βρῶμος stench. podo*brom*idrosis
bronch-	βρόγχος windpipe. *bronch*oscopy
bry-	βρύω be full of life. em*bry*onic
bucc-	*bucca* cheek. disto*bucc*al
cac-	κακός bad, abnormal. Cf. mal-. *cac*odontia, arthro*cac*e. (See also dys-)
calc-¹	*calx, calcis* stone (cf. lith-), limestone, lime. *calci*pexy
calc-²	*calx, calcis* heel. *calc*aneotibial
calor-	*calor* heat. Cf. therm-. *calor*imeter
cancr-	*cancer, cancri* crab, cancer. Cf. carcin-. *cancr*ology. (Also spelled chancr-)
capit-	*caput, capitis* head. Cf. cephal-. de*capit*ator
caps-	*capsa* (from capio; see cept-) container. en*caps*ulation
carbo(n)-	*carbo, carbonis* coal, charcoal. *carbo*hydrate, *carbon*uria
carcin-	καρκίνος crab, cancer. Cf. cancr-. *carcin*oma

cardi-	καρδία heart. lipo*cardi*ac
cary-	See kary-. *cary*okinesis
cat-	See cata-. *cat*hode
cata-	κατά (final *a* is dropped before words beginning with a vowel) down, negative. *cata*batic
caud-	*cauda* tail. *caud*ad
cav-	*cavus* hollow. Cf. coel-. con*cav*e
cec-	*caecus* blind. Cf. typhl-. *cec*opexy
cel-¹	See coel-. amphi*cel*ous
cel-²	See -cele. *cel*ectome
-cele	κήλη tumor, hernia. gastro*cele*
cell-	*cella* room, cell. Cf. cyt-. *cell*iferous
cen-	κοινός common. *cen*esthesia
cent-	*centum* hundred. Cf. hect-. Indicates fraction in metric system. [This exemplifies the custom in the metric system of identifying fractions of units by stems from the Latin, as centimeter, decimeter, millimeter, and multiples of units by the similar stems from the Greek, as hectometer, decameter, and kilometer.] *centi*meter, *centi*pede
cente-	κεντέω puncture. Cf. punct-. entero*cente*sis
centr-	κέντρον or *centrum* point, center. neuro*centr*al
cephal-	κεφαλή head. Cf. capit-. en*cephal*itis
cept-	*capio, -cipientis, -ceptus* take, receive. re*cept*or
cer-	κηρός or *cera* wax. *cer*oplasty, *cer*omel
cerat-	See kerat-. a*cerat*osis
cerebr-	*cerebrum*. *cerebr*ospinal
cervic-	*cervix, cervicis* neck. Cf. trachel-. *cervic*itis
chancr-	See cancr-. *chancr*iform
cheil-	χεῖλος lip. Cf. labi-. *cheil*oschisis
cheir-	χείρ hand. Cf. man-. macro*cheir*ia. (Also spelled chir-)
chir-	See cheir-. *chir*omegaly
chlor-	χλωρός green. a*chlor*opsia
chol-	χολή bile. Cf. bil-. hepato*chol*angeitis
chondr-	χόνδρος cartilage. *chondr*omalacia
chord-	χορδή string, cord. peri*chord*al
chori-	χόριον protective fetal membrane. endo*chori*on
chro-	χρώς color. poly*chro*matic
chron-	χρόνος time. syn*chron*ous
chy-	χέω, χυ- pour. ec*chy*mosis
-cid(e)	*caedo, -cisus* cut, kill. infanti*cide*, germi*cidal*
cili-	*cilium* eyelid. Cf. blephar-. super*cili*ary
cine-	See kine-. auto*cine*sis
-cipient	See cept-. in*cipient*
circum-	*circum* around. Cf. peri-. *circum*ferential
-cis-	*caedo, -cisus* cut, kill. ex*cis*ion
clas-	κλάω, κλασ- break. cranio*clas*t
clin-	κλίνω bend, incline, make lie down. *clin*ometer
clus-	*claudo, -clusus* shut. Ma*locclus*ion
co-	See con-. *co*hesion
cocc-	κόκκος seed, pill. gono*cocc*us
coel-	κοῖλος hollow. Cf. cav-. *coel*enteron. (Also spelled cel-)
col-¹	See colon-. *col*ic
col-²	See con-. *col*lapse
colon-	κόλον lower intestine. *colon*ic
colp-	κόλπος hollow, vagina. Cf. sin-. endo*colp*itis
com-	See con-. *com*masculation
con-	*con-* (becomes co- before vowels or h; col- before l; com- before b, m, or p; cor- before r) with, together. Cf. syn-. *con*traction
contra-	*contra* against, counter. Cf. anti-. *contra*indication
copr-	κόπρος dung. Cf. sterco-. *copr*oma
cor-²	κόρη doll, little image, pupil. iso*cor*ia
cor-¹	See con-. *cor*rugator
corpor-	*corpus, corporis* body. Cf. somat-. intra*corpor*al
cortic-	*cortex, corticis* bark, rind. *cortic*osterone
cost-	*costa* rib. Cf. pleur-. inter*cost*al
crani-	κρανίον or *cranium* skull. peri*crani*um
creat-	κρέας, κρεατ- meat, flesh. *creat*orrhea
-crescent	*cresco, crescentis, cretus* grow. ex*crescent*

cret-¹ *cerno, cretus* distinguish, separate off. Cf. crin-. dis*cret*e

cret-² See -crescent. ac*cret*ion

crin- κρίνω distinguish, separate off, secrete. Cf. cret-¹. endo*crin*ology

crur- *crus, cruris* shin, leg. brachio*crur*al

cry- κρύος cold. *cry*esthesia

crypt- κρίπτω hide, conceal. *crypt*orchism

cult- *colo, cultus* tend, cultivate. *cult*ure

cune- *cuneus* wedge. Cf. sphen-. *cune*iform

cut- *cutis* skin. Cf. derm(at)-. sub*cut*aneous

cyan- κίανος blue. antho*cyan*in

cycl- κύκλος circle, cycle. *cycl*ophoria

cyst- κύστις bladder. Cf. vesic-. nephro*cyst*itis

cyt- κύτος cell. Cf. cell-. plasmo*cyt*oma

dacry- δάκρυ tear. *dacry*ocyst

dactyl- δάκτυλος finger, toe. Cf. digit-. hexa*dactyl*ism

de- *de* down from. *de*composition

dec-¹ δέκα ten. Indicates multiple in metric system. Cf. dec-². *dec*agram

dec-² *decem* ten. Indicates fraction in metric system. Cf. dec-¹. *dec*ipara, *dec*imeter

dendr- δένδρον tree. neuro*dendr*ite

dent- *dens, dentis* tooth. Cf. odont-. inter*dent*al

derm(at)- δέρμα, δέρματος skin. Cf. cut-. endo*derm*, *derma*titis

desm- δεσμός band, ligament. syn*desm*opexy

dextr- *dexter, dextr-* right-hand. ambi*dextr*ous

di-¹ *di-* two. *di*morphic. (See also bi-²)

di-² See dia-. *di*uresis

di-³ See dis-. *di*vergent.

dia- διά (*a* is dropped before words beginning with a vowel) through, apart. Cf. per-. *dia*gnosis

didym- δίδυμος twin. Cf. gemin-. epi*didym*al

digit- *digitus* finger, toe. Cf. dactyl-. *digit*igrade

diplo- διπλόος double. *diplo*myelia

dis- *dis-* (*s* may be dropped before a word beginning with a consonant) apart, away from. *dis*location

disc- δίσκος or *discus* disk. *disc*oplacenta

dors- *dorsum* back. ventro*dors*al

drom- δρόμος course. hemo*drom*ometer

-ducent See duct-. ad*ducent*

duct- *duco, ducentis, ductus* lead, conduct. ovi*duct*

dur- *durus* hard. Cf. scler-. in*dur*ation

dynam(i)- δύναμις power. *dynam*oneure, neuro*dynam*ic

dys- δυσ- bad, improper. Cf. mal-. *dys*trophic. (See also cac-)

e- *e* out from. Cf. ec- and ex-. *e*mission

ec- ἐκ out of. Cf. e- *ec*centric

-ech- ἔχω have, hold, be. syn*ech*otomy

ect- ἐκτός outside. Cf. extra-. *ect*oplasm

ede- οἰδέω swell. *ede*matous

ef- See ex-. *ef*florescent

-elc- ἔλκος sore, ulcer. enter*elc*osis. (See also *helc-*)

electr- ἤλεκτρον amber. *electr*otherapy

em- See en-. *em*bolism, *em*pathy, *em*phlysis

-em- αἷμα blood. an*em*ia. (See also hem(at)-)

en- ἐν (*n* changes to *m* before *b, p,* or *ph*) in, on. Cf. in-². *en*celitis

end- ἔνδον inside. Cf. intra-. *end*angium.

enter- ἔντερον intestine. dys*enter*y

ep- See epi-. *ep*axial

epi- ἐπί (*i* is dropped before words beginning with a vowel) upon, after, in addition. *epi*glottis

erg- ἔργον work, deed. *energy

erythr- ἐρυθρός red. Cf. rub(r)-. *erythr*ochromia

eso- ἔσω inside. Cf. intra-. *eso*phylactic

esthe- αἰσθάνομαι, αἰσθη- perceive, feel. Cf. sens-. an*esthe*sia

eu- εὐ good, normal. *eu*pepsia

ex- ἐξ or *ex* out of. Cf. e-. *ex*cretion

exo- ἔξω outside. Cf. extra-. *exo*pathic

extra- *extra* outside of, beyond. Cf. ect- and exo-. *extra*cellular

faci- *facies* face. Cf. prosop-. brachio*faci*olingual

-facient *facio, facientis, factus, -fectus* make. Cf. poie-. cal*efacient*

-fact- See facient-. arte*fact*

fasci- *fascia* band. *fasci*orrhaphy

febr- *febris* fever. Cf. pyr-. *febr*icide

-fect- See -facient. de*fect*ive

-ferent *fero, ferentis, latus* bear, carry. Cf. phor-. ef*ferent*

ferr- *ferrum* iron. *ferr*oprotein

fibr- *fibra* fibre. Cf. in-¹. chondro*fibr*oma

fil- *filum* thread. *fil*iform

fiss- *findo, fissus* split. Cf. schis-. *fiss*ion

flagell- *flagellum* whip. *flagell*ation

flav- *flavus* yellow. Cf. xanth-. ribo*flav*in

-flect- *flecto, flexus* bend, divert. de*flect*ion

-flex- See -flect-. re*flex*ometer

flu- *fluo, fluxus* flow. Cf. rhe-. *flu*id

flux- See flu-. af*flux*ion

for- *foris* door, opening. per*for*ated

-form *forma* shape. Cf. -oid. ossi*form*

fract- *frango, fractus* break. re*fract*ive

front- *frons, frontis* forehead, front. naso*front*al

-fug(e) *fugio* flee, avoid. vermi*fuge*, centri*fug*al

funct- *fungor, functus* perform, serve, function. mal*funct*ion

fund- *fundo, fusus* pour. in*fund*ibulum

fus- See fund-. dif*fus*ible

galact- γάλα, γάλακτος milk. Cf. lact-. dys*galact*ia

gam- γάμος marriage, reproductive union. a*gam*ont

gangli- γάγγλιον swelling, plexus. neuro*gangli*itis

gastr- γαστήρ, γαστρός stomach. cholangio*gastr*ostomy

gelat- *gelo, gelatus* freeze, congeal. *gelat*in

gemin- *geminus* twin, double. Cf. didym-. quadri*gemin*al

gen- γίγνομαι, γεν-, γον- become, be produced, originate, or γεννάω produce, originate. cyto*gen*ic

germ- *germen, germinis* bud, a growing thing in its early stages. Cf. blast-. *germ*inal, ovi*germ*

gest- *gero, gerentis, gestus* bear, carry. con*gest*ion

gland- *glans, glandis* acorn. Cf. aden-. intra*gland*ular

-glia γλία glue. neuro*glia*

gloss- γλῶσσα tongue. Cf. lingu-. tricho*gloss*ia

glott- γλῶττα tongue, language. *glott*ic

gluc- See glyc(y)-. *gluc*ophenetidin

glutin- *gluten, glutinis* glue. ag*glutin*ation

glyc(y)- γλυκύς sweet. *glyc*emia, *glyc*yrrhizin. (Also spelled gluc-)

gnath- γνάθος jaw. ortho*gnath*ous

gno- γιγνώσκω, γνω- know, discern. dia*gno*sis

gon- See gen-. amphi*gon*y

grad- *gradior* walk, take steps. retro*grad*e

-gram γράφω, γραφ- + -μα scratch, write, record. cardio*gram*

gran- *granum* grain, particle. lipo*gran*uloma

graph- γράφω scratch, write, record. histo*graph*y

grav- *gravis* heavy. multi*grav*ida

gyn(ec)- γυνή, γυναικός woman, wife. andro*gyn*y, *gynec*ologic

gyr- γῦρος ring, circle. *gyr*ospasm

haem(at)- See hem(at)-. *haem*orrhagia, *haemat*oxylon

hapt- ἅπτω touch. *hapt*ometer

hect- ἑκτ- hundred. Cf. cent-. Indicates multiple in metric system. *hect*ometer

helc- ἔλκος sore, ulcer. *helc*osis

hem(at)- αἷμα, αἵματος blood. Cf. sanguin-. *hem*angioma, *hemat*ocyturia. (See also -em-)

hemi- ἡμι- half. Cf. semi-. *hemi*ageusia

hen- εἷς, ἑνός one. Cf. un-. *hen*ogenesis

hepat- ἧπαρ, ἧπατος liver. gastro*hepat*ic

hept(a)- ἑπτά seven. Cf. sept-². *hept*atomic, *hepta*valent

hered- *heres, heredis* heir. *hered*oimmunity

hex-¹ ἑξ six. Cf. sex-. *hex*yl-. An *a* is added in some combinations.

hex-² ἔχω, ἐχ- (added to σ becomes ἑξ-) have, hold, be. ca*chex*y

hexa- See hex-¹. *hexa*chromic

hidr- ἱδρώς sweat. hyper*hidr*osis

hist- ἱστός web, tissue. *hist*odialysis

hod- ὁδός road, path. *hod*oneuromere. (See also od- and -ode¹)

hom- ὁμός common, same. *hom*omorphic

horm- ὁρμή impetus, impulse. *horm*one

hydat- ὕδωρ, ὕδατος water. *hydat*ism

hydr- ὕδωρ, ὕδρ- water. Cf. lymph-. achlor*hydr*ia

hyp- See hypo-. *hyp*axial

hyper- ὑπέρ above, beyond, extreme. Cf. super-. *hyper*trophy

hypn- ὕπνος sleep. *hypn*otic

hypo- ὑπό (*o* is dropped before words beginning with a vowel) under, below. Cf. sub-. *hypo*metabolism

hyster- ὑστέρα womb, uterus. colpo*hyster*opexy

iatr- ἰατρός physician. ped*iatr*ics

idi- ἴδιος peculiar, separate, distinct. *idi*osyncrasy

il- See in-²,³. *il*linition (in, on), *il*legible (negative prefix)

ile- See ili- [ile- is commonly used to refer to the portion of the intestines known as the ileum]. *ile*ostomy

ili- *ilium (ileum)* lower abdomen, intestines [ili- is commonly used to refer to the flaring part of the hip bone known as the ilium]. *ili*osacral

im- See in-²,³. *im*mersion (in, on), *im*perforation (negative prefix)

in-¹ ἴς, ἰνός fiber. Cf. fibr-. *in*osteatoma

in-² *in* (*n* changes to *l, m,* or *r* before words beginning with those consonants) in, on. Cf. en-. *in*sertion

in-³ *in-* (*n* changes to *l, m,* or *r* before words beginning with those consonants) negative prefix. Cf. a-. *in*valid

infra- *infra* beneath. *infra*orbital

insul- *insula* island. *insul*in

inter- *inter* among, between. *inter*carpal

intra- *intra* inside. Cf. end- and eso-. *intra*venous

ir- See in-²,³. *ir*radiation (in, on), *ir*reducible (negative prefix)

irid- ἴρις, ἴριδος rainbow, colored circle. kerato*irid*ocyclitis

is- ἴσος equal. *is*otope

ischi- ἰσχίον hip, haunch. *ischi*opubic

jact- *iacio, iactus* throw. *jact*itation

ject- *iacio, -iectus* throw. in*ject*ion

jejun- *ieiunus* hungry, not partaking of food. gastro*jejun*ostomy

jug- *iugum* yoke. con*jug*ation

junct- *iungo, iunctus* yoke, join. con*junct*iva

kary- κάρυον nut, kernel, nucleus. Cf. nucle-. mega*kary*ocyte. (Also spelled cary-)

kerat- κέρας, κέρατος horn. *kerat*olysis. (Also spelled cerat-)

kil- χίλιοι one thousand. Cf. mill-. Indicates multiple in metric system. *kil*ogram

kine- κινέω move. *kine*matograph. (Also spelled cine-)

labi- *labium* lip. Cf. cheil-. gingivo-*labi*al

lact- *lac, lactis* milk. Cf. galact-. gluco*lact*one

lal- λαλέω talk, babble. glosso*lal*ia

lapar- λαπάρα flank. *lapar*otomy

laryng- λάρυγξ, λάρυγγος windpipe. *laryng*endoscope

lat- *fero, latus* bear, carry. Cf. -ferent. trans*lat*ion

later- *latus, lateris* side. ventro*later*al

lent- *lens, lentis* lentil. Cf. phac-. *lent*iconus

lep- λαμβάνω, ληπ- take, seize. cata*lep*tic

leuc- See leuk-. *leuc*inuria

leuk- λευκός white. Cf. alb-. *leuk*orrhea. (Also spelled leuc-)

lien- *lien* spleen. Cf. splen-. *lien*ocele

lig- *ligo* tie, bind. *lig*ate

lingu- *lingua* tongue. Cf. gloss-. sub*lingu*al

lip- λίπος fat. Cf. adip-. glyco*lip*in

lith- λίθος stone. Cf. calc-¹. nephro*lith*otomy

loc- *locus* place. Cf. top-. *loc*omotion

log- λέγω, λογ- speak, give an account, *log*orrhea, embryo*log*y

lumb- *lumbus* loin. dorso*lumb*ar

lute- *luteus* yellow. Cf. xanth-. *lute*oma

ly- λύω loose, dissolve. Cf. solut-. kerato*ly*sis

lymph- *lympha* water. Cf. hydr-. *lymph*adenosis

macr- μακρός long, large. *macr*omyeloblast

mal- *malus* bad, abnormal. Cf. cac- and dys-. *mal*function

malac- μαλακός soft. osteo*malac*ia

mamm- *mamma* breast. Cf. mast-. sub*mamm*ary

man- *manus* hand. Cf. cheir-. *man*iphalanx

mani- μανία mental aberration. *mani*graphy, kleptoma*mani*a

mast- μαστός breast. Cf. mamm-. hyper*mast*ia

medi- *medius* middle. Cf. mes-. *medi*frontal

mega- μέγας great, large. Also indicates multiple (1,000,000) in metric system. *mega*colon, *mega*dyne. (See also megal-)

megal- μέγας, μεγάλου great, large. acro*megal*y

mel- μέλος limb, member. sym*mel*ia

melan- μέλας, μέλανος black. hippo*melan*in

men- μήν month. dys*men*orrhea

mening- μῆνιγξ, μήνιγγος membrane. encephalo*mening*itis

ment- *mens, mentis* mind. Cf. phren-, psych-, and thym-. de*ment*ia

mer- μέρος part. poly*mer*ic

mes- μέσος middle. Cf. medi-. *mes*oderm

met- See meta-. *met*allergy

meta- μετά (*a* is dropped before words beginning with a vowel) after, beyond, accompanying. *meta*carpal

metr-¹ μέτρον measure. stereo*metr*y

metr-² μήτρα womb. endo*metr*itis

micr- μικρός small. photo*micr*ograph

mill- *mille* one thousand. Cf. kil-. Indicates fraction in metric system. *milli*gram, *milli*pede

miss- See -mittent. intro*miss*ion

-mittent *mitto, mittentis, missus* send. inter*mittent*

mne- μιμνήσκω, μνη- remember. pseudo*mne*sia

mon- μόνος only, sole. *mon*oplegia

morph- μορφή form, shape. poly*morph*onuclear

mot- *moveo, motus* move. vaso*mot*or

my- μῦς, μυός muscle. inoleio*my*oma

-myces μύκης, μύκητος fungus. myelo*myces*

myc(et)- See -myces. asco*myc*etes, strepto*myc*in

myel- μυελός marrow. polio*myel*itis

myx- μύξα mucus. *myx*edema

narc- νάρκη numbness. topo*narc*osis

nas- *nasus* nose. Cf. rhin-. palato*nas*al

ne- νέος new, young. *ne*ocyte

necr- νεκρός corpse. *necr*ocytosis

nephr- νεφρός kidney. Cf. ren-. para*nephr*ic

neur- νεῦρον nerve. esthesio*neur*e

nod- *nodus* knot. *nod*osity

nom- νόμος (from νέμω deal out, distribute) law, custom. taxo*nom*y

non- *nona* nine. *non*acosane

nos- νόσος disease. *nos*ology

nucle- *nucleus* (from *nux, nucis* nut) kernel. Cf. kary-. *nucle*ide

nutri- *nutrio* nourish. mal*nutri*tion

ob-   *ob* (*b* changes to *c* before words beginning with that consonant) against, toward, etc. *ob*tuse

oc-   See ob-. *oc*clude

ocul-   *oculus* eye. Cf. ophthalm-. *ocul*omotor

-od-   See -ode¹. peri*od*ic

-ode¹   ὁδός road, path. cath*ode*. (See also hod-)

-ode²   See -oid. nemat*ode*

odont-   ὀδούς, ὀδόντος tooth. Cf. dent-. orth*odont*ia

-odyn-   ὀδύνη pain, distress. gastr*odyn*ia

-oid   εἶδος form. Cf. form. hy*oid*

-ol   See ole-. cholester*ol*

ole-   *oleum* oil. *ole*oresin

olig-   ὀλίγος few, small. *olig*ospermia

omphal-   ὀμφαλός navel. peri*omphal*ic

onc-   ὄγκος bulk, mass. hemat*onc*ometry

onych-   ὄνυξ, ὄνυχος claw, nail. an*onych*ia

oo-   ὠόν egg. Cf. ov-. peri*oo*thecitis

op-   ὁράω, ὀπ- see. erythr*op*sia

ophthalm-   ὀφθαλμος eye. Cf. ocul-. ex*ophthalm*ic

or-   *os, oris* mouth. Cf. stom(at)-. intra*or*al

orb-   *orbis* circle. sub*orb*ital

orchi-   ὄρχις testicle. Cf. test-. *orchi*opathy

organ-   ὄργανον implement, instrument. *organ*oleptic

orth-   ὀρθός straight, right, normal. *orth*opedics

oss-   *os, ossis* bone. Cf. ost(e)-. *oss*iphone

ost(e)-   ὀστέον bone. Cf. oss-. en*ost*osis, *oste*anaphysis

ot-   οὖς, ὠτός ear. Cf. aur-. par*ot*id

ov-   *ovum* egg. Cf. oo-. syn*ov*ia

oxy-   ὀξύς sharp. *oxy*cephalic

pachy(n)-   παχύνω thicken. *pachy*derma, myo*pachyn*sis

pag-   πήγνυμι, παγ- fix, make fast. thoraco*pag*us

par-¹   *pario* bear, give birth to. primi*par*ous

par-²   See para-. *par*epigastric

para-   παρά (final *a* is dropped before words beginning with a vowel) beside, beyond. *para*mastoid

part-   *pario, partus* bear, give birth to. *part*urition

path-   πάθος that which one undergoes, sickness. psycho*path*ic

pec-   πήγνυμι, πηγ- (πηκ- before τ) fix, make fast. sym*pec*tothiene. (See also pex-)

ped-   παῖς, παιδός child. ortho*ped*ic

pell-   *pellis* skin, hide. *pell*agra

-pellent   *pello, pellentis, pulsus* drive. re*pellent*

pen-   πένομαι need, lack. erythrocyto*pen*ia

pend-   *pendeo* hang down. ap*pend*ix

pent(a)-   πέντε five. Cf. quinque-. *pent*ose, *penta*ploid

peps-   πέπτω, πεψ- (before σ) digest. brady*peps*ia

pept-   πέπτω digest. dys*pept*ic

per-   *per* through. Cf. dia-. *per*nasal

peri-   περί around. Cf. circum-. *peri*phery

pet-   *peto* seek, tend toward. centri*pet*al

pex-   πήγνυμι, πηγ- (added to σ becomes πηξ-) fix, make fast. hepato*pex*y

pha-   φημί, φα- say, speak. dys*pha*sia

phac-   φακός lentil, lens. Cf. lent-. *phac*osclerosis. (Also spelled phak-)

phag-   φαγεῖν eat. lipo*phag*ic

phak-   See phac-. *phak*itis

phan-   See phen-. dia*phan*oscopy

pharmac-   φάρμακον drug. *pharmac*ognosy

pharyng-   νάρυγξ, φαρυγγ- throat. glosso*pharyng*eal

phen-   φαίνω, φαν- show, be seen. phos*phen*e

pher-   φέρω, φορ- bear, support. peri*pher*y

phil-   φιλέω like, have affinity for. eosino*phil*ia

phleb-   φλέψ, φλεβός vein. peri*phleb*itis

phleg-   φλέγω, φλογ- burn, inflame. adeno*phleg*mon

phlog-   See phleg-. anti*phlog*istic

phob-   φόβος fear, dread. claustro*phob*ia

phon-   φωνή sound. echo*phon*y

phor-   See pher-. Cf. -ferent. exo*phor*ia

phos-   See phot-. *phos*phorus

phot-   φῶς, φωτός light. *phot*erythrous

phrag-   φράσσω, φραγ- fence, wall off, stop up. Cf. sept-¹. dia*phrag*m

phrax-   φράσσω, φραγ- (added to σ becomes φραξ-) fence, wall off, stop up. em*phrax*is

phren-   φρήν mind, midriff. Cf. ment-. meta*phren*ia, meta*phren*on

phthi-   φθίνω decay, waste away. ophthalmo*phthi*sis

phy-   φίω beget, bring forth, produce, be by nature. noso*phy*te

phyl-   φῦλον tribe, kind. *phyl*ogeny

-phyll   φύλλον leaf. xantho*phyll*

phylac-   φύλαξ guard. pro*phylac*tic

phys(a)-   φυσάω blow, inflate. *phys*ocele, *physa*lis

physe-   φυσάω, φυση- blow, inflate. em*physe*ma

pil-   *pilus* hair. e*pil*ation

pituit-   *pituita* phlegm, rheum. *pituit*ous

placent-   *placenta* (from πλακοῖς) cake. extra*placent*al

plas-   πλάσσω mold, shape. cine*plas*ty

platy-   πλατύς broad, flat. *platy*rrhine

pleg-   πλήσσω, πληγ- strike. di*pleg*ia

plet-   *pleo, -pletus* fill. de*plet*ion

pleur-   πλευρά rib, side. Cf. cost-. peri*pleur*al

plex-   πλήσσω, πληγ- (added to σ becomes πληξ-) strike. apo*plex*y

plic-   *plico* fold. com*plic*ation

pne-   πνοιά breathing. traumato*pne*a

pneum(at)-   πνεῦμα, πνεύματος breath, air. *pneum*odynamics, *pneumat*othorax

pneumo(n)-   πνεύμων lung. Cf. pulmo(n)-. *pneumo*centesis, *pneumon*otomy

pod-   πούς, ποδός foot. *pod*iatry

poie-   ποιέω make, produce. Cf. -facient. sarco*poie*tic

pol-   πόλος axis of a sphere. peri*pol*ar

poly-   πολύς much, many. *poly*spermia

pont-   *pons, pontis* bridge. *pont*ocerebellar

por-¹   πόρος passage. myelo*por*e

por-²   πῶρος callus. *por*ocele

posit-   *pono, positus* put, place. re*posit*or

post-   *post* after, behind in time or place. *post*natal, *post*oral

pre-   *prae* before in time or place. *pre*natal, *pre*vesical

press-   *premo, pressus* press. *press*oreceptive

pro-   πρό or *pro* before in time or place. *pro*gamous, *pro*cheilon, *pro*lapse

proct-   πρωκτός anus. entero*proct*ia

prosop-   πρόσωπον face. Cf. faci-. di*prosop*us

pseud-   ψευδής false. *pseud*oparaplegia

psych-   ψυχή soul, mind. Cf. ment-. *psych*osomatic

pto-   πίπτω, πτω- fall. nephro*pto*sis

pub-   *pubes, puber, puberis* adult. ischio*pub*ic. (See also puber-)

puber-   *puber* adult. *puber*ty

pulmo(n)-   *pulmo, pulmonis* lung. Cf. pneumo(n)-. *pulmo*lith, cardio*pulmon*ary

puls-   *pello, pellentis, pulsus* drive. pro*puls*ion

punct-   *pungo, punctus* prick, pierce. Cf. cente-. *puncti*form

pur-   *pus, puris* pus. Cf. py-. sup*pur*ation

py-   πύον pus. Cf. pur-. nephro*py*osis

pyel-   πύελος trough, basin, pelvis. nephro*pyel*itis

pyl-   πύλη door, orifice. *pyl*ephlebitis

pyr-   πῦρ fire. Cf. febr-. galacto*pyr*a

quadr-   *quadr* four. Cf. tetra-. *quadr*igeminal

quinque-   *quinque* five. Cf. pent(a)-. *quinque*cuspid

rachi-   ῥαχίς spine. Cf. spin-. encephalo*rachi*dian

radi-   *radius* ray. Cf. actin-. ir*radi*ation

re-   *re-* back, again. *re*traction

ren-   *renes* kidneys. Cf. nephr-. ad*ren*al

ret-   *rete* net. *ret*othelium

retro-   *retro* backwards. *retro*deviation

rhag-   ῥήγνυμι, ῥαγ- break, burst. hemor*rhag*ic

rhaph-   ῥαφή suture. gastror*rhaph*y

rhe-   ῥέω flow. Cf. flu-. diar*rhe*al

rhex- ῥήγνυμι, ῥηγ- (added to σ becomes ῥηξ-) break, burst. metror*rhex*is

rhin- ῥίς, ῥινός nose. Cf. nas-. basi*rhin*al

rot- *rota* wheel. *rot*ator

rub(r)- *ruber, rubri* red. Cf. erythro-. bili*rub*in, *rub*rospinal

salping- σάλπιγξ, σάλπιγγος tube, trumpet. *salping*itis

sanguin- *sanguis, sanguinis* blood. Cf. hem(at)-. *sanguin*eous

sarc- σάρξ, σαρκός flesh. *sarc*oma

schis- σχίζω, σχιδ- (before τ or added to σ becomes σχισ-) split. Cf. fiss-. *schis*torachis, rachi*schis*is

scler- σκληρός hard. Cf. dur-. *scler*osis

scop- σκοπέω look at, observe. endo*scop*e

sect- *seco, sectus* cut. Cf. tom-. *sect*ile

semi- *semi-* half. Cf. hemi-. *semi*flexion

sens- *sentio, sensus* perceive, feel. Cf. esthe-. *sens*ory

sep- σήπω rot, decay. *sep*sis

sept-¹ *saepio, saeptus* fence, wall off, stop up. Cf. phrag-. naso*sept*al

sept-² *septem* seven. Cf. hept(a)-. *sept*an

ser- *serum* whey, watery substance. *ser*osynovitis

sex- *sex* six. Cf. hex-¹. *sex*digitate

sial- σίαλον saliva. poly*sial*ia

sin- *sinus* hollow, fold. Cf. colp-. *sin*obronchitis

sit- σῖτος food. para*sit*ic

solut- *solvo, solventis, solutus* loose, dissolve, set free. Cf. ly-. dis*solut*ion

-solvent See solut-. dis*solvent*

somat- σῶμα, σώματος body. Cf. corpor-. psycho*somat*ic

-some See somat-. dictyo*some*

spas- σπάω, σπασ- draw, pull. *spas*m, *spas*tic

spectr- *spectrum* appearance, what is seen. micro*spectr*oscope

sperm(at)- σπέρμα, σπέρματος seed. *sperm*acrasia, *spermat*ozoon

spers- *spargo, -spersus* scatter. di*spers*ion

sphen- σφήν wedge. Cf. cune-. *sphen*oid

spher- σφαῖρα ball. hemi*spher*e

sphygm- σφυγμός pulsation. *sphygm*omanometer

spin- *spina* spine. Cf. rachi-. cerebro*spin*al

spirat- *spiro, spiratus* breathe. in*spirat*ory

splanchn- σπλάγχνα entrails, viscera. neuro*splanchn*ic

splen- σπλήν spleen. Cf. lien-. *splen*omegaly

spor- σπόρος seed. *spor*ophyte, zygo*spor*e

squam- *squama* scale. de*squam*ation

sta- ἵστημι, στα- make stand, stop. genesi*sta*sis

stal- στέλλω, σταλ- send. peri*stal*sis. (See also stol-)

staphyl- σταφυλή bunch of grapes, uvula. *staphyl*ococcus, *staphyl*ectomy

stear- στέαρ, στέατος fat. Cf. adip-. *stear*odermia

steat- See stear-. *steat*opygous

sten- στενός narrow, compressed. *sten*ocardia

ster- στερεός solid. chole*ster*ol

sterc- *stercus* dung. Cf. copr-. *sterc*oporphyrin

sthen- σθένος strength. a*sthen*ia

stol- στέλλω, στολ- send. dia*stol*e

stom(at)- στόμα, στόματος mouth, orifice. Cf. or-. ana*stom*osis, *stomat*ogastric

strep(h)- στρέφω, στρεπ- (before τ) twist. Cf. tors-. *strep*hosymbolia, *strep*tomycin. (See also stroph-)

strict- *stringo, stringentis, strictus* draw tight, compress, cause pain. con*strict*ion

-stringent See strict-. a*stringent*

stroph- στρέφω, στροφ- twist. ana*stroph*ic. (See also strep(h)-)

struct- *struo, structus* pile up (against). ob*struct*ion

sub- *sub* (*b* changes to *f* or *p* before words beginning with those consonants) under, below. Cf. hypo-. *sub*lumbar

suf- See sub-. *suf*fusion

sup- See sub-. *sup*pository

super- *super* above, beyond, extreme. Cf. hyper-. *super*motility

sy- See syn-. *sy*stole

syl- See syn-. *syl*lepsiology

sym- See syn-. *sym*biosis, *sym*metry, *sym*pathetic, *sym*physis

syn- σύν (*n* disappears before *s*, changes to *l* before *l*, and changes to *m* before *b*, *m*, *p*, and *ph*) with, together. Cf. con-. myo*syn*izesis

ta- See ton-. ec*ta*sis

tac- τάσσω, ταγ- (τακ- before τ) order, arrange. a*tac*tic

tact- *tango, tactus* touch. con*tact*

tax- τάσσω, ταγ- (added to σ becomes ταξ-) order, arrange. a*tax*ia

tect- See teg-. pro*tect*ive

teg- *tego, tectus* cover. in*teg*ument

tel- τέλος end. *tel*osynapsis

tele- τῆλε at a distance. *tele*ceptor

tempor- *tempus, temporis* time, timely or fatal spot, temple. *tempor*omalar

ten(ont)- τένων, τένοντος (from τείνω stretch) tight stretched band. *ten*odynia, *ten*onitis, *tenont*agra

tens- *tendo, tensus* stretch. Cf. ton-. ex*tens*or

test- *testis* testicle. Cf. orchi-. *test*itis

tetra- τετρα- four. Cf. quadr-. *tetra*genous

the- τίθημι, θη- put, place. syn*the*sis

thec- θήκη repository, case. *thec*ostegnosis

thel- θηλή teat, nipple. *thel*erethism

therap- θεραπεία treatment. hydro*therap*y

therm- θέρμη heat. Cf. calor-. dia*therm*y

thi- θεῖον sulfur. *thi*ogenic

thorac- θώραξ, θώρακος chest. *thorac*oplasty

thromb- θρόμβος lump, clot. *thromb*openia

thym- θυμός spirit. Cf. ment-. dys*thym*ia

thyr- θυρεός shield (shaped like a door θύρα). *thyr*oid

tme- τέμνω, τμη- cut. axono*tme*sis

toc- τόκος childbirth. dys*toc*ia

tom- τέμνω, τομ- cut. Cf. sect-. appendec*tom*y

ton- τείνω, τον- stretch, put under tension. Cf. tens-. peri*ton*eum

top- τόπος place. Cf. loc-. *top*esthesia

tors- *torqueo, torsus* twist. Cf. strep-. ex*tors*ion

tox- τοξικόν (from τόξον bow) arrow poison, poison. *tox*emia

trache- τραχεῖα windpipe. *trache*otomy

trachel- τράχηλος neck. Cf. cervic-. *trachel*opexy

tract- *traho, tractus* draw, drag. pro*tract*ion

traumat- τραῦμα, τραύματος wound. *traumat*ic

tri- τρεῖς, τρία or *tri-* three. *tri*gonid

trich- θρίξ, τριχός hair. *trich*oid

trip- τρίβω rub. en*trip*sis

trop- τρέπω, τροπ- turn, react. sito*trop*ism

troph- τρέφω, τροφ- nurture. a*troph*y

tuber- *tuber* swelling, node. *tuber*cle

typ- τύπος (from τύπτω strike) type. a*typ*ical

typh- τῦφος fog, stupor. adeno*typh*us

typhl- τυφλός blind. Cf. cec-. *typhl*ectasis

un- *unus* one. Cf. hen-. *un*ioval

ur- οὖρον urine. poly*ur*ia

vacc- *vacca* cow. *vacc*ine

vagin- *vagina* sheath. in*vagin*ated

vas- *vas* vessel. Cf. angi-. *vas*cular

vers- See vert-. in*vers*ion

vert- *verto, versus* turn. di*vert*iculum

vesic- *vesica* bladder. Cf. cyst-. *vesic*ovaginal

vit- *vita* life. Cf. bi-¹. de*vit*alize

vuls- *vello, vulsus* pull, twitch. con*vuls*ion

xanth- ξανθός yellow, blond. Cf. flav- and lute-. *xanth*ophyll

-yl- ὕλη substance. cacod*yl*

zo- ζωή life, ζῷον animal. micro*zo*aria

zyg- ζυγόν yoke, union. *zyg*odactyly

zym- ζύμη ferment. en*zym*e

Common Abbreviations, Acronyms, and Symbols

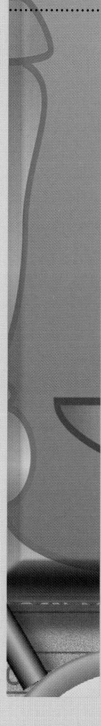

abd	abdomen
a.c.	before meals
ad lib	as desired
AgNO₃	silver nitrate
A/KA	above knee amputation
Anesth	anesthesia
A & P	anterior and posterior, auscultation and percussion
ASCVD	arteriosclerotic cardiovascular disease
ASHD	arteriosclerotic heart disease
A & W	alive and well
BE	barium enema
BID	twice a day
B/KA	below knee amputation
BM	bowel movement
BMR	basal metabolic rate
BP	blood pressure
BPH	benign prostatic hypertrophy
BUN	blood urea nitrogen
Bx	biopsy
C	centigrade
Ca	calcium
CA	carcinoma
cal	calorie
CBC	complete blood count
cc	cubic centimeter
CCU	Coronary Care Unit
CHF	congestive heart failure
cm	centimeter
CNS	central nervous system
CO₂	carbon dioxide
COPD	chronic obstructive pulmonary disease
CPR	cardiopulmonary resuscitation
C/S	cesarean section
CSF	cerebrospinal fluid
CT	computed tomography
CVA	cerebrovascular accident
cysto	cystoscopy
D & C	dilatation and curettage
disch	discharge
DJD	degenerative joint disease
DM	diabetes mellitus
DNA	deoxyribonucleic acid
DOA	dead on arrival
DOB	date of birth
DPT	diphtheria, pertussis, tetanus
DR	delivery room
Dx	diagnosis

ECG	electrocardiogram
EDC	estimated date of confinement
EEG	electroencephalogram
EENT	eye, ear, nose, and throat
EKG	electrocardiogram
ENT	ear, nose, and throat
EOM	extraocular movements
ER	emergency room
EUA	examination under anesthesia
expl lap	exploratory laparotomy
F	female
Fa or F	Fahrenheit
FB	foreign body
FBS	fasting blood sugar
FH	family history
FHT	fetal heart tones
FS	frozen section
FTG	full thickness graft
FU	follow up
FUO	fever of unknown origin
Fx	fracture
GB	gallbladder
GE	gastroenterology
GI	gastrointestinal
g	gram
GP	general practitioner
GTT	glucose tolerance test
gtt	drops
GU	genitourinary
GYN	gynecology
HCl	hydrochloric acid
HCVD	hypertensive cardiovascular disease
Hgb	hemoglobin
hs	at bedtime
Hx	history
ICU	Intensive Care Unit
I & D	incision and drainage
IM	intramuscular
inj	injection
int & ext	internal and external
I & O	intake and output
IP	inpatient
IPPB	intermittent positive pressure breathing
IT	inhalation therapy
IUD	intrauterine device
IV	intravenous
IVP	intravenous pyelogram
K	potassium
KJ	knee jerk
KUB	kidney, ureter, and bladder
L	left
L & A	light and accommodation
lat	lateral
LLQ	left lower quadrant
LMP	last menstrual period
LOM	limitation of motion
LUQ	left upper quadrant
M	male
MH	marital history
MRI	magnetic resonance imaging
MS	multiple sclerosis
NB	newborn
NP	neuropsychiatric
NPN	nonprotein nitrogen

N.P.O.	nothing by mouth
N & V	nausea and vomiting
OB	obstetrics
O.C.	oral contraceptive
OD	overdose
O.D.	right eye
OP	outpatient
O.R.	operating room
O.S.	left eye
O.U.	both eyes
Path	pathology
PBI	protein bound iodine
p.c.	after meals
PCCU	Postcoronary Care Unit
Peds	pediatrics
PERRLA	pupils equal, round, regular, react to light and accommodation
PFT	pulmonary function test
PH	past history
PID	pelvic inflammatory disease
PKU	phenylketonuria
PMR	paramedic run
PND	paroxysmal nocturnal dyspnea
PO	by mouth (per os)
PROM	premature rupture of membranes
pro time	prothrombin time
prn	when needed
Psych	psychiatry
pt	patient
PT	physical therapy
PU	peptic ulcer
Px	physical examination
q	every
qd	every day
qh	every hour
QID	four times a day
qn	every night
qns	quantity not sufficient
R	right
Ra	radium
R.A.	rheumatoid arthritis
RBC	red blood cell
REM	rapid eye movement
RHD	rheumatic heart disease
R/O	rule out
ROS	review of systems
R.R.	recovery room
Rx	prescription
SH	social history
sig	directions
SMR	submucous resection
SOB	shortness of breath
stat	immediately
STG	split thickness graft
subq	subcutaneous
SWD	short wave diathermy
T	temperature
T & A	tonsillectomy & adenoidectomy
tab	tablet
TB	tuberculosis
TIA	transient ischemic attack
TID	three times a day
TPR	temperature, pulse, respiration
TUR	transurethral resection
UA	urinalysis
UCHD	usual childhood diseases
UR	utilization review

URI	upper respiratory infection
UTI	urinary tract infection
VA	visual acuity
VD	venereal disease
VDRL	Venereal Disease Research Laboratory
VS	vital signs
Wass	Wassermann
WBC	white blood cell
WDWN	well developed and well nourished
WF	white female
WM	white male
WNL	within normal limits

Symbols

| $\bar{a}$ | before |
| $\bar{aa}$ | of each |

$\bar{c}$	with
$\bar{p}$	after
$\bar{s}$	without
ss	one half
↓	decreased
↑	increased
>	greater than
<	less than
c	birth
−	negative
+	positive
±	negative or positive (indefinite)
♂	male
♀	female
μ	micron
†	death
ℳ	minim
ʒ	dram
℥	ounce

Resources

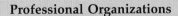

Professional Organizations

American Association of Medical Assistants
20 North Wacker Drive, Suite 1575
Chicago, IL 60606

American Association for Medical Transcription
PO Box 576187
Modesto, CA 95357

Professional Secretaries International
10502 NW Ambassador Drive
PO Box 20404
Kansas City, MO 64195-0404

Registered Medical Assistant
710 Higgins Road
Park Ridge, IL 60068

Office Materials

Colwell Company
275 Kenyon Road
Champaign, IL 61820

Control-o-Fax
Box 778
Waterloo, IA 50704
(800) 344-7777

Patient Care Systems
16 Thorndal Circle
Darien, CT 06820

VISIrecord Systems
160 Gold Star Boulevard
Worcester, MA 01606

Bibbero Systems, Inc.
1300 N. McDowell Boulevard
Petaluma, CA 94954

Glossary

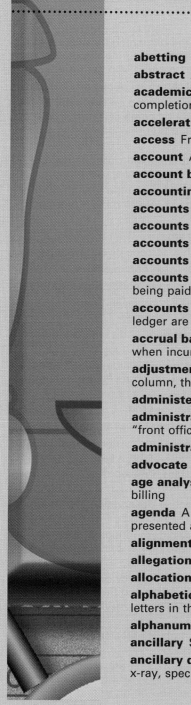

abetting Encouraging or supporting

abstract A written summary of the key points of a book, paper, or case history

academic degree A title conferred by a college, university, or professional school on completion of a program of study

accelerating Causing to act or move faster

access Freedom to obtain or make use of

account A single financial record

account balance The debit or credit balance remaining in an account

accounting equation Assets = Liabilities + Proprietorship (Capital)

accounts payable Debts incurred and not yet paid

accounts receivable Amounts owed to the creditor (physician)

accounts receivable control A summary of unpaid accounts

accounts receivable ledger The combined record of all patient accounts

accounts receivable ratio A formula for measuring how fast outstanding accounts are being paid

accounts receivable trial balance A method of determining that the journal and the ledger are in balance

accrual basis of accounting Income is recorded when earned, and expenses are recorded when incurred

adjustment column An account column, sometimes included to the left of the balance column, that is used for entering discounts

administering Instilling a drug into the body of a patient

administrative Having to do with management duties; in medical assisting, refers to all "front office" activities

administrative law Regulations set forth by government agencies

advocate A person who pleads the cause of another

age analysis A procedure for classifying accounts receivable by age from the first date of billing

agenda A list of the specific items under each division of the order of business that is to be presented at a business meeting

alignment The state of being in the correct relative position

allegation A statement of what a party to a legal action will undertake to prove

allocation Apportioned for a specific purpose or person

alphabetic filing Any system that arranges names or topics according to the sequence of letters in the alphabet

alphanumeric Filing systems made up of combinations of letters and numbers

ancillary Subordinate; auxiliary

ancillary diagnostic services Services that support patient diagnoses (e.g., laboratory or x-ray, specialists, or surgery)

anesthetic Agent that causes loss of sensation with or without loss of consciousness

annotating To furnish with notes, which are usually critical or explanatory

anthrax An acute infectious disease caused by a bacillus. Humans contract the disease from animal hair, hides, or waste matter

aphonia Loss of the ability to speak

aphrodisiacs Drugs that cause sexual arousal

appease To make peaceful or quiet

applications Software programs designed to perform specific tasks

appraisal Setting a value on, or judging as to quality

arbitration The hearing and determination of a cause in controversy by a person or persons either chosen by the parties involved or appointed under statutory authority

arbitrator A neutral person chosen to settle differences between two parties in controversy

artificial insemination The introduction of semen into the vagina or cervix by artificial means

assault An intentional, unlawful *attempt* of bodily injury to another by force or threat

assignment of benefits Statement authorizing the insurance company to pay benefits directly to the physician

attenuated Weakened, or change in, virulence of a pathogenic microorganism

augment To make greater (larger) or more effective (intense)

auscultation The act of listening for sounds within the body, normally with a stethoscope

authority The quality of being in command

autocratic Ruling with unlimited authority

avocational Pertaining to a subordinate occupation or a hobby

back-space key Key at upper right of keyboard with left arrow that deletes characters as it is struck

back up A tape or floppy disk for storage of files to prevent their loss in the event of hard disk failure

bacteria Single-celled microscopic organisms

balance The difference between the debit and credit totals

balance column The account column on the far right that is used for recording the difference between the debit and credit columns

balance sheet A financial statement for a specific date that shows the total assets, liabilities, and capital of the business

barrier A factor that restricts free movement

battery A willful and unlawful use of force or violence upon the person of another

beneficiary The person receiving the benefits of an insurance policy

bibliography A list of the works that are referred to in a text or that were consulted by the author in producing a text

biennially Occurring every 2 years

birthday rule The rule governing the hierarchy of coordination of benefits

body language Gestures and mannerisms that influence communication

bookkeeping The recording part of the accounting process

candid Frank; straightforward

capital purchase The purchase of a major item of furniture or equipment

capitation System of payment in which providers are paid a fixed per capita fee for each enrolled patient, not dependent on the services rendered

caption A heading, title, or subtitle under which records are filed

cash basis of accounting Income is recorded when received, and expenses are recorded when paid

cash flow statement A financial summary for a specific period that shows the beginning balance on hand, the receipts and disbursements during the period, and the balance on hand at the end of the period

cash payment journal A record of all cash paid out

cassette A magnetic tape wound on two reels and encased in a plastic or metal container; *microcassette* A very small cassette tape that may be used in a hand-held dictating unit

categorically Applied to a limited classification; placed in a specific division of a system of classification

catheterization The act of passing a tube through the body for removing fluids or injecting them into body cavities

caustic remark Biting wit

caustics Substances that corrode or eat away tissues

CD-ROM Compact disk–read only memory

censure The act of blaming or condemning sternly

cervical vertebrae The upper seven bones of the spinal column; the skeleton of the neck

chemotherapy The treatment of disease using chemical agents

cholera An acute, infectious, bacillus-caused disease involving the entire bowel; *chicken cholera*—cholera that affects chickens

chronologic In the order of time

circumvention Going around or avoiding

claim A demand to the insurer by the insured person for the payment of benefits under a policy

clarity The quality or state of being clear; the state of being clear or lucid

clinical Pertaining to actual observation and treatment of patients

coding Converting verbal descriptions of diseases, injuries, and procedures into numeric and alphanumeric designations

co-insurance/copayment A policy provision by which both the insured person and the insurer share in a specified ratio of the expenses resulting from an illness or injury

collection ratio A formula for measuring the effectiveness of the billing system

colloquialisms Expressions that are acceptable and correct in ordinary conversation or informal speeches but unsuitable for formal speech or writing

communicable Capable of being transmitted from one person to another

comorbidity A preexisting condition that will, because of its presence with a specific principal diagnosis, cause an increase in length of hospital stay by at least one day in approximately 75% of the cases

compensatory damages General or special damages without specific monetary value

complication A condition that arises during the hospital stay that prolongs the length of stay by at least one day in approximately 75% of the cases

compulsory Obligatory; enforced

computer A machine that is designed to accept, store, process, and give out information

concise Expressing much in a brief form

concurrently Occurring at the same time

confidential Containing information that requires authorization for disclosure

congruency The quality of agreeing

consultation report A report of the findings of the consulting physician to be sent to the referring physician

contagious Transmitted readily from one person to another by direct or indirect contact

contamination The act of soiling, staining, or polluting; especially the introduction of infectious materials or germs that produce disease

contingent Dependent on or conditioned by something else

continuation pages The second and following pages of a letter

continuity The quality or state of being continuous

contract law Enforceable promises

conversely Reversed in order

coordination of benefits The provision in an insurance contract that limits benefits to 100% of the cost

copay A flat fee payable by the insured in most health maintenance organization plans

correlation A mutual relationship

CPT-4 manual *Current Procedural Terminology* manual

CPU Central processing unit; the part of a computer system that processes information

credit The record of a payment received

credit balance The amount of advance payment or overpayment on an account (amount of receipts exceeding amount of charges)

credit column The account column to the right of the debit column that is used for entering funds received

crossover claim A claim for benefits under both Medicare and Medicaid

culminate To reach a high or decisive point

cursor A symbol appearing on the monitor that shows where the next character to be typed will appear

cursor-control keys Keys that have an arrow pointing up, down, left, or right that are used to move a cursor

cyanosis Bluish discoloration of the skin, extremities, and mucous membranes caused by a decreased level of oxygen transported to cells

daily journal The book in which all transactions are first recorded; the book of original entry, or general journal

daisy wheel A printing element made of plastic or metal used on some typewriters and impact printers that derives its name from its shape, which is like that of a daisy

database A collection of related files that serves as a foundation for retrieving information

debit The record of a charge or debt incurred

debit column The account column on the left that is used for entering charges

deceptive Misleading; having the power to deceive

deductible A statement in an insurance policy that the insuring company will pay the expenses incurred after the insured person has paid a specified amount

democratic Relating to social equality

demographics Relating to the statistical characteristics of populations, such as births, marriages, mortality, and health

deposition Oral testimony taken from a party or witness to the litigation and is not limited to parties named in the lawsuit

dictation The process of recording the spoken word onto a storage medium from which a printed copy will be produced

diction Choice of words to express ideas, especially with regard to correctness, clearness, or effectiveness

direct filing system A filing system in which materials can be located without consulting an intermediary source of reference

disability The condition resulting from illness or injury that makes an individual unable to be employed

disbursements Money (funds) paid out

disbursements journal A summary of amounts paid out

discernible A difference that can be seen between two or more things

discounts Subtractions from the patient's balance

discretion Quality of being discreet, tactful, or prudent

discrimination Different treatment on a basis other than individual merit

disk A magnetic surface that is capable of storing computer programs that sometimes is flexible (floppy disks) and sometimes is hard (hard disks)

disk drives Devices that load a program or data stored on a disk into a computer

dispensing Giving of drugs, in some type of bottle, box, or other container, to the patient. (Under the Controlled Substances Act of 1970, the definition of "dispense" includes the administering of controlled substances.)

disruption A breaking down or upset

dissection The process of cutting apart or separating tissues for anatomic study

disseminate To broadcast or spread over a considerable area

dot matrix printer An impact printer that forms characters using patterns of dots

draft A preliminary outline or writing that the author expects to amend or revise

editing The process of examining text to determine accuracy and clarity

electronic billing The submission of a claim via computer to computer

electronic mail (E-mail) Communications transmitted via computer using a telephone modem

emancipated minor A person under legal age who is self-supporting and living apart from parents or a guardian

embryology The science or study of the development of living organisms during the embryonic stage

empathy Intellectual and emotional awareness of another person's thoughts, feelings, and behavior

endorsement To express approval publicly and definitely

endorser Person who signs his or her name on the back of a check for the purpose of transferring title to another person

enter key Key that performs the same function as the return key on a typewriter

enunciation The act of pronouncing words distinctly

established patient A patient who has received care from the physician within the past 3 years or other specified period

ethics A set of moral principles or values

ethnic Pertaining to large groups of people classed according to cultural origin or background

etiology Classifying a claim according to the cause of the disorder

exemplary Serving as a warning

expediency A situation requiring haste or caution

expendable Concerning supplies or equipment that is normally used up or consumed in service

expert witness Professional who belongs to a certifying or qualifying organization and who is called to testify in court

expulsion Act of expelling or forcing out

externship The practice of receiving employment experience in qualified health care facilities under the cooperative supervision of the medical staff and the program instructor as part of the educational curriculum

extracurricular Relating to those activities that form part of the life of students but are not part of the courses of study

fallopian tubes The tubes that capture the expelled ova and transport them to the uterus; usual location of fertilization; also called the *oviducts*

fee profile Compilation of a physician's fees over a given period of time

fee schedule Compilation of preestablished fee allowances for given services or procedures

fee splitting Sharing a fee with another physician, laboratory, or drug company not based on services performed

feedback Letting people know how you feel about them at a given moment

felony A crime of a graver nature than one designated as a misdemeanor; generally, an offense punishable by imprisonment in a penitentiary

fiscal agent An organization under contract to the government as well as some private plans to act as financial representative in handling insurance claims from providers of health care; also referred to as **fiscal intermediary**

fiscal intermediary An organization that handles claims from hospitals, nursing facilities, intermediate and long-term care facilities, and home health agencies

flagged Using something to signal or attract attention

flagging A way of bringing attention to a blank space for possible correction in a transcribed page (also called tagging, carding or marking)

floppy disk (diskette) A thin disk (diskette) of magnetic material capable of storing a large amount of information

flourishing Achieving success

fonts Sets of printing type that are of one size and style

footnotes Comments placed at the bottom of a page that would be distracting if placed within the main text

format Shape, size, and general makeup of a publication, such as a resumé; to magnetically create tracks on a disk where information will be stored; to initialize a disk

freestanding emergency center An emergency facility not associated with a hospital

fringe benefit A benefit granted by an employer that involves a money cost but does not affect the basic wage rates of employees

galley proofs Printer's proofs taken from composed type before page composition

general journal The book of original entry in bookkeeping

genetic Pertaining to the branch of biology dealing with heredity and variation among related organisms

gesture The use of motions as a means of expression

ghost surgery A situation in which a patient has consented to have surgery done by one surgeon but, without the patient's knowledge or consent, the surgery is actually performed by another surgeon

group policy A policy that covers a group (e.g., all employees of one company) under a master contract

group practice The provision of services by a group of at least three practitioners

grouper Computer software program that is used by the fiscal intermediary in all cases to assign discharges to the appropriate DRGs using the following information abstracted from the inpatient bill: patient's age, sex, principal diagnosis, principal procedures performed, and discharge status

hard copy The readable paper copy or printout of information

hardware Computer components that perform four main functions

harmonious All parts are agreeably related or in accord

harmony Having an atmosphere of cordiality

HCFA Health Care Financing Administration; the authority that administers Medicare

HCPCS Acronym for HCFA's Common Procedure Coding System, used in determining Medicare fees

health maintenance organization (HMO) An organization that provides comprehensive health care to an enrolled group for a fixed periodic payment

hemiplegia Paralysis of one side of the body

histologist One who specializes in the study of the minute structure, composition, and function of the tissues

ICD manual *International Classification of Diseases* manual

immunology Science that deals with the phenomena and causes of immunity and immune responses

impartiality The quality of treating or affecting all equally

in balance Total ending balances of patient ledgers equal total of accounts receivable control

indemnity A benefit paid by an insurer for a loss insured under a policy

indicator strip A charted strip that is inserted into the dictation unit and on which the dictator marks the beginning and end point of each document and any corrections to be made

indirect filing system A filing system in which an intermediary source of reference, such as a card file, must be consulted to locate specific files

individual policy A policy usually held by a person who does not qualify for a group policy

infectious Capable of causing infection

inflection Change in pitch or loudness of the voice

informed consent A consent, verbal or written, in which there is understanding of what treatment is to be undertaken and of the risks involved, why it should be done, and alternative methods of treatment available (including no treatment) and their attendant risks

infraction Breaking the law, a minor offense of the rules

innovation Act of introducing something new or novel

input Information entered into and used by the computer

insubordination Refusing to submit to authority

integral Essential; being an indispensable part of a whole

interaction A two-way communication

intercom (intercommunication system) A direct telephone line from one station to another

intermittent Coming and going at intervals, not continuous

intrinsic Inward; indwelling

inventory A list of articles in stock, with the description and quantity of each

invoice A paper describing a purchase and the amount due

invulnerable Incapable of being injured or harmed

keyboarding The process of entering characters into the memory of a word processor

laissez faire Management style of "hands off" when dealing with employees

legend Heading or title of a figure

letter-quality printer A printer that resembles a typewriter and that may be either mechanical or electronic

liability Subject to some adverse action

ligation Something that binds

listening An active process of receiving information and examining one's reaction to the messages received

litigation Contest in a court of justice for the purpose of enforcing a right

litigious Tending to engage in lawsuits

living will A document in which an individual expresses wishes regarding medical treatment at or near the end of life

main memory Section of the computer where information and instructions are stored

major diagnostic category (MDC) Broad clinical category that is differentiated from all others based on body system involvement and disease etiology

maker (of a check) Any individual, corporation, or legal party who signs a check or any type of negotiable instrument

maladies Diseases or disorders of the body

malfeasance The doing of an act that is wholly wrongful and unlawful

malpractice Professional misconduct, improper discharge of professional duties, or failure to meet the standard of care by a professional that results in harm to another

mandated Having a formal order from a superior to an inferior source

mandatory In the nature of a mandate or command; obligatory

manipulative Treating or operating with the hands in a skillful manner

manuscript Written or typewritten document, as distinguished from printed copy

matrix Something in which something else originates, develops, takes shape, or is contained; a base upon which to build

medically indigent Able to take care of ordinary living expenses but cannot afford medical care

member physician A physician who has agreed to accept the contracts of an insurer; this usually includes accepting the insurance benefits as payment in full

meticulous Extremely careful of small details

microfilming Photographic records in reduced size on film

microorganism An organism of microscopic or ultramicroscopic size (also called *microbe*)

millennia Thousands of years (*mille* = thousands)

misdemeanor A crime less serious than a felony

misfeasance The improper performance of a lawful act

modem Acronym for modulator demodulator; a device that enables data to be transmitted over telephone lines

monitor To listen to a matter transmitted by telephone as a third party; a device used to display computer-generated information; a video screen; a CRT

monograph Learned treatise on a small area of knowledge; a written account of a single thing or class of things

mons veneris The rounded, elevated area overlying the symphysis pubis that is covered with hair after puberty

motivation Process of inciting a person to some action or behavior

mouse Pointing device that controls the cursor

mysticism The experience of seeming to have direct communication with God or ultimate reality

mythology A branch of knowledge that deals with the interpretation of myths

negligence The doing of some act that a reasonable or prudent physician would not do, or the failure to do some act that such a person would or should do

negotiable Legally transferable to another party

neophyte A new convert or novice

new patient A patient who has not received any professional services from the physician in the past 3 years or other specified period

nominal Existing in name only

noncommittal Not revealing any specific attitude or opinion

nonconsensual Not having received consent

nonfeasance The failure to do something that should have been done

non-par Nonparticipating provider

nonparticipating provider A physician who does not accept assignment under Medicare or the Blue Plans

no-show A person who fails to keep an appointment without giving advance notice of that failure

numeric filing The filing of records, correspondence, or cards by number

objective Something toward which effort is directed; an aim or end of action

objective information Perceptible to the external senses (e.g., conclusions reached by a physician after listening to body sounds with a stethoscope)

obliteration To remove from existence; destroy

observation An inference from what has been seen or heard

office policy manual An informational guide for employees.

oral hygiene Proper care of mouth and teeth resulting in clean teeth and an absence of unpleasant breath.

order of business List of the different divisions of business in the order in which each is to be addressed at a business meeting

orientation The determination or adjustment of one's intellectual or emotional position with reference to circumstances

OUTfolder A folder used to provide space for the temporary filing of materials

OUTguide A heavy guide that is used to replace a folder that has been temporarily moved from the filing space

outliers (atypical cases) Cases involving an extremely long stay (day outlier) or extraordinarily high costs (cost outlier) when compared with most discharges classified in the same DRG

output Information that is processed by the computer and transmitted to a monitor, printer, or other device

overaccentuate Greatly emphasize

overutilization Excessive use

oviducts The pair of tubes in the female that carry the egg from the ovary to the uterus; fallopian tubes

packing slip An itemized list of objects in a package

pandemic Affecting the majority of the people in a country or a number of countries

par Participating provider

paradox A statement that seems to be contradictory and yet is perhaps true

parlance Manner or mode of speech

participating provider A physician who accepts assignment under Medicare or the Blue Plans

pathologic Altered or caused by disease

payables Amounts owed to others

payee Person named on a draft or check as the recipient of the amount shown

payer Person who writes a check in favor of the payee

pediatrician A physician who specializes in the care of children

peer review organization (PRO) An entity that is composed of a substantial number of licensed doctors of medicine and osteopathy engaged in the practice of medicine or surgery in the area, or an entity that has available to it the services of a sufficient number of physicians engaged in the practice of medicine or surgery, to ensure the adequate peer review of the services provided by the various medical specialties and subspecialties

pejorative Having negative connotations; a depreciatory word

perception A mental image

percussion The act of striking a part of the body with short, sharp blows as an aid in diagnosing the condition of the underlying parts by the sound obtained

perfusion The passing of a fluid through spaces

periodicals Journals published with a fixed interval (greater than 1 day) between its issues or numbers

periphery The external surface or boundary of a body

perjured testimony Telling what is false when sworn to tell the truth

personal inventory A complete summary of pertinent information about oneself

petty cash fund A fund maintained from which to pay small unpredictable cash expenditures

phagocytosis The engulfing of microorganisms, other cells, and foreign particles by phagocytes

philosophy The general laws that furnish the rational explanation of anything

phonetic Alteration of ordinary spelling that better represents the sounding of a word

physical impairment A lessening of physical capabilities

pitch The vibratory frequency of a tone or sound

placenta The vascular structure that develops within the uterus during pregnancy and through which a fetus receives nourishment

POMR Problem-oriented medical record

portfolio A set of documents either bound in book form or loose in a folder

posting The act of transferring information from one record to another

power of attorney A legal statement in which a person authorizes another person to act as his or her attorney or agent. The authority may be limited to the handling of certain procedures. The person authorized to act as the agent is known as an *attorney in fact*

practitioner One who practices a profession

preamble An introductory portion; a preface

preauthorization Permission by the insurance carrier obtained prior to giving certain treatment to a patient

precepts Practical rules guiding behavior or technique

preexisting condition A physical condition of an insured person that existed prior to the issuance of the insurance policy

premium The periodic payment required to keep a policy in force

prepaid plan A plan that provides all covered services to a policyholder for payment of a monthly fee

prescribe To issue a prescription for the patient; to direct, designate, or order use of a remedy

principal diagnosis That condition that after study is determined to be chiefly responsible for occasioning the admission of the patient to the hospital

principal procedure One that was performed for definitive treatment rather than for diagnostic or exploratory purposes, or one necessary to take care of a complication. It is that procedure most related to the principal diagnosis

printout The output from a printer, also called *hard copy*

privileged communication Information disclosed to a physician during the relationship between physician and patient that is confidential and should not be revealed without the express consent of the patient, unless required to do so by law

probationary Pertaining to a trial or a period of trial to ascertain fitness for a job

procrastination The intentional putting off of doing something that should be done

professional courtesy Reduction or absence of fee to professional associates

professional standards review organization (PSRO) A group of physicians working with the government to review cases for hospital admission and discharge under government guidelines; sometimes referred to as peer review

proficiency Competency as a result of training and practice

progress notes Records of patient visits, telephone calls, progress, and treatment that are inserted into the patient's chart

pronunciation The act or manner of pronouncing words

proofreading Checking a document for spelling, sentence structure, punctuation, capitalization, style, and format

Prospective Payment Assessment Commission (ProPAC) A 15-member commission of independent experts with experience and expertise in the provision and financing of health care who are appointed to review and provide recommendations on the annual inflation factor, DRG recalibration, and new and existing medical and surgical procedures and services

protozoa Primitive animal organisms, each of which consists of a single cell

provider One who provides medical service (e.g., a physician)

prudent Marked by wisdom or circumspection

public domain The realm embracing property rights that belong to the community at large and that are subject to appropriation by anyone

puerperal fever The fever that accompanies an infection of the birth canal following delivery of a child; childbed fever

puerperium The period between childbirth and the return of the uterus to its normal size

punitive Inflicting punishment

purulent Consisting of or containing pus

pustule A raised pus-filled area or sac

putrefaction Decomposition of animal matter that results in a foul smell

quackery The pretension of possessing medical skill to cure disease

rabies An acute infectious disease of the nervous system caused by a virus, usually communicated to humans through animal bite

random access memory (RAM) The computer's temporary memory that stores data and programs that are input

read-only memory (ROM) Memory that can be altered only by changing the physical structure of the computer chip and that is used to store information that is essential to the operation of the computer

receipts Money received

receivables Amounts owing from others

reciprocity A mutual exchange of privileges

reconciliation (of bank statement) The process of proving that the bank statement and the checkbook balance are in agreement

recruitment The supplying of new members or help

reentry student One who has been away from formal education or employment for several years and who is now preparing to reenter the workplace

regional Pertaining to a region or territory; local

rehabilitation Restoration of normal form and function after injury or illness

reprints Reproductions of printed matter

reputable Honorable; having a good reputation

res ipsa loquitur The thing speaks for itself

resident A graduate and licensed physician receiving training in a specialty in a hospital

respondeat superior Let the master answer

response Something constituting a reply or reaction

responsible person One who is responsible for payment, usually the patient if an adult

résumé A *selective* summary of one's education and employment record tailored to the position being sought

rete mucosum The innermost layer of the epidermis (*rete* = network of nerves or vessels)

retention schedule A listing of dates until which records are to be kept, based on statutes of limitation, tax regulations, and other factors

revoke To annul by recalling or taking back

rider A legal document that modifies the protection of a policy

rural Pertaining to the country, as distinguished from a city or town

salutation Expression of greeting (e.g., *good morning*)

scanner An input device that converts printed matter into a computer-readable format

screen The act of determining to whom a telephone call is to be directed

self-concept A mental picture of one's self

seminar A group of students meeting regularly and informally with a professor to discuss ideas and problems

sequential Succeeding or following in order or as a result; **sequentially** Following one another in an orderly plan

service benefit plan A plan that agrees to pay for certain surgical and medical services and that is not restricted to a fee schedule

shelf filing A system that uses open shelves (rather than cabinets) for storing records

site A designated place or point

socioeconomic Relating to a combination of social and economic factors

software The programming necessary to direct the hardware of a computer system; computer programs

sole community hospital (SCH) Those hospitals that, by reason of factors such as isolated location, weather conditions, travel conditions or absence of other hospitals are the sole source of inpatient hospital services reasonably available to individuals in a geographic area

solo private practice One physician practicing alone

spermatozoa The mature male sex cells or germ cells

stat report An immediate report (from the Latin *statim,* meaning "at once")

statement A request for payment

statement of income and expense A summary of all income and expenses for a given period

statute of limitations The time limit within which an action may legally be brought upon a contract

statutory body A part of the legislative branch of a government

steepling Upward position of hands together with fingertips touching

stethoscope An instrument for listening to sounds within the body

subject filing Arranging records alphabetically by names of topics or things rather than by names of individuals

subjective information Findings perceptible only by the affected person (the patient) (e.g., pain experienced in a specific area under certain circumstances)

subpoena A writ commanding a person to appear in court

subscriber A person named as principal in an insurance contract

subscripts Symbols or numbers written immediately below another character

subsidize To aid or promote something (such as a private enterprise) with public money

substantiated Having been established as true by proof of competent evidence; verified

superbill A combination charge slip, statement, and insurance reporting form

superscripts Symbols or numbers written immediately above another character

suspend To debar temporarily from a privilege

suspension The act of interrupting or discontinuing temporarily, but with an expectation or purpose of resumption

swine erysipelas A contagious disease affecting young swine in Europe

synopsis A summary of the main points of a longer text

syphilitic chancre The primary sore of syphilis

tab The projection on a file folder or guide on which the caption is written

Tax Equity and Fiscal Responsibility Act (TEFRA) Signed into federal law in 1982; contains provisions for major changes in Medicare reimbursement

tedious Tiresome because of length or dullness

telecommunications The science and technology of communication by transmission of information from one location to another via telephone, television, or telegraph

teller A bank employee who is assigned the duty of waiting on the bank's customers

third-party check A check written to the order of the person offering payment and unknown to the payee, who is a third party in the process

third-party payer Someone other than the patient, spouse, or parent who is responsible for paying all or part of the patient's medical costs

tickler (file) A chronologic file used as a reminder that something must be taken care of on a certain date

tort An act that brings harm to a person or damage to property, caused negligently or intentionally

transaction The occurrence of a financial event or condition that must be recorded

transcription Listening to recorded dictation and translating it into written form

transmitter The part of a telephone into which one speaks

treason A crime against the United States

treatise Systematic exposition or argument in writing

trespass To exceed the bounds of what is lawful, right, or just

triage Responding to requests for immediate care and treatment after evaluating the urgency of the need and prioritizing the treatment; to sort or to choose; to determine priority of need for treatment

trial balance A method of checking the accuracy of accounts

uniform hospital discharge data set (UHDDS) A minimum data set required to be collected for each Medicare patient on discharge

unit Each part of a name that is used in indexing

urban Characteristic of or pertaining to a city or town

usual, customary, and reasonable A formula for determining medical insurance benefits payable

vagina Collapsible muscular tube extending from the vaginal opening to the cervix in the female

venereal Due to or propagated by sexual intercourse

virulent Exceedingly pathogenic, noxious, or deadly

vivisection Operation or cutting on a living animal for research purposes

weight (DRG) An HCFA-derived figure intended to reflect the relative resource consumption of each DRG. The payment rate is multiplied by the appropriate DRG weight to determine the reimbursement amount for each patient

word processing System used to process written communications

Index

Note: Page numbers in *italics* refer to illustrations; page numbers followed by (t) refer to tables.

Multimedia CD-ROM
Single User License Agreement

1. NOTICE. WE ARE WILLING TO LICENSE THE MULTIMEDIA PROGRAM PRODUCT TITLED "CD-ROM TO ACCOMPANY THE ADMINISTRATIVE MEDICAL ASSISTANT, 4TH EDITION" ("MULTIMEDIA PROGRAM") TO YOU ONLY ON THE CONDITION THAT YOU ACCEPT ALL OF THE TERMS CONTAINED IN THIS LICENSE AGREEMENT. PLEASE READ THIS LICENSE AGREEMENT CAREFULLY BEFORE OPENING THE SEALED DISK PACKAGE. BY OPENING THAT PACKAGE YOU AGREE TO BE BOUND BY THE TERMS OF THIS AGREEMENT. IF YOU DO NOT AGREE TO THESE TERMS WE ARE UNWILLING TO LICENSE THE MULTIMEDIA PROGRAM TO YOU, AND YOU SHOULD NOT OPEN THE DISK PACKAGE. IN SUCH CASE, PROMPTLY RETURN THE UNOPENED DISK PACKAGE AND ALL OTHER MATERIAL IN THIS PACKAGE, ALONG WITH PROOF OF PAYMENT, TO THE AUTHORIZED DEALER FROM WHOM YOU OBTAINED IT FOR A FULL REFUND OF THE PRICE YOU PAID.

2. **Ownership and License.** This is a license agreement and NOT an agreement for sale. It permits you to use one copy of the MULTIMEDIA PROGRAM on a single computer. The MULTIMEDIA PROGRAM and its contents are owned by us or our licensors, and are protected by U.S. and international copyright laws. Your rights to use the MULTIMEDIA PROGRAM are specified in this Agreement, and we retain all rights not expressly granted to you in this Agreement.

   • You may use one copy of the MULTIMEDIA PROGRAM on a single computer.

   • After you have installed the MULTIMEDIA PROGRAM on your computer, you may use the MULTIMEDIA PROGRAM on a different computer only if you first delete the files installed by the installation program from the first computer.

   • You may not copy any portion of the MULTIMEDIA PROGRAM to your computer hard disk or any other media other than printing out or downloading nonsubstantial portions of the text and images in the MULTIMEDIA PROGRAM for your own internal informational use.

   • You may not copy any of the documentation or other printed materials accompanying the MULTIMEDIA PROGRAM.

   Neither concurrent use on two or more computers nor use in a local area network or other network is permitted without separate authorization and the payment of additional license fees.

3. **Transfer and Other Restrictions.** You may not rent, lend, or lease this MULTIMEDIA PROGRAM. You may not and you may not permit others to (a) disassemble, decompile, or otherwise derive source code from the software included in the MULTIMEDIA PROGRAM (the "Software"), (b) reverse engineer the Software, (c) modify or prepare derivative works of the MULTIMEDIA PROGRAM, (d) use the Software in an on-line system, or (e) use the MULTIMEDIA PROGRAM in any manner that infringes on the intellectual property or other rights of another party.

   However, you may transfer this license to use the MULTIMEDIA PROGRAM to another party on a permanent basis by transferring this copy of the License Agreement, the MULTIMEDIA PROGRAM, and all documentation. Such transfer of possession terminates your license from us. Such other party shall be licensed under the terms of this Agreement upon its acceptance of this Agreement by its initial use of the MULTIMEDIA PROGRAM. If you transfer the MULTIMEDIA PROGRAM, you must remove the installation files from your hard disk and you may not retain any copies of those files for your own use.

4. **Limited Warranty and Limitation of Liability.** For a period of sixty (60) days from the date you acquired the MULTIMEDIA PROGRAM from us or our authorized dealer, we warrant that the media containing the MULTIMEDIA PROGRAM will be free from defects that prevent you from installing the MULTIMEDIA PROGRAM on your computer. If the disk fails to conform to this warranty, you may, as your sole and exclusive remedy, obtain a replacement free of charge if you return the defective disk to us with a dated proof of purchase. Otherwise the MULTIMEDIA PROGRAM is licensed to you on an "AS IS" basis without any warranty of any nature.

   WE DO NOT WARRANT THAT THE MULTIMEDIA PROGRAM WILL MEET YOUR REQUIREMENTS OR THAT ITS OPERATION WILL BE UNINTERRUPTED OR ERROR-FREE. WE EXCLUDE AND EXPRESSLY DISCLAIM ALL EXPRESS AND IMPLIED WARRANTIES NOT STATED HEREIN, INCLUDING THE IMPLIED WARRANTIES OF MERCHANTABILITY AND FITNESS FOR A PARTICULAR PURPOSE.

   WE SHALL NOT BE LIABLE FOR ANY DAMAGE OR LOSS OF ANY KIND ARISING OUT OF OR RESULTING FROM YOUR POSSESSION OR USE OF THE MULTIMEDIA PROGRAM (INCLUDING DATA LOSS OR CORRUPTION), REGARDLESS OF WHETHER SUCH LIABILITY IS BASED IN TORT, CONTRACT OR OTHERWISE AND INCLUDING, BUT NOT LIMITED TO, ACTUAL, SPECIAL, INDIRECT, INCIDENTAL OR CONSEQUENTIAL DAMAGES. IF THE FOREGOING LIMITATION IS HELD TO BE UNENFORCEABLE, OUR MAXIMUM LIABILITY TO YOU SHALL NOT EXCEED THE AMOUNT OF THE LICENSE FEE PAID BY YOU FOR THE MULTIMEDIA PROGRAM. THE REMEDIES AVAILABLE TO YOU AGAINST US AND THE LICENSORS OF MATERIALS INCLUDED IN THE MULTIMEDIA PROGRAM ARE EXCLUSIVE.

   Some states do not allow the limitation or exclusion of implied warranties or liability for incidental or consequential damages, so the above limitations or exclusions may not apply to you.

5. **United States Government Restricted Rights.** The MULTIMEDIA PROGRAM and documentation are provided with Restricted Rights. Use, duplication, or disclosure by the U.S. Government or any agency or instrumentality thereof is subject to restrictions as set forth in subdivision (c)(1)(ii) of the Rights in Technical Data and Computer Software clause at 48 C.F.R. 252.277-7013, or in subdivision (c)(1) and (2) of the Commercial Computer Software-Restricted Rights Clause at 48 C.F.R. 52.277-19, as applicable. Manufacturer is the W.B. Saunders Company, the Curtis Center, Suite 300, Independence Square West, Philadelphia, PA 19106.

6. **Termination.** This license and your right to use this MULTIMEDIA PROGRAM automatically terminate if you fail to comply with any provisions of this Agreement, destroy the copy of the MULTIMEDIA PROGRAM in your possession, or voluntarily return the MULTIMEDIA PROGRAM to us. Upon termination you will destroy all copies of the MULTIMEDIA PROGRAM and documentation.

7. **Miscellaneous Provisions.** This Agreement will be governed by and construed in accordance with the substantive laws of the Commonwealth of Pennsylvania. This is the entire agreement between us relating to the MULTIMEDIA PROGRAM, and supersedes any prior purchase order, communications, advertising or representations concerning the contents of this package. No change or modification of this Agreement will be valid unless it is in writing and is signed by us.